OVERWHELMING ANTIFUNGAL SUCCESS

Neutrophil phagocytizes *Candida albicans.*

* Results of a multicenter, open-label, randomized clinical trial using Diflucan 100 mg/day for 7 days; clotrimazole 50 mg/day for 14 days. Results reflect complete resolution (clinical cure) or substantial (clinical) improvement of baseline signs and symptoms of infection and therapy for 5 days with Diflucan or 10 days with clotrimazole.

† Endoscopic cure results of a multicenter, prospective, randomized, double-blind trial comparing Diflucan 100 to 200 mg/day; ketoconazole 200 to 400 mg/day. Endoscopic cure means complete resolution of esophageal lesions at end-of-cure endoscopic examination. Not all patients underwent endoscopy at initiation and completion of therapy.

‡ Open-label trial. Diflucan 100 to 200 mg/day. "Overall" includes cases of candidemia, disseminated candidiasis, peritonitis, urinary tract infections, and pneumonia. The "urinary tract" data is a subset of the overall systemic candidiasis efficacy data. Results reflect complete resolution (clinical cure) or substantial (clinical) improvement of baseline signs and symptoms of infection.

§ Open-label randomized trial. Results reflect cure (CSF culture negative and either absence of disease, or disappearance or improving signs/symptoms) and quiescent (CSF culture positive, stable or improving signs/symptoms). Diflucan, 400-mg loading dose on the first day and 200 mg thereafter or amphotericin B, at least 0.3 mg/kg/day. Three risk factors that may predict a negative outcome for AIDS patients with cryptococcal meningitis are abnormal mental status, CSF with antigen titer >1:1024, and CSF WBC <20 cells per cubic millimeter.

‖ Multicenter comparative study. Results reflect successful maintenance without culture-confirmed relapse and without toxicity necessitating discontinuance as evaluated at a median of 279 days for Diflucan and 140 days for amphotericin B. Diflucan, 200 mg/day; amphotericin B, 1 mg/kg/week.

Excellent clinical success in oropharyngeal, esophageal, and systemic candidiasis, and cryptococcal meningitis

	OROPHARYNGEAL[1*] $P < .001$		ESOPHAGEAL[2†] (endoscopic cures) $P < .001$	
MUCOSAL CANDIDIASIS	DIFLUCAN (212/221) Cured 81% Improved 15%	96%	DIFLUCAN (58/64)	91%
	clotrimazole (72/91) Cured 65% Improved 14%	79%	ketoconazole (34/65)	52%
	OVERALL[1‡]		URINARY TRACT[1‡]	
SYSTEMIC CANDIDIASIS	DIFLUCAN (189/219) Cured 63% Improved 23%	86%	DIFLUCAN (30/38) Cured 53% Improved 26%	79%
	ACUTE THERAPY[3§] $P = .39$ (NS)		MAINTENANCE TO PREVENT RELAPSE[1,4‖] $P < .001$	
CRYPTOCOCCAL MENINGITIS	DIFLUCAN (78/131) Cured 34% Quiescent 26%	60%	DIFLUCAN (103/111)	93%
	amphotericin B (42/63) Cured 40% Quiescent 27%	67%	amphotericin B (52/78)	67%

Extensive penetration to key tissues, organs, and fluids

Distribution throughout the body approximates that of total body water after oral or IV dosing.[1] Oral bioavailability of Diflucan is >90% and unaffected by agents that increase gastric pH.[1]

Excellent clinical safety

In over 4,000 patients who received Diflucan for at least 7 days, the most common adverse events were nausea (3.7%), headache (1.9%), skin rash (1.8%), vomiting (1.7%), abdominal pain (1.7%), and diarrhea (1.5%).[1] Rare incidents of serious hepatotoxicity have been reported, but the causal relationship to Diflucan is uncertain.[1]

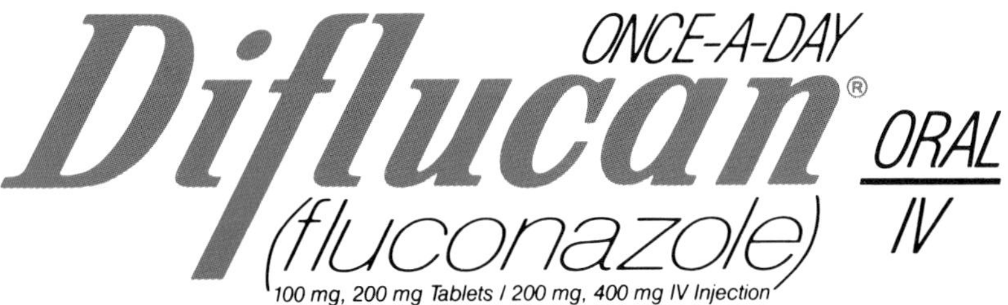

Overwhelming antifungal success

Please see brief summary of prescribing information on last page of this advertisement.

NATIONAL DIRECTORY of AIDS CARE 1994-95

The Authoritative Reference for Health Care Providers, Community Support Systems and Consumers

Edited By:
Lori Hullfish
Kathy Wolden

FIFTH ANNUAL EDITION

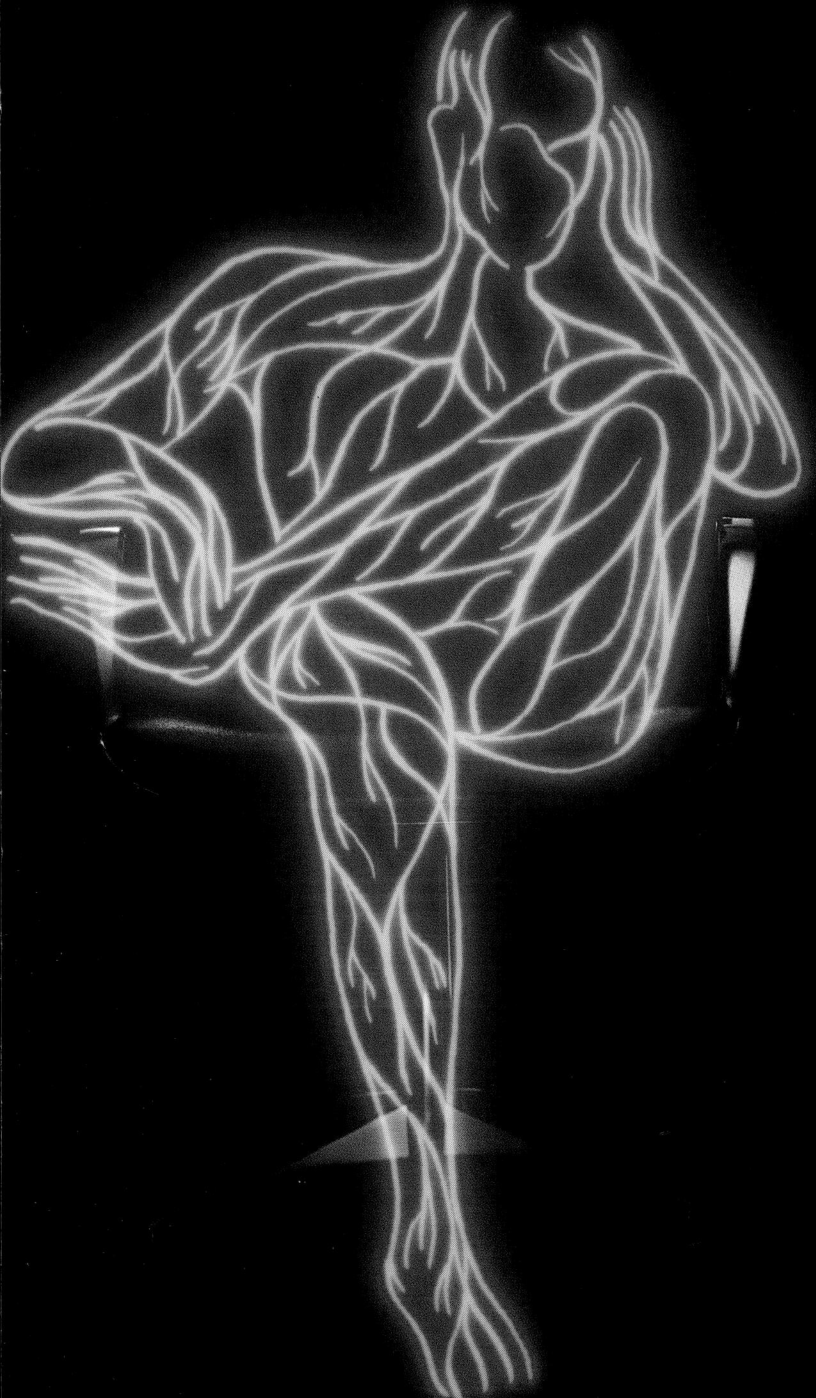

MYCOBUTIN® (rifabutin capsules) 150 mg

BRIEF SUMMARY

CONTRAINDICATIONS

Rifabutin is contraindicated in patients who have had clinically significant hypersensitivity to this drug, or to any other rifamycins.

WARNINGS

MYCOBUTIN prophylaxis must not be administered to patients with active tuberculosis. Tuberculosis in HIV-positive patients is common and may present with atypical or extrapulmonary findings. Patients are likely to have a nonreactive purified protein derivative (PPD) despite active disease. In addition to chest X-ray and sputum culture, the following studies may be useful in the diagnosis of tuberculosis in the HIV-positive patient: blood culture, urine culture, or biopsy of a suspicious lymph node.

Patients who develop complaints consistent with active tuberculosis while on MYCOBUTIN prophylaxis should be evaluated immediately, so that those with active disease may be given an effective combination regimen of anti-tuberculosis medications. Administration of single-agent MYCOBUTIN to patients with active tuberculosis is likely to lead to the development of tuberculosis that is resistant both to MYCOBUTIN and to rifampin.

There is no evidence that MYCOBUTIN is effective prophylaxis against *Mycobacterium tuberculosis*. Patients requiring prophylaxis against both *M. tuberculosis* and *Mycobacterium avium* complex may be given isoniazid and MYCOBUTIN concurrently.

PRECAUTIONS

Because MYCOBUTIN may be associated with neutropenia, and more rarely thrombocytopenia, physicians should consider obtaining hematologic studies periodically in patients receiving MYCOBUTIN prophylaxis.

Information for patients

Patients should be advised of the signs and symptoms of both MAC and tuberculosis, and should be instructed to consult their physicians if they develop new complaints consistent with either of these diseases. In addition, since MYCOBUTIN may rarely be associated with myositis and uveitis, patients should be advised to notify their physicians if they develop signs or symptoms suggesting either of these disorders.

Urine, feces, saliva, sputum, perspiration, tears, and skin may be colored brown-orange with rifabutin and some of its metabolites. Soft contact lenses may be permanently stained. Patients to be treated with MYCOBUTIN should be made aware of these possibilities.

Drug Interactions

In 10 healthy adult volunteers and 8 HIV-positive patients, steady-state plasma levels of zidovudine (ZDV), an antiretroviral agent which is metabolized mainly through glucuronidation, were decreased after repeated MYCOBUTIN dosing; the mean decrease in C_{max} and AUC was 48% and 32%, respectively. *In vitro* studies have demonstrated that MYCOBUTIN does not affect the inhibition of HIV by ZDV.

Steady-state kinetics in 12 HIV-positive patients show that both the rate and extent of systemic availability of didanosine (ddI), was not altered after repeated dosing of MYCOBUTIN.

MYCOBUTIN has liver enzyme-inducing properties. The related drug rifampin is known to reduce the activity of a number of other drugs, including dapsone, narcotics (including methadone), anticoagulants, corticosteroids, cyclosporine, cardiac glycoside preparations, quinidine, oral contraceptives, oral hypoglycemic agents (sulfonylureas), and analgesics. Rifampin has also been reported to decrease the effects of concurrently administered ketoconazole, barbiturates, diazepam, verapamil, beta-adrenergic blockers, clofibrate, progestins, disopyramide, mexiletine, theophylline, chloramphenicol, and anticonvulsants. Because of the structural similarity of rifabutin and rifampin, MYCOBUTIN may be expected to have some effect on these drugs as well. However, unlike rifampin, MYCOBUTIN appears not to affect the acetylation of isoniazid. When rifabutin was compared with rifampin in a study with 8 healthy normal volunteers, rifabutin appeared to be a less potent enzyme inducer than rifampin. The significance of this finding for clinical drug interactions is not known. Dosage adjustment of drugs listed above may be necessary if they are given concurrently with MYCOBUTIN. Patients using oral contraceptives should consider changing to nonhormonal methods of birth control.

Carcinogenesis, Mutagenesis, Impairment of Fertility:

Long term carcinogenicity studies were conducted with rifabutin in mice and in rats. Rifabutin was not carcinogenic in mice at doses up to 180 mg/kg/day, or approximately 36 times the recommended human daily dose. Rifabutin was not carcinogenic in the rat at doses up to 60 mg/kg/day, about 12 times the recommended human dose.

Rifabutin was not mutagenic in the bacterial mutation assay (Ames Test) using both rifabutin-susceptible and resistant strains. Rifabutin was not mutagenic in *Schizosaccharomyces pombe P_1* and was not genotoxic in V-79 Chinese hamster cells, human lymphocytes *in vitro*, or mouse bone marrow cells *in vivo*.

Fertility was impaired in male rats given 160 mg/kg (32 times the recommended human daily dose).

Pregnancy:

Pregnancy Category B: Reproduction studies have been carried out in rats and rabbits given rifabutin using dose levels up to 200 mg/kg (40 times the recommended human daily dose). No teratogenicity was observed in either species. In rats, given 200 mg/kg/day, there was a decrease in fetal viability. In rats, at 40 mg/kg/day (8 times the recommended human daily dose), rifabutin caused an increase in fetal skeletal variants. In rabbits, at 80 mg/kg/day (16 times the recommended human daily dose), rifabutin caused maternotoxicity and increase in fetal skeletal anomalies. There are no adequate and well-controlled studies in pregnant women. Because animal reproduction studies are not always predictive of human response, rifabutin should be used in pregnant women only if the potential benefit justifies the potential risk to the fetus.

Nursing Mothers:

It is not known whether rifabutin is excreted in human milk. Because many drugs are excreted in human milk and because of the potential for serious adverse reactions in nursing infants, a decision should be made whether to discontinue nursing or discontinue the drug, taking into account the importance of the drug to the mother.

Pediatric Use:

Safety and effectiveness of rifabutin for prophylaxis of MAC in children have not been established. Limited safety data are available from treatment use in 22 HIV-positive children with MAC who received MYCOBUTIN in combination with at least two other antimycobacterials for periods from 1 to 183 weeks. Mean doses (mg/kg) for these children were: 18.5 (range 15.0 to 25.0) for infants one year of age; 8.6 (range 4.4 to 18.8) for children 2 to 10 years of age; and 4.0 (range 2.8 to 5.4) for adolescents 14 to 16 years of age. There is no evidence that doses greater than 5 mg/kg daily are useful. Adverse experiences were similar to those observed in the adult population, and included leukopenia, neutropenia and rash. Doses of MYCOBUTIN may be administered mixed with foods such as applesauce.

ADVERSE REACTIONS

MYCOBUTIN was generally well tolerated in the controlled clinical trials. Discontinuation of therapy due to an adverse event was required in 16% of patients receiving MYCOBUTIN compared to 8% of patients receiving placebo in these trials. Primary reasons for discontinuation of MYCOBUTIN were rash (4% of treated patients), gastrointestinal intolerance (3%), and neutropenia (2%).

The following table enumerates adverse experiences that occurred at a frequency of 1% or greater, among the patients treated with MYCOBUTIN in studies 023 and 027.

CLINICAL ADVERSE EXPERIENCES REPORTED IN ≥1% OF PATIENTS TREATED WITH MYCOBUTIN		
ADVERSE EVENT	MYCOBUTIN (n = 566) %	PLACEBO (n = 580) %
BODY AS A WHOLE		
Abdominal Pain	4	3
Asthenia	1	1
Chest Pain	1	1
Fever	2	1
Headache	3	5
Pain	1	2
DIGESTIVE SYSTEM		
Anorexia	2	2
Diarrhea	3	3
Dyspepsia	3	1
Eructation	3	1
Flatulence	2	1
Nausea	6	5
Nausea and Vomiting	3	2
Vomiting	1	1
MUSCULOSKELETAL SYSTEM		
Myalgia	2	1
NERVOUS SYSTEM		
Insomnia	1	1
SKIN AND APPENDAGES		
Rash	11	8
SPECIAL SENSES		
Taste Perversion	3	1
UROGENITAL SYSTEM		
Discolored Urine	30	6

CLINICAL ADVERSE EVENTS REPORTED IN <1% OF PATIENTS WHO RECEIVED MYCOBUTIN

Considering data from the 023 and 027 pivotal trials, and from other clinical studies, MYCOBUTIN appears to be a likely cause of the following adverse events which occurred in less than 1% of treated patients: flu-like syndrome, hepatitis, hemolysis, arthralgia, myositis, chest pressure or pain with dyspnea, and skin discoloration.

The following adverse events have occurred in more than one patient receiving MYCOBUTIN, but an etiologic role has not been established: seizure, paresthesia, aphasia, confusion, and non-specific T wave changes on electrocardiogram.

When MYCOBUTIN was administered at doses from 1050 mg/day to 2400 mg/day, generalized arthralgia and uveitis were reported. These adverse experiences abated when MYCOBUTIN was discontinued.

The following table enumerates the changes in laboratory values that were considered as laboratory abnormalities in studies 023 and 027.

PERCENTAGE OF PATIENTS WITH LABORATORY ABNORMALITIES		
LABORATORY ABNORMALITIES	MYCOBUTIN (n = 566) %	PLACEBO (n = 580) %
Chemistry:		
Increased Alkaline Phosphatase[1]	<1	3
Increased SGOT[2]	7	12
Increased SGPT[2]	9	11
Hematology:		
Anemia[3]	6	7
Eosinophilia	1	1
Leukopenia[4]	17	16
Neutropenia[5]	25	20
Thrombocytopenia[6]	5	4

INCLUDES GRADE 3 OR 4 TOXICITIES AS SPECIFIED:

[1]all values > 450 U/L
[2]all values > 150 U/L
[3]all hemoglobin values < 8.0 g/dL
[4]all WBC values < 1,500/mm³
[5]all ANC values < 750/mm³
[6]all platelet count values < 50,000/mm³

The incidence of neutropenia in patients treated with MYCOBUTIN was significantly greater than in patients treated with placebo (p = 0.03). Although thrombocytopenia was not significantly more common among MYCOBUTIN treated patients in these trials, MYCOBUTIN has been clearly linked to thrombocytopenia in rare cases. One patient in study 023 developed thrombotic thrombocytopenic purpura, which was attributed to MYCOBUTIN.

CAUTION: Federal law prohibits dispensing without prescription.

Manufactured by:
FARMITALIA CARLO ERBA
ASCOLI PICENO, ITALY

For:
ADRIA LABORATORIES
COLUMBUS, OHIO 43216

References: **1.** U.S. Department of Health and Human Services, Public Health Services, Centers for Disease Control and Prevention. Recommendations on prophylaxis and therapy for disseminated *Mycobacterium avium* complex for adults and adolescents infected with human immunodeficiency virus. *MMWR Morb Mortal Wkly Rep.* 1993;42(No. RR-9):14-20. **2.** Chaisson RE, Moore RD, Richman DD, et al. Incidence and natural history of *Mycobacterium avium*-complex infections in patients with advanced human immunodeficiency virus disease treated with zidovudine. *Am Rev Respir Dis.* 1992;146:285-289. **3.** Havlik JA Jr, Horsburgh CR Jr, Metchock B, Williams PP, Fann SA, Thompson SE III. Disseminated *Mycobacterium avium* complex infection: clinical identification and epidemiologic trends. *J Infect Dis.* 1992;165:577-580. **4.** Horsburgh CR Jr. *Mycobacterium avium* complex infection in the acquired immunodeficiency syndrome. *N Engl J Med.* 1991;324:1332-1338. **5.** Data on file, Pharmacia. **6.** Chabner BA. Oncology. In: Wyngaarden JB, Smith LH, Bennett JC, eds. *Cecil Textbook of Medicine.* 19th ed. Philadelphia: W.B. Saunders Co; 1992:1022. **7.** Nightingale SD, Cameron DW, Gordin FM, et al. Two controlled trials of rifabutin prophylaxis against *Mycobacterium avium* complex infection in AIDS. *N Engl J Med.* 1993;329:828-833.

Keep one step ahead of MAC

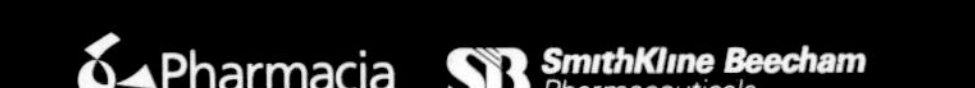

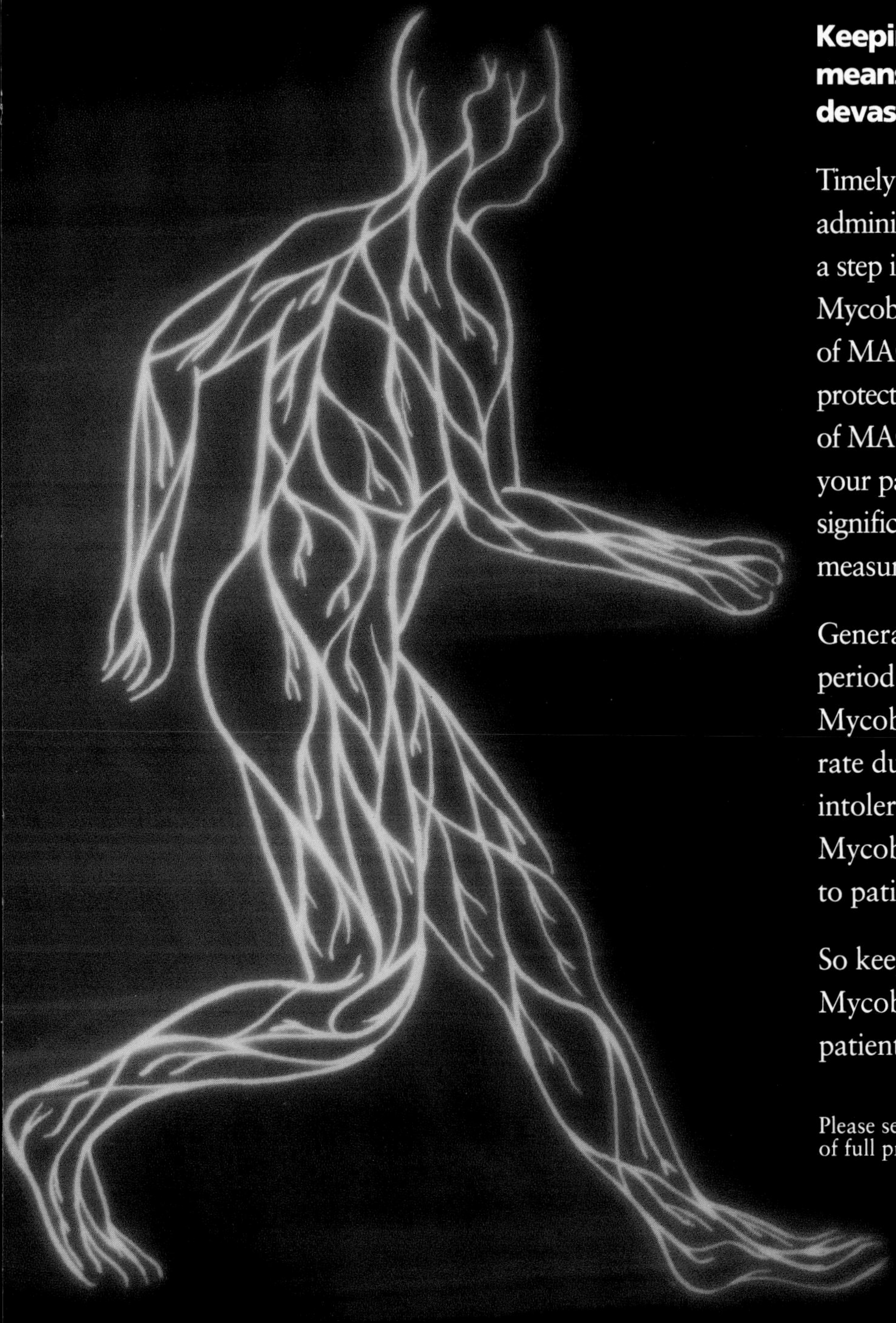

Keeping one step ahead of MAC* means keeping one step ahead of its devastating symptoms.

Timely MAC prophylaxis with a once-daily administration of 300 mg of Mycobutin is a step in the right direction. That's because Mycobutin is proven to reduce the incidence of MAC bacteremia. Mycobutin also protects against the most recognized features of MAC-related morbidity...and maintains your patient's baseline level of activity significantly longer than placebo, as measured by Karnofsky scores.[7]

Generally well tolerated during the trial period compared with placebo, Mycobutin had a higher discontinuation rate due to rash (4%), gastrointestinal intolerance (3%), and neutropenia (2%).[5] Mycobutin must not be administered to patients with active tuberculosis.

So keep a step ahead of MAC with Mycobutin. You'll be helping *your* AIDS patients at risk for MAC *feel better longer*.

Please see adjacent page for brief summary of full prescribing information.

300 mg
once daily†

Prevent MAC Now!

Mycobutin®
150mg (rifabutin capsules)

**Mycobacterium avium* complex.
†Rifabutin, structurally related to rifampin, may reduce the activity of drugs affected by its liver enzyme inducing properties.

TIMELY PROPHYLAXIS HELPS AIDS PATIENTS FEEL BETTER LONGER

Pharmacia Adria   SB SmithKline Beecham Pharmaceuticals

Publisher:

NC Directories
1211 Locust Street
Philadelphia, PA 19107

A listing of a health care or service agency in this Directory does not necessarily imply an endorsement by the publishers/authors.

CREATING REIMBURSEMENT SOLUTIONS

PROCRIT®
EPOETIN ALFA

Ortho Biotech Inc. is helping to create reimbursement solutions through our unsurpassed patient financial support programs.* We invite you to take advantage of our comprehensive reimbursement services.

PROCRITline™ 1-800-553-3851
Assists with third-party billing issues and facilitates reimbursement.

Cost Sharing Program 1-800-441-1366
Limits costs associated with long-term therapy.

Financial Assistance Program (FAP™) 1-800-447-3437
Offers PROCRIT at no charge to qualifying noninsured, low-income patients.

Reimbursement Assurance Program 1-800-553-3851
Ensures that if reimbursement is denied, the amount of PROCRIT administered while awaiting the reimbursement decision will be replaced to the purchasing physician or home healthcare organization. Additional PROCRIT will be provided if patients qualify for the FAP™ for ongoing therapy.

Ortho Biotech Customer/Medical Services and Support 1-800-325-7504

*Available only to qualifying nondialysis patients.

TABLE of CONTENTS

DIRECTORY STAFF

1994-95
NATIONAL
DIRECTORY
of AIDS

ISBN: 0-925133-39-6
5th ANNUAL EDITION

PUBLISHER:
Joseph Braden

EDITORS:
Lori Hullfish
Kathy Wolden

ADVERTISING MANAGER:
Joseph Braden

CIRCULATION MANAGER:
Kelly Collins

EDITORIAL OFFICE:
1800 Byberry Road
800 Masons Mill Business Park
Huntingdon Valley, PA 19006
(215) 938-5511

CIRCULATION & ADVERTISING OFFICE:
1211 Locust Street
Philadelphia, PA 19107
(215) 545-7222

HOW TO USE

Section One: National Organizations and Hotlines

In this section, only toll-free 800 numbers for hotlines that can be dialed nationwide are listed. Hotlines accessible only within specific states are found at the beginning of each state listing in Section II.

The listing of national organizations in this section includes a variety of HIV/AIDS-related organizations, professional associations and national foundations.

Section Two: State, County and Local Services (by state)

In this section, listings for care providing organizations and services are presented by state in alphabetical order. A map displaying counties and major cities and towns introduces each state section.The following categories appear in each state section for statewide organizations: State Health Departments; Statewide Services; Hotlines (toll-free, 800 and non-800); Education

The following categories appear by county for organizations which provide countywide and locally oriented services: Community Services; County Health Departments; Home Health Care (including home care agencies, hospice services and visiting nurse associations); Medical Services (including hospitals, health centers and clinics); Testing Sites

Section III: Federal Agencies & Programs

This section provides a map of the ten Department of Health and Human Services (DHHS) regions and listings for Medicaid Regional AIDS Coordinators, Social Security AIDS Coordinators, Human Resource and Service Administration (HRSA) Education and Training Centers and Ryan White funded care programs.

The Bureau of Health Professionals administers the Regional Education and Training Centers (ETC). These centers train community primary care providers to incorporate strategies for HIV prevention into their clinical practice, and to manage and counsel clients and their support systems. ETCs also train individuals to serve as instructors in their local areas.

The Ryan White Comprehensive AIDS Resources Emergency (CARE) Act of 1990 mandates funds for the provision of services for people infected with the HIV virus. The Act directs assistance to: metropolitan areas with the largest numbers of cases of AIDS to meet emergency service needs (Title I); all states to improve the quality, availability and organization of health care and support services for HIV positive individuals and their families (Title II); all states to support early intervention services (Title III); support a series of specified general provisions including evaluations and reports, research and services for children with HIV (Title IV)

The Human Resource and Service Administration is responsible for Title I and Title II programs which are managed by the BHRD. The Bureau of Health Care Delivery Assistance (also part of HRSA) participates with the Centers for Disease Control (CDC) to carry out the requirements of Title III.

The purpose of the HHS's Pediatric/Family Demonstration Program is to develop national models of care for children, adolescents, women and families infected with HIV. The program focuses primarily on developing systems of care for children who have HIV or AIDS and participating pediatric programs have begun to provide women access to specialized medical, testing and counseling services, as well as related psychosocial services such as foster care, respite care and financial and transportation services.

The National Institute of Allergy and Infectious Diseases (NIAID) funds the AIDS Clinical Trials Groups, AIDS Clinical Trials Units, Community Programs for Clinical Research on AIDS, the Division of AIDS Treatment Research Initiative and the newly formed AIDS Clinical Infrastructure for Minority Institutions Program.

The goal of these programs is to conduct clinical trials that will provide guidance to physicians in the selection of therapies for their patients and lead to the approval of new drugs. The NAIAD Clinical Trials Information Service can be reached at 800-874-2572. This computerized service provides information on various study options, eligibility requirements, exclusion criteria, study locaton and duration, and names and telephone numbers of contacts at each study site.

Community-based clinical trials are coordinated through the American Foundation for AIDS Research (AMFAR) and NIAID. These trials work to expand the number of experimental drugs for actual use. The process has a shorter drug approval time than that of the Food & Drug Administration. Patients participate in the trials and receive medical care at the same location.

Section IV: Clinical Trials and Research Sites

This section provides listings of clinical trials for AIDS therapies and clinical research projects located at hospitals, medical centers, universities and community-based sites throughout the U.S. Most are funded by the National Institute of Allergy and Infectious Diseases (NIAID), a unit of the National Institutes of Health and the research arm of the U.S. Public Health Service, Department of Health and Human Services.The goal of these programs is to conduct clinical trials that will provide guidance to physicians responsible for selecting appropriate therapies for AIDS patients and also provide information that will contribute to the approval of new drugs.

The AIDS Clinical Trials Information Service may be contacted at 800-874-2572.

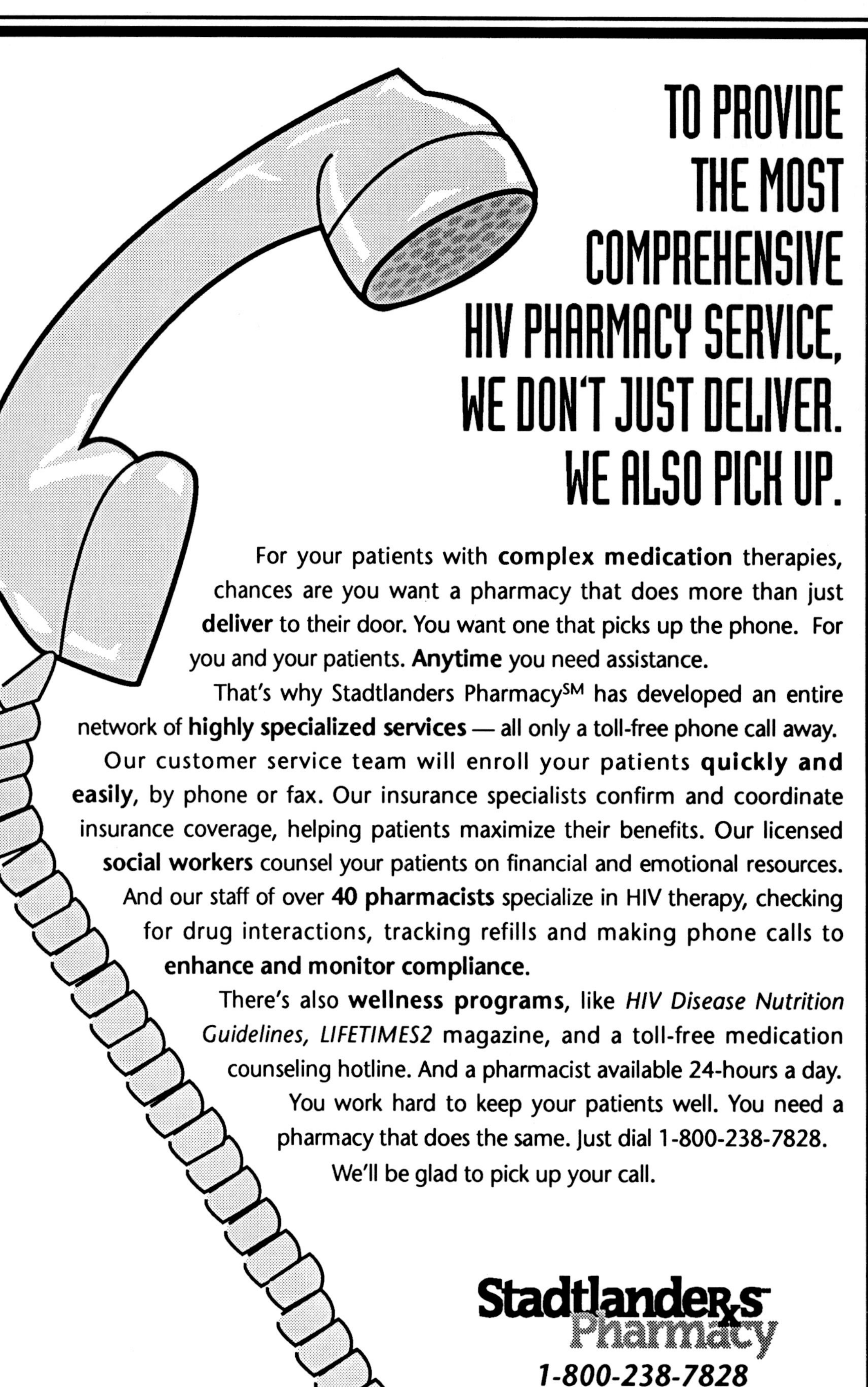
TO PROVIDE
THE MOST
COMPREHENSIVE
HIV PHARMACY SERVICE,
WE DON'T JUST DELIVER.
WE ALSO PICK UP.
For your patients with complex medication therapies, chances are you want a pharmacy that does more than just deliver to their door. You want one that picks up the phone. For you and your patients. Anytime you need assistance.
That's why Stadtlanders Pharmacy℠ has developed an entire network of highly specialized services — all only a toll-free phone call away.
Our customer service team will enroll your patients quickly and easily, by phone or fax. Our insurance specialists confirm and coordinate insurance coverage, helping patients maximize their benefits. Our licensed social workers counsel your patients on financial and emotional resources. And our staff of over 40 pharmacists specialize in HIV therapy, checking for drug interactions, tracking refills and making phone calls to enhance and monitor compliance.
There's also wellness programs, like HIV Disease Nutrition Guidelines, LIFETIMES2 magazine, and a toll-free medication counseling hotline. And a pharmacist available 24-hours a day.
You work hard to keep your patients well. You need a pharmacy that does the same. Just dial 1-800-238-7828.
We'll be glad to pick up your call.
Stadtlanders
Pharmacy
1-800-238-7828

AIDS Action Council
1875 Connecticut Ave. NW
Suite 700
Washington, DC 20009
Telephone: (202)-986-1300 Fax: (202)-986-1345
Lobbies for AIDS services, AIDS public policy analysis, education

AIDS Coalition to Unleash Power
135 W 29th Street
10th Floor
New York, NY 10001
Telephone: (212)-564-2437
Education Services, Policy Analysis and Recommendations

AIDS Healthcare Foundation
1800 N. Argyle Avenue
3rd Floor
Los Angeles, CA 90028
Telephone: (000)-021-3462
Information, referrals to clinic sites

AIDS National Interfaith Network
132 W. 31st Street
17th Floor
New York, NY 10001
Telephone: (212)-239-0700

Alcohol and Drug Abuse Services Administration
1300 1st Street, NE
Washington, DC 20002-3314
Telephone: (202)-727-0713
AIDS education, coordination of drug programs.

Amer. Alliance for Health, Phys. Ed., Recreation and Dance
Assoc for Adv of Hlth Ed.
1900 Association Drive
Reston, VA 22091
Telephone: (703)-476-3440
Contact: Martin A. Connor - Acquisitions Editor; Reiko Philpotts - Publications Editor
Education Services, Publication Dissemination, Information Production Services

American Association for Respiratory Care
11030 Ables Lane
Dallas, TX 75229
Telephone: (214)-243-2272
Contact: Sam Giordano - Executive Director; Sherry Milligan - Asst. Executive Director
Education, Videorecordings, Newsletter

American Association of Physicians for Human Rights
273 Church Street
P.O. Box 14366
San Francisco, CA 94114-0366
Telephone: (415)-255-4547
Contact: Ben Schate - Executive Director
Support for Lesbian and Gay Physicians, Newsletter, Referrals, Counseling

American Association of Women
2210 Wilshire Blvd., #174
Santa Monica, CA 90403-5784
Telephone: (310)-395-0244 Fax: (310)-395-1718
Education, Referrals, Research, Speakers Bureau, Transportation, Volunteers

American Bar Association
750 N. Lake Shore Drive
Chicago, IL 60611
Telephone: (312)-988-5158
Referral services

American Cancer Society
901 N. University Avenue
Little Rock, AR 72207-6355
Telephone: (501)-666-5409 Fax: (501)-666-0068
Contact: Liz Larkins
Educational Target: Persons with AIDS diagnosed with cancer.

American Cancer Society
77 East Monroe
Chicago, IL 60603
Telephone: (312)-372-0471 Fax: (312)-372-0910
Information, education, referrals

American Civil Liberties Union Foundation AIDS PROJECT-ACLU
National Headquarters
132 West 43rd Street
New York, NY 10036
Telephone: (212)-944-9800
Contact: Norman Dorsen - President; Ira Glasser - Executive Director; William B. Rubenstein - Director & Staff Counsel

American Civil Liberties Union, National Office
122 Maryland Avenue, NE
Washington, DC 20002
Telephone: (202)-544-1681

American Federation of Home Health Agencies
1320 Fenwick Ln, Ste 100
Silver Spring, MD 20910
Telephone: (301)-588-1454 Fax: (301)-588-4732
Toll-Free: (800)-234-4211
Contact: Anne Howard

American Foundation for AIDS Research
733 3rd Avenue
12th Floor
New York, NY 10017-3204
Telephone: (212)-682-7440
Contact: Robert Brown

Publishes: Facts About AIDS
American Health Foundation
320 East 43rd Street
New York, NY 10017
Telephone: (212)-953-1900 Fax: (212)-687-2339
Contact: Jeff Rossos

AIDS Research
American Holistic Medical Association
4101 Lake Boone Trail
Suite 201
Raleigh, NC 27607-2506
Telephone: (919)-787-5146
Newletter and Journal Production, Referrals, Alternative Therapies

American Hospital Association
840 North Lake Shore Drive
Chicago, IL 60611
Telephone: (312)-280-6000
Toll-Free: (800)-242-2626
Publications on AIDS/HIV

American Indian AIDS Institute
333 Valencia Street
#400
San Francisco, CA 94103-3547
Telephone: (415)-626-7639 Fax: (415)-626-1737
Contact: Liz Hansen
Information, Education, Referrals, Prevention for Native Americans

American Institute for Teen AIDS Prevention
P.O. Box 136116
Fort Worth, TX 76136-0862
Telephone: (817)-237-0230
Contact: Duane Crumb - Director
Education, Publications Dissemination and Production, Videorecordings

American Management Association, Publications Division
PO Box 1026
Saranac Lake, NY 12983
Telephone: (518)-891-1500 Fax: (518)-891-3653
Publisher of: AIDS, The Workplace Issues

American Psychiatric Association
AIDS Task Force
1400 K Street, NW
Washington, DC 20005
Telephone: (202)-682-6104 Fax: (202)-789-1874
Contact: Carol Svoboda
Materials and policies on care of PWAs/PWARCs.

American Psychological Association
AIDS Office
750 First St., NE
Washington, DC 20002
Telephone: (202)-336-5500
Material and policies on care of PWAs/PWARCs.; AIDS newsletter & database

Association for the Care of Children's Health
7910 Woodmont Avenue
Suite 300
Bethesda, MD 20814
Telephone: (301)-654-6549 Fax: (301)-986-4553
Contact: Karen Lawrence - Ph.D., LCSW
Education, training, family center care for AIDS/HIV

BIOSIS (Biosciences Information Service)
2100 Arch Street
Philadelphia, PA 19103-1399
Telephone: (800)-523-4806
Databases, Electronic Media

Foundation Center/National Foundations Database
79 5th Avenue
New York, NY 10003
Telephone: (212)-620-4230 Fax: (212)-691-1828
Contact: Martha Keens - Vice-President
Databases, Electronic Media

Healing Alternatives Foundation
1748 Market Street
San Francisco, CA 94102
Telephone: (415)-626-4053 Fax: (415)-626-0451
Nutritional, Foreign & Experimental Products; AIDS/HIV Treatment Library

Health Resources and Services Administration
Office of AIDS Services
5600 Fischer Lane
Rockville, MD 20857
Telephone: (301)-443-6745
Grants on educational and training centers and AIDS service projects

Hofstra Law Association, Hofstra University
School of Law
Hempstead, NY 11550
Telephone: (516)-463-5916
Publisher of Review on AIDS and Employment Law

Lambda Legal Defense and Education Fund, Inc.
666 Broadway, 12th Fl
New York, NY 10012-2317
Telephone: (212)-995-8585
Contact: Mike Isbell
Test case litigation

Nat. Assoc. of Children's Hospitals and Related Institutions
401 Wythe Street
Alexandria, VA 22314
Telephone: (703)-684-1355
Referral Services, Publication Production, Directories

National AIDS Network
Telephone: (415)-565-3616
Education & Support Services

National AIDS/Pre-AIDS Epidemiological Network
333 East Huron
Chicago, IL 60611-3004
Telephone: (312)-943-6600
Contact: Kathy Pietschmann, RN
Counseling, testing

National Association of Social Workers
750 First St., NE
Ste. 700
Washington, DC 20002
Telephone: (202)-408-8600

National Association of State Boards of Education
AIDS Education Project
1012 Cameron Street
Alexandria, VA 22314
Telephone: (703)-684-4000
Contact: Katherine Fraser - Co-Director
AIDS Publications and Technical Assistance to Schools, Education

National Cancer Institute
9000 Rockville Pike
Clinical Center
Bethesda, MD 20892
Telephone: (301)-496-8959
Protocols for HIV

National Center for Health Education, Resource Bank
72 Spring Street
Suite #208
New York, NY 10012
Telephone: (212)-334-9470 Fax: (212)-334-9845
Contact: M. Ninjo - Administrative Assistant
Education services, publications on AIDS

National Coalition of Hispanic HHS Org. (COSSMHO)
1501 Sixteenth St NW
Washington, DC 20036-1401
Telephone: (202)-387-5000 Fax: (202)-797-4353
Spanish: AIDS directory of Organizations, newsletter, educational materials.

National Community AIDS Partnership
1140 Connecticut Ave. NW
Suite 901
Washington, DC 20036-4001
Telephone: (202)-429-2820 Fax: (202)-429-2814
Contact: Paula Van Ness
Fund raising to support HIV prevention and care

National Community AIDS Partnership
1140 Connecticut Ave NW
Suite 901
Washington, DC 20036
Telephone: (202)-429-2820

National Council of Churches
475 Riverside Drive
New York, NY 10115
Telephone: (212)-870-2511
AIDS task force, education, service and support programs

National Council of La Raza
900 Wilshire Blvd., #1520
Los Angeles, CA 90017-4716
Telephone: (213)-489-3428 Fax: (213)-489-1167
Civil rights, research, non-profit

National Council on Alcoholism & Drug Addiction
944 Market, #300
3rd Floor
San Francisco, CA 94102-4010
Telephone: (415)-296-9900
Contact: Maggi Hoogs
Substance abuse services, AIDS/HIV education

National Council on Alcoholism & Drug Dependence
1922 The Alameda
#212
San Jose, CA 95126-1430
Telephone: (408)-241-5577 Fax: (408)-241-2159
Contact: Mary Ellen Shell
Helpline; drug, alcohol & tobacco resource center, youth education

National Council on Alcoholism,NCH Multicultural AIDS Projct
1446 Martin Luther King Pkwy.
Des Moines, IA 50314
Telephone: (515)-244-2297 Fax: (515)-244-2297
Contact: Preston Daniels - Director
Minority Grantees, HIV prevention and risk-prevention education

National Education Association, Health Information Network
1201 16th Street, NW
Washington, DC 20036-3290
Telephone: (202)-833-4000 Fax: (202)-822-7775
Education Services, Training, Workshops, Seminars

National Foundation for Infectious Diseases
4733 Bethesda Avenue
Suite 750
Bethesda, MD 20815
Telephone: (301)-656-0003
Contact: William E. Small
Meetings, Conferences, Training, Workshops, Seminars, Book, Monograph,Pamphlets

National Funeral Directors Association
11121 W. Oklahoma Avenue
Milwaukee, WI 53227-4096
Telephone: (414)-541-2500
Funeral Assistance, Information, Journal Publication

National Hemophilia Foundation, National Center for AIDS
Soho Building
110 Greene Street, Rm 303
New York, NY 10012
Telephone: (212)-219-8180 Fax: (212)-431-0906
Toll-Free: (800)-424-2634
Contact: Alan P. Brownstein - MSW
Education, training, library services, information & hemophilia HIVinformation network

National Hospice Organization
1901 N. Fort Meyer Drive
Suite 307
Arlington, VA 22209
Telephone: (703)-243-5900
Contact: John J. Mahoney - President
Hospice Information and Locations, Referrals, Education, Publication Production

National Institute for Occupational Safety and Health
4676 Columbia Pky.
Cincinnati, OH 45226
Telephone: (513)-533-8328
Information on AIDS

National Institute of Allergy & Infectious Disease
9000 Rockville Pike
Clinical Center, Bldg. 10, 11-N228
Bethesda, MD 20892
Telephone: (301)-496-7196
Research

National Institute of Allergy and Infectious Disease
AIDS Treatment & Evaluation Units
Bldg.31 #7A50
Bethesda, MD 20892
Telephone: (301)-496-5717
National toll free hotline 1-800 TRIALS-A

National Institute of Allergy and Infectious Disease (NIAID)
AIDS Treatment & Evaluation Units
Bldg. 31 #7A50
Bethesda, MD 20892
Telephone: (301)-496-5717 Fax: (301)-402-0120
Contact: Judy Murphy
AIDS education

National Institute of Justice, AIDS Clearinghouse
Rockville, MD 20850
Toll-Free: (800)-458-5231
Information on legal issues

National Institutes of Health
9000 Rockville Pike
Clinical Center
Bethesda, MD 20892
Telephone: (301)-496-9565
Contact: Candace Curtz
Clinical trials information, research information, protocols

National Institutes of Health, Clinical Center
Patient Referral Service
Building 10, Room 1C-255
Bethesda, MD 20892
Telephone: (301)-496-4891
Research, clinical care, and support. AIDS health information protocols.

National Jewish Center for Immunology & Respiratory Medicine
1400 Jackson Street
Denver, CO 80206-2762
Telephone: (303)-398-1907
Contact: Jim Joneschonbrun - HIV Coordinator
Medical Services, Education, Information Dissemination, Referrals, Research

National League for Nursing
350 Hudson Street
4th Floor
New York, NY 10014-4504
Telephone: (212)-989-9393 Fax: (212)-727-3715
Toll-Free: (800)-669-1656
Contact: Florence Sandiford
Database for nursing information

National Library of Medicine/AIDSLINE
8600 Rockville Pike
Rockville, MD 20894
Telephone: (301)-496-6193
Free online database on AIDS/HIV, part of MEDLARS ManagementSection

National Mental Health Association
1021 Prince Street
Alexandria, VA 22314-2971
Telephone: (703)-684-7722
Contact: Beth Kempter - Editor
Newsletter and Periodical Production and Dissemination

National Minority AIDS Council
300 I St. NE, #400
Washington, DC 30002-4389
Telephone: (202)-544-1076 Fax: (202)-544-0378
Contact: Cheryl McClellan
Model of education and leadership, advocacy, minority sensitive programs.

National Native American AIDS Prevention Center
3515 Grand Avenue
Suite 100
Oakland, CA 94610
Telephone: (510)-444-2051 Fax: (510)-444-1593
Contact: Executive Director
Education and prevention

National Native American AIDS Prevention Center
3515 Grand Avenue
Suite 100
Oakland, CA 94610
Telephone: (510)-444-2051 Fax: (510)-444-1593
Contact: Ron Rowell - Executive Director
Computer Bulletin Board, Conferences, Training, Hotline, Newsletter

National School Boards Association
1680 Duke Street
Alexandria, VA 22314
Telephone: (703)-838-6722
Clearinghous for AIDS policies/education curricula. AIDS training, publications

National Urban League
500 East 62nd Street
New York, NY 10021
Telephone: (212)-310-9000
Provides AIDS education to affiliated organizations

National Women's Health Network
1325 G Street, NW
Washington, DC 20005-3189
Telephone: (202)-347-1140
Counseling, Education, Workshops, Newsletter

Planned Parenthood Federation of America
810 7th Avenue
New York, NY 10019
Telephone: (212)-541-7800
Contact: Susan Newcomer - Education Director
Counseling, Testing Sites, Education, Database, Publication, Policy Analysis

Pride Institute
14400 Martin Drive
Eden Prairie, MN 55344-2031
Telephone: (612)-934-7554 Fax: (612)-934-8764
Contact: David Lewis - Director of Admissions
Alcohol/drug abuse rehab treatment for Lesbians, Gays, Bisexuals.

Project Inform
1965 Market Street
Suite 220
San Francisco, CA 94103
Telephone: (800)-822-7422 Fax: (415)-558-0684
Contact: Martin Delaney - Director
Hotline: Medical information on AIDS

PWA Coalition Newsline

New York, NY
Telephone: (212)-645-4538
Contact: Chris Babbock; Diane Cross

PWA Health Group
150 West 26th Street
Suite 201
New York, NY 10010-1003
Telephone: (212)-255-0520
Experimental Drug Treatments

Robert Wood Johnson Foundation
Route 1, N. and College Road, E.
PO Box 2316
Princeton, NJ 08543-2316
Telephone: (609)-452-8701

Scientific American, Incorporated/ Medicine Database
415 Madison Avenue
New York, NY 10017-1179
Telephone: (212)-754-0805 Fax: (212)-980-3062
Contact: Toby Bilanow
Databases, Electronic Media

US Department of Health and Human Services, Nat. Inst./Hlth
National Library/Medicine
8600 Rockville Pike
Bethesda, MD 20894
Telephone: (301)-496-4000
Education Services, Free Online Database (AIDSLINE), Electronic Media,Library Services

US Department of Health and Human Services, Public Health Services
Rockville, MD
Telephone: (301)-496-2351

US Department of Health and Human Services, Public Health Services
Public Inquiries Branch
5600 Fishers Lane
Rockville, MD 20857
Telephone: (301)-443-2403
Books, Monographs, Pamphlets, Brochures

US Dept. of Health and Human Services, AIDS Research Program
Building 31, Rm. 11-A-48
9000 Rockville Pike
Bethesda, MD 20892
Telephone: (301)-496-5615
Contact: Samuel Broder, MD - Dir., Natl. Cancer Institute
AIDS Treatment, Evaluation Services, Hotlines, Referral Services, Research,Drug

US Dept. of Health and Human Services, Office for Civil Rights
50 United Nations Plaza
Room 322
San Francisco, CA 94102-4912
Telephone: (415)-556-8586 Fax: (415)-556-5165
Contact: Virginia Apodaca
Federal agency to ensure non-discrimination in health care & social services.

ALABAMA

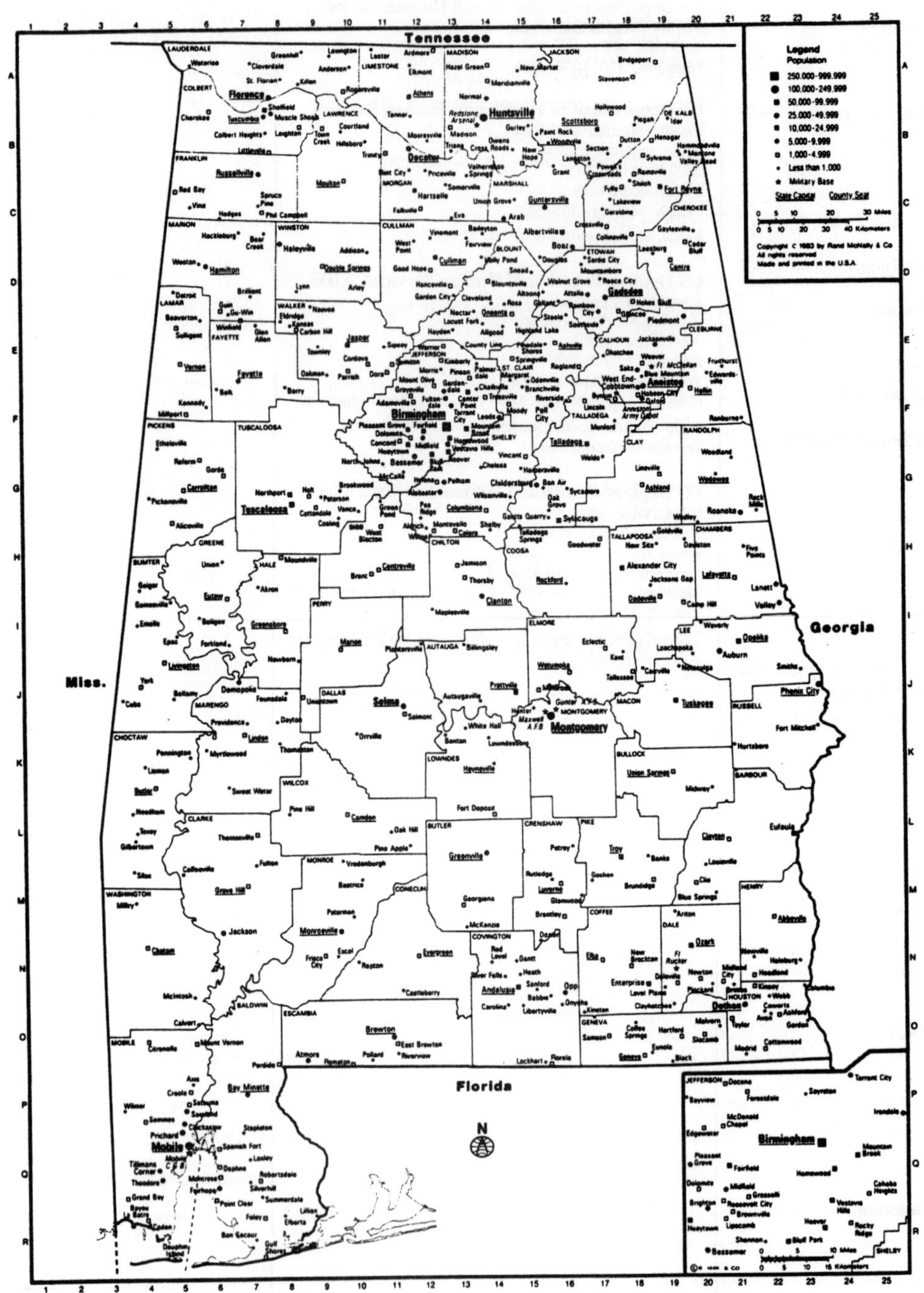

From City/County Planning Atlas Copyright 1989 by Reed McNally & Company, R.L. 90-S-28

Alabama

General Services

Education

AIDS Information Center, College of Community Health Science
Health Sciences Library
P.O. Box 870378
Tuscaloosa, AL 35487-0378
Telephone: (205)-348-1364
Contact: Barbara P. Doughty
Information on AIDS to Health Care Professionals in West Alabama

Alabama Academy of Family Physcians
19 South Jackson Street
Montgomery, AL 36102
Telephone: (205)-263-6441 Fax: (205)-269-5200
Contact: Holley Midgley
Public and Physician Awareness Programs

Alabama AIDS Symposium, Inc., Alabama Dept. of Public Health
AIDS Education Field Services Section
2451 Fillingim Street
Mobile, AL 36617
Telephone: (205)-471-7322
Contact: Joan B. Huffstutler, M.Ed. - Chief, AIDS Education
Holds Annual Statewide AIDS Symposium on AIDS/HIV prevention

Alabama Dental Association
836 Washington Avenue
Montgomery, AL 36104-3893
Telephone: (205)-265-1684 Fax: (205)-262-6218
Contact: Dr. Hiram Johnson
AIDS Educational Programs

Alabama Public Health Association, Inc. (ALPHA)
P.O. Box 2343
Montgomery, AL 36102
Telephone: (205)-613-5273 Fax: (205)-240-3377
Contact: Winkler Sims - President
Educational Meetings, Education and Training Programs for Public Health Workers

American Red Cross, Alabama Territory
P.O. Box 1207
Birmingham, AL 35201-1207
Telephone: (205)-328-3087
Contact: James Long - Field Service Manager
Community Service, Education

American Red Cross, Colbert County Chapter
120 West 5th Street
Tuscumbia, AL 35674-2412
Telephone: (205)-383-3721
Contact: Rebecca Stainback - Director
Blood Bank, AIDS Brochures and Audiovisuals

American Red Cross, Covington County Chapter
110 Crescent Street
Andalusia, AL 36420
Telephone: (205)-222-4231
Contact: Joy Cooke - Chapter Manager
Service to military families, disaster relief, blood collection, education

American Red Cross, Dallas County Chapter
P.O. Box 652
Selma, AL 36702-0652
Telephone: (205)-874-4641
Contact: Howard R. Tinsley
AIDS Education, Youth Counseling

American Red Cross, Jackson County Chapter
Courthouse
Broad Street
Scottsboro, AL 35768
Telephone: (205)-574-9382
Contact: Sandra Venable - Chapter Manager
Speakers, videos, and current pamphlets on AIDS

American Red Cross, Limestone County Chapter
P.O. Box 712
107 West Elm Street
Athens, AL 35611-0712
Telephone: (205)-232-6820
Contact: Hazel White
Serving Persons in Athens and Limestone County; Education, Resources

American Red Cross, Madison County Chapter
1101 Washington Street
Huntsville, AL 35801-5417
Telephone: (205)-536-0084 Fax: (205)-539-5914
Contact: Mary Elizabeth Marr - Health Education Spec.; Gail Williams, R.N. - HIV/AIDS Coordinator
Education, HIV instructor training, resource referral, video library

American Red Cross, Mobile Bay Area Chapter
P.O. Box 1764
Mobile, AL 36633-1764
Telephone: (205)-438-2571 Fax: (205)-433-2741
Contact: Dean Owens, R.N.
Public and Worksite Education, Facilitator Training

American Red Cross, Montgomery County Chapter
364 South Ripley Street
Montgomery, AL 36104
Telephone: (205)-834-8680
Contact: Marilyn Hall
AIDS education for schools and community groups upon request

American Red Cross, Pike County Chapter
315 West Walnut Street
Troy, AL 36081-2039
Telephone: (205)-566-0632 Fax: (205)-566-0419
Contact: Ralph E. Fowee
Education at Schools, Clubs, Community Groups; Printed Materials, Audiovisuals

American Red Cross, Shelby County Service Center
509 D Highway 119
Alabaster, AL 35007-9747
Telephone: (205)-663-4290
Contact: Margo Fallin; Sally Olson -
Visual aids, teacher, parent and student guides, printed materials andcourses

American Red Cross, Southeast Region
P.O. Box 11003
Birmingham, AL 35202-1003
Telephone: (205)-715-2101
Contact: John E. Evans - Regional Chairman
Covering seven states in Southeast U.S., AIDS instructions

American Red Cross, Tuscaloosa County Chapter
1100 15th Street, East
Tuscaloosa, AL 35404
Telephone: (205)-758-3608
Contact: Madge Noland
Education of Public for Prevention of AIDS, Videos, Written Materials

Assn. for Practitioners in Infection Control, Alabama Chap.
Baptist Med Ctr-Montclair
800 Montclair Road
Birmingham, AL 35213
Telephone: (205)-592-5411
Contact: Leigh Champion - President
Speakers

H. Grady Bradshaw Chambers County Library
3419 20th Avenue
Valley, AL 36854
Telephone: (205)-768-2161
Contact: Anne K. Alsobrook
AIDS programs, support information

Carraway Northwest Medical Center
P.O. Box 130
Winfield, AL 35594
Telephone: (205)-487-4234 Fax: (205)-487-6187
Contact: Sheri White, R.N. - Infection Control Coord.
AIDS programs presented to civic organizations in the community

Cooperative Health Manpower Education Program
VA Medical Center
Bldg.9, 2400 Hospital Road
Tuskegee, AL 36083
Telephone: (205)-727-0550
Contact: Sceiva Holland - Executive Director
Statewide Education for Community, Health Care Providers, and Minorities

Foundation for Women's Health in Alabama
225-A Arlington Avenue
Birmingham, AL 35205
Telephone: (205)-877-2538
Contact: Debra Cook - President
Programs to raise the awareness of women about health care issues

Guntersville City Schools
P.O. Box 129
Guntersville, AL 35976
Telephone: (205)-582-2743
Contact: Gayle Moore; Lawayne Vanzandt -
AIDS Prevention by Education; Films, Presentations for Students and Community

Health and Welfare Ministries, The United Methodist Church
P.O. Box 777
Calera, AL 35040
Telephone: (205)-668-0358 Fax: (205)-226-7954
Contact: Phillip Huckaby
Furnish films and teach in training events. Present an annual update on AIDS.

Health Education Linkage Programs (HELP)
901 13th Street South
University of Alabama
Birmingham, AL 35294
Telephone: (205)-582-0292
Education, special classes for minorities, group sessions

Helen Keller Memorial Hospital
P.O. Box 610
Sheffield, AL 35660
Telephone: (205)-386-4196
Contact: Jane Barnett, R.N.
Student, patient and community education

March of Dimes, Dothan
200 Honeysuckle Road
Suite C
Dothan, AL 36301
Telephone: (205)-792-0149
Contact: Lisa Goodman
Public awareness, resource information; pamphlets on HIV+ babies

March of Dimes, Montgomery
2143 Eastern Boulevard
Suite 18
Montgomery, AL 36117
Telephone: (205)-277-6910
Contact: Linda Alred
Public awareness and resource information

Marion County AIDS Prevention Subcommittee
Marion County Health Council
P.O. Box 158
Hamilton, AL 35570-0158
Telephone: (205)-921-3118
Contact: Ann Couch, R.N.
AIDS speakers bureau, resource information, public awareness

Planned Parenthood of Alabama, Inc., Huntsville
813 Franklin Street
Suite C
Huntsville, AL 35801
Telephone: (205)-539-2746 Fax: (205)-536-3228
Contact: Kay Thrash, C.R.N.P. - Clinic Director
Free telephone information system, AIDS education and referral for testing

Southern Christian Leadership Conference, Wings of Hope Program
1702 Noble Street
Anniston, AL 36201
Telephone: (205)-237-6731
Contact: James Ford - Director
Conducts Red Cross certified HIV/AIDS training for adults and teenagers

United Way Information Line
407 Noble Street
Anniston, AL 36201
Telephone: (205)-237-4636 Fax: (205)-236-2356
Contact: Priscilla Studdard
Refer people in need to appropriate agency

University of Alabama, Student Health Services
P.O. Box 870360
Tuscaloosa, AL 35487-0360
Telephone: (205)-348-3878
Contact: Dr. George Wilson
Education, Referrals, and Counseling for U of AL Students; Pamphlets, Videos

University of Montevallo Health Services
Station #6275
Montevallo, AL 35115
Telephone: (205)-665-6275
Contact: Jeanette Merijanian, RN, MPH
Counseling, referral, AIDS educational materials, program consultants, videos

University of Southern Alabama Library

Mobile, AL 36688
Telephone: (205)-460-7025
Contact: Jerry Wright - Reference Librarian
AIDS resource materials, books, brochures, videotapes, films

Washington County Health Council
P.O. Box 280
Chatom, AL 36518-0280
Telephone: (205)-847-2295
Contact: Sara H. Hazen
Assists with educational programs for general public concerning AIDS;volunteers

Wilcox County Department of Education
Highway 221
Camden, AL 36726
Telephone: (205)-682-4922 Fax: (205)-682-4409
Contact: Mary Whiting, R.N. - School Nurse
HIV/AIDS education to students in Wilcox County; community workshops

State Health Departments

Alabama AIDS Network, Alabama Department of Public Health
2451 Fillingim Street
Mobile, AL 36617
Telephone: (205)-471-7322 Fax: (205)-471-7884
Contact: Joan B. Huffstutler, M.Ed. - Chief, AIDS Education
Coordinates Area AIDS Educ. and Services; Branch Offices at County Health Depts

Alabama Department of Public Health, Public Health Area I
Madison County Health Dept.
P.O. Box 467, 304 Eustis Street
Decatur, AL 35602-1628
Telephone: (205)-353-7021
Contact: Diana Quirk - AIDS Social Worker
HIV Testing, Counseling, Home Care Services, Referrals, Education, SpeakersCase Management, HIV Clinic.

Alabama Department of Public Health, Public Health Area II
Public Health II
P.O. Box 70190
Tuscaloosa, AL 35407
Telephone: (205)-554-4451 Fax: (205)-556-2701
Contact: Glenn Collins - Disease Control Coord.
Coordinates Area AIDS Educ. and Services; Branch Offices at County Health Depts

Alabama Department of Public Health, Public Health Area III
P.O. Box 1059
Pelham, AL 35124
Telephone: (205)-939-2754 Fax: (205)-987-3353
Contact: Jill Lowman, R.N. - Area AIDS Coordinator; Melinda G. Rowe, M.D. - Asst.State Health Officer
Coordinates Area AIDS Educ. and Services; Branch Offices at County Health Depts

Alabama Department of Public Health, Public Health Area IV
P.O. Box 2648
Anniston, AL 36202
Telephone: (205)-236-3274 Fax: (205)-237-7974
Contact: Jane Haney, R.N.
Coordinates Area AIDS Educ. and Services; Branch Offices at County Health Depts

Alabama Department of Public Health, Public Health Area V
500 Eastern Blvd.
Suite 310
Montgomery, AL 36117
Telephone: (205)-242-5133 Fax: (205)-213-0497
Contact: Brenda Cummings, L.G.S.W. - Area AIDS Coordinator
Coordinates Area AIDS Educ. and Services; Branch Offices at County Health Depts

Alabama Department of Public Health, Public Health Area VII
Mobile County Health Dept
PO Box 2867, 251 N. Bayou
Mobile, AL 36652
Telephone: (205)-690-8167 Fax: (205)-690-8951
Contact: Alfreda King, M.C. - Area AIDS Coordinator; Vivian DeVivo, M.Ed. - Dir.Community Hlth.Svcs.; Alternate tel. 205-690-8816/10
Coordinates Area AIDS Educ. and Services

Alabama Dept. of Public Health, Bureau of Health Promotion & Info.
434 Monroe Street
Room 644
Montgomery, AL 36130-1701
Telephone: (205)-242-2848
Contact: Laurie Eldridge - Dir., Risk Surveillance
Annual AIDS knowledge and opinion surveys

Alabama Dept. of Public Health, Division of Home-Based Services
434 Monroe Street
Suite 406
Montgomery, AL 36130-1701
Telephone: (205)-613-5341 Fax: (205)-240-3376
Contact: Mary Jane Winkler - Dir., Community-Based Services
Home health, home and community-based services including IV therapy

Statewide Services

Alabama Association of County Health Councils
P.O. Box 99
University Station
Birmingham, AL 35294-0001
Telephone: (205)-386-2793
Contact: William J. Parkhurst; Vee Stalker -
Health Forum, Project Planning, Advocacy, Health Resources Evaluation

Alabama Department of Human Resources, Personnel Division
Gordon Persons Adm. Bldg.
50 North Ripley Avenue
Montgomery, AL 36130-1801
Telephone: (205)-242-1793 Fax: (205)-242-8339
Contact: Debbie Milner - AIDS Coordinator
Public assistance, food assistance, adult and child protective services, more

Alabama Department of Public Health, Public Health Area VI
P.O. Box 879
Spanish Fort, AL 36527
Telephone: (205)-621-9103 Fax: (205)-621-9427
Contact: Charles Mitchell - Public Health Representitive
Coordinates Area AIDS Educ. and Services; Branch Offices at County Health Depts

Alabama Department of Public Health, Public Health Area VIII
Jefferson County Health Dept
Box 2648, 1400 6th Ave, S
Birmingham, AL 35202
Telephone: (205)-933-9110

Contact: Loretta Myricks, M.P.H. - Area AIDS Coordinator; Jim Alosi - State Public Health Rep.; Ann Atkinson, L.G.S.W. - Social Worker
Coordinates Area AIDS Education and Services

Alabama Medicaid Agency
2500 Fairlane Drive
Montgomery, AL 36130-0001
Telephone: (205)-277-2710 Fax: (205)-272-6364
Contact: John Anderson
Medicaid; Branches in Birmingham, Opelika, Decatur, Dothan, Gadsden,Mobile, Tuscaloo

Alabama Primary Health Care Association, Inc.
6013 East Shirley Lane
Suite A
Montgomery, AL 36117
Telephone: (205)-271-7068 Fax: (205)-271-7069
Contact: Ray Overton - Executive Director; Emmanuel Uchem - Director Special Projects
Coordinate the training of primary care providers in community health centers

Alabama State Department of Education
Gordon Persons Building
50 N. Ripley St., Rm. 3318
Montgomery, AL 36130-3901
Telephone: (205)-242-8083 Fax: (205)-242-0482
Education Curriculum, Policies, and Guidelines for Students and Staff

Alabama State Nurses' Association
360 N. Hull Street
Montgomery, AL 36104-3658
Telephone: (205)-262-8321 Fax: (205)-262-8578
Speakers Bureau, Nurse Consultants

Health Educators Association of Alabama
Shelton State Community College
202 Skyland Boulevard
Tuscaloosa, AL 35405
Telephone: (205)-391-2294
Contact: Susan Thomas - President
Continuing Education Workshops for Health Educators, Annual Meetings, Speakers

Autauga County

County Health Depts

Autauga County Health Department
153 West Fourth Street
Prattville, AL 36067-3011
Telephone: (205)-361-3743 Fax: (205)-361-3718
HIV Testing, Counseling, Home Care Services, Referrals, Education, Speakers

Baldwin County

County Health Depts

Baldwin County Health Department
72 Fairhope Avenue
Fairhope, AL 36532-3421
Telephone: (205)-928-5504
Contact: Deborah Pennington
HIV Testing, Counseling, Home Care Services, Referrals, Education, Speakers

Baldwin County Health Department, Branch Office
257 Hand Avenue
Bay Minette, AL 36507-4823
Telephone: (205)-937-0217
HIV Testing, Counseling, Home Care Services, Referrals, Education, Speakers

Baldwin County Health Department, Branch Office
104 West Wilson Blvd.
Foley, AL 36535-2680
Telephone: (205)-943-2342
Contact: Charles Watterson
HIV Testing, Counseling, Home Care Services, Referrals, Education, Speakers

Medical Services

Mercy Medical
P.O. Box 1090
Daphne, AL 36526
Telephone: (205)-626-2694 Fax: (205)-626-0315
Contact: Kay McLeod, L.C.S.W. - Dir.of Social Work & Adm.
AIDS patients may receive in-patient and/or homecare services

Barbour County

County Health Depts

Barbour County Health Department
178 East Cottonwood Road
Eufaula, AL 36027-1619
Telephone: (205)-687-4808 Fax: (205)-793-5366
Contact: Joanne Holland - Office Manager
HIV Testing, Counseling, Home Care Services, Referrals, Education, Speakers

Barbour County Health Department, Branch Office
North Midway Street
Clayton, AL 36016
Telephone: (205)-775-8324
Contact: Peggy Blakeney
HIV Testing, Counseling, Home Care Services, Referrals, Education,Speakers, Literature

Home Health Care

Vital Care of Eufaula
146 East Broad Street
Eufaula, AL 36027
Telephone: (205)-687-3591
Contact: Jim Scarborough
At-home therapies including total parenteral nutrition and IV antibiotics

Bibb County

County Health Depts

Bibb County Health Department
105 Church Street
Centreville, AL 35042-1207
Telephone: (205)-926-9702
Contact: Kim Ingrham
HIV Testing, Counseling, Home Care Services, Referrals, Education, Speakers

Blount County

County Health Depts

Blount County Health Department
1004 Second Avenue, East
Oneonta, AL 35121-2508
Telephone: (205)-274-2120
Contact: Kathy Burtram, R.N.
HIV Testing, Counseling, Home Care Services, Referrals, Education, Speakers

Bullock County

County Health Depts

Bullock County Health Department
103 Conecuh Avenue, West
P.O. Box 030
Union Springs, AL 36089-1317
Telephone: (205)-738-3030
HIV Testing, Counseling, Home Care Services, Referrals, Education, Speakers

Butler County

County Health Depts

Butler County Health Department
201 South Conecuh Street
Greenville, AL 36037-2713
Telephone: (205)-382-3154
Contact: Susan Sims
HIV Testing, Counseling, Home Care Services, Referrals, Education, Speakers

Calhoun County

Community Services

Agency for Substance Abuse Prevention
1302 Noble Street
Suite 3-B
Anniston, AL 36201
Telephone: (205)-237-8131 Fax: (205)-236-5186
AIDS video for the public and substance abuse programs for schools, community

All Saints Interfaith Center of Concern
1029 West 15th Street
Anniston, AL 36201
Telephone: (205)-236-7793
Emergency financial aid, food, clothing, transportation

Partnerships, Inc.
P.O. Box 314
1302 Noble St., Suite 2F
Anniston, AL 36202
Telephone: (205)-238-8336
Contact: Josephine Ayers
Provides HIV/AIDS info in a one-act, 30-45 minute audience participationperformance

County Health Depts

Calhoun County Health Department
309 East Eighth Street
Anniston, AL 36201-5731
Telephone: (205)-237-7523
Contact: Donna Rawlings
HIV Testing, Counseling, Home Care Services, Referrals, Education, Speakers

Home Health Care

Alabama Hospice Organization
P.O. Box 2581
Anniston, AL 36202
Telephone: (205)-236-5334 Fax: (205)-231-4558
Contact: Jeannie Stanko
Some hospices (not all) provide terminally ill care to AIDS patients

Option Care
311 East 11th Street
Anniston, AL 36202
Telephone: (205)-238-1508 Fax: (205)-492-7979
Contact: Lynn Lacher - Marketing; Scott Godfrey - C.E.O.
In-home IV therapies including TPN hydration, pain control, antibiotic

Medical Services

AIDS Services Center
P.O. Box 1392
Anniston, AL 36202
Telephone: (205)-835-0923 Fax: (205)-835-0923
Contact: Deborah Wade
Full service outpatient medical

Northeast Alabama Regional Medical Center
400 East 10th Street
P.O. Box 2208
Anniston, AL 36201
Telephone: (205)-235-5864
Contact: Miranda Jair, RN
Education, Speakers, HIV Testing, Counseling, Referrals

Testing Sites

AIDS Services Center Inc.
608 Martin Luther King Drive
Hobson City, AL 36201
Telephone: (205)-835-0923
Contact: Deborah Wade
HIV testing and counseling, medical evaluation and follow-up

Chambers County

County Health Depts

Chambers County Health Department
18 Alabama Avenue, East
Lafayette, AL 36862-1745
Telephone: (205)-864-8834
Contact: Frances Brown
HIV Testing, Counseling, Home Care Services, Referrals, Education, Speakers

Chambers County Health Department, Branch Office
3205 22nd Avenue
Valley, AL 36854-3020
Telephone: (205)-768-2196
HIV Testing, Counseling, Home Care Services, Referrals, Education, Speakers

Cherokee County

County Health Depts

Cherokee County Health Department
833 Cedar Bluff Road
Centre, AL 35960-1005
Telephone: (205)-927-3132
Contact: Cathy Lee
HIV Testing, Counseling, Home Care Services, Referrals, Education, Speakers

Medical Services

Baptist Medical Center, Cherokee
400 Northwood Drive
Centre, AL 35960-1023
Telephone: (205)-927-5531 Fax: (205)-927-1412
Contact: Velma Howell, R.N.
Community education, literature, testing

Chilton County

Community Services

Chilton County Emergency Assistance Center
1212 Fifth Avenue, North
Clanton, AL 35045
Telephone: (205)-755-9467
Contact: Levern Babb - Director
Provide emergency assistance to Chilton County families in need

County Health Depts

Chilton County Health Department
101 Fifth Street, North
Clanton, AL 35045-3442
Telephone: (205)-755-1287
HIV Testing, Counseling, Home Care Services, Referrals, Education, Speakers

Choctaw County

County Health Depts

Choctaw County Health Department
315 East Pushmataha Street
Butler, AL 36904-2533
Telephone: (205)-459-4026
Contact: Barbara Shoemaker - Clinic Supervisor
HIV Testing, Counseling, Home Care Services, Referrals, Education, Speakers

Clarke County

County Health Depts

Clarke County Health Department
140 Clark Street
Grove Hill, AL 36451
Telephone: (205)-275-3772
HIV Testing, Counseling, Home Care Services, Referrals, Education, Speakers

Clay County

County Health Depts

Clay County Health Department
208 North Second E Street
Ashland, AL 36251
Telephone: (205)-354-2181
Contact: Ruth Little
HIV Testing, Counseling, Home Care Services, Referrals, Education, Speakers

Cleburne County

County Health Depts

Cleburne County Health Department
Brockford Road
Heflin, AL 36264-1605
Telephone: (205)-463-2296
Contact: Carolee Warneke
HIV Testing, Counseling, Home Care Services, Referrals, Education, Speakers

Home Health Care

East Alabama Vital Care
601 Ross Street
Heflin, AL 36264
Telephone: (205)-463-2188 Fax: (205)-463-2377
Contact: William Wright
At-home therapies including total parenteral nutrition and IV antibiotic

Coffee County

County Health Depts

Coffee County Health Department
167 North & County Rd. 48
Enterprise, AL 36331-2554
Telephone: (205)-347-9574
Contact: Peggy Searcy
IV Testing, Counseling, Home Care Services, Referrals, Education, Speakers

Colbert County

County Health Depts

Colbert County Health Department
1000 Jackson Highway, S.
Sheffield, AL 35660-5761
Telephone: (205)-383-1231
Contact: Ronnie Moore
HIV/STD Testing, Counseling, Home Care Services, Referrals, Education,Speakers

Conecuh County

County Health Depts

Conecuh County Health Department
526 Belleville Street
Evergreen, AL 36401-3005
Telephone: (205)-578-1952
Contact: Debra Lett
HIV Testing, Counseling, Referrals, Education, Speakers

Coosa County

County Health Depts

Coosa County Health Department
Jackson Street
Rockford, AL 35136
Telephone: (205)-377-4364
Contact: Linda Wheeler
HIV Testing, Counseling, Home Care Services, Referrals, Education, Speakers

Coosa County Health Department, Satellite Office
Main Street, Highway 9
Goodwater, AL 35072
Telephone: (205)-839-6727
Contact: Linda Wheeler
HIV Testing, Counseling, Home Care Services, Referrals, Education, Speakers

Covington County

County Health Depts

Covington County Health Department
County Road 56
P.O. Box 186
Andalusia, AL 36420-4533
Telephone: (205)-222-1560
Contact: Sarah Martha Batchelor
HIV Testing, Counseling, Home Care Services, Referrals, Education, Speakers

Home Health Care

Vital Care of Covington County
405 North Main
Opp, AL 36467
Telephone: (205)-493-4541
Contact: Ted Roquemore
At-home therapies including total parenteral nutrition and IV antibiotic

Crenshaw County

County Health Depts

Crenshaw County Health Department
206 Fourth Street, East
Luverne, AL 36049-1560
Telephone: (205)-335-6568
HIV Testing, Counseling, Home Care Services, Referrals, Education, Speakers

Home Health Care

Community Health Care
Highway 331 South
Luverne, AL 36049
Telephone: (205)-335-6622 Fax: (205)-335-5667
Contact: Tom Ray
At-home therapies including total parenteral nutrition and IV antibiotic

Cullman County

Community Services

Cullman Regional Medical Center
401 Arnold Street, N.E.
Cullman, AL 35055
Telephone: (205)-734-1210
Contact: Marti Smith
Education for employees and community education

County Health Depts

Cullman County Health Department and AIDS Task Force
P.O. Box 1678
500 Logan Avenue, NW
Cullman, AL 35055
Telephone: (205)-734-1030
Contact: Sondra Nassetta
HIV Testing, Counseling, Home Care Services, Referrals, Education, Speakers

Dale County

County Health Depts

Dale County Health Department
200 Katherine Avenue
Ozark, AL 36361
Telephone: (205)-774-5146
HIV Testing, Counseling, Home Care Services, Referrals, Education, Speakers

Dallas County

Community Services

Legal Services Corp. of Alabama, Selma Regional Office
1114 Church Street
P.O. Box 954
Selma, AL 36701
Telephone: (205)-875-3770
Contact: Carolyn Gaines-Varner
Free legal assistance in civil matters for those individuals who qualify

County Health Depts

Dallas County Health Department
108 Church Street
Selma, AL 36702-0330
Telephone: (205)-874-2550
Contact: Joyce Conn
HIV Testing, Counseling, Home Care Services, Referrals, Education, Speakers

De Kalb County

County Health Depts

DeKalb County Health Department
500 Grand Avenue, South
Fort Payne, AL 35967-1716
Telephone: (205)-845-1931
Contact: Becky Gilbreath
HIV testing, counseling, referrals, education, speakers

Elmore County

County Health Depts

Elmore County Health Department
Highway 231 North
Wetumpka, AL 36092
Telephone: (205)-567-1171 Fax: (205)-567-1186
Contact: Elizabeth Bass
HIV Testing, Counseling, Home Care Services, Referrals, Education, Speakers

Escambia County

County Health Depts

Brewton County Health Department
P.O. Box 66
Brewton, AL 36426
Telephone: (205)-867-5765 Fax: (205)-867-5179
Contact: Tina Findley
HIV Testing, Counseling, Home Care Services, Referrals, Education, Speakers

Escambia County Health Department
204 Sowell Street
Brewton, AL 36426-2034
Telephone: (205)-867-5765 Fax: (205)-867-5179
Contact: Tina Findley
HIV Testing, Counseling, Home Care Services, Referrals, Education, Speakers

Escambia County Health Department, Branch Office
P.O. Box 1390
Highway 31
Atmore, AL 36504
Telephone: (205)-368-9188 Fax: (205)-368-9189
Contact: Helen Byrd, R.N.
HIV Testing, Counseling, Home Care Services, Referrals, Education, Speakers

Home Health Care

Greenlawn Vital Care, Inc.
406 Medical Park Drive
Atmore, AL 36502
Telephone: (205)-368-3189 Fax: (205)-368-4459
Contact: Jim Justice
At-home therapies including total parenteral nutrition and IV antibiotic

Etowah County

Community Services

Legal Services Corp. of Alabama, Gadsden Regional Office
802 Chestnut Street
Gadsden, AL 35901
Telephone: (205)-543-2435
Contact: Ruth Ezellter
Free legal assistance in civil matters for those individuals who qualify

County Health Depts

Etowah County Health Department
109 South 8th Street
Gadsden, AL 35902
Telephone: (205)-547-6311
Contact: Shelva Lee
HIV Testing, Counseling, Home Care Services, Referrals, Education, Speakers

Home Health Care

HNS Accucare
605 South Third Street
Gadsden, AL 35901
Telephone: (205)-549-1911 Fax: (305)-549-0101
Contact: Hugh Campbell
Home infusion therapy, attendants, nurses, pentamidine, pharmacy, counseling

Option Care
Route 7
3863 Piedmont Highway
Gadsden, AL 35903
Telephone: (205)-492-7192 Fax: (208)-492-7979
Toll-Free: (800)-729-7192
Contact: Lynn Lacher - Marketing; Scott Godfrey - C.E.O.
In-home IV therapies including TPN hydration, pain control, antibiotic

Physicians Choice Homecare Service
173 Lakeshore Drive
Gadsden, AL 35906
Telephone: (205)-442-9834
Contact: Alice Edwards - Administrator
Private Visiting Nurse Agency and Private Duty Nurse Service

Medical Services

Gadsen Regional Medical Center
1007 Goodyear Avenue
Gadsden, AL 35999
Telephone: (205)-494-4000
Contact: Diana Adrian, R.N. - Nurse Epidemiologist
Individual & family counseling, education to health care & emergency personnel

Fayette County

County Health Depts

Fayette County Health Department
211 First Street, N.W.
Fayette, AL 35555-2550
Telephone: (205)-932-5260
Contact: Donna Dodd
HIV Testing, Counseling, Home Care Services, Referrals, Education, Speakers

Franklin County

County Health Depts

Franklin County Health Department
300 E. Limestone Street
Russellville, AL 35653-2448
Telephone: (205)-332-2700
Contact: Robert Hudson - Program Manager
HIV Testing, Counseling, Home Care Services, Referrals, Education, Speakers

Medical Services

Northwest Medical Center
Highway 43 Bypass
P.O. Box 1089
Russellville, AL 35653
Telephone: (205)-332-1611
Contact: Rebecca Michael, RN, BSN - Director, Inservice Educ.
Health care facility for both in-patient and out-patient care

Geneva County

County Health Depts

Geneva County Health Department
606 S. Academy Street
P.O. Box 386
Geneva, AL 36340-2527
Telephone: (205)-684-2257
HIV Testing, Counseling, Home Care Services, Referrals, Education, Speakers

Greene County

County Health Depts

Greene County Health Department
412 Morrow Avenue
Eutaw, AL 35462-1109
Telephone: (205)-372-9361
HIV Testing, Counseling, Home Care Services, Referrals, Education, Speakers

Testing Sites

West Alabama Health Services, Inc.
P.O. Box 711
Eutaw, AL 35462-0711
Telephone: (205)-372-9225 Fax: (205)-372-9513
Contact: Bradley R. Ware, M.D.
Testing, Counseling

Hale County

County Health Depts

Hale County Health Department
1102 N. Centerville St.
Greensboro, AL 36744-1303
Telephone: (205)-624-3018
HIV Testing, Counseling, Home Care Services, Referrals, Education, Speakers

Henry County

County Health Depts

Henry County Health Department
505 Kirkland Street
Abbeville, AL 36310-2736
Telephone: (205)-585-2660
Contact: Ms. Lisa Smith - RN
HIV Testing, Counseling, Home Care Services, Referrals, Education, Speakers

Henry County Health Department, Branch Office
2 Cable Street
Headland, AL 36345-2136
Telephone: (205)-693-2220
Contact: Jenie Farret
HIV Testing, Counseling, Home Care Services, Referrals, Education, Speakers

Houston County

Community Services

Legal Services Corp. of Alabama, Dothan Regional Office
161 South Oates Street
Dothan, AL 36301
Telephone: (205)-793-7932
Contact: Ishmael Jaffree
Free legal assistance in civil matters for those individuals who qualify

Wiregrass AIDS Outreach, Inc.
P.O. Box 6138
Dothan, AL 36302-6138
Telephone: (205)-794-4357
Contact: Karen Sprenger
Volunteer Support Group; Nutritional, Emotional, Social and Medical Counseling

Home Health Care

Vital Care of Dothan
509 West Main Street
Dothan, AL 36301
Telephone: (205)-792-5132
Contact: Sid Beasley
At-home therapies including Total Parenteral Nutrition, IV antibiotic

Jackson County

County Health Depts

Jackson County Health Department & AIDS Prevention Committee
609 South Broad Street
P.O. Box 398
Scottsboro, AL 35768
Telephone: (205)-259-4161 Fax: (205)-259-1330
Contact: Nancy Hodges, R.N. - Secretary; Robert Colvin, R.N. - President, AIDS Prev Comm
HIV Testing, Counseling, Home Care Services, Referrals, Education, Speakers

Jefferson County

Community Services

Birmingham AIDS Outreach, Inc.
P.O. Box 550070
Birmingham, AL 35255-0070
Telephone: (205)-322-4197
Contact: Patricia Todd - Executive Director
Education, Support Services, Referrals, Information, Support Group, Counseling, buddy/PWA program

Children's Aid Society
3600 8th Avenue, South
Suite 300
Birmingham, AL 35222
Telephone: (205)-251-7148 Fax: (205)-202-3828
Contact: Joyce Greathouse - Executive Director
Permanency planning for children with AIDS/HIV infected parents

Travelers Aid Society of Birmingham, Alabama, Inc.
3600 8th Avenue, South
Suite 110-W
Birmingham, AL 35222-3292
Telephone: (205)-322-5426
Contact: Donna Henley - Social Worker
Emergency Assistance, Transportation Help to Medical Facilities for Ill People

County Health Depts

Jefferson County Health Department
1400 Sixth Avenue, South
Birmingham, AL 35233-1598
Telephone: (205)-933-9110
Contact: Linda DeMarco
HIV Testing, Counseling, Home Care Services, Referrals, Education, Speakers

Jefferson County Health Department, Branch Office
Northern Health Center
2817 30th Avenue, North
Birmingham, AL 35207-4599
Telephone: (205)-323-4548
HIV Testing, Counseling, Home Care Services, Referrals, Education, Speakers

Jefferson County Health Department, Branch Office
Eastern Health Center
5720 1st Avenue, South
Birmingham, AL 35212-2599
Telephone: (205)-591-5180
Contact: Dr. Freenor
HIV Testing, Counseling, Home Care Services, Referrals, Education, Speakers

Jefferson County Health Department, Branch Office
Western Health Center
1700 Avenue E, Ensley
Birmingham, AL 35218-1543
Telephone: (205)-788-3321 Fax: (205)-781-6136
HIV Testing, Counseling, Home Care Services, Referrals, Education, Speakers

Jefferson County Health Department, Branch Office
Bessemer Health Center
2201 Arlington Avenue
Bessemer, AL 35020-4299
Telephone: (205)-424-6001 Fax: (205)-426-1410
Contact: Harriet Williams
HIV Testing, Counseling, Home Care Services, Referrals, Education, Speakers

Jefferson County Health Department, Branch Office
Morris Health Center P.O. Box 272
586 Morris Majestic Road
Morris, AL 35116
Telephone: (205)-647-0572
HIV Testing, Counseling, Home Care Services, Referrals, Education, Speakers

Jefferson County Health Department, Branch Office
Leeds Health Center
210 Park Drive
Leeds, AL 35094-1846
Telephone: (205)-699-2442
HIV Testing, Counseling, Home Care Services, Referrals, Education, Speakers

Home Health Care

Olsten Kimberly Quality Care Infusion Therapy Services
2200 Woodcrest Place
Suite 120
Birmingham, AL 35233
Telephone: (205)-324-7644
Contact: Paula Shoemaker
IV antibiotics, chemotherapy, internal

Medical Services

Birmingham Health Care for the Homeless Coalition, Inc.
P.O. Box 11523
Birmingham, AL 35202
Telephone: (205)-323-5311 Fax: (205)-250-7743
Contact: Audrey Johnson
Assist homeless HIV infected persons, respite care, AIDS counseling, testing

Pediatric AIDS Care Team (PACT)
751 Childrens Hosp.Towers
1600 Seventh Ave., South
Birmingham, AL 35294-0011
Telephone: (205)-939-9400
Contact: Tara Dortchal - Program Coordinator
Care for all HIV/AIDS infected family members at a single clinic site

University of Alabama, Birmingham Drug Free Program
3015 7th Avenue South
Birmingham, AL 35233
Telephone: (205)-934-5060
Contact: Tony Morris
Chemical dependence treatment, outreach program, counseling, HIV testing, referrals & education programs

Testing Sites

Planned Parenthood of Alabama, Inc.
1211 27th Place, South
Birmingham, AL 35205-1800
Telephone: (205)-322-2121 Fax: (205)-322-2162
Contact: Angela Lee; Larry Rodick
Couneling, Education, HIV testing

University of Alabama, Birmingham Methadone Program
3015 7th Avenue, South
Birmingham, AL 35233
Telephone: (205)-934-5060 Fax: (205)-323-6976
Contact: Linda Garner
HIV testing/counseling for IV drug abusers and their families

University of Alabama, Birmingham Outpatient Clinic
Byrd Building
908 South 20th Street
Birmingham, AL 35294-2050
Telephone: (205)-934-1917 Fax: (205)-934-8490
Contact: Richard Taylor, R.N., M.S. - Nurse Coordinator; Susan P. Wilder, L.B.S.W. - Social Service Coord.
AIDS Testing & Treatment, Counseling for Patients & Families

Lamar County

County Health Depts

Lamar County Health Department
207 Columbus Avenue, West
Vernon, AL 35592
Telephone: (205)-695-9195
HIV Testing, Counseling, Home Care Services, Referrals, Education, Speakers

Lauderdale County

Community Services

Legal Services Corp. of Alabama, Florence Regional Office
412 South Court Street
P.O. Box 753
Florence, AL 35631
Telephone: (205)-767-2122
Contact: Floyd Sherrod - Attorney
Legal Representation for PWAs and HIV+

County Health Depts

Lauderdale County Health Department
200 W. Tennessee Street
Florence, AL 35630-5420
Telephone: (205)-764-7453
HIV Testing, Counseling, Home Care Services, Referrals, Education, Speakers

Medical Services

Riverbend Center for Mental Health
635 West College Street
P.O. Box 941
Florence, AL 35630
Telephone: (205)-764-3431
Contact: Cindy Ardis - Intake Info Referral Spec
Seminars, educational presentations, psychiatric services, testing & evaluation

Lawrence County

County Health Depts

Lawrence County Health Department
640 East Street, North
Moulton, AL 35650-1292
Telephone: (205)-974-1141 Fax: (205)-974-5587
Contact: Peggy Shelton - Office Manager
HIV Testing, Counseling, Home Care Services, Referrals, Education, Speakers

Lee County

Community Services

Lee County AIDS Outreach
P.O. Box 1971
Auburn, AL 36830
Telephone: (205)-887-5244
Contact: Kate Kellenberger - Project Director
Education, Referrals, Services and Support to PWAs and Families, Support Group

County Health Depts

Lee County Health Department
1930 Pepperell Parkway
Opelika, AL 36802-1301
Telephone: (205)-745-5765 Fax: (205)-745-5784
Contact: Melinda Mara - Office Manager
HIV Testing, Counseling, Home Care Services, Referrals, Education, Speakers

Medical Services

Action AIDS
PO Box 871
Huntsville, AL 36801
Telephone: (205)-533-2437
Contact: Fran Spluak - Clinic Manager
Full service HIV clinic

Limestone County

County Health Depts

Limestone County Health Dept. and AIDS Prevention Committee
P.O. Box 889
310 West Elm Street
Athens, AL 35611-0889
Telephone: (205)-232-3200 Fax: (205)-232-6632
Contact: Martha Camp - Nurse Supervisor
HIV Testing, Counseling, Home Care Services, Referrals, Education, Speakers

Lowndes County

County Health Depts

Lowndes County Health Department
Highway 21
Tuskeena Street
Hayneville, AL 36040-0035
Telephone: (205)-548-2564 Fax: (205)-548-2566
HIV Testing, Counseling, Home Care Services, Referrals, Education, Speakers

Macon County

Community Services

AIDS Ministerial Alliance
2508 Old Montgomery Road
Tuskegee Inst., AL 36088
Telephone: (205)-727-2864
Contact: Rev. T. W. Billups
Ministering to the sick, education and information, support groups, speakers

County Health Depts

Macon County Health Department
608 North Dibble Street
Tuskegee, AL 36083-1509
Telephone: (205)-727-1800 Fax: (205)-727-7100
Contact: Wanda A. Wilson - Office Manager
HIV Testing, Counseling, Home Care Services, Referrals, Education, Speakers

Madison County

Community Services

Legal Services of North-Central Alabama, Inc.
2000-C Vernon Street
P.O. Box 2465
Huntsville, AL 35804
Telephone: (205)-536-9645 Fax: (205)-536-1544
Contact: Tom Keith - Director
Free legal assistance in civil matters for individuals who qualify

Samaritan Family Services
2400 Bob Wallace
Suite 103
Huntsville, AL 35805
Telephone: (205)-533-6220
Contact: Felicia Fontaine; Janet Pierce -
Counseling for HIV+, family & friends; grief & bereavement support

County Health Depts

Madison County Health Department
P.O. Box 467
304 Eustis Avenue
Huntsville, AL 35804-0425
Telephone: (205)-539-3711
Contact: Dr. Lawrence Roby
HIV Testing, Counseling, Home Care Services, Referrals, Education, Speakers

Home Health Care

Hospice of Huntsville
806 Governors Drive
Suite 202
Huntsville, AL 35801
Telephone: (205)-536-1889
Contact: Nancy Kramer
Physical, emotional, and spiritual support to terminally ill AIDS patients

Nutritional/Parenteral Home Care, Inc.
805 Madison Street
Suite 1-D
Huntsville, AL 35801
Telephone: (205)-534-4663 Fax: (205)-534-0252
Contact: Sharon Mckeeman
Total parenteral feedings, eteral feedings, IV hydration, IV chemotherapy

Olsten Kimberly Quality Care
721 Clinton Avenue W. 3-A
Huntsville, AL 35801
Telephone: (205)-533-4453 Fax: (205)-533-4166
Contact: Louise Meryman - Dir. Clinical Services
Nursing services, IV therapy or care to the ventilator dependent client

Marengo County

County Health Depts

Marengo County Health Department
209 North Main Street
Linden, AL 36748-0877
Telephone: (205)-295-4205
Contact: Sharyn Cooke, R.N.
HIV Testing, Counseling, Home Care Services, Referrals, Education, Speakers

Marion County

County Health Depts

Marion County Health Department
1501 Military Street, S.
Hamilton, AL 35570
Telephone: (205)-921-3118
Contact: Ann Couch, R.N.
HIV Testing, Counseling, Home Care Services, Referrals, Education, Speakers

Marshall County

County Health Depts

Marshall County Health Department
2067 Gunter Avenue
P.O Drawer 339
Guntersville, AL 35976-1111
Telephone: (205)-582-3174
Contact: Pat Franklin
HIV Testing, Counseling, Home Care Services, Referrals, Education, Speakers

Home Health Care

Hospice of Marshall County, Inc.
501 Blount Avenue
Guntersville, AL 35976
Telephone: (205)-582-2111
Contact: Anne L. Walker - Executive Director
Physical, emotional, and spiritual support to terminally ill AIDS patients

Mobile County

Community Services

Children's Rehabilitation Services, Hemophilia Program
1870 Pleasant Avenue
Mobile, AL 36617
Telephone: (205)-479-8617
Contact: Madalyn Rochford, R.N.
Provide counseling for hemophiliacs and their families regarding HIV issues

Independent Living Center, Mobile
5304-B Overlook Road
Mobile, AL 36618
Telephone: (205)-460-0301 Fax: (205)-460-0302
Contact: Michael Davis; Ann Robertson -
AIDS information, referral, case management, printed materials

Legal Services Corp. of Alabama, Mobile Regional Office
601 Van Antwerp Building
103 Dauphin Street
Mobile, AL 36602
Telephone: (205)-433-6560
Contact: Christopher Knight
Represent income eligible people with HIV/AIDS in a variety of legal problems

Mobile AIDS Fund, Inc.
271 Morgan Avenue
Mobile, AL 36606
Telephone: (205)-478-6911
Contact: Grace Willis - Director
Provide funds for PWA's for living expenses, medicine, doctor's visits,etc.

Mobile AIDS Support Services
107 N. Anne Street
Mobile, AL 36604
Telephone: (205)-433-6277 Fax: (205)-432-2437
Contact: LaDawn Harrison - Director
Counseling, Support Groups, Advocacy, Referrals, Transportation, EducationCommunity outreach

Mobile County Department of Human Resources
P.O. Box 1906
Mobile, AL 36633-1906
Telephone: (205)-694-2744
Contact: Katherine Coumanis, PhD
Public assistance, food assistance, adult and child protective services

Mothers of AIDS Patients/South Alabama
c/o 1255 Peabody Drive
Mobile, AL 36618
Telephone: (205)-342-9208
Contact: Bernadette Devery - Support Supervisor
Support, information and assistance for families of persons with AIDS, ARC,HIV

Service Center of Catholic Social Services
555 Dauphin Street
Mobile, AL 36602
Telephone: (205)-434-1500
Contact: Sister Judith Vander Grinten
Assistance with food, clothing, furniture, etc.; limited financial assistance

County Health Depts

Mobile County Health Department
251 North Bayou Street
P.O. Box 2867
Mobile, AL 36652
Telephone: (205)-690-8158
Contact: Alfreda King
HIV testing, counseling, literature referrals, education, speakers

Home Health Care

I.V. Services, Inc.
32-D Tacon Street
Mobile, AL 36607
Telephone: (205)-479-2300
Contact: Bob Barillari
Home infusion therapy, attendants, nurses, pentamidine, pharmacy, counseling

Medical Services

HIV/AIDS High Risk Clinic
251 North Bayou Street
Mobile, AL 36603
Telephone: (205)-690-8167 Fax: (205)-690-8853
Contact: Alfreda King
Medical and dental services, case management, and mental health counseling

Mobile Mental Health Center, Inc., Anchorage/Phoenix House
406 Government Street
Mobile, AL 36602
Telephone: (205)-431-0755
Contact: Fred Conrad
Case management, supportive day treatment and supported employment

University of Southern Alabama Student Health Service
Health Service Building
Suite 1100
Mobile, AL 36689
Telephone: (205)-460-7151 Fax: (203)-460-7617
Contact: Richard H. Esham, M.D.
Educational resources as well as out-patient HIV evaluation and management

University of Southern Alabama, Division of Infectious Diseases
472 Cancer Center Clinical Bldg.
Mobile, AL 36688-0001
Telephone: (205)-460-7220 Fax: (205)-460-7637
Contact: Keith Ramsey, M.D.; G. Lynn Marks, M.D. -
Treatment of Infectious Disease Patients, Education of Public

Monroe County

County Health Depts

Monroe County Health Department
P.O. Box 609
301 W. Claiborne Street
Monroeville, AL 36460-0609
Telephone: (205)-575-3109
Contact: Gerrie McMillian
HIV Testing, Counseling, Home Care Services, Referrals, Education, Speakers

Montgomery County

Community Services

Baptist Medical Center
2105 East South Boulevard
Montgomery, AL 36111
Telephone: (205)-286-2964
Contact: William Larry Davidson - Pastor
Coordinate AIDS presentations, confidential counseling, other limited services

Legal Services Corp. of Alabama, Central Office
500 Bell Building
207 Montgomery Street
Montgomery, AL 36104
Telephone: (205)-264-1471 Fax: (205)-264-1474
Contact: Merceria Ludgood
Free legal assistance in civil matters for those who qualify

Legal Services Corp. of Alabama, Montgomery Regional Office
600 Bell Building
207 Montgomery Street
Montgomery, AL 36104
Telephone: (205)-832-4570
Toll-Free: (800)-844-5342
Contact: James O. Smith
Free legal assistance in civil matters for those individuals who qualify

Montgomery AIDS Outreach, Inc.
1209 Mulberry Street
P.O. Box 5213
Montgomery, AL 36130-0001
Telephone: (205)-269-1002 Fax: (205)-269-2621
Contact: Jacquelyn Stancil - Administrator
Support to PWAs, PWARCs, HIV+; Support Groups, Buddies, Speakers, Education

St. Jude Social Services Center
2048 West Fairview Avenue
Montgomery, AL 36108-4198
Telephone: (205)-269-1983
Contact: Dorothy H. Brundidge; Sister Theresita Sabol -
Emergency Services: Rent, Utility and Medical Bills, Medicine, Food, Clothes

County Health Depts

Montgomery County Health Department, Branch Office
Primary Care Center
88 West South Blvd.
Montgomery, AL 36105-3144
Telephone: (205)-281-8008 Fax: (205)-286-0835
Contact: Rhonda Taylor - Social Worker
Testing, follow-up medical care for HIV positive

Montgomery County Health Department, Branch Office
Specialty Clinic
800-B West South Blvd.
Montgomery, AL 36111-2401
Telephone: (205)-284-3553 Fax: (205)-284-3653
Contact: Charlena Freeman - Social Worker
Coordinator clinic with Montgomery Community AIDS Outreach

Montgomery County Health Department, Branch Office
Maternity Clinic
800-A West South Blvd.
Montgomery, AL 36111-2401
Telephone: (205)-286-0907 Fax: (205)-284-3653
Contact: Geri Moore - Social Worker
HIV Testing, Counseling, Home Care Services, Referrals, Education, Speakers

Home Health Care

Adams Drugs Vital Care, Inc.
2229 East South Boulevard
Montgomery, AL 36111
Telephone: (205)-281-1671
Contact: Michael Vinson
At-home therapies including total parenteral nutrition, IV antibiotic

Medical Services

Health Services, Inc.
1000 Adams Avenue
Montgomery, AL 36104
Telephone: (205)-263-2301 Fax: (205)-263-0881
General medicine & primary care, dental

Morgan County

Community Services

Shoals Area Services
P.O. Box 1628
Decatur, AL 35602-1628
Telephone: (205)-353-7021
Assist persons with AIDS and provide HIV/AIDS education to the community

County Health Depts

Morgan County Health Department
510 Cherry Street, N.E.
P.O. Box 1628
Decatur, AL 35601-1970
Telephone: (205)-353-7021
Contact: Diana Quirk - Medical Social Worker
HIV Testing, Counseling, Home Care Services, Referrals, Education, Speakers

Home Health Care

Hospice of Morgan County, Inc.
P.O. Box 2745
Decatur, AL 35602
Telephone: (205)-350-5585
Contact: Carolyn Dobson Cole - Executive Director
Total care concept designed to keep patient with life-limiting illness at home

Intracare-Vital Care
1517 Moulton Street West
Decatur, AL 35602
Telephone: (205)-355-7900
Contact: Sandie Smith
Parental & Enteral Feedings, Chemotherapy, RPT Services, IV Antibiotic Therapy

Perry County

County Health Depts

Perry County Health Department
206 Pickens Street
Marion, AL 36756-1818
Telephone: (205)-683-6153
HIV Testing, Counseling, Home Care Services, Referrals, Education, Speakers

Perry County Health Department, Satellite Office
Thomaston Road
Uniontown, AL 36786
Telephone: (205)-683-6153 Fax: (205)-683-4509
Toll-Free: (800)-683-8084
Contact: Ashvin Kiparikh
HIV testing, counseling, home care services, referrals, education,speakers

Home Health Care

Vital Care of Marion
313 Washington Street
Marion, AL 36756
Telephone: (205)-683-9355 Fax: (205)-683-9621
Contact: Roy Bamett
At-home therapies including Total Parenteral Nutrition, IV antibiotic

Pickens County

County Health Depts

Pickens County Health Department
Hospital Drive
Carrollton, AL 35447
Telephone: (205)-367-8157
Contact: Epsiz Drewry
HIV Testing, Counseling, Home Care Services, Referrals, Education, Speakers

Pike County

County Health Depts

Pike County Health Department
306 South Three Notch St.
Troy, AL 36081-1910
Telephone: (205)-566-2860
HIV Testing, Counseling, Home Care Services, Referrals, Education, Speakers

Randolph County

County Health Depts

Randolph County Health Department
527 Price Street
Roanoke, AL 36274-2196
Telephone: (205)-863-8981 Fax: (205)-869-8975
Contact: Kathy Green - Nurse/Supervisor
HIV Testing, Counseling, Home Care Services, Referrals, Education, Speakers

Russell County

County Health Depts

Russell County Health Department
1320 Broad Street
Phoenix City, AL 36868-0548
Telephone: (205)-297-0251
HIV Testing, Counseling, Home Care Services, Referrals, Education, Speakers

Saint Clair County

County Health Depts

St. Clair County Health Department
205 19th Street, North
Pell City, AL 35125-1641
Telephone: (205)-338-3357
Contact: Karen Sullidan
HIV Testing, Counseling, Home Care Services, Referrals, Education, Speakers

St. Clair County Health Department, Satellite Office
411 N. Gadsden Highway
Ashville, AL 35953-0249
Telephone: (205)-594-7944
Contact: Karen Sullivan
HIV Testing, Counseling, Home Care Services, Referrals, Education, Speakers

Shelby County

Community Services

Shelby Emergency Assistance, Inc.
620 Valley Street
Montevallo, AL 35115
Telephone: (205)-665-1942
Contact: Carol H. Schulz - Executive Director
Assist with emergency food, clothing, advocacy, financial assistance, etc.

County Health Depts

Shelby County Health Department
110 Mildred Street
PO Box 976
Columbiana, AL 35051-9331
Telephone: (205)-669-3920
Contact: Jill Lowman
HIV Testing, Counseling, Home Care Services, Referrals, Education, Speakers

Shelby County Health Department, Branch Office
3160 Highway 31, South
PO Box 846
Pelham, AL 35124-2022
Telephone: (205)-664-2470
HIV testing, counseling, referrals, education, speakers

Sumter County

County Health Depts

Sumter County Health Department
318 Washington Street
Livingston, AL 35470
Telephone: (205)-652-7972
Contact: Carolyn Patrenos - RN
HIV Testing, Counseling, Home Care Services, Referrals, Education, Speakers

Home Health Care

Vital Care Inc.
P.O. Box 1249
110 Lafayette Street
Livingston, AL 35470
Telephone: (800)-447-4095 Fax: (205)-652-6111
Contact: Keith C. Conner, R.Ph.
At-home therapies including total parenteral nrition, IV antibiotic

Medical Services

Sumter County Mental Health Center
P.O. Box 1470
Livingston, AL 35470
Telephone: (205)-652-6731
Contact: David O'Haren - Clinical Director
Outpatient services to AIDS victims and their families

Talladega County

Community Services

Alabama Inst. for the Deaf & Blind, E.H. Gentry Tech. Facility
P.O. Box 698
Talladega, AL 35160
Telephone: (205)-761-3409
Contact: Marilyn M. Loftis - Social Worker
Vocational training for the sensory, physically, emotionally or drugimpaired; AIDS education, social services, referral for HIV/AIDS testing

County Health Depts

Talladega County Health Department
510 West South Street
Talladega, AL 35160-2449
Telephone: (205)-362-2593 Fax: (205)-362-0529
Contact: Jane Haney
HIV Testing, Counseling, Home Care Services, Referrals, Education, Speakers

Talladega County Health Department, Branch Office
109 S. Anniston Avenue
P.O. Box 2430
Sylacauga, AL 35150-2430
Telephone: (205)-249-3807
Contact: Vivian King
HIV Testing, Counseling, Home Care Services, Referrals, Education, Speakers

Tallapoosa County

County Health Depts

Tallapoosa County Health Department
202 Lafayette Street, W.
Dadeville, AL 36853-1327
Telephone: (205)-825-9203 Fax: (205)-825-6546
Contact: Jan LaFollette - Office Manager
HIV Testing, Counseling, Home Care Services, Referrals, Education, Speakers

Tallapoosa County Health Department, Branch Office
124 Airport Circle
Alexander City, AL 35010-9805
Telephone: (205)-329-0531
Contact: Carol Fields - RN
HIV Testing, Counseling, Home Care Services, Referrals, Education, Speakers

Home Health Care

Vital Care of Alexander City
2003 Cherokee Road
Alexander City, AL 35010
Telephone: (205)-234-2538 Fax: (205)-234-0042
Contact: Jimmy Jackson
At-home therapies including Total Parenteral Nutrition, IV antibiotic

Tuscaloosa County

Community Services

Legal Services Corp. of Alabama, Tuscaloosa Regional Office
SECOR Bank Building
Suite 426
Tuscaloosa, AL 35401
Telephone: (205)-758-7503 Fax: (205)-758-6041
Contact: Sue Thompson
Free legal assistance in civil matters for those individuals who qualify

County Health Depts

Tuscaloosa County Health Department
1101 Jackson Avenue
PO Box 03009
Tuscaloosa, AL 35401-3299
Telephone: (205)-345-4131
HIV Testing, Counseling, Home Care Services, Referrals, Education, Speakers

West Alabama District Health Department
1101 Jackson Avenue
Tuscaloosa, AL 35401-3299
Telephone: (205)-345-4131 Fax: (205)-759-4039
HIV Testing, Counseling, Home Care Services, Referrals, Education, Speakers

Walker County

Community Services

Walker County Department of Human Resources
1901 Highway 78 East
P.O. Box 1772
Jasper, AL 35502-1772
Telephone: (205)-387-5400 Fax: (205)-221-9746
Contact: Emilie Johnson
In-house social services, referral contract services, financial services

County Health Depts

Walker County Health Department
705 20th Avenue, East
Jasper, AL 35502-3207
Telephone: (205)-221-9775
Contact: Jeanie Hudson
HIV Testing, Counseling, Home Care Services, Referrals, Education

Home Health Care

Griffin Vital Care, Inc.
6th Avenue West
Sipsey, AL 35584
Telephone: (205)-648-9696 Fax: (205)-648-9642
Toll-Free: (800)-525-1805
Contact: Steve Griffin
At-home therapies including total parenteral nutrition, IV antibiotic

Washington County

County Health Depts

Washington County Health Department
Court and Granade Avenues
Chatom, AL 36518
Telephone: (205)-847-2245
Contact: Ann Overstreet
HIV Testing, Counseling, Home Care Services, Referrals, Education, Speakers

Wilcox County

County Health Depts

Wilcox County Health Department
107 Union Street
Camden, AL 36726-1728
Telephone: (205)-682-4515
Contact: Sara Evans
HIV Testing, Counseling, Home Care Services, Referrals, Education, Speakers

Winston County

County Health Depts

Winston County Health Department & AIDS Prevention Committee
P.O. Box 57
Highway 195 South
Double Springs, AL 35553-0057
Telephone: (205)-489-2101
Contact: Carol Davis, R.N.
HIV Testing, Counseling, Home Care Services, Referrals, Education

Winston County Health Department, Branch Office
1001 20th Street
Haleyville, AL 35565-1047
Telephone: (205)-486-2479
HIV Testing, Counseling, Home Care Services, Referrals, Education

ALASKA

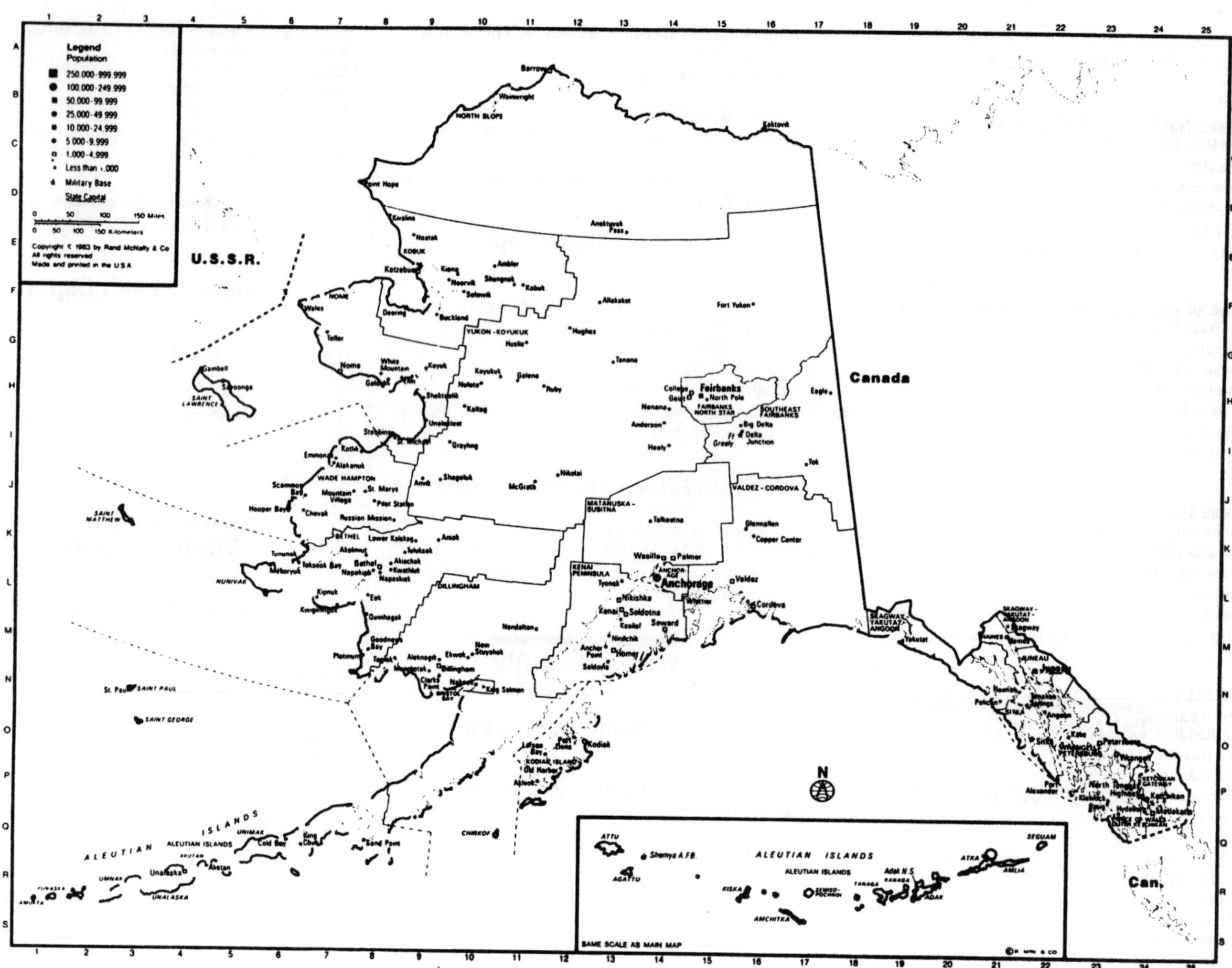

From City/County Planning Atlas Copyright 1989 by Reed McNally & Company, R.L. 90-S-28

Alaska

General Services

Education

Alaska Native Health Board, AIDS Program
1345 Rudakof Circle
Suite 206
Anchorage, AK 99508-6103
Telephone: (907)-337-0028
AIDS Resources for Health Boards and Corporations Targeting Alaska Natives,AIDS training

Dept. of Education, HIV Prevention Program
801 West 10th Street
Suite 200
Juneau, AK 99801
Telephone: (907)-465-2841
Contact: Rocky Plotnick-Weller
Support to School Districts & PTAs in Designing/Implementing AIDS/HIV Curricula

Nome Hospital
Community Health Office
P.O. Box 966
Nome, AK 99762
Telephone: (907)-443-3311 Fax: (907)-443-3139
Contact: Chris Larson - Director of Health Education
AIDS education and awareness programs

WAMI Program, Rural Health AIDS Education and Training Program
118 Red Building
P.O. Box 756740
Fairbanks, AK 99775-6740
Telephone: (907)-474-6020
AIDS Education for Rural Health Providers

Yukon Kuskokwim Health Corp., AIDS Program
P.O. Box 528
Bethel, AK 99559-0528
Telephone: (907)-543-3321 Fax: (907)-543-5277
Health Education to the Yukon Kuskokwim Delta Region

State Health Departments

Alaska Department of Health and Social Services
P.O. Box 110610
Juneau, AK 99811
Telephone: (907)-465-3090 Fax: (907)-586-1877
Contact: Peter Nakamura
Referrals

State of Alaska, AIDS/STD Program
PO Box 240249
3601 C Street, Suite 576
Anchorage, AK 99524-0249
Telephone: (907)-561-4406 Fax: (907)-562-7802
Training for counselors, technical assistance to various agencies

Statewide Services

Alaska State Commission for Human Rights
800 A Street, Suite 204
Anchorage, AK 99501-3669
Telephone: (907)-276-7474 Fax: (907)-278-8588
Legal services, discrimination complaints

Alaska State Housing Finance Corp.
Cedar Park West Juneau
Juneau, AK 99801
Telephone: (907)-586-3750 Fax: (907)-463-4967
Housing

Alaskan AIDS Assistance Association (4A's)
730 I St. #100
Anchorage, AK 99501
Telephone: (907)-276-4880
Food, housing, legal and financial assistance, education and support/carecase management

Aleutian Islands County

Testing Sites

Iliuliuk Family and Health Services
Box 144
Unalaska, AK 99685-0144
Telephone: (907)-581-1201
HIV testing, STD services

St. Paul Clinic
PO Box 148
St. Paul, AK 99660-9999
Telephone: (907)-546-2310 Fax: (907)-546-2268
HIV testing, STD services, education

Aleutians East County

Testing Sites

Sand Point Clinic
P.O. Box 172
Sand Point, AK 99661-0172
Telephone: (907)-383-3151
HIV testing and counseling, STD services, education

Anchorage County

Community Services

Alaska Legal Services
1016 W. 6th Avenue
Suite 200
Anchorage, AK 99501-1963
Telephone: (907)-272-9431
Legal Services

First Christian Church
3031 Latouche Street
Anchorage, AK 99508-4203
Telephone: (907)-272-0615
Contact: Rev. Wesley Veatch
Christian church clergy, counseling, HIV task force

McKinnel House Salvation Army
546 East 15th Street
Anchorage, AK 99501
Telephone: (907)-276-1609
Shelter, family services, food service, prescription vouchers

S.T.O.P. AIDS Project
520 East 4th Street
Anchorage, AK 99501-2624
Telephone: (907)-278-5019 Fax: (907)-276-3637
Contact: Gean Perry Crawford
Outreach, Prevention Education, HIV Antibody Testing for IV DrugUsers/Partners

Home Health Care

Home Health Care
PO Box 196604
Anchorage, AK 99519-6604
Telephone: (907)-261-3173
Home Health Care

Hospice of Anchorage
3605 Artic Blvd
#555
Anchorage, AK 99503
Telephone: (907)-561-5322
Home Health Care, Hospice

Medical Services

Alaska Regional Hospital
PO Box 143889
Anchorage, AK 99514-3889
Telephone: (907)-276-1131 Fax: (907)-264-1143
Medical Services

Anchorage Neighborhood Health Center
1217 East 10th Avenue
Anchorage, AK 99501-4003
Telephone: (907)-257-4600
Contact: Patty Donnelly
Primary care, HIV counseling and testing

Charter North Hospital
2530 DeBarr Drive
Anchorage, AK 99508-2996
Telephone: (907)-258-7575
Substance Abuse

Clitheroe Center
2207 Spenard Road
Anchorage, AK 99503
Telephone: (907)-243-1181 Fax: (907)-248-7483
Residential outpatient, halfway house

North Star Hospital
1650 South Bragaw Street
Anchorage, AK 99508-3467
Telephone: (907)-277-1522
Substance Abuse

Providence Hospital
PO Box 196604
Anchorage, AK 99519-6604
Telephone: (907)-562-2211
Medical Services

Testing Sites

Veterans Administration Outpatient & Regional Office
2925 DeBarr Road
Anchorage, AK 99508
Telephone: (907)-257-4700
Counseling, HIV testing

Bethel County

Community Services

Division of Public Assistance
P.O. Box 365
Bethel, AK 99559-0365
Telephone: (907)-543-2686 Fax: (907)-543-5912
Provides Food, Medical Services, and Cash to Eligible Persons

Dillingham County

Medical Services

Bristol Bay Area Health Corp.
P.O. Box 130
Dillingham, AK 99576-0130
Telephone: (907)-842-5201
Contact: John R. Bich - Counseling; Vivian Echzarria, PhD - Education
Medical services, counseling, education, pamphlets and videos

Fairbanks North Star County

Community Services

Family Focus
P.O. Box 74450
Fairbanks, AK 99707-4450
Telephone: (907)-452-5802
Housing for runaway teens, AIDS education

Interior AIDS Association
1514 Cushman St.
Suite 212
Fairbanks, AK 99707-1248
Telephone: (907)-452-4222
Education, Assistance, Emotional Support, Intervention, Counseling

Public Assistance
675 7th Avenue
Station G
Fairbanks, AK 99701-4526
Telephone: (907)-451-2850
Aid to families with dependent children, food stamps, Medicaid

Home Health Care

Hospice of Tanana Valley
P.O. Box 82770
Fairbanks, AK 99708
Telephone: (907)-474-0311
Contact: Mary Kay Brown
Hospice, Intervention, Counseling

Testing Sites

Fairbanks Health Center
800 Airport Way
Fairbanks, AK 99701-6092
Telephone: (907)-452-1776 Fax: (907)-451-4424
Contact: Nurse Manager
Confidential or Anonymous HIV Testing Site with Counseling, Referrals

Juneau County

Community Services

Holy Trinity Episcopal Church
325 Gold Street
Juneau, AK 99801-1126
Telephone: (907)-586-3532
Counseling, education

Dixie A Hood
222 Seward Suite 210
Juneau, AK 99801
Telephone: (907)-586-2200
Contact: Dixie Hood - MA, MFCC
Counseling

Home Health Care

Hospice of Juneau
3200 Hospital Drive
Suite 100
Juneau, AK 99801
Telephone: (907)-463-3113
Hospice Care, Emergency Services

Medical Services

Bartlett Memorial Hospital
3260 Hospital Drive
Juneau, AK 99801-7808
Telephone: (907)-586-2611 Fax: (907)-463-4919
Medical services, community funded care program

SEARHC Medical/Dental
3245 Hospital Drive
Juneau, AK 99801-7809
Telephone: (907)-463-4040 Fax: (907)-463-4032
Contact: Ron Baines - AIDS Coordinator
Medical & dental care for Native Americans, HIV testing & counseling

Kenai Peninsula County

Community Services

Central Peninsula Counseling Services
215 Fidalgo Street
Suite 102
Kenai, AK 99611-7751
Telephone: (907)-283-7501
Contact: David C. Wagner - Ed.D.
Counseling

Salvation Army
P.O. Box 2814
Kenai, AK 99611-2814
Telephone: (907)-283-3879
Emergency Assistance: Counseling, Limited Food, Clothing

State of Alaska, Department of Health & Social Services
601 East Pioneer Avenue
#122
Homer, AK 99603-7626
Telephone: (907)-235-6132
Food stamps, Medicaid, AFDC, general relief assistance, medical & adultpublic assistance

Medical Services

Kenai Health Center
210 Fidalgo Street
Room 102
Kenai, AK 99611-7750
Telephone: (907)-283-4871
Information on HIV Antibody Testing, STD Services, Pamphlets, Public Education

North Star Health Clinic
PO Box 1429
Adtec Dorm
Seward, AK 99664-1429
Telephone: (907)-224-3490 Fax: (907)-224-2085
Contact: Rhonda Johnson - Clinic Coordinator
HIV Counseling and Testing, STD, TB

Seward General Hospital

Seward, AK 99664
Telephone: (907)-224-5205 Fax: (907)-224-7248
AIDS/HIV testing, counseling, patient education

Testing Sites

Homer Hospital
4300 Bartlett Street
Homer, AK 99603-7005
Telephone: (907)-235-8101 Fax: (907)-235-3980
Testing, AIDS/HIV awareness, education

Manillaq Assn. Health Center
P.O. Box 170
Kotzebue, AK 99572
Telephone: (907)-442-3311 Fax: (907)-442-2133
Confidential HIV Testing with Counseling, TB Testing

North Pacific Medical Center
104 Center
Kodiak, AK 99605
Telephone: (907)-486-4183 Fax: (907)-486-4233
Confidential/Anonymous HIV Testing with Counseling

Seward Health Center
P.O. Box 810
Seward, AK 99664-0810
Telephone: (907)-224-5567 Fax: (907)-224-2385
HIV Antibody Testing, STD Medical Services, Pamphlets, Public EducationOutreach, Information, Conferences

Ketchikan Gateway County

Community Services

Division of Public Assistance
618 Dock Street
Ketchikan, AK 99901-6530
Telephone: (907)-225-2135
Food assistance, medical services, cash to eligible persons

Salvation Army
P.O. Box 5157
Ketchikan, AK 99901-0157
Telephone: (907)-225-5277
Emergency assistance: counseling, limited food, clothing

Medical Services

Ketchikan Health Center
3054 Fifth Ave.
Ketchikan, AK 99901-5775
Telephone: (907)-225-4350 Fax: (907)-247-0978
HIV antibody testing, STD medical services, pamphlets, confidentialcounseling & referral

Kodiak Island County

Community Services

Division of Public Assistance
307 Center Street
Kodiak, AK 99615-3000
Telephone: (907)-486-3783 Fax: (907)-486-3116
Provides food, medical services, and cash to eligible persons; medicaidassistance

Medical Services

Kodiak Island Hospital
1915 E Rezanos Drive
Kodiak, AK 99615
Telephone: (907)-486-3281
Contact: Ilva Fox
Medical services, HIV testing & counseling

Testing Sites

Kodiak Health Center
316 Mission Road
Room 207
Kodiak, AK 99615-6326
Telephone: (907)-486-3319
STD services, pamphlets, public education, HIV testing pre & postcounseling

Kodiak Island Medical Association
1818 Rezanof East
Kodiak, AK 99615
Telephone: (907)-486-6065 Fax: (907)-486-2248
Confidential/Anonymous HIV Testing with Counseling

Nome County

Community Services

Division of Public Assistance
Front Street
Old Federal Building
Nome, AK 99762-0221
Telephone: (907)-443-2237 Fax: (907)-443-2307
Food stamps, Medicaid, referrals to other agencies

Medical Services

Norton Sound Health Corp., Nome Health Center
P.O. Box 1710
Nome, AK 99762-1710
Telephone: (907)-443-3221 Fax: (907)-443-3139
Toll-Free: (800)-487-3318
HIV testing, STD services, pamphlets, public education, counseling

North Slope County

Medical Services

Barrow PHS Hospital
1296 F Agvik Street
Barrow, AK 99723
Telephone: (907)-852-4611
Medical Services

Northwest Arctic County

Community Services

Division of Public Assistance
P.O. Box 1210
Kotzebue, AK 99752-1210
Telephone: (907)-442-3451
Provides food, medical services, and cash to eligible persons; medicaidprogram, energy assistance

Medical Services

Manillaq Medical Center
P.O. Box 43
Kotzebue, AK 99752
Telephone: (907)-442-3321
Medical services, HIV testing, counseling, referrals

Sitka County

Medical Services

Sitka Community Hospital
209 Moller Avenue
Sitka, AK 99835
Telephone: (907)-747-3241 Fax: (907)-747-1758
Medical services & HIV testing

Testing Sites

Sitka Health Center
210 Moller Street
Sitka, AK 99835-7100
Telephone: (907)-747-3255
HIV Antibody Testing, STD Medical Services, Pamphlets, Public Education

Valdez-Cordova County

Medical Services

Valdez Hospital
911 Meals Ave
Valdez, AK 99686-0550
Telephone: (907)-835-2249 Fax: (907)-835-3735
Medical services & HIV testing

Testing Sites

Cordova Community Hospital
P.O. Box 160
Cordova, AK 99574-0160
Telephone: (907)-424-8116
HIV testing, counseling, community awarneness, education programs

Wrangell-Petersburg County

Community Services

Division of Public Assistance
P.O. Box 1089
Petersburg, AK 99833-1089
Telephone: (907)-772-3393
Contact: Kathleen Mason
Provides Food, Medical Services, and Cash to Eligible Persons

Medical Services

Wrangell Hospital
310 Bennett Street
Wrangell, AK 99929
Telephone: (907)-874-3356
Medical Services, HIV testing

Testing Sites

Petersburg Health Center
P.O. Box 377
Petersburg, AK 99833
Telephone: (907)-772-4611 Fax: (908)-772-4617
HIV testing and counseling, STD services, TB testing

Petersburg Hospital
PO Box 589
Petersburg, AK 99833
Telephone: (907)-772-4291
Counseling & testing

Yukon-Koyukuk County

Community Services

Four Rivers Counseling Service
P.O. Box 229
McGrath, AK 99627
Telephone: (907)-524-3867
Medical Services, Counseling

Medical Services

Yukon-Koyukuk Mental Health Program
P.O. Box 17
Galena, AK 99741-0017
Telephone: (907)-656-1617 Fax: (907)-656-1581
Toll-Free: (800)-478-1618
Counseling

ARIZONA

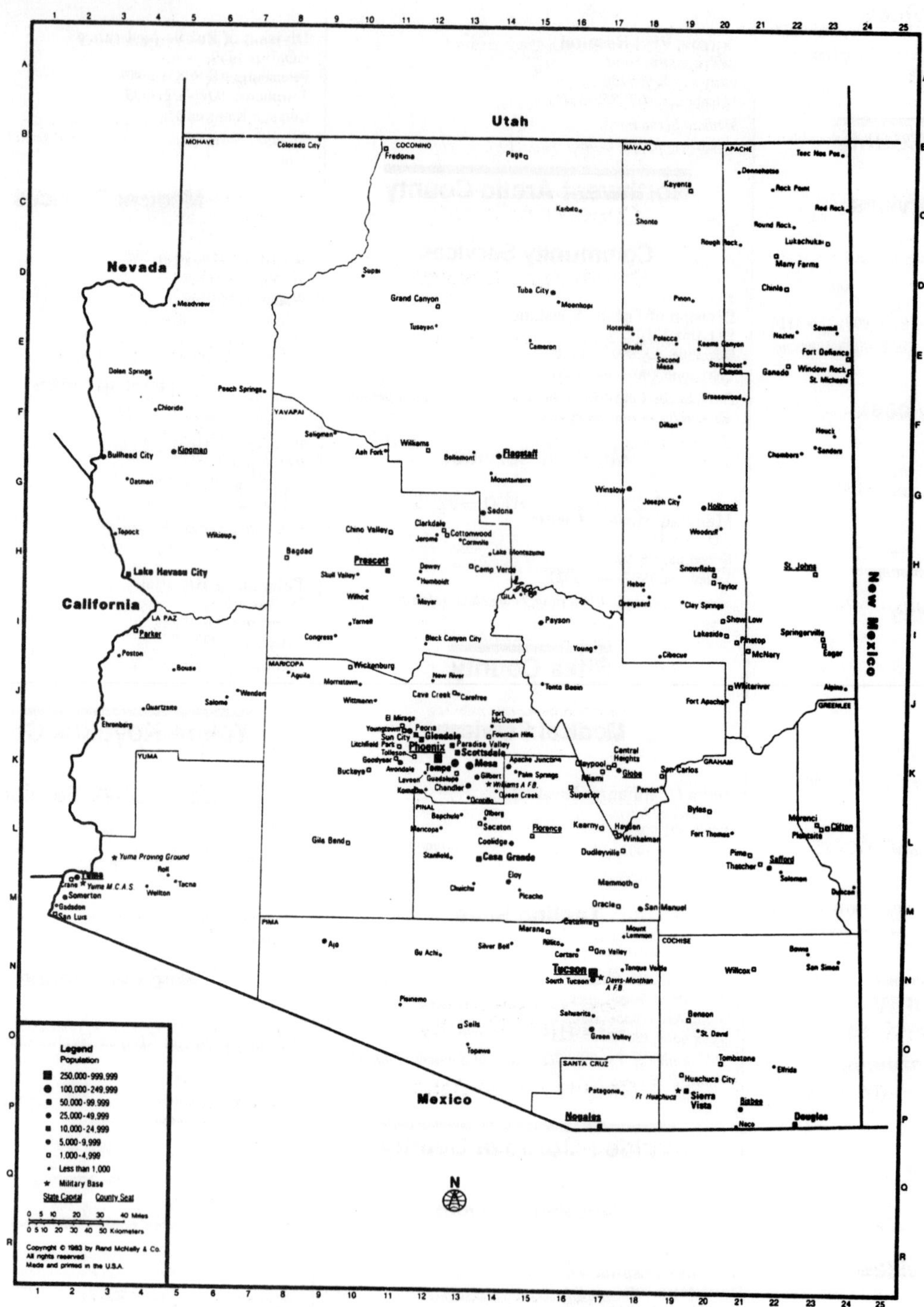

From City/County Planning Atlas Copyright 1989 by Reed McNally & Company, R.L. 90-S-28

Arizona

General Services

Education

AIDS Education Projects (University of Arizona)
1601 North Tucson Blvd.
Building #16
Tucson, AZ 85716-4206
Telephone: (602)-323-2437
Contact: Pam Reidbuffy, PhD
Comprehensive curriculum & training for health care professionals.

American Red Cross
1325 N. Beaver
Flagstaff, AZ 86001
Telephone: (602)-773-2523
Educational programs; printed and video materials available.

Arizona Spanish Speaking Community Information and Referral
The Annex
1515 East Osborne
Phoenix, AZ 85014
Telephone: (602)-263-8856
Information on HIV infection and AIDS in Spanish & English/Referrals

St. Joseph's Hospital/Medical Education/Infection Control
350 W. Thomas Road
Phoenix, AZ 85013-4496
Telephone: (602)-285-3249
Presentations to medical & general community; medical & ethical aspects of AIDS

State Health Departments

Arizona Department of Health Services
3815 North Black Cannon Hwy.
Phoenix, AZ 85015
Telephone: (602)-230-5819
Statistics & research

Statewide Services

Intertribal Council of Arizona/AIDS Project HIV/STD
4205 N. 7th Avenue
Suite 200
Phoenix, AZ 85013-
Telephone: (602)-248-0071
Minority Coalition

State Department of Insurance Consumer Affairs
2910 North 44th Street
Suite 210
Phoenix, AZ 85018
Telephone: (602)-255-4783
Information regarding insurance guidelines for discrimination claims.

Apache County

County Health Depts

Apache County Health Department
PO Box 697
St. Johns, AZ 85936-0697
Telephone: (602)-337-4364
Contact: Don Forster - Director
Confidential HIV testing, counseling, referrals

Coconino County

Community Services

AIDS Outreach of Northern Arizona
PO Box 183
Flagstaff, AZ 86002-0183
Telephone: (602)-525-1199
Contact: Lee Broderick
Referral & support for people with AIDS, ARC or HIV; AIDS hotline

County Health Depts

Coconino County Health Department
2500 North Fort Valley Rd
Flagstaff, AZ 86001-9332
Telephone: (602)-779-5164
Contact: George J. Graham - Director; Bee Torrey -
HIV testing/counseling

Graham County

County Health Depts

Graham County Health Department
826 W. Main Street
Safford, AZ 85546-2899
Telephone: (602)-428-0110
Contact: Neil Kames - Director
HIV testing & counseling

Greenlee County

County Health Depts

Greenlee County Health Department
PO Box 936
Clifton, AZ 85533-0936
Telephone: (602)-865-2601
Contact: Barbara Brutcher - Administrator
HIV Testing

La Paz County

County Health Depts

La Paz County Health Department
916 12th Street
Parker, AZ 85344-5714
Telephone: (602)-669-6155
Contact: Bill Myers - Director

Maricopa County

Community Services

Arizona AIDS Project (AAP)
4460 N. Central Street
Phoenix, AZ 85012-1815
Telephone: (602)-420-9396
Volunteers assist people with AIDS, counseling, case management, referrals

Catholic Social Services
325 East Southern STE 115
Tempe, AZ 85282
Telephone: (602)-894-1871
Contact: Ann Ryan
Foster care

Christo AIDS Ministry (CAM)
1029 E. Turney
Phoenix, AZ 85064
Telephone: (602)-265-2831
Contact: Fred Pattison
Spiritual guidance for AIDS patients, families & friends; emergency food, other

City of Phoenix Council
c/o City Council Offices
251 W. Washington Street
Phoenix, AZ 85003
Telephone: (602)-262-7492
Contact: Rachel LaMaide
Advisory to Phoenix City Council on AIDS policy & education.

Hemophilia Association
555 W. Catalina Drive
Suite #17
Phoenix, AZ 85013-4427
Telephone: (602)-266-8427
Contact: Michael Rosenthal
Education and counseling for hemophilia patients and families; grantservices, support groups

Human Resource Center
1250 S. 7th Avenue
Phoenix, AZ 85007-3996
Telephone: (602)-258-8011
Contact: Lupe Cavazos
Information & referral service; some emergency food, clothing, rent & utilities, AIDS program

Legal Services
305 South Second Street
P.O. Box 21538
Phoenix, AZ 85036
Telephone: (602)-258-3434
Contact: Joan Boyer
Help for low-income persons with legal issues involving access to health care.

Mesa Community Council
225 E Main Street
Suite 301
Mesa, AZ 85202-1414
Telephone: (602)-834-7777
Contact: Dr. Guy Spiesman
Referrals for AIDS/HIV testing; food and clothing for homeless

Phoenix Urban League
1402 South 7th Street
Phoenix, AZ 85007-
Telephone: (602)-254-5611

Contact: Sylvester White

Tri-City Behavioral Health Center
1255 W Baseline, Ste 296
Mesa, AZ 85202-5822
Telephone: (602)-730-1103
Contact: Tonya Jensen
Counseling services/support groups

County Health Depts

County Health Department AIDS Service-Education/Surveillance
1825 E. Roosevelt
Phoenix, AZ 85006
Telephone: (602)-258-6381
Contact: Heidi Hutchins - HIV/AIDS Coordinator
Provides epidemiological & statistical data, educational services, HIVtesting; individual counseling, primary care clinic

Maricopa County Department of Public Health
2225 North 16th Street
Phoenix, AZ 85006-1823
Telephone: (602)-252-1678 Fax: (602)-259-9087
Contact: Jeanne Frieden - AIDS Project Manager
HIV surveillance, counseling and referrals, partner notification

Home Health Care

Caremark Connection Network
1725 West 1st Street
Tempe, AZ 85281-2439
Telephone: (602)-277-8585
Contact: Steve Grady - Sales Director; Cathy Smeed - Branch Manager
Clinical Support and Infusion Therapies: Nutrition, Antimicrobials, Chemo.,Hematopoe, AIDS program education IV

East Valley Samaritan Hospice
2222 S. Dobson
Suite 401
Mesa, AZ 85202-4712
Telephone: (602)-835-0711 Fax: (602)-730-6078
Contact: Sandra Hancin
Coordinated & individualized home-care program for terminally ill.

Homedco Infusion
2202 East University
Suite B
Phoenix, AZ 85034
Telephone: (602)-392-2260
Experienced in providing quality infusion therapy to home HIV/AIDS patients.

Hospice of the Valley
2601 East Thomas Road
Suite 100
Phoenix, AZ 85016
Telephone: (602)-264-4827
Contact: Joan Lowell
Skilled nursing care, home health aides, social work, pastoral counseling.AIDS terminal care.

Lutheran Healthcare Hospice
Mesa Lutheran Hospital
325 E. Elliot Street
Chandler, AZ 85225
Telephone: (602)-497-5335 Fax: (602)-499-8250
Contact: Linda Cumberland
Medicare hospice; volunteers provide emotional and spiritual support toterminally ill and their families

Maricopa City Health Department
2601 East Roosevelt
Phoenix, AZ 85006-3642
Telephone: (602)-267-5011
Home Health Care

nmc HOMECARE
3844 E. University, Suite 4
Phoenix, AZ 85034
Telephone: (602)-437-4480
Fax: (602)-437-4552
Contact: Phil McCarty
National JCAHO-Accredited company providing a full range of Infusion and Respiratory therapies and specializing in the care of HIV/AIDS patients.National Case Manager is also available at 800-445-1188

Medical Services

Good Samaritan Medical Center
1111 E. McDowell Road
P.O. Box 52174
Phoenix, AZ 85062-2174
Telephone: (602)-239-2000
Toll-Free: (602)-239-2084
Contact: Dr. McKeller. I.D. Division
Comprehensive medical services.

Phoenix Indian Medical Center
4212 N. 16th Street
Phoenix, AZ 85016-5389
Telephone: (602)-263-1200 Fax: (602)-263-1648
Free medical services for members of an Indian tribe.

Phoenix Veteran's Administration Medical Center
650 East Indian School Road
Phoenix, AZ 85012
Telephone: (602)-277-5551 Fax: (602)-222-6435
Toll-Free: (800)-761-7000
Qualified veterans. Contact HIV Coordinator for further information.

Testing Sites

Arizona State University
Student Health Center
Tempe, AZ 85287-2104
Telephone: (602)-965-3346
Confidential HIV antibody testing; counseling & education for ASU students.

Planned Parenthood of Central and Northern Arizona
5651 N. 7th Street
Phoenix, AZ 85014-2500
Telephone: (602)-277-7526
AIDS/HIV testing, AIDS presentations to business/employees, schools, andreligious organizations

Mohave County

County Health Depts

Mohave County Health Department
305 West Beale
Kingman, AZ 86401-5881
Telephone: (602)-753-0748 Fax: (602)-753-0777
Contact: Terri Williams - Nurse Manager
HIV testing, counseling

Navajo County

County Health Depts

Navajo County Health Department
PO Box 639
Holbrook, AZ 86025-0639
Telephone: (602)-524-6825 Fax: (602)-524-1907
Contact: Maxine McKee - Director

Pima County

Community Services

Department of Economic Security
400 w. Congress St. #420
Tucson, AZ 85701-1723
Telephone: (602)-628-5428
Contact: Linda Blessing,D.P.A.
Social Services

People with AIDS Coalition of Tucson (PACT)
P.O. Box 2488
Tucson, AZ 85702-2488
Telephone: (602)-322-9808
Contact: Jerome Beillard - Director
HIV & AIDS infected peer counseling, social activities, referral.

Shanti Foundation of Tucson
602 N. 4th Avenue
Tucson, AZ 85705-8449
Telephone: (602)-622-7107
Contact: Ann Maley - Office Manager
Volunteer service organization/emotional support - illness and/or grief.

Tucson AIDS Project (TAP)
151 South Tucson Blvd
#252
Tucson, AZ 85716-5523
Telephone: (602)-322-6226 Fax: (602)-327-9557
Emotional and practical support for HIV/AIDS infected, education, information.

County Health Depts

Pima County Health Department
150 West Congress
Tucson, AZ 85701-
Telephone: (602)-740-8554
Contact: Christopher Brown
HIV testing, counseling, education, HIV surveillance

Home Health Care

Caremark Connection Network
3450 S Broadmont
Suite 100
Tucson, AZ 85713-5245
Telephone: (602)-624-0500
Contact: Debbie Kelly - Ops. Manager
Clinical Support and Infusion Therapies: Nutrition, Antimicrobials, Chemo.,Hematopoe, AIDS IV therapy

nmc HOMECARE
1141 West Grant Rd, Suite 100
Tuscon, AZ 85705
Telephone: (602)-798-1498
Fax: (602)-798-1634

Contact: Cindy Dorr

National JCAHO-Accredited company providing a full range of Infusion and Respiratory therapies and specializing in the care of HIV/AIDS patients. National Case Manager is also available at 800-445-1188

Medical Services

Arizona Cancer Center
1501 North Campbell Ave
Tucson, AZ 85724
Telephone: (602)-626-6372
Out patient clinic

Kino Community Hospital
2800 East Ajo Way
Tucson, AZ 85713-6204
Telephone: (602)-294-4471   Fax: (602)-741-6817
Contact: Dr. Leonard Ditmanson
Medical, Mental Health

Veterans Medical Center
Medical Service 111
Tucson, AZ 85723
Telephone: (602)-792-1450
Free HIV clinic, nursing care for veterans

Pinal County

Testing Sites

Pinal County Health Department
188 South Main Street
Coolidge, AZ 85228-4439
Telephone: (602)-723-9541
HIV Testing

Yavapai County

County Health Depts

Yavapai County Health Department
930 Division Street
Prescott, AZ 86301
Telephone: (602)-771-3130   Fax: (602)-771-3369
Anonymous HIV testing and counseling.

Home Health Care

nmc HOMECARE
1000 Willow Creek Road, Suite L
Prescott, AZ 86301
Telephone: (602)-771-0167
Fax: (602)-771-0354
Contact: Phil McCarty

National JCAHO-Accredited company providing a full range of Infusion and Respiratory therapies and specializing in the care of HIV/AIDS patients. National Case Manager is also available at 800-445-1188

O.P.T.I.O.N. Care of Yavapai County
811 Ainsworth
Suite 100
Prescott, AZ 86301-1641
Telephone: (602)-771-5276
Contact: Larry Anderson, RPh - Owner, Valorie Salzman, RN - Patient Coordinator
Home IV and Nutritional Services, AIDS IV therapy

Yuma County

County Health Depts

Yuma County Health Department
201 Second Avenue
Yuma, AZ 85364-2213
Telephone: (602)-329-2220   Fax: (602)-329-2226
Contact: Becky Smith - HIV Department Head
HIV testinf/STD nutrition immunization

ARKANSAS

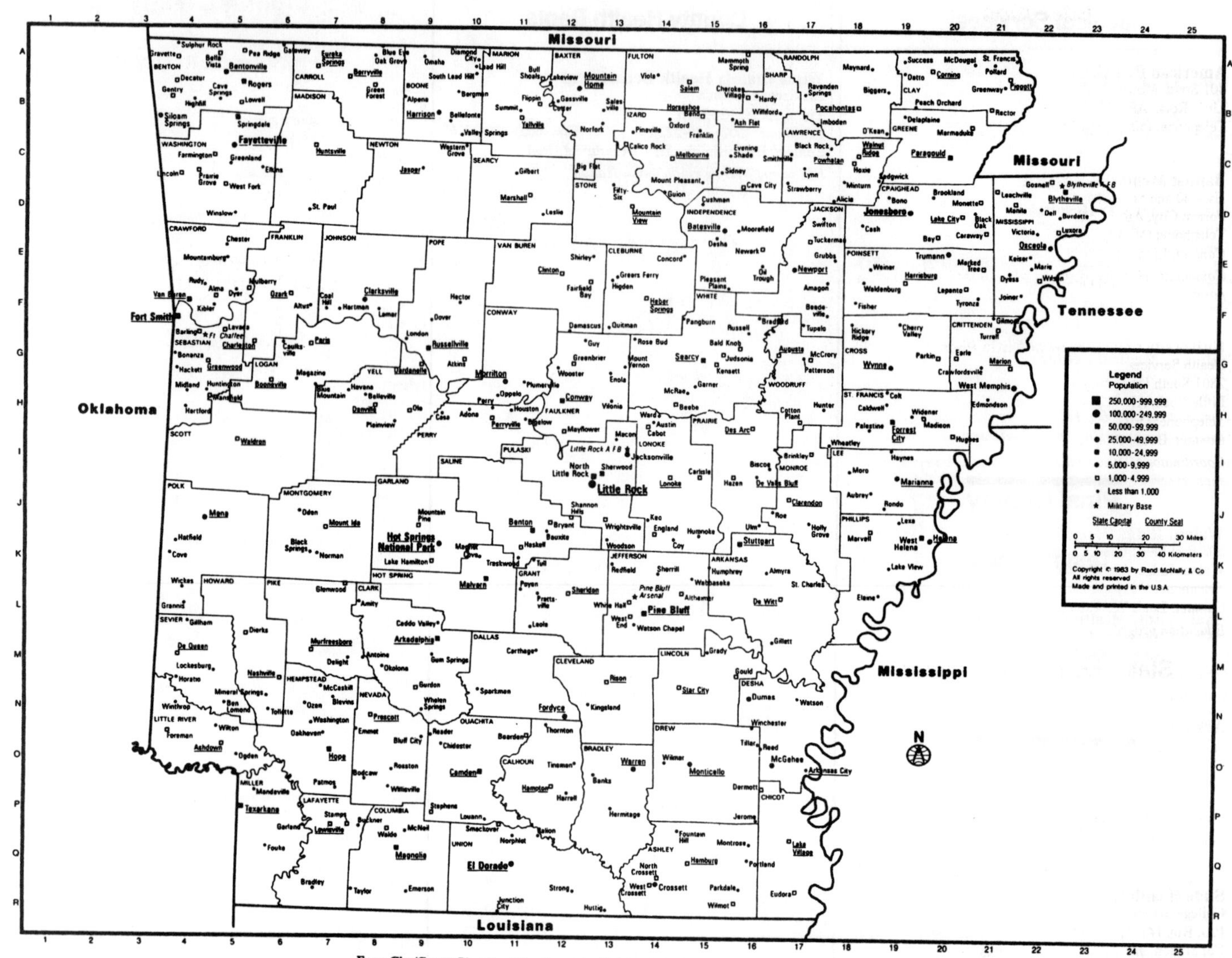

From City/County Planning Atlas Copyright 1989 by Reed McNally & Company, R.L. 90-S-28

Arkansas

General Services

Education

American Red Cross
401 South Monroe
Little Rock, AR 72204
Telephone: (501)-666-0351

Baptist Memorial Hospital
Hwy 40 and State 284
Forrest City, AR 72335
Telephone: (501)-633-2020
Contact: Linda Hall, R.N.
Community Health forums are utilized for educational purposes.

University of Arkansas at Little Rock
Health Services
2801 South University
Little Rock, AR 72204
Telephone: (501)-569-3188 Fax: (501)-569-3588
Contact: Bobbi Prior
Coordinator AIDS educaation programs for campus, provide support servicesfor campus & surrounding community

Walnut Ridge Public Schools
508 East Free Street
Walnut Ridge, AR 72476
Telephone: (501)-886-6623
Contact: Lucia W. Allen - Librarian
Education programs on HIV/AIDS

State Health Departments

Arkansas State Department of Health, AIDS/HIV Division
4815 West Markham
Little Rock, AR 72205
Telephone: (501)-661-2292 Fax: (501)-661-2082
Contact: Lola Turman
Three-day HIV counselor training course, HIV testing

State Health Department
College Station Clinic
P.O. Box 147
Col Station, AR 72053
Telephone: (501)-490-1604
Contact: Pearl Holmes
Counseling, testing

Statewide Services

Arkansas AIDS Foundation
123A Vanburen
Little Rock, AR 72205
Telephone: (501)-663-7833
Contact: Gene Holloway
Free HIV testing

Arkansas Department of Health
4815 West Markham Street
Little Rock, AR 72205-3867
Telephone: (501)-661-2408 Fax: (501)-661-2082
Contact: AIDS Prevention Program
Three day HIV counselor training course. Hotline 1-800-445-7720

Arkansas Department of Human Services
250 Shopping Way
West Memphis, AR 72301
Telephone: (501)-732-5170
Contact: Hubert Gray
Children & family services, food stamps, presentations, Medicaid assistance

State Department of Education
Arch Ford Building
4 Capitol Mall
Little Rock, AR 72201
Telephone: (501)-371-2941
Contact: Jean Wilhout

Arkansas County

County Health Depts

County Health Unit
1570 S. Madison Avenue
P.O. Box 151
Dewitt, AR 72042-0151
Telephone: (501)-946-2934 Fax: (501)-946-2662
Testing, referrals, follow-up contact

County Health Unit
711 N. College
P.O. Box 455
Stuttgart, AR 72160
Telephone: (501)-673-6601
Government programs, home health care

Ashley County

County Health Depts

County Health Unit
1300 West 5th Avenue
Crossett, AR 71635
Telephone: (501)-364-2115
HIV testing, referrals, counseling

County Health Unit
205 E. Jefferson
Hamburg, AR 71646
Telephone: (501)-853-5525
Home care

Baxter County

County Health Depts

County Health Unit
Baxter County Hospital
P.O. Box 308
Mtn Home, AR 72653
Telephone: (501)-425-3072 Fax: (501)-424-6646
HIV, STD, TB testing

Boone County

Home Health Care

North Arkansas Medical Center
620 North Willow
Harrison, AR 72601
Telephone: (501)-365-2035 Fax: (501)-365-2430
Contact: Arlene Betki, RN - Director of Nursing
Home care, in/outpatient care, occupational/physical therapy

Bradley County

County Health Depts

County Health Unit
North Bragg Street
Warren, AR 71671
Telephone: (501)-226-8440 Fax: (501)-226-7828
Contact: Wanda Taulbee - RN
HIV testing, pre & post counseling, home health

Calhoun County

County Health Depts

County Health Unit
First & Hunt
P.O. Box 236
Hampton, AR 71744
Telephone: (501)-798-2808
HIV testing

Carroll County

County Health Depts

County Health Unit
104 Spring Street
Berryville, AR 72616
Telephone: (501)-423-2923 Fax: (501)-423-5315
HIV testing, screening, counseling

Chicot County

County Health Depts

County Health Unit
846 Highway 65 & 82
Lake Village, AR 71653
Telephone: (501)-265-2236 Fax: (501)-265-5445
HIV testing

County Health Unit
600 Pecan Street
Dermott, AR 71638
Telephone: (501)-538-3336
Testing

County Health Unit
2420 Highway 65 North
Eudora, AR 71640
Telephone: (501)-355-2356
Testing

Clark County

County Health Depts

County Health Unit
605 South 10th Street
Arkadelphia, AR 71923
Telephone: (501)-246-4471 Fax: (501)-246-9619
Testing, home health

Clay County

County Health Depts

County Health Unit
Front & Cherry Streets
Piggott, AR 72454
Telephone: (501)-598-3390
HIV testing, counseling

County Health Unit
18 Huddle Plaza Mall
Highway 67 N
Corning, AR 72422
Telephone: (501)-857-6281
Testing, counseling

Cleburne County

County Health Depts

County Health Unit
918 South 9th Street
Heber Springs, AR 72543
Telephone: (501)-362-7581 Fax: (501)-362-4684
HIV testing

Cleveland County

County Health Depts

County Health Unit
501 E. Magnolia
P.O. Box 446
Rison, AR 71665
Telephone: (501)-325-6311 Fax: (501)-325-6301
HIV testing

Columbia County

County Health Depts

County Health Unit
207 West Calhoun
P.O. Box 177
Magnolia, AR 71753
Telephone: (501)-235-3754
Contact: Diane Pittman
HIV testing

Conway County

County Health Depts

County Health Unit
100 Hospital Drive
Morrilton, AR 72110
Telephone: (501)-354-4652

Craighead County

Community Services

Salvation Army
P.O. Box 726
Jonesboro, AR 72401
Telephone: (501)-932-3785
Contact: Capt. Elen Hill
Support for homeless

County Health Depts

County Health Unit
2920 McClellan Drive
Jonesboro, AR 72401
Telephone: (501)-933-4585 Fax: (501)-933-6416
Contact: Cheryl Sipa
Testing & counseling

County Health Unit
2920 McClellan Drive
Jonesboro, AR 72401
Telephone: (501)-933-4585
Testing, counseling

Medical Services

Methodist Hospital
3024 Stadium Blvd
Jonesboro, AR 72401
Telephone: (501)-972-7000 Fax: (501)-932-4149
Contact: Janet Johnson
Acute care facility

St. Bernards Regional Medical Center
Matthews Street
Jonesboro, AR 72401
Telephone: (501)-972-4493
Contact: Pam Tedderor, Jane McDaniel -

Crawford County

County Health Depts

County Health Unit
105 Pointer Trail West
Van Buren, AR 72956
Telephone: (501)-474-6391
Contact: Betsy Rhyne - Office Administration
AIDS/HIV testing; individual counseling; offer referral sources for otherservices

Crittenden County

Medical Services

East Arkansas Regional Mental Health
105 West Harrison
West Memphis, AR 72301
Telephone: (501)-735-6923 Fax: (501)-735-6941
Contact: Betty Getner
Mental health counseling

Cross County

County Health Depts

County Health Unit
704 Canal Street
Wynne, AR 72396
Telephone: (501)-238-2101 Fax: (501)-238-4569
Contact: Pat Edwards - Administrator
AIDS/HIV testing; individual counseling; referrals; in-home health visits;hospice program for terminally ill

Dallas County

County Health Depts

County Health Unit
209 North Clifton
Fordyce, AR 71742
Telephone: (501)-352-7197 Fax: (501)-352-2911
Contact: Karen Archer - Administrator
AIDS/HIV testing; counseling; referrals

Desha County

County Health Depts

County Health Unit
100 E. Oak St
McGehee, AR 71654
Telephone: (501)-222-3910
Contact: Paula Chesser, RN - Coordinator
AIDS/HIV testing; individual counseling; offers referral sources for otherinformation

County Health Unit
Hwy 65 South
Dumas, AR 71639
Telephone: (501)-382-2377 Fax: (501)-382-5015
Contact: Marty Chambers - Administrator
AIDS/HIV testing; counseling; referrals

Drew County

County Health Depts

County Health Unit
940 Scogin Drive
Monticello, AR 71655
Telephone: (501)-367-6234
Contact: Mary Beth Woods - Administrator
AIDS/HIV testing, counseling; referrals

County Health Unit, Area VII
129 East Jackson
Monticello, AR 71655
Telephone: (501)-367-6202
Referrals for AIDS/HIV services, testing and counseling

Faulkner County

County Health Depts

Faulkner County Health Unit
811 N Creek Drive
Conway, AR 72032
Telephone: (501)-327-6505   Fax: (501)-450-4941
Contact: Elese Brown, RN - Administrator
AIDS/HIV testing; counseling; referrals

Franklin County

County Health Depts

County Health Unit
111 West Spring Street
Ozark, AR 72949
Telephone: (501)-667-2555
Contact: Bessie L. Hobbs - Office Administrator
AIDS/HIV testing; individual counseling; offer referral sources for otherservices

Fulton County

County Health Depts

County Health Unit
Hospital Grounds
P.O. Box 939
Salem, AR 72576
Telephone: (501)-895-3300   Fax: (501)-895-4340
Contact: Gwen Montgomery - Administrator
AIDS/HIV testing; counseling

Garland County

County Health Depts

County Health Unit
115 Market, Suite 200
Hot Springs, AR 71901
Telephone: (501)-624-3394
Contact: Frances Gray
Home care service

Grant County

County Health Depts

Grant County Health Unit
609 East Centre
Sheridan, AR 72150
Telephone: (501)-942-3157
Referrals, counseling, home care & HIV testing

Greene County

Medical Services

Arizona AIDS Project (AAP)
900 West King Highway
Paragould, AR 72450
Telephone: (501)-239-7000   Fax: (501)-239-7400
Contact: Dr. Jack Richmond
Keycare hospital-general medical services

Hempstead County

County Health Depts

County Health Unit
808 West 5th
Hope, AR 71801
Telephone: (501)-777-2191
HIV/STD testing

Hot Spring County

County Health Depts

County Health Unit
2204 East Sullenberger
Malvern, AR 72104
Telephone: (501)-332-6974
AIDS/HIV testing

Howard County

County Health Depts

County Health Unit
410 West Henderson
Nashville, AR 71852
Telephone: (501)-845-2208
HIV testing, counseling, homecare, referrals

County Health Unit, Area V
421 North Main Street
Nashville, AR 71852
Telephone: (501)-845-4512   Fax: (501)-845-5477
STD/HIV testing, family planning, child services

Independence County

County Health Depts

County Health Unit
1792 Myers Street
Batesville, AR 72501
Telephone: (501)-793-8848
Contact: Nancy Martin
HIV testing & counseling

Izard County

County Health Depts

County Health Unit
P.O. Box 604
Melbourne, AR 72556
Telephone: (501)-368-7790
HIV testing, counseling; homecare, referrals

Jackson County

County Health Depts

Jackson County Health Unit
Courthouse Annex
PO Box 130
Newport, AR 72112
Telephone: (501)-523-8968
Contact: Maryann McCoy
HIV testing, counseling

Jefferson County

County Health Depts

County Health Unit
2306 Rike Drive
P.O. Box 7267
Pine Bluff, AR 71611-7267
Telephone: (501)-535-2142
Referral services

Medical Services

Jefferson Regional Medical Center
1515 West 42nd
Pine Bluff, AR 71603
Telephone: (501)-541-7100   Fax: (501)-541-7204
Contact: Katherine Williams, RN - Infection Control Coord.
Medical services

Johnson County

County Health Depts

Johnson County Health Unit
6 Professional Park Drive
Clarksville, AR 72830
Telephone: (501)-754-2949
Contact: Jo Wise - Program Coordinator
Referrals, testing, counseling

Lafayette County

County Health Depts

County Health Unit
1105 Chestnut
P.O. Box 367
Lewisville, AR 71845
Telephone: (501)-921-5744
HIV testing, home care, referrals & counseling

Lawrence County

County Health Depts

County Health Unit
Hwy 25 West
P.O. Box 405
Walnut Ridge, AR 72476
Telephone: (501)-886-3201 Fax: (501)-886-1722
Contact: Linda Clarke
Pre- and post counseling

County Health Unit, Area XI
388 Walnut Ridge
P.O. Box 388
Walnut Ridge, AR 72476
Telephone: (501)-886-3153
Referrals, home care, counseling

Lee County

County Health Depts

County Health Unit
141 North Hicky Street
P.O. Box 668
Marianna, AR 72360
Telephone: (501)-295-7780 Fax: (501)-295-7788
Contact: Evelynn E. Vanderford
HIV counseling, HIV blood test; home health

Lincoln County

County Health Depts

County Health Unit
101 West Wiley Street
Star City, AR 71667
Telephone: (501)-628-5121
Home care, screening, referrals

Little River County

County Health Depts

County Health Unit
150 Keller Street
Ashdown, AR 71822
Telephone: (501)-898-3831
Referrals, home care, counseling

Logan County

County Health Depts

County Health Unit
100 E. Academy Street
P.O. Box 509
Paris, AR 72855
Telephone: (501)-963-6126
HIV testing, counseling, referrals, homecare

Testing Sites

County Health Unit
461 East 5th Street
Booneville, AR 72927
Telephone: (501)-675-2593
HIV testing, counseling, referrals, homecare

Lonoke County

County Health Depts

County Health Unit
320 South Washington
England, AR 72046
Telephone: (501)-842-3436
HIV testing, counseling, referrals, homecare

County Health Unit
614 N Grant, P.O. Box 1203
Cabot, AR 72023-2656
Telephone: (501)-843-7561
HIV testing, counseling

County Health Unit
311 Court Street
P.O. Box 172
Lonoke, AR 72086
Telephone: (501)-676-2268
Contact: Rosa Hignight
Testing, counseling, referral

Miller County

Testing Sites

County Health Unit
1007 Jefferson Street
Texarkana, AR 75502
Telephone: (501)-773-2108 Fax: (501)-772-2852
HIV testing, counseling, referral, follow-up, care clinic

Monroe County

Testing Sites

County Health Unit
306 West King Drive
Brinkley, AR 72021
Telephone: (501)-734-1461 Fax: (501)-734-1024
Contact: Gloria Lloyd
HIV testing

Nevada County

County Health Depts

County Health Unit
482 Hale Avenue
P.O. Box 360
Prescott, AR 71857
Telephone: (501)-887-2004
Contact: Janet Thompsom
HIV testing & counseling.

Pike County

Testing Sites

County Health Unit
Pike County Health Unit
P.O. Box 413
Murfreesboro, AR 71958
Telephone: (501)-285-3154 Fax: (501)-285-2707
Contact: Irene Chambers
HIV testing & counseling

Poinsett County

County Health Depts

County Health Unit
610 Walnut Street
Trumann, AR 72472
Telephone: (501)-483-5761
Contact: Diana Milligan
HIV pre-counseling, testing, post-counseling, referrals

County Health Unit
102 Liberty
Marked Tree, AR 72365
Telephone: (501)-358-3615
Contact: Lisa Southward
HIV testing, counseling, referrals

Polk County

County Health Depts

County Health Unit
222 Hornbeck
Mena, AR 71953
Telephone: (501)-394-5324
Contact: Mary Cannell
HIV testing & counseling.

Pope County

County Health Depts

County Health Unit, Area III
1708 West C Place
Russellville, AR 72801
Telephone: (501)-968-3254
Contact: Delores Brown
HIV testing, counseling

Prairie County

County Health Depts

County Health Unit
Main Street
P.O. Box 249
Des Arc, AR 72040
Telephone: (501)-256-4430
Contact: Donna Speight
HIV testing, counseling

Pulaski County

Community Services

Family Service Center
P.O. Box 5431
N. Little Rock, AR 72119
Telephone: (501)-372-4842 Fax: (501)-372-6565
Contact: Linda Hale - Data Coordinator
Upgrading program, support group.

Ryan White Center
2422 West 10th Street
Little Rock, AR 72202
Telephone: (501)-376-6299
Contact: Shelly Crump
Medical services, case management & counseling

County Health Depts

County Health Unit
Eastgate Clinic, Apt 60
Eastgate Terrace
N. Little Rock, AR 72114
Telephone: (501)-753-8973
Contact: Gwen Bourquin RN
Testing, education, referrals

County Health Unit
5 Computer Drive South
Albany, AR 72205
Telephone: (501)-776-5650 Fax: (501)-776-5654
Contact: Marsha Shay
Pre & post HIV counseling, testing, referrals

County Health Unit
2800 Willow Street
N. Little Rock, AR 72114
Telephone: (501)-758-1540
Contact: Geraldine Rambo - RN
HIV testing

County Health Unit, Area VIII
200 South University Avenue
Suite 310
Little Rock, AR 72205
Telephone: (501)-661-2195
Contact: Zenobia Harris
Supervisor, referrals

Pulaski Central County Health Unit
Mall Health Unit
200 S University, Ste 300
Little Rock, AR 72205
Telephone: (501)-664-6764
Contact: Cathy Messick
Family planning

Home Health Care

Caremark Homecare Branch Network
2201 Brookwood Drive
Suite 118
Little Rock, AR 72202
Telephone: (501)-666-0287
Contact: Jennifer McMinn
Home infusion

Medical Services

Doctor's Hospital
6101 West Capitol
Little Rock, AR 72205
Telephone: (501)-661-4000 Fax: (501)-661-3979
Contact: Michelle Fraleigh - Director of Nursing
AIDS treatment

Memorial Hospital
#1 Pershing Circle
N. Little Rock, AR 72114
Telephone: (501)-771-3000
Contact: Marge Branscum - Infectious Control Risk Mgr
Medical Services, physical therapy

Veteran's Admin. Hospital McClellan
4300 West 7th Street
Little Rock, AR 72205
Telephone: (501)-661-1202
Contact: Dr. Thomas Munson
HIV/AIDS clinical service and general medical services

Testing Sites

County Health Unit
Pulaski-Central Clinic
3915 West 8th Street
Little Rock, AR 72204
Telephone: (501)-562-2464
Contact: Mark Barns
AIDS screening, referrals

Randolph County

County Health Depts

Randolph County Health Unit
1304 Pace Road
Pocahontas, AR 72455
Telephone: (501)-892-5239
HIV testing, counseling, education

Saint Francis County

County Health Depts

County Health Unit
413 N. Division Street
P.O. Box 956
Forrest City, AR 72335
Telephone: (501)-633-1340
Contact: Ms. Bonnie Dodson - RN
In home services, referral, HIV testing

County Health Unit, Area IX
P.O. Box 788
Forrest City, AR 72335-0788
Telephone: (501)-633-6812
Contact: Ms. Louise Dennis - Manager Regional Office
AIDS education staff for county health units

Scott County

County Health Depts

County Health Unit
440 Featherston
P.O. Box 808
Waldron, AR 72958
Telephone: (501)-637-2165

Searcy County

County Health Depts

County Health Unit
HC 89, Box 55
Marshall, AR 72650
Telephone: (501)-448-3374
Contact: Royann Hudsten - RN
HIV testing, counseling, referrals

Sebastian County

County Health Depts

County Health Unit
3112 South 70th Street
Ft. Smith, AR 72903
Telephone: (501)-452-6600 Fax: (501)-452-8600
Counseling & testing-HIV

Sevier County

County Health Depts

County Health Unit
304 N 4th
DeQueen, AR 71832
Telephone: (501)-642-2535

Sharp County

County Health Depts

County Health Unit
P.O. Box 37
Ash Flat, AR 72513
Telephone: (501)-994-7364

Stone County

County Health Depts

County Health Unit
Blanchard Avenue
Route 73, Box 204 HC
Mountain View, AR 72560
Telephone: (501)-269-3308
Contact: Lily Roberts - RN
HIV testing, referral, education, home health care

Union County

County Health Depts

County Health Unit
620 West Grove
El Dorado, AR 71730
Telephone: (501)-863-5101
Contact: Susan Blake
HIV testing, counseling & referrals

Van Buren County

County Health Depts

County Health Unit
Quality Drive
P.O. Box 452
Clinton, AR 72031
Telephone: (501)-745-2485
Contact: Ms. Connies Barnes - RN
HIV testing, counseling, referrals

Washington County

Medical Services

Washington County HIV Clinic
1100 N Woolsey
Fayetteville, AR 72703
Telephone: (501)-521-5580 Fax: (501)-521-5584
Contact: Dr. Linda McGhee - Director
Only residents of Washington County are eligible

White County

County Health Depts

County Health Unit
101 Windwood Drive
Suite 5
Beebe, AR 72012
Telephone: (501)-882-5128

County Health Unit
3216 East Race Street
Searcy, AR 72143
Telephone: (501)-268-6102
HIV testing, counseling & education

Woodruff County

County Health Depts

County Health Unit
502 North Third Street
P.O. Box 542
Augusta, AR 72006
Telephone: (501)-347-5915
Contact: Nell Jones
HIV testing, counseling & education

Yell County

County Health Depts

County Health Unit
403 Atlanta Street
P.O. Box 628
Danville, AR 72833
Telephone: (501)-495-2741
Contact: Chris Bonting
HIV testing, education & counseling

County Health Unit
619 North 5th Street
Dardanelle, AR 72834
Telephone: (501)-229-3509
HIV testing, counseling, education

CALIFORNIA

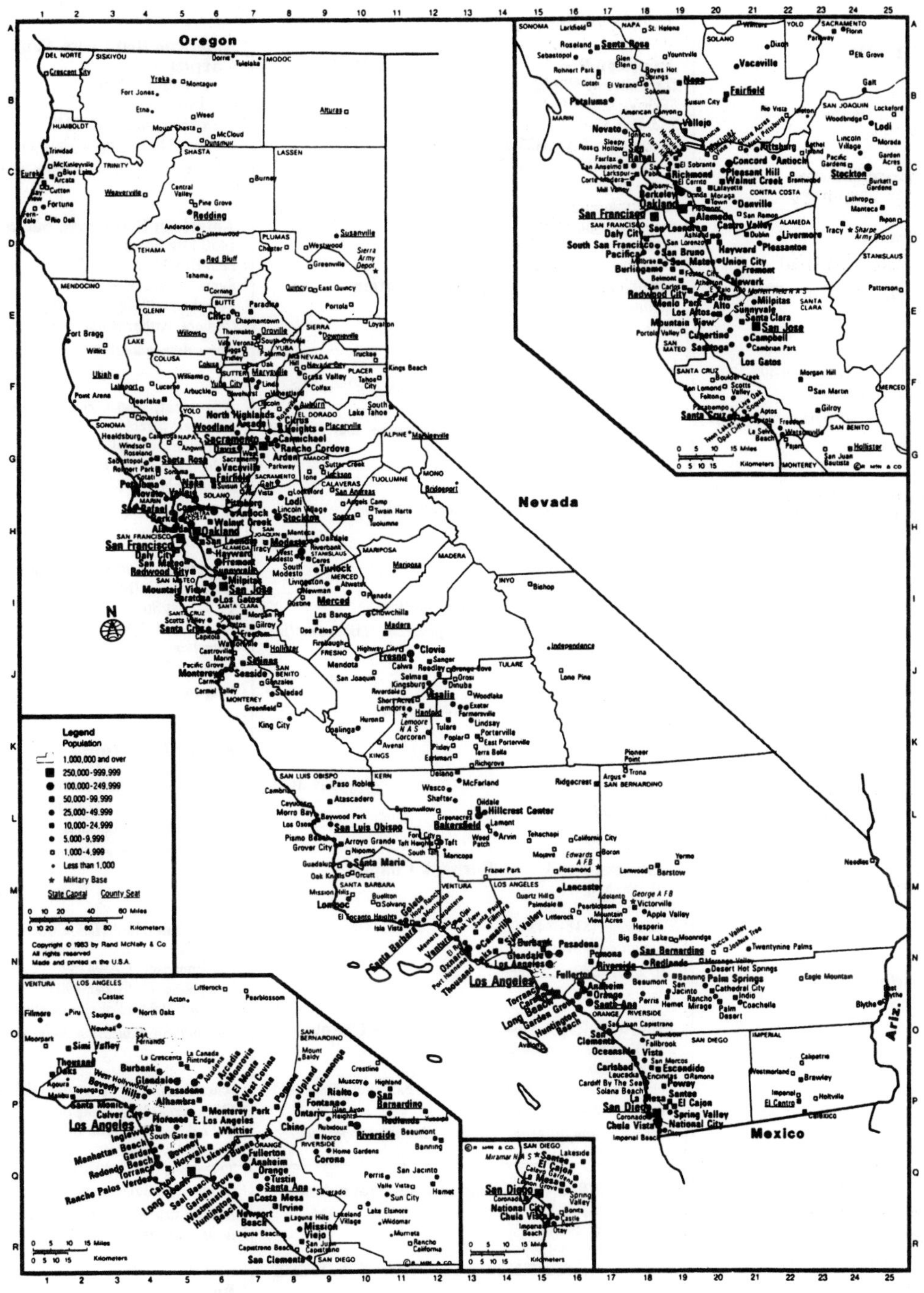

From City/County Planning Atlas Copyright 1989 by Reed McNally & Company, R.L. 90-S-28

California

General Services

Education

AIDS Education & Training Center
USC, 1975 Zonal Avenue
Mail Code KAM200
Los Angeles, CA 90033
Telephone: (213)-342-1846
Contact: Dr. Jerry Gates
HIV training for medical staff members

AIDS Foundation of San Diego, Local AIDS Assistance Contract
4080 Centre St
San Diego, CA 92103-2698
Telephone: (619)-686-5000 Fax: (619)-497-5252
Contact: Diane Bonne - Assoicate Director
AIDS Education and Prevention Projects, Seminars, Support Groups, Hotline,Social services

AIDS Information BBS (voice)
PO Box 421528
San Francisco, CA 94142
Telephone: (415)-626-1245 Fax: (415)-626-9415
Contact: Ben Gardiner
Information

AIDS Project of the East Bay
565 16th Street
Oakland, CA 94612
Telephone: (510)-834-8181 Fax: (510)-834-0442
Contact: Valerie Papayamann - Executive Director
AIDS Education and Prevention Projects, Support Groups, Literature Distribution

AIDS Response Program, Gay and Lesbian Center of Orange Cty.
12832 Garden Grove Blvd.
Suite A
Garden Grove, CA 92643
Telephone: (714)-534-0961 Fax: (714)-534-5491
Contact: Donna Yutzy
Support Groups, Counseling, Referrals, Education, Speakers Bureau, Training

AIDS Treatment News
PO Box 411256
San Francisco, CA 94141-1256
Telephone: (415)-255-0588 Fax: (413)-255-4659
Toll-Free: (800)-873-2812
Contact: Editor & Publisher
Biweekly publication covering standards, trials and experiments

American Foundation for AIDS Research, West Coast Office
5900 Wilshire Boulevard
Suite 2300
Los Angeles, CA 90036-5032
Telephone: (213)-857-5900
Fund raising for AIDS research

American Red Cross
868 E. Santa Clara
Ventura, CA 93001
Telephone: (805)-339-2234 Fax: (805)-339-0311
General information, courses on AIDS

American Red Cross
2707 State Street
Santa Barbara, CA 93101
Telephone: (805)-687-1331 Fax: (805)-682-4655
Contact: Diane Lantz
AIDS education community/workplace presentations, special programs for jr.high & high school

American Red Cross Sacramento, AIDS Educ. for Emerg. Workers
8928 Volunteer Lane
P.O. Box 160167
Sacramento, CA 95826-3221
Telephone: (916)-368-3137 Fax: (916)-368-3224
Contact: Rebecca Livingston
AIDS Education and Prevention Projects for Emergency Workers, guide book

American Red Cross, AIDS Prevention Education
Greater Long Beach Chapt.
3150 E. 29th Street
Long Beach, CA 90804
Telephone: (310)-595-6341 Fax: (310)-424-2821
Contact: Stan Schwartz
Prevention Education, Videos, Information, and Referral services

American Red Cross, Antelope Valley
42335 N. 50th Street
#201
Lancaster, CA 93534-3227
Telephone: (805)-948-4729
Contact: Fran Stewart - Executive Director
AIDS/HIV education & awareness program, classes on AIDS prevention;training for business

American Red Cross, Arcadia Chapter
376 W. Huntington Drive
P.O. Box 660
Arcadia, CA 91066
Telephone: (818)-447-2193 Fax: (818)-445-4147
Educational services

American Red Cross, Burbank Chapter
1001 W. Magnolia Blvd.
Burbank, CA 91506
Telephone: (818)-842-5295 Fax: (818)-845-6270
Contact: Gay Weston
AID information classes

American Red Cross, Inland Empire Chapter
202 West Rialto Avenue
San Bernardino, CA 92408
Telephone: (909)-888-1481 Fax: (909)-888-1485
Contact: Christopher A. Smith
Peer education program, outreach, literature, referrals

American Red Cross, Napa Chapt, Napa Assoc for Prev. of AIDS
575 Jefferson Street
Napa, CA 94559-3299
Telephone: (707)-257-2900 Fax: (707)-257-2902
Contact: Jane Hilsbeck
AIDS Education and Prevention Projects, Support Activities, Training

American Red Cross, Pomona Valley Chapter
675 N. Park Avenue
P.O. Box 559
Pomona, CA 91768-0599
Telephone: (909)-622-1348 Fax: (909)-629-4176
Contact: Jeanette Bollock - Director
AIDS education programs; speakers

American Red Cross, Rio Hondo Chapter
6707 S. Friends Avenue
Whittier, CA 90608-0683
Telephone: (310)-945-3944
Contact: Samantha Ridout
Referrals, education

American Red Cross, Santa Clara Valley Chapter
2731 North 1st Street
San Jose, CA 95134
Telephone: (408)-292-6242 Fax: (408)-297-3519
Contact: Dr. Lawrence Naiman
Counseling, referrals, AIDS education videos

American Red Cross, Santa Monica Chapter
1450 11th Street
P.O. Box 1008
Santa Monica, CA 90406-2902
Telephone: (310)-394-3773 Fax: (310)-451-3226
Contact: Arthur Rojas - Health Educator
Prevention education

American Red Cross, Silverado Chapter
473 Main Street
St. Helena, CA 94574
Telephone: (707)-963-2717 Fax: (707)-963-2353
Contact: Nancy Jocobo
AIDS education classes

American Red Cross, Valley Chapter, West San Gabriel, Valley Services
17 S. First Street
Alhambra, CA 91801
Telephone: (818)-289-4414 Fax: (818)-458-1456
Contact: Ray Hughes
Literature, referral

Asian AIDS Project
300 4th Street, Rm 401
San Francisco, CA 94107-1239
Telephone: (415)-227-0946 Fax: (415)-227-0945
Contact: Mr. Vince Sales
Education and prevention programs for the Asian community.

Asian Pacific AIDS Coalition
Dept. 513, P.O.Box 597004
San Francisco, CA 94159
Telephone: (415)-243-8909 Fax: (415)-243-8628
Contact: Public Policy Coordinator
Information, Education, Referrals

Association of Asian/Pacific Community Health Organizations (Aapcho)
1212 Broadway Suite 730
Oakland, CA 94612
Telephone: (510)-272-9536 Fax: (510)-272-0817
Contact: Judith Rogers
Adminstration Services, Education, Information Dissemination, Database

Bay View Hunter's Point Foundation/MAPA
5815 Third Street
San Francisco, CA 94124
Telephone: (415)-822-7500 Fax: (415)-822-7093
AIDS workshops designed specifically for ethnic communities.

Berry Creek Health Center
P.O. Box 40
10 Townhill Way
Berry Creek, CA 95916
Telephone: (916)-589-2285 Fax: (916)-589-2287
Contact: Alma Thorton - Manager
Counseling, referrals, education, literature

Beverly Foundation
70 South Lake # 750
Pasadena, CA 91101-2601
Telephone: (818)-792-2292 Fax: (818)-792-6117
Contact: Dr. Carroll Wendlands - President; ; - 1
Provide education, & materials for nursing facilities on long term care

California AIDS Clearinghouse
4 Carbonero Way
Los Angeles, CA 90028
Telephone: (213)-993-7415 Fax: (213)-993-7419
Contact: Roberta Wilson - Assistant Coordinator
Databases (electronic media for public use), educational materials, literature

California Associaton of AIDS Agencies
926 J. Street # 803
Sacramento, CA 95814
Telephone: (916)-447-7199 Fax: (916)-447-5302
AIDS information and resources

California Medical Association, AIDS Task Force
P.O. Box 7690
San Francisco, CA 94120-7690
Telephone: (415)-882-5186 Fax: (415)-882-3390
Contact: Staff Coordinator
Information, Education, Referrals

California Nurses Association, AIDS Education and Training
Train the Trainer Program
1855 Folsom St., Ste. 670
San Francisco, CA 94103
Telephone: (415)-864-4141 Fax: (415)-431-1011
Contact: Project Director - Allen Harris, RN, C; Board Director -
AIDS Education and Prevention Projects for Trainers of Health Care Providers

California Partner's Study (Male/Female)
San Francisco Hospital OBGYN
Ward 6D
San Francisco, CA 94110
Telephone: (415)-550-6896 Fax: (415)-206-5322
Contact: Sarah Glass - Field Director
Research Projects, Support Groups, Referrals, Support for Partners

California Rural Indian Health Board, Inc.
650 Howe Ave
Suite 200
Sacramento, CA 95825-3223
Telephone: (916)-929-9761 Fax: (916)-929-7246
Toll-Free: (800)-274-4288
Contact: Larry Murillo
AIDS Education for Health Services Workers Dealing with Native Americans

Cara a Cara, El Centro del Pueblo
1157 Lehoyne
Los Angeles, CA 90026
Telephone: (213)-483-6335 Fax: (213)-483-5523
Contact: Robert Aguayo
AIDS education, counseling, outreach

Center for Health Training
2229 Lombard Street
San Francisco, CA 94123-2703
Telephone: (415)-929-9100 Fax: (415)-929-9464
AIDS Education for Professionals, Education for Migrant Populations

Community Health Centers of Kern County, Kerns AIDS Project
601 California Avenue
Bakersfield, CA 93304
Telephone: (805)-324-9808 Fax: (805)-324-6301
Contact: Fenton Karnes
AIDS Education and Prevention Projects

Comprehensive AIDS Resource, Education Program
411 E. 10th St, #202
Long Beach, CA 90813
Telephone: (310)-491-9905
Contact: Ralph Brooks
Nurse case management, Education, Buddy Programs

CORE Program
7740 1/2 Santa Monica Blvd.
West Hollywood, CA 90046-6220
Telephone: (213)-656-8201 Fax: (213)-656-4925
Contact: Ralph Mayo
Prevention education; 213-484-9389 for Spanish speaking

Correctional Education Division Hall of Justice
211 West Temple
Room 808
Los Angeles, CA 90012
Telephone: (213)-974-5096 Fax: (213)-974-0999
Contact: Larry Agnew
AIDS education, counseling

Education Programs Associates
1 W. Campbell Avenue
Suite 40
Campbell, CA 95008
Telephone: (408)-374-3720
Contact: Susan Kaklins
Resource center for education materials; administrative office & HIVincluded

El Centro Human Services Corp., Milagros AIDS Project
972 South Goodrich Blvd.
Los Angeles, CA 90022-4187
Telephone: (213)-725-1337 Fax: (213)-728-9629
Contact: Xavier Aguilera
AIDS Education and Prevention Projects

FAME
2248 South Hobart Blvd.
Los Angeles, CA 90018-2143
Telephone: (213)-737-0897
Contact: Peggy Hill - AIDS Project Director

Families Who Care
6475 E. Pacific Coast Hwy
Suite 202
Long Beach, CA 90803-4296
Telephone: (714)-498-6366 Fax: (714)-821-5559
Support, Referral, Networking, Education, Speakers, Training, Advocacy

Family Survival Caregiver
425 Bush Street
San Francisco, CA 94108-3708
Telephone: (415)-434-3388 Fax: (415)-434-3508
Contact: Kathleen Kelley
Education for Caregivers, Legal Referrals, Information, Counseling, Respite

Girls and Boys Club
2740 Mountain View Road
P.O. Box 4703
El Monte, CA 91732
Telephone: (818)-442-5470
Contact: Jack Gutowski
HIV education

Greater Los Angeles Council on Deafness, Inc.
AIDS Educ. for the Deaf
616 S. Westmoreland Ave.
Los Angeles, CA 90005
Telephone: (213)-383-2220 Fax: (213)-383-3808
Contact: Mary M Meyer - Agency Director
AIDS Education and Prevention Projects for the Deaf/Hard-of-Hearing, Videotapes

Health ETC - Health Education and Training Center
Project TECLA
675 E. Santa Clara Street
San Jose, CA 95112
Telephone: (408)-977-4562
AIDS Education and Prevention Projects for Latinos

Hemophilia Council of California
7700 Edgewater Drive
Suite 710
Oakland, CA 94621
Telephone: (415)-568-7074 Fax: (510)-568-2048
Contact: Jackie Eweberg - Health Manager
Health education, information and referral for the Hemophiliac community.Information on Blood transfusions, HIV, education

Institute of Advanced Study of Human Sexuality
1523 Franklin Street
San Francisco, CA 94109-2918
Telephone: (415)-928-1133
Contact: Ted McIlvenna
Certificate Programs in AIDS Education

Kairos Support For Care Givers
114 Douglas Street
San Francisco, CA 94114-1920
Telephone: (415)-861-0877
Support Groups for Caregivers, Resource Library, Workshops

Kaiser Permanente
4647 Zion Ave
San Diego, CA 92120
Telephone: (619)-528-3028 Fax: (619)-528-7632
Contact: Patrick Graham - Health Ed. Specialist
HIV prevention education

Korean Health Education, Information & Referral Center
981 S. Western Ave. #404
Los Angeles, CA 90006-1005
Telephone: (213)-732-5648 Fax: (213)-732-3857
Contact: Laura Jeon
Education, seminars, presentations, referral services, research

KPOO Radio
P.O. Box 425000
San Francisco, CA 94142
Telephone: (415)-346-5373
Special broadcast - public service announcements

Krames Communications Department, AIDS/BUS
1100 Grundy Lane
San Bruno, CA 94066
Telephone: (415)-742-0400 Fax: (415)-742-9265
Publications on AIDS in the Workplace

Labor Occupational Health Program, Univ. of Calif., Berkeley
AIDS Labor Educ. Project
2515 Channing Way

Berkeley, CA 94720
Telephone: (510)-642-5507 Fax: (510)-643-5698
Contact: Robin Bakerector
AIDS Education and Prevention Projects for Health Care Workers and Employees

Last Gasp
2180 Bryant Street
San Francisco, CA 94110-2128
Telephone: (415)-824-6636 Fax: (415)-824-1836
Contact: Ron Tucker
Producer of Comic Book: Strip AIDS USA

Long Beach AIDS Network, Inc.
600 Cedar Avenue
Long Beach, CA 90802
Telephone: (310)-495-2330 Fax: (310)-983-1421
Contact: Nan Corby - Executive Director
Education and Organization Coordination, Resource Identification, Speakers

Long Beach-Harbor-Southeast Unit
936 Pine Avenue
Long Beach, CA 90813
Telephone: (310)-437-0791 Fax: (310)-495-1782
Contact: Carol Chesser - Director
Education, fund raising

Maternity Center Valley Presbyterian Hospital
15225 Vanowen Street
Suite 205
Van Nuys, CA 91405
Telephone: (818)-902-5794
Contact: Mary Esther
On-Site Education and Training Programs, Seminars

Mobilization Against AIDS (MAA)
584-B Castro
San Francisco, CA 94114
Telephone: (415)-863-4670 Fax: (415)-863-4740
Picketing, petitioning, pressuring governmental departments to fight AIDS.

Nechama: A Jewish Response to AIDS
6505 Wilshire Boulevard
Suite 608
Los Angeles, CA 90048
Telephone: (213)-653-8313
Education, Advocacy, Information, Referrals, Training Program

Nipomo Community Medical Center, AIDS Education & Information Project
P.O. Box 430
150 Tejas Place
Nipomo, CA 93444
Telephone: (805)-929-3211 Fax: (805)-929-6440
Contact: Isabel Ruiz - Director
AIDS Education and Prevention Projects for Hispanic Farm Workers and Teenagers

North San Joaquin Valley Health Development Council
1101 Standiford Avenue
Suite B-4
Modesto, CA 95350
Telephone: (209)-577-3103
Contact: Executive Director
AIDS education

Northeast Los Angeles County Unit
50 North Hill Avenue
Pasadena, CA 91106
Telephone: (213)-681-4507 Fax: (818)-568-2888
Educational services

Orange County AIDS Outreach
1725 West 17th Street
Santa Ana, CA 92706
Telephone: (714)-834-7926 Fax: (714)-834-8741
HIV/AIDS education, prevention and outreach, TB testing

Orange County Health Care, AIDS Community Education Project
1725 W. 17th Street
Santa Ana, CA 92706-2316
Telephone: (714)-834-8733 Fax: (714)-834-8741
Contact: Andrea Hollatz-Brown
Education and prevention projects for Hispanic/Latino community; generalpopulation, HIV testing (834-8787), early intervention program (834-2095)

People with AIDS Speakers Bureau
126 East Haley A17
Santa Barbara, CA 93101
Telephone: (805)-963-3636 Fax: (805)-963-9086
Contact: Derek Gordon
AIDS counseling & assistance, speakers for public presentations for groups,schools/No fee

Perinatal HIV Reduction and Education Demonstration Project
University of California
3130 20th St., Room 352
San Francisco, CA 94143-0001
Telephone: (415)-476-6117 Fax: (415)-647-7611
Contact: Project Coordinator
Risk prevention education and demonstration activity

Pilipino AIDS Education Project
965 Mission Street
Suite #500
San Francisco, CA 94103-2912
Telephone: (415)-882-9291
Contact: Edward Ysmeal
English/Tagalog Prevention and Education, Counseling Referrals

Planned Parenthood of Shasta-Diablo, AIDS Educ & Prev. Proj.
2185 Pachelo Street
Concord, CA 94520
Telephone: (510)-676-0505 Fax: (510)-676-2184
Contact: Heather Saunders Estes - Agency Director
AIDS Education and Prevention Projects, Training

Polaris Research and Development
185 Berry Street
#6400
San Francisco, CA 94107-1729
Telephone: (415)-777-3229 Fax: (415)-512-9625
Contact: Noel Day
Develops AIDS Training, Education, and Prevention Materials

Rand E. Publishing
P.O. Box 2008
Saratoga, CA 95070-2008
Telephone: (408)-866-6303 Fax: (408)-954-0767
Contact: Robert Reed
Publisher of: The AIDS Catalog, Complete AIDS Resources

Sacramento AIDS Foundation
920 20th Street
Sacramento, CA 95814-4119
Telephone: (916)-448-2437 Fax: (916)-448-3568
Contact: Beth Colmanor - Communication Director
AIDS education and prevention projects, regional presentations, homehealth; outreach

Sacramento County AIDS Educ. Task Force & Prevention Unit
3701 Branch Center Road
Sacramento, CA 95827-3822
Telephone: (916)-366-2922 Fax: (916)-366-2388
Group support, community outreach, education

San Bernardino County Public Health Department
Community AIDS Educ. Proj
799 East Rialto Avenue
San Bernardino, CA 92415-0010
Telephone: (909)-386-8157 Fax: (909)-383-3212
Contact: Ms. Beverly Durden
AIDS Education and Prevention Projects, Training, Information, Referrals

San Francisco AIDS Foundation, Deaf Services, TDD Phone
25 Van Ness Avenue, Suite 660
San Francisco, CA 94142-6182
Telephone: (415)-864-6606 Fax: (415)-552-1583
Education, Resources, Referrals

San Francisco AIDS Foundation, Northern California Services
P.O. Box 426182
San Francisco, CA 94142-6182
Telephone: (415)-864-4376 Fax: (415)-487-3098
Toll-Free: (800)-367-2437
Contact: Lyn Paleo - Executive Director
AIDS Education and Prevention Projects for Northern California, Hotline

San Luis Obispo County AIDS Task Force
P.O. Box 1489
San Luis Obispo, CA 93406
Telephone: (805)-781-5540 Fax: (805)-781-1235
Contact: Marsha Bollinger
Information forum, education

Santa Barbara County Health Care Services, AIDS Services
Tri-Counties AIDS Project
300 San Antonio Road
Santa Barbara, CA 93110
Telephone: (805)-681-5365 Fax: (805)-681-5424
Contact: Valwyn Hooper - Agency Director
AIDS Education and Prevention Projects, Training, Workshops, Seminars, Speakers

Santa Cruz AIDS Project
911 Center Street, #A
Santa Cruz, CA 95060-3807
Telephone: (408)-427-3900 Fax: (408)-427-0398
Contact: John Leopold - Executive Director
AIDS education for general community and the Latino community.

South Bay Free Clinic, Mental Health Center
710 Pier Avenue
Hermosa Beach, CA 90254
Telephone: (310)-379-1940 Fax: (310)-379-0450
Contact: Stewart Sokol
Education, prevention, speakers

Stiggall and Associates
21450 Bear Creek Road
Los Gatos, CA 95030
Telephone: (408)-354-0821
Contact: Lynne Muccigrosso
Program development, sexuality education/AIDS, resource materials.

STOP AIDS Project, Inc.
201 Sanchez Street
San Francisco, CA 94114
Telephone: (415)-621-7177
National Resource Center supporting peer-led interactive Stop-AIDS discussions.

Tarzana Treatment Center (Free Men, Inc.)
AIDS Educ. and Prev. Proj
18646 Oxnard Street
Tarzana, CA 91356
Telephone: (818)-996-1051 Fax: (818)-345-3778
HIV/AIDS prevention education

The Urban League of San Diego
4261 Market Street
San Diego, CA 92102-4651
Telephone: (619)-266-6166 Fax: (619)-263-3660
Contact: AIDS Educator
AIDS Awareness Project

The Women's AIDS Project
8240 Santa Monica Blvd.
West Hollywood, CA 90046-5914
Telephone: (213)-650-1508
Contact: Executive Director
AIDS Education and Prevention Projects

Tri City Community Health
161 Thunder Drive
Suite 212
Vista, CA 92083-5297
Telephone: (619)-631-5030 Fax: (619)-724-9596
Contact: Kelly McCleary
HIV/AIDS education and prevention programs.

UCLA Family Planning Clinic, AIDS Education and Prevention Project
1010 Veteran Avenue
Los Angeles, CA 90024-1683
Telephone: (310)-825-2753 Fax: (310)-825-0288
Contact: Lupe Samaniego - Director
HIV testing, AIDS education, outreach

United Cerebral Palsy Association
100 View Street
Suite 102
Mountain View, CA 94041-1342
Telephone: (415)-969-4711
Contact: Jane Lefferdink - Executive Director
Education & presentations, AIDS library

Valley Comm Hlth Cen, Livermore/Amador Valley AIDS Educ Prog
4361 Railroad Avenue
Pleasanton, CA 94566
Telephone: (510)-462-1755 Fax: (510)-462-1650
Contact: Amy Sims Candido - Executive Director
AIDS education and prevention projects, HIV testing

Valley Community Clinic
5648 Vineland Avenue
North Hollywood, CA 91601-2028
Telephone: (818)-763-8836 Fax: (818)-763-7231
Contact: Marsha Marcoe
AIDS education & prevention projects; medical services

West Oakland Health Center, AIDS Community Education Project
700 Adeline Street
Oakland, CA 94607
Telephone: (510)-835-9610
Contact: Dwayne Fisher
AIDS Education and Prevention Projects

Western AIDS Education and Training Center
Univ of CA-San Francisco
5110 E. Clinton Wy, S 115
Fresno, CA 93727-2098
Telephone: (209)-252-2851 Fax: (209)-454-8012
Contact: E. Michael Reyes, M.D. Fax:209-454-8012

Western AIDS Etc.
5110 East Clinton Way
Suite 115
Fresno, CA 93727-2098
Telephone: (209)-252-2851 Fax: (209)-454-8012
Contact: E. Michael Reyes, M.D.
Resource center; materials for AIDS educators

Hotlines

Community Helpline
P.O. Box 2503
Palos Verdes, CA 90274-2503
Telephone: (310)-541-2525 Fax: (310)-544-2730
Contact: Marlys Kinnel

State Health Departments

California Department of Health Services AIDS Activities
714/744 P Street
Sacramento, CA 94234-7320
Telephone: (916)-445-0553 Fax: (916)-323-4642
Contact: Vanessa Baird - AIDS Care Unit

Statewide Services

California Association of AIDS Agencies
926 J. Street
Suite 803
Sacramento, CA 95814-4108
Telephone: (916)-447-7199 Fax: (916)-447-5302
Contact: Geni Cowan
Organizational development, technical assistance, membership services &newsletters

California Dept. of Health Services, Office of AIDS
830 S Street
Sacramento, CA 95814
Telephone: (916)-323-7415
Contact: Wayne Sauseda
HIV testing and counseling

Multicultural Liaison Board, California AIDS Intervention Training Ctr
507 Divisadero
Suite B
San Francisco, CA 94117
Telephone: (415)-922-6135 Fax: (415)-922-3932
Contact: Pat Norman
Collaboration with communities of color and inpartnership with State Officeof AIDS; develops recommendations and policies for providing education andprevention services for people of color

Multicultural Liaison Board, Special Services for Groups
1313 W. 8th Street
Suite 201
Los Angeles, CA 90017
Telephone: (213)-353-6039 Fax: (213)-413-1539
Contact: Dean Goishi - API Intervention Team
Collaboration with communities of color and in partnership with StateOffice of AIDS; develops recommendations and policies forproviding education and preventionservices for people of color

Social Service Agency
1725 Technology Drive
San Jose, CA 95110-1305
Telephone: (408)-441-5460 Fax: (408)-441-7913
Contact: Ken Borelli - Chairman
Public Assistance, Medi-Cal, GA, SSI Advocacy, In Home Support Services

Alameda County

Community Services

AIDS Project of the East Bay (Pacific Center)
565 16th Street
Oakland, CA 94612
Telephone: (510)-834-8181 Fax: (510)-834-0442
Contact: Valerer Papayaman
AIDS education services, support groups, workshops, food bank.

The Center for AIDS Services
5720 Shattuck Avenueay
Oakland, CA 94609
Telephone: (510)-655-3435 Fax: (510)-655-2543
Contact: Jerry Dednung
Emotional support, massages, food bank

Center for Independent Living
2539 Telegraph Avenue
Berkeley, CA 94704
Telephone: (510)-841-4776 Fax: (510)-841-6168
Contact: Michael Winter
Support services, benefits, counseling, employment

Children's Quilt Project
PO Box 11343
Suite 186
Berkeley, CA 94701-7343
Telephone: (415)-548-3843 Fax: (510)-548-3843
Contact: Diane Dehler - Executive Director
Homeless & children with AIDS

Disability Rights Education and Legal Defense Fund
2212 6th Street
Berkeley, CA 94710
Telephone: (510)-644-2629 Fax: (510)-841-8645
Legal Assistance and Litigation Support Services, Education

East Oakland Recovery Center
9702 East 14th Street
Oakland, CA 94621
Telephone: (415)-568-2432 Fax: (510)-568-2432
Contact: Willy Porter
Substance abuse, AIDS education

Horizon Services
1403 164th Avenue
San Leandro, CA 94578
Telephone: (510)-278-8654 Fax: (510)-278-5321
Contact: Lee Gibbs
Substance abuse program, HIV testing, education

Kapuna West Inner City Child Family AIDS Network
3220 Sacramento Street
Berkeley, CA 94702
Telephone: (415)-843-5577 Fax: (510)-843-5477
Contact: John Bilroskey
Support services, counseling, education, prevention services, outreach

Oakland Community Counseling
2647 East 14th Street
Suite 420
Oakland, CA 94619
Telephone: (510)-261-9595 Fax: (510)-261-1794
Contact: James Small
Support Services, Counseling

Pacific Center
2712 Telegraph Avenue
Berkeley, CA 94705
Telephone: (415)-548-8283 Fax: (510)-548-2938
Contact: Akya Windwood
Support Services, Counseling

Southern Alameda County AIDS Services
Tri-City Health Center
38355 Logan Drive
Fremont, CA 94536
Telephone: (510)-794-8848 Fax: (510)-794-9921
Contact: Andy Rose
HIV speakers bureau, case management, support groups, benefits

County Health Depts

Alameda County Health Dept., HIV/AIDS Services Division
499 5th Street, 1st Floor
Oakland, CA 94607
Telephone: (510)-268-2639 Fax: (510)-268-4205
Contact: Gene Richards
HIV testing & counseling

Home Health Care

Caremark
21353 Cabot Blvd.
Hayward, CA 94545
Telephone: (510)-732-8800 Fax: (510)-832-8801
Contact: Dan Starnes
Clinical support & infusion therapies: 33Nutrition, anticromatics, chemo

Critical Care America
1105 Atlantic Ave, #101
Alameda, CA 94501
Telephone: (510)-522-1492
Coordinate & integrate all clinical, psychosocial services for HIV+

Critical Care America
1105 Atlantic Avenue
Suite 101
Alameda, CA 94501
Telephone: (510)-748-5460 Fax: (510)-748-5468
Contact: Charlton Blackbuene
Coordinate & integrate all clinical & psychosocial services for HIV+

Curaflex Infusion Services
3506 Breakwater Court
Hayward, CA 94545
Telephone: (800)-444-1338 Fax: (510)-782-9589
Contact: Armel Crocker
Home IV therapy: TPN, Enteral, IV Antibiotics, Aerosolized/IV Pentamidine

Homedco Infusion
2547 Barrington Court
Hayward, CA 94545
Telephone: (510)-786-1860 Fax: (510)-786-2184
Toll-Free: (800)-824-8400
Contact: Jim Anderson
Home infusion therapy for HIV/AIDS patients

Hope Hospice
6500 Dublin Blvd
Suite 100
Dublin, CA 94568
Telephone: (510)-829-8770 Fax: (510)-829-0868
Contact: Joanne Howard
Support & counseling, home care, bereavment counseling

Mount Diablo Home Health Care
477 Devlin Road
Napa, CA 94588
Telephone: (707)-252-2078
Contact: Joyce Gammon
Home Health Care

nmc HOMECARE
3521 Investment Blvd,
Bldg G Suite 2
Hayward, CA 94545
Telephone: (510)-732-5488
Fax: (510)-732-5823
Contact: Pam Pressel
National JCAHO-Accredited company providing a full range of Infusion and Respiratory therapies and specializing in the care of HIV/AIDS patients. National Case Manager is also available at 800-445-1188

Northern California Visiting Nurse Association, Inc.
1900 Powell Street
3rd Floor
Emeryville, CA 94608
Telephone: (510)-596-4800 Fax: (510)-653-2226
Contact: Keith Kertland
Home Health Care

Vesper Hospice and Home Care
311 MacArthur
San Leandro, CA 94577
Telephone: (510)-632-4390 Fax: (510)-632-3334
Contact: Susan Graham
Health Care, Medical Referrals, Home Health Care, Hospice

Medical Services

14th Street Clinic
1124 East 14th Street
Oakland, CA 94606
Telephone: (510)-533-0800 Fax: (510)-533-0300
Contact: Susan Sky
Substance Abuse Intervention, Education, Prevention Services

AIDS Minority Health Initiative
1440 Broadway, Suite 403
Oakland, CA 94612
Telephone: (510)-763-1872 Fax: (510)-763-3132
Contact: Adelbert Campbell
Health Care, Medical Referrals, Case Mgt

Alta Bates-Herrick Medical Center
Adult Hemophilia Program
3031 Telegraph Avenue, Suite 101
Berkeley, CA 94705
Telephone: (510)-204-1522 Fax: (510)-843-0802
Contact: Brad Lewis, MD
Treatment for individuals with coagulation disorders

Berkeley Community Health Project, Berkeley Free Clinic
2339 Durant
Berkeley, CA 94704
Telephone: (510)-548-2570 Fax: (510)-548-1730
Contact: Victor Martinez
Health Care, Medical Referrals, Education, Prevention Services

California Children Services, Alameda County
499 5th Street
Oakland, CA 94609
Telephone: (510)-268-2666 Fax: (510)-268-7939
Contact: Marge Deichman
Diagnostic Testing, Medical Treatment, Medical Support Services, Counseling

California Children Services, HIV Children Program
Sonoma County
370 Administration Drive
Santa Rosa, CA 94501
Telephone: (707)-524-7330 Fax: (707)-524-7345
Contact: Program Coordinator
Diagnostic Testing, Medical Treatment/Support Services, Financial Assistance

East Bay AIDS Center, University of California
Student Health Service
3031 Telegraph Ste 325
Berkeley, CA 94705
Telephone: (415)-540-1870 Fax: (510)-848-9764
Contact: Carol Brosgart
Medical care HIV patients

HAART
15400 Foothill Boulevard
San Leandro, CA 94578
Telephone: (510)-357-4202 Fax: (510)-357-4070
Contact: Anne Bolla
Methadone maintenance and detox

Maxim Health Care
1970 Bradway, Ste 310
Oakland, CA 94612
Telephone: (415)-921-8360
Toll-Free: (800)-959-3747
Contact: Scott Rausch
Medical services, nursing, home care

Over 60 Health Clinic
1860 Alcatraz
Berkeley, CA 94703
Telephone: (415)-644-6060 Fax: (510)-644-6177
Contact: Marty Lynch
Health Care, Medical Referrals

Summit Medical Center
Immunology Clinic
350 Hawthorne Avenue
Oakland, CA 94609
Telephone: (510)-655-4000 Fax: (510)-420-6760
Contact: Irwin Hansen
Health Care, Medical Referrals

West Berkeley Health Center
2031 6th Street
Berkeley, CA 94710
Telephone: (510)-644-6939 Fax: (510)-841-6897
Contact: Jenny Rucklehaus
Education, Prevention, Referrals, Health Care, Substance Abuse Intervention

Testing Sites

Alameda County CD Bureau
499 5th Street
Room 304
Oakland, CA 94607
Telephone: (510)-268-2727
Contact: Tim Livermore, MD
HIV testing

Berkeley Health & Human Services
2180 Milvia St, 3rd FL
Berkeley, CA 94704
Telephone: (510)-644-6500 Fax: (510)-644-6494
Contact: Laura Anderson - Mgr. of Health Promotion
Anonymous HIV Testing

California Partners Study
140 Warren Hall
University of California
Berkeley, CA 94720
Telephone: (415)-476-5325
Contact: Nancy Padian
AIDS transmission research, confidential testing, education.

Central Health Center
470 27th Street
Oakland, CA 94612
Telephone: (510)-271-4263 Fax: (510)-271-4205
Contact: Regina Stewart-Budd
Anonymous HIV Testing

Eastern Alameda Health Center
2449 88th Avenue
Oakland, CA 94605
Telephone: (510)-577-5666 Fax: (510)-635-3582
Contact: Frankie Lee
Anonymous HIV testing, family planning, health clinic, immunizations

Newark Health Center
6066 Civic Terrace Avenue
Newark, CA 94560
Telephone: (415)-795-2414 Fax: (510)-795-2414
Contact: Frances Way, RN
Anonymous HIV testing, counseling, referrals

Planned Parenthood Alameda/San Francisco, Hayward Center
1866 B Street
Hayward, CA 94541
Telephone: (510)-733-1814 Fax: (510)-537-6024
Contact: Pat Hughes
HIV/STD testing

Planned Parenthood Alameda/San Francisco, MacArthur Center
482 W. MacArthur
Oakland, CA 94609
Telephone: (510)-601-4700 Fax: (510)-547-7446
Contact: Margie White
Anonymous HIV Testing

Tiburcio Vasquez Health Center
33255 9th Street
Union City, CA 94587
Telephone: (510)-471-5907 Fax: (510)-471-9051
Contact: Joel Garcia
HIV testing, counseling, referrals

Alpine County

County Health Depts

Alpine County Health Department
260 Montgomery Street
P.O. Box 545
Markleeville, CA 96120
Telephone: (916)-694-2146 Fax: (916)-694-2770
Contact: Diane Lattanzio, RN, PhN - Health Director
AIDS testing, task force, education, counseling

Amador County

County Health Depts

Amador County Health Department
1001 Broadway
Suite 206
Jackson, CA 95642
Telephone: (209)-223-6407 Fax: (209)-223-1562
Contact: James B. McClenahan
HIV testing, case management

Home Health Care

Amador Home Health Agency
635 Caourt Street
Jackson, CA 95642
Telephone: (209)-223-3866 Fax: (209)-223-3882
Contact: Eileen Sweet - Director, RN
Home Health Care

Medical Services

Amador County Alcohol/Drug Services
1001 Broadway, Suite 103
Jackson, CA 95642
Telephone: (209)-223-6556
Contact: Sheila Zeszotek
Drug treatment, AIDS education program

Sutter Amador Hospital
810 Court Street
Jackson, CA 95642
Telephone: (209)-223-6600 Fax: (209)-223-6652
Contact: Mike Kilpatrick - Human Resource Director
Medical Services

Butte County

County Health Depts

Butte County Health Department
18 County Center Drive
Suite B
Oroville, CA 95965
Telephone: (916)-538-7581
Contact: Mayama Morehart, MD - AIDS Coord.; Chester L. Ward, MD - AIDS Task Force
Education, AZT Drug Program, AIDS Task Force, Community Services

Butte County Public Health Department
695 Oleander Avenue
Chico, CA 95926
Telephone: (916)-891-2865 Fax: (916)-891-8743
Contact: Lonna Bartlett - AIDS Education Project Coord.
AIDS Education and Prevention Projects

Home Health Care

California Health Professionals, Inc.
2060 3rd Street
Suite B
Oroville, CA 95965-3416
Telephone: (916)-533-9500 Fax: (916)-533-0679
Home Health Care

California Health Professionals, Inc.
1390 Ridewood Drive
Chico, CA 95926
Telephone: (916)-895-3003 Fax: (916)-895-1703
Contact: Barbra Hanna
Home health nursing

Enloe Hospital Home Health Agency
5th and Esplanade
Chico, CA 95926
Telephone: (916)-891-7395 Fax: (916)-899-2008
Contact: Christain Lundbert
Home care

Enloe Hospital Hospice
5th and Esplanade
Chico, CA 95926
Telephone: (916)-891-7420 Fax: (916)-899-2021
Hospice

Feather River Home Health Agency
P.O. Box 1990
6283 Clark Road
Paradise, CA 95969
Telephone: (916)-872-3378 Fax: (916)-877-8448
Home Health Care

Paradise Hospice and Homecare
P.O. Box 2287
1295 Billie Road
Paradise, CA 95969
Telephone: (916)-877-8755 Fax: (916)-877-4801
Hospice, home care

Calaveras County

County Health Depts

Calaveras County Health Department
Government Center
San Andreas, CA 95249
Telephone: (209)-754-6460 Fax: (209)-754-6459
Contact: AIDS Coordinator
Anonymous AIDS/HIV testing

Home Health Care

ABC Home Health
134 E St. Charles
P.O. Box 519
San Andreas, CA 95249
Telephone: (209)-754-5107 Fax: (209)-754-1000
Toll-Free: (800)-542-4299
Contact: Linda Perry
Home Health Care

Colusa County

County Health Depts

Colusa County Health Department
P.O. Box 610
Colusa, CA 95932
Telephone: (916)-458-5177 Fax: (916)-458-4136
Contact: Martha Dragoo - AIDS Coordinator
HIV testing, counseling, education

Home Health Care

Colusa Community Hospital Home Health Agency
P.O. Box 331
199 East Webster Street
Colusa, CA 95932
Telephone: (916)-458-2075 Fax: (916)-458-2847
Contact: Georgeanne Hulbert
Home Health Care

Contra Costa County

Community Services

Alcoholics Anonymous
PO Box 416
Concord, CA 94520-0416
Telephone: (415)-932-6770 Fax: (510)-932-6770
Serves district 14

Compassionate Friends
2343 Mallard Drive
Walnut Creek, CA 94596
Telephone: (510)-284-2273
Contact: Anne Piper
Nationwide Network of Parents Who Have Lost a Child, Support Group, Information

Contra Costa County AIDS Project
2280 Diamond Blvd.
Suite 350
Concord, CA 94520
Telephone: (510)-356-2437 Fax: (510)-356-8805
Contact: Bob Rybicki
Counseling, referrals, legal referrals, fund raisers

Resource Opportunities, Inc.
1600 Riviera Avenue
Suite 320
Walnut Creek, CA 94596
Telephone: (510)-934-7373
Contact: Ione Harris
Medical Case Management, Vocational Rehab., Life Care Plans, Expert Testimony

Home Health Care

John Muir Medical Center Home Care Services
1399 Ygnacio Valley Road
Suite 14
Walnut Creek, CA 94598
Telephone: (510)-939-4220 Fax: (510)-937-3706
Contact: Sandra Baughn
Home health care

Premier
1390 S. Main Street
Suite 300
Walnut Creek, CA 94596
Telephone: (510)-932-2500 Fax: (510)-943-6938
Toll-Free: (800)-678-6703
Contact: Edi Klecker, RN - Vice President
Infusion therapy, wound care, pediatric, maternal, newborn; casemanagement, ventilator care, psychiatric nursing, rehab, live-in, homemaker

Medical Services

California Children Services, HIV Children Program
Contra Costa County
595 Center Ave, Suite 110
Martinez, CA 94553
Telephone: (510)-313-6100 Fax: (510)-313-6115
Contact: Robin Thomas - Program Coordinator
Rehabilitationfor physcially handicapped, treatmentfor children withcatastrophic conditions

Testing Sites

Planned Parenthood Alameda/Shastal Diablo
101 Broadway
Richmond, CA 94804
Telephone: (510)-232-1250 Fax: (510)-232-6837
Contact: Erin Harr Yee
Anonymous HIV Testing

El Dorado County

County Health Depts

El Dorado County Health Department
931 Spring Street
Placerville, CA 95667
Telephone: (916)-621-6100 Fax: (916)-626-4713
Contact: Michael Ungeheuer, RN - AIDS Coordinator
AIDS Services, AZT Drug Program

El Dorado County Health Department (Branch Office)
1360 Johnson Blvd.
Suite 107
S. Lake Tahoe, CA 96150
Telephone: (916)-573-3155
Toll-Free: (800)-573-3333
Contact: Chuck Newport - AIDS Coordinator
AIDS Education and Prevention Projects

Home Health Care

Barton Memorial Hospital
2450-2489 Lake Tahoe Blvd.
S. Lake Tahoe, CA 96150
Telephone: (916)-541-3420 Fax: (916)-541-2653
Contact: Terry Kirschenheider
Home care for HIV patients

Visiting Nurse Association
670 Placerville Drive
#3-C
Placerville, CA 95667-4200
Telephone: (916)-626-4960
Home Health Care

Fresno County

Community Services

Central Valley AIDS Team
625 North Palm
Fresno, CA 93728
Telephone: (209)-264-2436 Fax: (209)-265-4716
Contact: Tim Reese - Director
AIDS education and prevention projects, workshops, training, speakersbureau, client services & presidental aid

Resource Opportunities, Inc.
1713 Tulare Street
Suite 102
Fresno, CA 93721
Telephone: (209)-266-4444 Fax: (209)-266-4464
Contact: District Manager
Medical Case Management, Vocational Rehab., Life Care Plans, Expert Testimony

County Health Depts

Fresno County Health Department
PO Box 11867
1221 Fulton Mall
Fresno, CA 93775
Telephone: (209)-445-3434 Fax: (209)-445-3170
Contact: Betty Carmona RN - AIDS Project Director
Anonymous and confidential HIV testing, counseling, risk assesment, pre andpost test counseling, consultations for employers on policies

Home Health Care

nmc HOMECARE
4180 W. Alamos
Fresno, CA 93722
Telephone: (209)-276-8600
Fax: (209)-276-8645
Contact: Jan Coon
National JCAHO-Accredited company providing a full range of Infusion and Respiratory therapies and specializing in the care of HIV/AIDS patients. National Case Manager is also available at 800-445-1188

Medical Services

BAART
2851 South Orange
Fresno, CA 93725
Telephone: (209)-268-6261 Fax: (209)-268-7518
Contact: Sue Ewart
Walk-in clinic for health care & educational services

Central Valley Indian Health, Inc.
20 North De Witt
Suite 10
Clovis, CA 93612
Telephone: (209)-299-2578 Fax: (209)-299-0245
Contact: Claudine Nunezirector - AIDS Counsler
HIV testing & conseling; pre natal services; other STD's treated

Valley Medical Center
445 S. Cedar
Special Services, Dept. of Medicine
Fresno, CA 93702
Telephone: (209)-453-4435 Fax: (209)-453-4367
Contact: Priscilla Javed - Nurse

Outpatient case management, coordinate care with other agencies

Testing Sites

California Children Services, HIV Children Program
Fresno County
1221 Fulton Mall
Fresno, CA 93721
Telephone: (209)-445-3300 Fax: (209)-445-3370
Contact: Nancy Hatcherinator
Diagnostic Testing, Medical Treatment, Medical Support Services, Counseling

Sequoia Community Health Foundation, Inc.
2790 South Elm Avenue
Fresno, CA 93706
Telephone: (209)-233-5747 Fax: (209)-485-2769
Contact: Bertha Selix - Director
HIV testing, referrals, primary & health care services

Glenn County

Testing Sites

Orland Family Health Center
1211 Cortina Drive
Orland, CA 95963
Telephone: (916)-865-5544 Fax: (916)-865-9209
Contact: ; ; - h
HIV testing and counseling

Humboldt County

Community Services

AIDS Task Force
529 I Street
Eureka, CA 95501
Telephone: (707)-445-6200 Fax: (707)-445-6097
Contact: Peggy Falk - Program Director
Education, client services, volunteers

Kings View Humboldt Alcohol and Drug Programs
720 Wood Street
Eureka, CA 95501-4482
Telephone: (707)-445-6250 Fax: (707)-445-7287
Counseling

Medical Services

California Children Services, HIV Children Program-Humboldt County
712 4th Street
Eureka, CA 95501
Telephone: (707)-445-6212 Fax: (707)-441-5686
Contact: Roberta James - Program Coordinator
Diagnostic Testing, Medical Treatment, Medical Support Services, Counseling

Eureka Mental Health Department
720 Wood Street
Eureka, CA 95501
Telephone: (707)-445-7203 Fax: (707)-445-7287
Contact: Valerie Hunter - Clinical Director
Mental health and social services; AIDS, alcohol and drug counseling

Imperial County

County Health Depts

Imperial County Department of Health Services
935 Broadway
El Centro, CA 92243
Telephone: (619)-339-4438 Fax: (619)-352-9933
Contact: Dr. Begley
HIV testing and counseling

Inyo County

Medical Services

Inyo-Mono County Medical Society
c/o Northern Inyo Hosp.
150 Pioneer Lane
Bishop, CA 93514
Telephone: (619)-873-5811 Fax: (619)-873-2868
Contact: Dr. Michael Dillon
Medical Referrals

Kern County

Community Services

American Red Cross, Kern Chapter
239 18th Street
Bakersfield, CA 93301
Telephone: (805)-324-6427 Fax: (805)-321-0744
Contact: Connie Reese
Referral service; counseling

Girl Scouts-Joshua Tree Council
1831 Brundage Lane
Bakersfield, CA 93303
Telephone: (800)-225-4475

Kern County Economic Opportunity Corp.
300 19th Street
Bakersfield, CA 93301-4502
Telephone: (805)-327-9789
Contact: Caroline Carter - AIDS Project Director

Salvation Army Lancaster Corps
45001 N. Beach
P.O. Box 951
Lancaster, CA 93554
Telephone: (805)-948-3418
Contact: Capt. Ken Hood
General assistance services

County Health Depts

Kern County AIDS Task Force, Kern County Health Department
1700 Flower Street
Bakersfield, CA 93305-4198
Telephone: (805)-861-3631 Fax: (805)-861-2018
Contact: David K. Martin, PHN-BSN
HIV testing & counseling; case management

Home Health Care

Caremark Connection Network
3101 Sillect Avenue, #109
Suite 109
Bakersfield, CA 93308
Telephone: (805)-325-8326 Fax: (805)-325-6509
Contact: Susan Eaton
Clinical Support & Infusion Therapies: nutrition, antimicrobials,chemo., hematopoe

O.P.T.I.O.N Care
3400 Unicorn Road
Suite 113
Bakersfield, CA 93308
Telephone: (805)-399-8866 Fax: (805)-399-8897
Contact: Bill Redman
Home IV and Nutritional Services

Medical Services

California Children Services, HIV Children Program
Kern County
1700 Flower Street
Bakersfield, CA 93305
Telephone: (805)-861-3657 Fax: (805)-861-0179
Contact: Cheryl Collins - Program Coordinator
Diagnostic Testing, Medical Treatment, Medical Support Services, Counseling

Testing Sites

Kern Medical Center
1830 Flower Street
Bakersfield, CA 93305
Telephone: (805)-326-2000 Fax: (805)-326-2181
Contact: Dr. Navin Amin
HIV testing; counseling

Kings County

Community Services

Kern County Department of Human Services
P.O. Box 511
Bakersfield, CA 93202
Telephone: (805)-631-6000
Income Assistance

Testing Sites

Kings County AIDS Project, Department of Public Health
330 Campus Drive
Hanford, CA 93230
Telephone: (209)-584-1401 Fax: (209)-582-0927
Contact: Don Nichols
AIDS Education and Prevention Projects, Test Site, Support Services

Lassen County

Community Services

Westwood Family Practice
201 3rd Street
Westwood, CA 96137
Telephone: (916)-256-3152 Fax: (916)-256-2061
Counseling, referrals

Home Health Care

Lassen Volunteer Hospice
1306 Riverside Drive
Susanville, CA 96130
Telephone: (916)-257-7094 Fax: (916)-257-6015
Contact: Dottie Larimar - 916-257-5563
Respite care

Northeastern Home Health
1306 Riverside Drive
Susanville, CA 96130
Telephone: (916)-257-6191 Fax: (916)-257-8965
Home care

Medical Services

Big Valley Medical Center
100 North Market Street
Bieber, CA 96009
Telephone: (916)-294-5241 Fax: (916)-294-5392
Medical Services

Lassen Family Practice
1306 Riverside Drive
Susanville, CA 96130
Telephone: (916)-257-5563 Fax: (916)-257-6015
Medical services, testing, counseling & referrals

Los Angeles County

Community Services

The Actor's Fund of America
4727 Wilshire Blvd.
Suite 310
Los Angeles, CA 90010-4202
Telephone: (213)-933-9244
Financial assistance to those in entertainment field

AFL-CIO Legal Immigration Assistance Program
515 South Shatto Place
1st Floor
Los Angeles, CA 90020
Telephone: (213)-381-2170 Fax: (213)-738-8359
Legal Services, AIDS Waiver Assistance, Referrals

AID for AIDS
8235 Santa Monica Blvd.
Suite 200
West Hollywood, CA 90046
Telephone: (213)-656-1107
Contact: Walt Hanna
Emergency rent, food, medication, etc. for AIDS/ARC patients

Aid for AIDS
8235 Santa Monica Blvd.
Suite 200
West Hollywood, CA 90046-5914
Telephone: (213)-656-1107 Fax: (213)-650-4323
Contact: Walter Hanna
Financial Assistance, Vitamins, Referrals

All Saints Church AIDS Services Center
126 W. Delmar Blvd
Pasadena, CA 91105-1802
Telephone: (818)-796-5633 Fax: (818)-796-8198
Counseling

American Cancer Society
2975 Wilsire Boulevard
Suite 200
Los Angeles, CA 90010
Telephone: (213)-386-6102
Referrals

American Red Cross, Claremont Chapter
2065 N. Indian Hill Blvd.
P.O. Box 250
Claremont, CA 91711
Telephone: (909)-624-0074 Fax: (909)-624-6399
Contact: Pat Bortseheller
Education & prevention information, disaster services

Asian American Drug Abuse Program, Inc.
5318 S. Crenshaw Blvd.
Los Angeles, CA 90043
Telephone: (213)-293-6284
Prevention, outpatient & impatient programs, AIDS committee

Asian Health Project/T.H.E. Clinic
3860 West M.L. King Blvd.
Los Angeles, CA 90008
Telephone: (213)-295-6571 Fax: (213)-295-6577
Contact: Sylvia Drew Ivie
Education, Referrals, Testing, Materials in Asian/Pacific Languages

Assistance League Family Agency
5607 Fernwood Avenue
Los Angeles, CA 90028
Telephone: (213)-469-5893 Fax: (213)-469-5896
Counseling

Being Alive
4222 Santa Monica Blvd.
#105
Los Angeles, CA 90029
Telephone: (213)-667-3262 Fax: (213)-667-2735
Contact: Dana Gorbea-Leon
HIV support group, referrals

Being Alive/Long Beach
1734 E. Broadway Avenue
Long Beach, CA 90802
Telephone: (310)-495-3422
Contact: Robert Edborg
Speakers, Counseling, Information, Referrals, Recreation, Advocacy, Newsletter

Bet Tzedek Legal Services
145 S. Fairfax Avenue
#200
Los Angeles, CA 90036
Telephone: (213)-939-0506
Legal aid for low income

Black C.A.R.E. (Community AIDS Resistance through Education)
101 N. La Brea, Suite 100
Inglewood, CA 90301
Telephone: (310)-671-1222
Contact: Cecilia Freeman
Outreach Program, Prevention, Education, Referrals

Black C.A.R.E. Project
1283 Franz Hall
Los Angeles, CA 90024-1563
Telephone: (310)-825-9858 Fax: (310)-206-5895
Contact: Dr. Vickie Mays
Community AIDS research, education, HIV testing

Casa De Las Amigas, Inc.
160 N. El Molino Avenue
Pasadena, CA 91101-1805
Telephone: (818)-792-2770
Contact: Corey Graves - Director
Recovery home for women, 90 day residential

Christ Chapel of Long Beach
3935 E. 10th Street
Long Beach, CA 90804
Telephone: (310)-438-5303
Contact: Rick McCabe
AIDS food store

Coalition for Humane Immigrants' Rights of Los Angeles
c/o United Way
621 South Virgil Avenue
Los Angeles, CA 90005-4046
Telephone: (213)-736-1300 Fax: (213)-487-2187
Contact: Karen Mack
Legal Services; Education and Training Sessions on Immigration and AIDS

El Centro del Pueblo
1157 LeMoyne Street
Los Angeles, CA 90026-4209
Telephone: (213)-483-6335 Fax: (213)-483-5523
Contact: Executive Director
AIDS prevention, youth counseling, job training, drug abuse programs

Family Counseling Services
314 E. Mission Drive
San Gabriel, CA 91776
Telephone: (818)-285-2139 Fax: (818)-285-2180
Contact: Roberta Trujillo - Executive Officer
Individual and family couseling

Focus Center for Education and Development
2829 North Glenoaks Blvd
Burbank, CA 91504-2604
Telephone: (818)-563-5500 Fax: (818)-846-3148
Contact: Bridge Focus
Counseling

Foothill Family Service
118 S. Oak Knoll Avenue
Pasadena, CA 91101-2667
Telephone: (818)-795-6907 Fax: (818)-795-7080
Contact: Acting Executive Director
Counseling services

Gay and Lesbian Adolescent Social Services
650 N. Robertson Blvd.
Suite A
West Hollywood, CA 90069-5613
Telephone: (310)-358-8727 Fax: (310)-358-8721
Toll-Free: (800)-429-4294
Contact: Michele D. Kipke - Project Director
Counseling, education, job training

Hemophilia Council of California, Los Angeles Basin/Adjacent County
1000 E. Walnut Street
Suite 220
Pasadena, CA 91106-1452
Telephone: (818)-796-5710 Fax: (818)-796-6838
Contact: George Tobdell - Executive Director
Education & psychosocial services for hemophiliacs & transfusion recipients

Hemophilia Foundation of Southern California
33 South Catalina Avenue
Suite 102

Pasadena, CA 91106
Telephone: (818)-793-6192 Fax: (818)-796-5605

Hollywood Sunset Community Clinic, Cara A Cara
3324 Sunset Blvd.
Los Angeles, CA 90026-2190
Telephone: (213)-661-6752 Fax: (213)-660-1408
Contact: Theresa Pauda - Agency Director, Michael Puente - Project Coord.
HIV testing, AIDS education

Homestead Hospice & Shelter Board - Headquarters
3731 Wilshire Blvd.
PO Box 931179
Los Angeles, CA 90010
Telephone: (213)-466-5411 Fax: (213)-388-3905
Residential facilities for people with AIDS

Jewish Family and Children Service of Long Beach
3801 E. Willow Street
Long Beach, CA 90815
Telephone: (310)-427-7916 Fax: (310)-427-7910
Contact: Judy Shultz - Temporary Director
Counseling & support services

Jewish Family Service of Los Angeles and Big Brothers Assoc.
6505 Wilshire Boulevard
#417
Los Angeles, CA 90048-4990
Telephone: (213)-852-1234 Fax: (213)-655-1978
Contact: David Levy
AIDS counseling

Jewish Family Services of Santa Monica
1424 Fourth Street, #303
Santa Monica, CA 90401-2371
Telephone: (310)-393-0732 Fax: (310)-395-0434
Counseling, information, referrals

Joint Efforts, Project HOPE
505 S. Pacific Avenue
Suite 205
San Pedro, CA 90731-2656
Telephone: (310)-831-2358 Fax: (310)-831-2356
Contact: Armita Ayala
Prevention, Education, Out-Patient Drug Treatment, Crisis Counseling, Workshops

L.A. City Attorney's Office - HIV/AIDS Discrimination Unit
200 North Main St, R 1600
City Hall East
Los Angeles, CA 90012-3320
Telephone: (213)-485-4579 Fax: (213)-237-0402
Contact: David Schulman - City AIDS Attorney
Legal Services, AIDS Discrimination Cases, Referrals

La Casa De San Gabriel Community Center
203 E. Mission Drive
San Gabriel, CA 91776
Telephone: (818)-286-2144
Contact: Cheryl Prentice - Executive Director
Emergency Assistance, referrals, childcare

Legal Aid Foundation of Long Beach
110 Pine Avenue
Long Beach, CA 90802
Telephone: (310)-435-3510
Legal Services

Legal Aid Foundation of Los Angeles
1636 W. Eighth Street
Suite 313
Los Angeles, CA 90017-2117
Telephone: (213)-389-3581 Fax: (213)-380-4319
Legal aid for low income

Los Angeles Free Clinic, Project ABLE
8405 Beverly Blvd
Los Angeles, CA 90048-3476
Telephone: (213)-653-8622
Contact: Dick Thor - Project Coordinator
AIDS Education and Prevention Projects, Support Projects.

Los Angeles Shanti Foundation
1616 N. La Brea Avenue
Hollywood, CA 90028
Telephone: (213)-962-8197 Fax: (213)-962-8299
Contact: Eve Rubell
HIV counseling, emotional & educational support

MCC/LA
5879 Washington Boulevard
Culver City, CA 90232
Telephone: (213)-930-1600 Fax: (213)-930-1067
Worship services, spiritual counseling

Metropolitan Community Church
1231 Locust Avenue
Long Beach, CA 90813
Telephone: (310)-432-3641 Fax: (310)-436-1184
Contact: Rev. Phil Crum
Spiritual Counseling, Support Group, Household Services, Information, Referrals

Minority AIDS Project
5149 W Jefferson Blvd
Los Angeles, CA 90016-3836
Telephone: (213)-936-4949 Fax: (213)-936-7943
Contact: Bishop Carl Bean - Director
Education,counseling, financial & housing assistance

Mothers of AIDS Patients
P.O. Box 1763
Lomita, CA 90717
Telephone: (310)-542-3019 Fax: (310)-214-0833
Contact: Janet McMahon
Support Groups, Counseling, Referral Information, Speakers

Neighborhood Youth Association
3877 Grandview Boulevard
Los Angeles, CA 90066-4494
Telephone: (310)-390-6641 Fax: (310)-391-1948
Special Community Services, AIDS counseling

Para Los Ninos
845 E. 6th Street
Los Angeles, CA 90021-1069
Telephone: (213)-623-8446 Fax: (213)-623-8716
Day & child care for needy families

Pasadena Council on Alcoholism and Drug Dependency
131 N. El Molino Avenue
#320
Pasadena, CA 91101-1873
Telephone: (818)-795-9127 Fax: (818)-795-0979
Contact: David Klein - Director
Referrals & limited case management

Project AHEAD (AIDS Health Education & Assistance Directory)
2017 East 4th Street
Long Beach, CA 90814
Telephone: (310)-434-4455 Fax: (310)-433-6428
Contact: Hal Hall
Referrals to the Providence & Lily shelters and the AIDS Hotel.

Project Andel Food
P.O. Box 69-616
Los Angeles, CA 90069
Telephone: (213)-850-0877 Fax: (213)-650-2944
Meal delivery program for homebound people with AIDS

Project Info, Inc.
9401 S. Painter Avenue
Whittier, CA 90605-2729
Telephone: (310)-698-9436 Fax: (310)-693-9524
Outpatient drug counseling

San Fernando Valley Child Guidance Clinic
9650 Zelzah Avenue
Northridge, CA 91325-2003
Telephone: (818)-993-9311 Fax: (818)-993-8206
Contact: Roy Marshall - Executive Director
Counseling for children & their families

San Fernando Valley Unit
14602 Victory Boulevard
Van Nuys, CA 91411-1621
Telephone: (818)-989-5555 Fax: (818)-994-5498
Contact: Diane Shapiro
HIV counseling, support group

Santa Anita Family Service
605 S. Myrtle Avenue
P.O. Box 570
Monrovia, CA 91016-0570
Telephone: (818)-359-9358
Social services

Santa Anita Family Service
527 E. Rowland
Covina, CA 91723
Telephone: (818)-966-1755
Contact: Sandra Broyard
HIV counseling

Southern California Youth and Family Center
101 North La Brea Avenue
Suite 100
Inglewood, CA 90301
Telephone: (310)-671-1222 Fax: (310)-671-0687
Contact: Gayle Nathieson - Executive Director
Counseling for teen mothers

St. Augustine by the Sea
1227 Fourth Street
Santa Monica, CA 90401-1350
Telephone: (310)-395-0977 Fax: (310)-451-8960
Contact: John Giloy
Counseling, fellowship, memorial services

Suicide Prevention Center, AIDS Support Services Program
626 South Kingsley Drive
Los Angeles, CA 90056
Telephone: (213)-381-5111 Fax: (213)-380-8923
Contact: Allison Barr - Agency Director
24 hour crisis intervention services,1-800-333-4444.

Toberman Settlement
131 N. Grand Avenue
San Pedro, CA 90731-2097
Telephone: (310)-832-1145
Contact: Howard Uller
AIDS education, support groups, counseling

Uhuru Counseling Center
8732 S. Western Avenue
Los Angeles, CA 90047
Telephone: (213)-751-3152
Substance abuse programs

United Cambodian Community
11859 Rosecrans Avenue
Norwalk, CA 90650-4102
Telephone: (310)-868-0706 Fax: (310)-864-0773
Contact: Robert Gulden
Education, Counseling, and Referrals in Southeast Asian Languages

Watts Health Foundation SLACAP
4116 E. Compton Blvd
Compton, CA 90221
Telephone: (310)-639-3068 Fax: (310)-638-4795
Contact: Wendell Carmicheal
AIDS education, outreach, testing & counseling, transportation

Women and AIDS Risk Network (WARN)
5601 W. Slausen Ave # 200
Culver City, CA 90230
Telephone: (310)-641-7795 Fax: (310)-649-4347
Toll-Free: (800)-427-1792
Contact: Ruth Slaughter
AIDS education, referral, support groups, crisis counseling

County Health Depts

Los Angeles County
600 South Commonwealth
6th Floor
Los Angeles, CA 90005
Telephone: (213)-351-8001 Fax: (213)-738-0825
Contact: John Schunhoff
Educational programs

Los Angeles County DHS, Department of Mental Health
2415 W. 6th Street
Los Angeles, CA 90057
Telephone: (213)-738-4961 Fax: (213)-386-1297
Contact: A. Crowell - PHG
Mental health care for HIV patients

Home Health Care

Critical Care America
16160 Stagg Street
Van Nuys, CA 91406
Telephone: (818)-780-3161 Fax: (818)-780-4172
Contact: Iris King
Coordinate & integrate all clinical & psychosocial services for HIV+

Homestead Hospice & Shelter
940 Atlantic Avenue
Long Beach, CA 90813
Telephone: (310)-432-2000
Contact: Bobbi Mations, RN
Hospice, In-Home Care

Homestead Hospice & Shelter
PO Box 931179
Los Angeles, CA 90093
Telephone: (213)-466-5411 Fax: (213)-388-3905
Housing & care for HIV patients

Homestead Hospice & Shelter Board - Pioneer Home
7402 Haskell Avenue
Van Nuys, CA 91406-3204
Telephone: (818)-787-2403 Fax: (818)-787-3008
Contact: Vicky Thorpe - House Manager
HIV support, HIV counseling

Hospital Home Health Care Agency-California
2601 Airport Drive
Suite 110
Torrance, CA 90505-6193
Telephone: (310)-530-3800 Fax: (310)-325-4792
Contact: Director of Hospice
Hospice, home care, care management

Integrated Care Systems
16160 Stagg Street
Van Nuys, CA 91406-1713
Telephone: (818)-780-3161
Infusion therapies in home

Lifeline Homecare
12130 S. Paramount Blvd.
Downey, CA 90242
Telephone: (310)-861-5305 Fax: (310)-861-6469
Contact: Lyn Boland
In-home care, social services, advocacy, information, referrals

Memorial Medical Center
2801 Atlantic Avenue
Long Beach, CA 90801
Telephone: (310)-933-0812 Fax: (310)-933-3134
Contact: Audrey Deveikis
Home care, hospice, intermittent basis with nursing care

Modern Home Care Pharmacy
720 S Glendale Ave
Glendale, CA 91205
Telephone: (818)-761-3739 Fax: (818)-551-0650
Contact: Peggy Pillion
HIV home care

nmc HOMECARE
2826 E. Foothill Blvd
Pasadena, CA 91107
Telephone: (818)-578-8694
Fax: (818)-578-8698
National JCAHO-Accredited company providing a full range of Infusion and Respiratory therapies and specializing in the care of HIV/AIDS patients. National Case Manager is also available at 800-445-1188

nmc HOMECARE
43423 Division St, Suite 205
Lancaster, CA 93535
Telephone: (805)-948-0660
Fax: (805)-948-7221
Contact: Sharon Doty
National JCAHO-Accredited company providing a full range of Infusion and Respiratory therapies and specializing in the care of HIV/AIDS patients. National Case Manager is also available at 800-445-1188

nmc HOMECARE
320/318 West Cerritos
Glendale, CA 91204
Telephone: (818)-502-0003
Fax: (818)-502-0722
Contact: Sharon Doty
National JCAHO-Accredited company providing a full range of Infusion and Respiratory therapies and specializing in the care of HIV/AIDS patients. National Case Manager is also available at 800-445-1188

nmc HOMECARE
20765 Superior Street
Chatsworth, CA 91311
Telephone: (818)-700-1266
Fax: (818)-700-1681
Contact: Mike Voelker
National JCAHO-Accredited company providing a full range of Infusion and Respiratory therapies and specializing in the care of HIV/AIDS patients. National Case Manager is also available at 800-445-1188

California, Los Angeles CountyOlsten Kimberly Quality Care
6222 Wilshire Blvd.
Suite 450
Los Angeles, CA 90048
Telephone: (213)-650-1800 Fax: (213)-930-4848
Home health care, home nursing service, case management, education,training, support, advocacy

East San Gabriel Valley
345 E Rowland Street
Covina, CA 91723
Telephone: (818)-967-9311 Fax: (818)-339-5847
Counceling, support, home care for HIV patients, home visits

Olsten Kimberly Quality Care
4001 Atlantic Ave
#440
Long Beach, CA 90807-2202
Telephone: (714)-963-9390 Fax: (310)-984-9423
Contact: Linda Davis
Home Health Care/Hospice

St. Mary Medical Center
1050 Linden Avenue
Long Beach, CA 90813
Telephone: (310)-435-4441 Fax: (310)-491-9867
Contact: Jennifer Andrews
Home care, hospice, intermittent basis with nursing care & daily volunteers

Visiting Nurse Association of Long Beach
3295 Pacific Avenue
Long Beach, CA 90807
Telephone: (310)-426-8856 Fax: (310)-988-9474
Contact: Susanne Fairman - Executive Director
Case management, home health care, hospice services, counseling, referrals

East San Gabriel Valley
345 E Rowland Street
Covina, CA 91723
Telephone: (818)-967-9311 Fax: (818)-339-5847
Counceling, support, home care for HIV patients, home visits

Visiting Nurse Association, Pasadena & Alhambra Branch
100 E. Huntingdon Drive
Alhambra, CA 91801
Telephone: (818)-458-1400
Contact: Clara Aguilera - Director
Skilled nursing

Visiting Nurse Association, Pomona-West End
170 W. San Jose
P.O. Box 908
Claremont, CA 91711-1208
Telephone: (909)-624-3574 Fax: (909)-624-8904
Contact: Karen Green
Home care for AIDS patients

Medical Services

Ahisma Care Center
67000 Sepulveda
Vaan Nuys, CA 91411
Telephone: (818)-908-2088 Fax: (818)-908-2077
Contact: Sue Eldred - Clinical Coordinator
Lic. skilled nursing facility and in-pt.hospice for chronic illness,agressive HIV/AIDS therapy

American Indian Free Clinic, Main Artery Program
1330 S. Long Beach Blvd.
Compton, CA 90221
Telephone: (310)-537-0103
Alcohol & HIV referral services

Behavioral Health Services, Inc.
279 W. Beach Avenue
Inglewood, CA 90302
Telephone: (310)-673-5750
Contact: Robert Douglas
Counseling for alcoholics

Children's Hospital/Adolescent Medicine
4650 Sunset Boulevard
Los Angeles, CA 90027
Telephone: (213)-669-2112 Fax: (213)-913-3691
Contact: Marvin Belzer
HIV counseling

Department of Health Services, California Children Services
19720 E. Arrow Hwy.
Covina, CA 91724-1022
Telephone: (818)-858-2100
Case management, HIV support groups, testing program for pediatricpatients and families

Didi Hirsch Community Mental Health Center
4760 S. Sepulveda Blvd.
Culver City, CA 90230
Telephone: (310)-390-8896 Fax: (310)-398-5690
Mental health services, crisis counseling

East Valley Community Health Center, Inc.
420 South Glendora Avenue
West Covina, CA 91790
Telephone: (818)-919-5724 Fax: (818)-919-6972
Contact: Heather Gummrector - Coordinator
Case management services, HIV counseling & testing, mental healthcounseling, HIV medical services

Hollywood Health Center
1462 N. Vine Street
Hollywood, CA 90028
Telephone: (213)-461-9355 Fax: (213)-461-7257
Contact: James Houck
Testing, counseling, medical services

La Clinica Familia Alsamed
133 N. Sunol Drive
Los Angeles, CA 90063-1429
Telephone: (213)-266-1122 Fax: (213)-266-3034
Medical Services

Les Kelley Family Health Center
1255 15th Street
Santa Monica, CA 90404-1101
Telephone: (310)-319-4700 Fax: (310)-393-5659
Contact: Yvonne Dangels
Primary care: referrals

Little House
9718 Harvard
Bellflower, CA 90706
Telephone: (310)-925-0806
Contact: Betty Boring
Recovery program for alcohol

Long Beach Asian Pacific Mental Health Program
1975 Long Beach Blvd.
Long Beach, CA 90806
Telephone: (310)-599-9401 Fax: (310)-599-3439
Contact: Lucy Riveria
Mental Health Evaluation and Screening, Psychotherapy, Crisis Intervention

Michael S. Gottlieb Medical Group
9201 Sunset Boulevard
Suite 414
West Hollywood, CA 90069
Telephone: (310)-273-3633 Fax: (310)-273-1398
Contact: MD
Medical Services

Pacific Clinics
909 S. Fair Oaks Ave.
Pasadena, CA 91105
Telephone: (818)-795-8471 Fax: (818)-449-4925
Contact: Maria Montes
Mental health care services

Pacific Hospital of Long Beach
2776 Pacific Avenue
Long Beach, CA 90806
Telephone: (310)-595-1911
Contact: Asst. Dir. Cardio-Pul. Svcs.
Medical Services, Education, Support, Information, Referrals, Research, Testing

Pasadena Mental Health Center
1495 N. Lake Avenue
Pasadena, CA 91104-2398
Telephone: (818)-798-0907
Contact: Nina Sorkin - Executive Director
Counseling & referral programs

Plaza Community Center Clinic
3700 Princeton Street
Los Angeles, CA 90023-1895
Telephone: (213)-268-1107 Fax: (213)-262-7332
Contact: Marie Talabera
Health care, substance abuse program

St. Mary Medical Center, Comprehensive AIDS Program
1050 Linden Avenue
Long Beach, CA 90813
Telephone: (310)-491-9050
Contact: Jennifer Andrews
Study of In-Home AIDS Care Cost, Case Management

Sherman Oaks Community Hospital
4929 Van Nuys Blvd.
Sherman Oaks, CA 91403-1777
Telephone: (818)-907-4573 Fax: (818)-907-2812
Contact: Denise O'Niel - Clinical Coordinator
HIV counseling,HIV support

US Veterans Admin. Medical Center, Infectious Disease Dept.
Sawtelle & Wilshire Blvd.
Building 500 Rm 4669
Los Angeles, CA 90073
Telephone: (310)-824-4480 Fax: (310)-824-6681
Case Management, Counseling, Medical Services, Testing, Information

Van Ness Recovery House
1919 North Beachwood Dr.
Los Angeles, CA 90068-4019
Telephone: (213)-463-4266 Fax: (213)-962-6721
Alcohol-Drug Residential Treatment Program for Gays and Lesbians, Referrals

West County Medical Clinic
900 E. Market Street
Long Beach, CA 90805-5924
Telephone: (310)-428-4222
Contact: Render Gray Fimon
Testing, Counseling, Case Management, Education, Treatment Research, Support

Testing Sites

American Red Cross, Los Angeles Chapter
2700 Wilshire Boulevard
P.O. Box 57930
Los Angeles, CA 90057
Telephone: (213)-739-5200 Fax: (213)-380-0362
Toll-Free: (800)-675-5799

HIV testing & counseling, tissue services

California State University--Long Beach
Student Health Center
1250 Bellflower Boulevard
Long Beach, CA 90840
Telephone: (310)-985-4771 Fax: (310)-985-4932
Contact: Mary Byron - Coordinator
Confidential HIV testing

The Center
2017 E. 4th Street
Long Beach, CA 90814
Telephone: (310)-434-4455 Fax: (310)-433-6428
Testing, counseling, referrals

Clinica Mrs. Oscar A. Romero
2675 W. Olympic Boulevard
Los Angeles, CA 90006
Telephone: (213)-389-0288 Fax: (213)-383-2260
Contact: Oscar Lopez
HIV testing, counseling

East Los Angeles Health Task Force
630 South St. Louis Str.
Los Angeles, CA 90023
Telephone: (213)-261-2171 Fax: (213)-261-0246
Contact: Executive Director
Medical-HIV testing-edcational, drug abuse

El Proyecto del Barrio, Inc.
8902 Woodman Avenue
Arleta, CA 91331
Telephone: (818)-830-7033 Fax: (818)-830-7280
Contact: Adrian Gonalez - Executive Director
HIV testing & counseling levels 1, 2, 3

Los Angeles County, USC Hospital, AIDS Services
1200 N. State Street
Los Angeles, CA 90033-4525
Telephone: (213)-226-7504
Contact: Chief of Infectious Disease
Infectious disease testing & counseling

Olive View Medical Center
14445 Olive View Drive
Sylmar, CA 91342
Telephone: (818)-364-1555 Fax: (818)-364-4573
Contact: Sharon Mitsuyaso, RN - HIV Coordinator
HIV testing, diagnosis and treatment, counseling, referrals

Planned Parenthood World Population Los Angeles
1920 Marrengo Street
Los Angeles, CA 90033-1317
Telephone: (213)-223-4462 Fax: (213)-225-5844
Toll-Free: (800)-230-7526
HIV testing, support groups

Ruth Temple Health Center
3834 S. Western Avenue
Los Angeles, CA 90062-1004
Telephone: (213)-730-3838
Contact: Hampton Oeslonde, M.D.
Confidential testing & counseling

South Bay Free Clinic
1807 Manhattan Beach Blvd
Manhattan Beach, CA 90266
Telephone: (213)-376-3000
Contact: Stewart Sokol
Anonymous HIV testing

South Bay Free Clinic
742 West Gardena Blvd.
Gardena, CA 90247
Telephone: (310)-376-3000
Contact: Stewart Sokol
Anonymous HIV Testing

Curtis R. Tucker Health Center
123 West Manchester
Inglewood, CA 90301
Telephone: (310)-419-5376
Contact: Carolyn Dong
HIV testing, counseling, referrals

Madera County

Community Services

Madera Counseling Center
14277 Road 28
Madera, CA 93638-5715
Telephone: (209)-673-3508 Fax: (209)-673-4407
Contact: Ed Thompson
Mental health, IV drug abuse services & alcohol abuse

Madera County Welfare Department
629 East Yosemite Avenue
Madera, CA 93637
Telephone: (209)-675-7841
Contact: Debbie Williams
Child & adult services, in-home supportive services

County Health Depts

Madera County Health Department
14215 Road 28
Madera, CA 93638-5715
Telephone: (209)-675-7893 Fax: (209)-674-7262
Contact: Ann Harris
HIV testing and counseling

Marin County

Community Services

Access Group
4 Cielo Lane, # 4D
Novato, CA 94949-6379
Telephone: (415)-883-6111
Contact: Daniel Barnes
Evaluation program for HIV referrals

AIDS Interfaith of Marin/Spectrum
1000 Sir Francis Dr. Blvd
Suite # 12
San Anselmo, CA 94960
Telephone: (415)-457-1129 Fax: (415)-457-2838
Pastoral counseling

Babcock Memorial Endowment
305 San Anselmo Avenue
Suite # 219
San Anselmo, CA 94960
Telephone: (415)-453-0901
Short-term finanical assistance for medical costs, including HIV

Center for Attitudinal Healing
19 Main Street
Tiburon, CA 94920
Telephone: (415)-435-5022 Fax: (415)-435-5085
Contact: Douglas Ellis
Provides support groups for people with AIDS/ARC

Center for Attitudinal Healing
19 Main Street
Tiburon, CA 94920
Telephone: (415)-435-5022 Fax: (415)-435-5085
Support Groups for AIDS/ARC Utilizing the Principles of Attitudinal Healing

County Alcohol and Drug Program
150 Suite C 1682 Novato Blvd.
Novato, CA 94947
Telephone: (415)-899-8660 Fax: (415)-899-8656
Contact: Joe Mazza
Information and referrals.

Human Rights Commission of Marin
Room 423 Civic Center
San Rafael, CA 94903
Telephone: (415)-499-6185 Fax: (415)-499-6108
Contact: Pat Maguire
Receives and investigates complaints of abuse.

Marin AIDS Political Action Committee (MAPAC)
PO Box 2424
Mill Valley, CA 94942
Telephone: (415)-383-1471
Contact: Paul Albritton
Promotes responsible health-policies regarding HIV/AIDS issues

Marin AIDS Project
1660 2nd Street
San Rafael, CA 94901
Telephone: (415)-457-2487 Fax: (415)-457-5687
Contact: Jan Gorewitz
Provides free direct services to HIV/AIDS clients families & friends

Marin Services for Women
444 Magnolia Avenue
Larkspur, CA 94939
Telephone: (415)-924-5995
Private, non-profit substance abuse recovery for women, Referrals for HIV

Home Health Care

Clarke Home Nursing Service
371 Bel Marin Keys Blvd.
Suite 110
Navato, CA 94948
Telephone: (415)-382-6868 Fax: (415)-382-6844
Home care including AIDS patients

Hospice of Marin
150 Nellen Avenue
Corte Madera, CA 94925
Telephone: (415)-927-2273
Contact: Carol Hannon - Health

Jenkins Nursing Service
901 East Street, #100
San Rafael, CA 94901
Telephone: (415)-454-6774 Fax: (415)-454-5185
Contact: Judith Jenkins
Registered nurses, licenses vocational nurses, certified home aides,companions, case management

North Bay Nursing Services
25 Bellam Blvd.
Suite # 250

San Rafael, CA 94901
Telephone: (415)-485-0155 Fax: (415)-485-3813
Contact: Katherine Shotwell
Home care, registered nurses

Medical Services

California Children Services, HIV Children Program
55 North Gate Drive
Suite B
San Rafael, CA 94903-4156
Telephone: (415)-499-6877 Fax: (415)-499-6396
Contact: Gretchen Antill
Diagnostic Testing, Medical Treatment, Medical Support Services, Counseling

Project Pentamidine
976 Vernal Avenue
Mill Valley, CA 94941-4445
Telephone: (415)-388-2105 Fax: (415)-388-4745
Contact: Jack Erdmann
Medical services, low-cost Pentamidine accessable nationwide

Testing Sites

Marin County AIDS Program
20 N San Pedro Road
Suite 2002
San Rafael, CA 94903-4158
Telephone: (415)-499-7804 Fax: (415)-499-3621
Contact: Jon Green
AIDS brug assistance, HIV antibody testing

Mariposa County

County Health Depts

Mariposa County Health Department
P.O. Box 5
Mariposa, CA 95338
Telephone: (209)-966-3689 Fax: (209)-966-4929
Contact: Juanita Smith
HIV testing, counseling

Mendocino County

County Health Depts

Mendocino County Public Health Department
890 North Bush Street
Court House
Ukiah, CA 95482
Telephone: (707)-463-4134 Fax: (707)-463-4138
Contact: Rosalie Anchordogvy - RN; Frank McGarvey -
Prevention, education, HIV testing, pre-post referral, case management

Merced County

County Health Depts

Merced County Department of Health
240 E. 15th Street
PO Box 471
Merced, CA 95341-0471
Telephone: (209)-385-7710 Fax: (209)-385-7887
Toll-Free: (800)-649-6849
Contact: Karen Resner - AIDS Project Director
HIV testing, counseling, serveillance, case management, outreach, education

Testing Sites

Merced Family Health Centers, Inc.
727 West Childs Avenue
PO Box 858
Merced, CA 95341-0471
Telephone: (209)-384-3064 Fax: (209)-383-0136
Confidential testing; spanish speaking

Modoc County

Medical Services

Modoc Medical Center
228 McDowell Street
Alturas, CA 96101
Telephone: (916)-233-5131 Fax: (916)-233-5884
Contact: Adminstrator
Medical services, visiting nurse

Surprise Valley Medical Center
745 Main Street
Cedarville, CA 96104
Telephone: (916)-279-6111 Fax: (916)-279-2680
Medical services, HIV testing, some general care

Mono County

Community Services

Mono County Alcohol and Drug Program
P.O. Box 2619
Mammoth Lakes, CA 93546-2619
Telephone: (619)-934-8221 Fax: (619)-924-5413
Contact: Alma Lones
Drug Treatment, Community Services, referrals

Medical Services

Mono County Group
P.O. Box 677
Bridgeport, CA 93517
Telephone: (619)-932-7011
Contact: Jack Bertman - Director
Referrals to public health clinics

Testing Sites

Mono County Health Department
PO Box 3329
Mamouth, CA 93546
Telephone: (619)-924-5410 Fax: (619)-934-1684
Contact: Sue Briston - AIDS Coordinator;
Aids services, HIV testing & counseling; referrals to other services

Monterey County

Community Services

Monterey County AIDS Project
P.O. Box 2081
Monterey, CA 93942
Telephone: (408)-424-5550 Fax: (408)-424-9615
Contact: Francisco Perez
Educational food, counseling, emergency assistance for services arebilingual

County Health Depts

Monterey County Health Department
1270 Natividad Road
Salinas, CA 93906
Telephone: (408)-755-4975 Fax: (408)-757-9586
Contact: Dr. Melton
Testing, counseling & education; alcohol and drug program

Home Health Care

Critical Care America
20 Lower Ragsdale Drive
Monterey, CA 93940
Telephone: (408)-373-1111 Fax: (408)-655-6466
Contact: Dora Thurman
HIV pharmacy & home nursing agency

Medical Services

California Children Services
Monterey County
1270 Natividad Road
Salinas, CA 93906
Telephone: (408)-755-4522
Contact: Kathie Yoshiyama - Program Coord.
Diagnostic Testing, Medical Treatment, Medical Support Services, Counseling

Community Hospital of the Monterey Peninsula
23845 Holman Hwy
Monterey, CA 93940
Telephone: (408)-625-4972
Contact: Mary Dugom
Medical care for HIV patients, HIV testing

Community Human Services Methadone Clinic
1101 F North Main
Salinas, CA 93906
Telephone: (408)-424-4828
Contact: Woody Bellector - Project Coord.
Methadone maintenance & detox

Napa County

County Health Depts

Napa County Health Department
2281 Elm Street
Napa, CA 94559
Telephone: (707)-253-4227 Fax: (707)-253-4155
Contact: Kristie Brandt
HIV testing, counseling, referrals, free condoms, bilingual

Medical Services

California Children Services, HIV Children Program
2281 Elm Street
Napa, CA 94559
Telephone: (707)-253-4391 Fax: (707)-253-4155
Contact: Mary Herzog - Program Coordinator
Diagnostic Testing, Medical Treatment, Medical Support Services, Counseling

Queen of the Valley Hospital
P.O. Box 2340; 1000 Trancas Street
Napa, CA 94558
Telephone: (707)-252-4411 Fax: (707)-224-7087
Home care services, general medical and surgical

Nevada County

Community Services

Nevada County Council on Alcoholism
139-1/2 Mill Street
Grass Valley, CA 95945
Telephone: (916)-273-9541
Education

County Health Depts

Nevada County Health Department
HEW Complex
10433 Willow Valley Road
Nevada City, CA 95959
Telephone: (916)-265-1450
Contact: Susie Fatheree - Health Officier
AIDS services, AZT drug program

Home Health Care

Hospice of the Foothills
12059 Neveda City Highway
Room 200
Grass Valley, CA 95945
Telephone: (916)-272-5739
Contact: Dennis Fournier
Hospice care, nursing care for terminally ill AIDS patients

Sierra Nevada Memorial Home Care, Inc.
P.O. Box 1029
10066 Joereschke Dr.
Grass Valley, CA 95945
Telephone: (916)-274-6350 Fax: (916)-274-9023
Contact: Sharon Turner
Home Health Care

Visiting Nurse Association
12509 Nevada City Highway
#104
Grass Valley, CA 95945-9307
Telephone: (916)-272-4218 Fax: (916)-272-7739
Home Health Care

Medical Services

Nevada County Mental Health Department
Substance Abuse Program
10433 Willow Valley Road
Nevada City, CA 95959
Telephone: (916)-265-5811
Contact: Doug Bond - Program Manager
Drug Treatment, Community Services

Tahoe Forest Hospital Home Health Department
P.O. Box 759
10122 Pine Avenue
Truckee, CA 96160
Telephone: (916)-587-6011 Fax: (916)-587-2532
Contact: Larry Loc
Home care, trauma center, HIV testing, HIV patient care

Orange County

Community Services

AIDS Service Foundation
17982 Sky Park, Suite J
Irvine, CA 92714-6303
Telephone: (714)-852-1010
Social service, mental health, case management, support groups

Al-Anon Information Service Office of Orange County
2098 S. Grand Avenue
Suite F
Santa Ana, CA 92705
Telephone: (714)-545-1102
Support groups for families & friends of alcoholics

Brea Dept. of Human Resources
1 Civic Center Plaza
Brea, CA 92621
Telephone: (714)-671-4422 Fax: (714)-990-2258
Contact: Judy Campos
Housing subsidies, assistance with disability & income requirements

Episcopal Service Alliance
317 East Santa Anna Blvd.
Santa Ana, CA 92701-4517
Telephone: (714)-953-9170
Partial financial assistance for gasoline, utilities, food bank etc.

Episcopal Service Alliance
311 W. South Street
Anaheim, CA 92801-4517
Telephone: (714)-776-7510
Contact: Mary Doman
Partial financial assistance for gasoline, utilities, food bank etc.

Food Distribution Center
426-A W. Almond Street
Orange, CA 92666-1338
Telephone: (714)-771-1343
Clearinghouse for surplus food distribution to 200+ community serviceorganizations.

Garrett-Norris & Rushforth, Attorneys at Law
414 W. Fourth Street
Suite L
Santa Ana, CA 92701-4563
Telephone: (714)-543-1200
Legal Services

Gay and Lesbian Community Services Center - Orange County
12832 Garden Grove Blvd.
Suite B
Garden Grove, CA 92643-2002
Telephone: (714)-534-0961 Fax: (714)-534-5491
Contact: Donna Yutzy - Executive Director
AIDS Education and Prevention Projects, Counseling, Support Services

Jewish Family Service of Orange County
23421 S. Pointe Dr, #155
Laguna Hills, CA 92653-1512
Telephone: (714)-951-9377 Fax: (714)-939-1772
Counseling on sliding fee basis; insurance accepted; food bank, some financial.

Legal Aid Society of Orange County
525 Main Street, #A
Huntington Beach, CA 92648-5133
Telephone: (714)-536-8864 Fax: (714)-969-1683
Contact: Barbara Youngblood
Legal Services

Legal Aid Society of Orange County
250 E. Cypress
Anaheim, CA 92805
Telephone: (714)-533-7490
Toll-Free: (800)-834-5001
Legal Services

Legal Aid Society of Orange County
902 N. Main Street
Santa Ana, CA 92701-3507
Telephone: (714)-835-8806 Fax: (714)-547-9527
Legal Services

Lutheran Social Services
215 N. Lemon
Fullerton, CA 92632-2028
Telephone: (714)-738-1058 Fax: (714)-534-6450
Contact: Roger Moore
Counseling; food bank, assistance with rent, bustickets, clothing

Narcotics Anonymous
217 N. Main Street
Santa Ana, CA 92705-4869
Telephone: (714)-776-8581
Self-help for drug users, HIV support groups

North Orange County Community Clinic
300 W. Romneya Street
Anaheim, CA 92801-2406
Telephone: (714)-774-2782 Fax: (714)-535-5407
Primary care, nutritional counseling, x-ray, medical referrals.

Orange County HCA/North Regional Alcoholism Team
211 W. Commonwealth Avenue
Suite 204
Fullerton, CA 92632-1810
Telephone: (714)-447-7099
Crisis intervention, assessment, evaluation, therapy

Orange County HCA/South Alchoholism Services
3115 Redhill Avenue
Costa Mesa, CA 92626-4515
Telephone: (714)-850-8423
Contact: Director
Crisis intervention, assessments, evaluation, therapy

Share Our Selves
1550 Superior Ave
Costa Mesa, CA 92627-3653
Telephone: (714)-642-3451 Fax: (714)-650-6976
Food bank available on once-a-week basis, clothing, limited financial aid.

Home Health Care

Abbey-Foster Infusion Care
1821 W. Lincoln Avenue
Anaheim, CA 92801-6731
Telephone: (714)-972-4872 Fax: (714)-491-0472
Home Health Care/Hospice

American Cancer Society/Orange County Unit
3631 S. Harbor Blvd.
Suite 200
Santa Ana, CA 92704-6951
Telephone: (714)-751-0441
Home health care for persons with Karposi's Sarcoma only.

Caremark Connection Network
One Wrigley Drive
Irvine, CA 92718-2711
Telephone: (714)-380-9360 Fax: (714)-380-0935
Toll-Free: (800)-223-6142
Contact: Cliff Oliver - Branch Mgr.

Clinical support and infusion therapies: nutrition, antimicrobials,chemotherapy, hematopoeti

Coordinated Home Care Services, Inc.
13800 Arizona Street
Suite 101
Westminster, CA 92683-3943
Telephone: (714)-895-6962 Fax: (714)-897-0962
Contact: Virginia Barton
Home Health Care/Hospice

Critical Care America
3550 Hyland Avenue
Costa Mesa, CA 92626
Telephone: (714)-754-4200 Fax: (714)-754-1639
Contact: Pamela Weathington
Coordinate & integrate all clinical & psychosocial services for HIV+,infusion services, dietery counseling

Curaflex Infusion Services
16580 Harbor Blvd
Suite D
Fountain Valley, CA 92708
Telephone: (800)-388-2872 Fax: (714)-531-5040
Contact: George Schram - General Manager
Home IV therapy: TPN, Enteral, IV Antibiotics, Aerosolized/IV Pentamidine

Healthdyne Home Infusion Therapy Inc.
18 Technology Drive
Suites 110-111
Irvine, CA 92718
Telephone: (714)-727-4010
Contact: Joel Ajopian
Home Infusion Therapy, In-home Nursing and Attendant Care, P.T. Services, Pentamidine

Homedco Infusion
5555 Corporate Drive
Suite D
Cypress, CA 90630
Telephone: (714)-995-4545 Fax: (714)-828-9417
Contact: Daniel Cole
Experienced in providing quality home infusion therapy to HIV/AIDS patients

Homedco Infusion
5555 Corporate Ave
Cyprus, CA 90630
Telephone: (805)-966-6468 Fax: (714)-828-9417
Toll-Free: (800)-821-1456
Contact: Pat Devlin
Home infusion therapy to HIV/AIDS patients

Integrated Care Systems
3550 Hyland Avenue
Suite 4
Costa Mesa, CA 92626
Telephone: (714)-754-4200 Fax: (714)-654-1639
Superior, quality traditional and innovative infusion therapies in home

nmc HOMECARE
1815 E. Wilshire Blvd, Suite 906
Santa Ana, CA 92705
Telephone: (714)-285-1891
Fax: (714)-285-0221
Contact: Sharon Doty
National JCAHO-Accredited company providing a full range of Infusion and Respiratory therapies and specializing in the care of HIV/AIDS patients. National Case Manager is also available at 800-445-1188

nmc HOMECARE
731 E. Ball Road
Anaheim, CA 92805
Telephone: (714)-776-3390
Fax:(714)-776-3898
Contact: Pam Weatherly
National JCAHO-Accredited company providing a full range of Infusion and Respiratory therapies and specializing in the care of HIV/AIDS patients. National Case Manager is also available at 800-445-1188

Visiting Nurse Association of Orange County
1337 Braden Court
Orange, CA 92668-1123
Telephone: (714)-771-1209 Fax: (714)-288-4666
Home care, hospice, intermittent basis with nursing care and dailyvolunteers

Medical Services

Critical Care America
7755 Center Acenue
Suite 600
Huntingdon Beach, CA 92647
Telephone: (714)-379-0242 Fax: (714)-379-0244
Contact: Jot Hollenbeck - Senior Vice President
Coordinate & integrate all clinical & psychosocial services for HIV+

Orange Cty Health Care Agency/Mental Health Services
211 W. Commonwealth Ave
Fullerton, CA 92632-1810
Telephone: (714)-447-7000 Fax: (714)-447-7003
Contact: Rochelle Pierr

South Laguna Mental Health Services
30818 South Coast Hiway
South Laguna, CA 92677-2505
Telephone: (714)-499-1877

Testing Sites

Huntington Beach Community Clinic
17692 Beach Blvd # 200
Huntington Bch, CA 92647-6810
Telephone: (714)-847-4222
Contact: Jackie Cherewick
TB & HIV Antibody Testing/Call for appointment

Laguna Beach Community Clinic
460 Ocean Avenue
Laguna Beach, CA 92651
Telephone: (714)-494-0761 Fax: (714)-497-4591
Contact: Joan Corbin
FREE anonymous HIV antibody testing.

Orange Co HCA/Epidemiology/Diseases Control Division
1719 West 17th Street
Santa Ana, CA 92706-2316
Telephone: (714)-834-8025 Fax: (714)-834-8196
Contact: Dr. Penny Weinmuller
HIV testing, referrals, medical & public health resources

Orange County Center for Health, Inc.
503 North Anaheim Blvd
Anaheim, CA 92805-2648
Telephone: (714)-956-1900 Fax: (714)-956-9198
Contact: Marcia Vickey
Confidential HIV testing

Orange County Health Care Agency
725 West 17th Street
Santa Ana, CA 92701
Telephone: (714)-834-7991 Fax: (714)-824-2657
Contact: Project Coordinator
HIV testing, AZT program, medical, social and dental services.

Orange County Health Care Agency
1719 W. 17th
P.O. Box 6128
Santa Ana, CA 92701
Telephone: (714)-834-8025 Fax: (714)-834-8196
Contact: AIDS Coordinator
HIV testing for residents of Santa Ana, Anaheim and Garden Grove

Orange County Health Care Agency
1725 W. 17th Street
Santa Ana, CA 92706
Telephone: (714)-834-8787 Fax: (714)-834-7958
Contact: Dr. Jody Meador
Free, anonymous and confidential HIV testing

Planned Parenthood
1801 North Broadway
Santa Ana, CA 92706
Telephone: (714)-973-1733 Fax: (714)-973-1409
Toll-Free: (800)-752-6633
Confidential HIV antibody testing, by appt. only

Placer County

Community Services

Placid County AIDS Task Force
11484 B Avenue
Auburn, CA 95603
Telephone: (916)-889-7141 Fax: (916)-889-7192
Contact: AIDS Coordinator
Testing & counseling

Home Health Care

ABC Home Health Services Inc.
11795 Education Street
Suite 236
Auburn, CA 95602-2432
Telephone: (916)-823-5408 Fax: (916)-823-5431
Home Health Care

Auburn Faith Hospice
P.O.Box 8992
11815 Education Street
Auburn, CA 95602-8992
Telephone: (916)-823-9691 Fax: (916)-889-0721
Contact: Temeca LaMair - Hospice Supervisor
Volunteers assist AIDS patients

Auburn Faith Visiting Nurse Association
11760 Atwood Road
Suite 6
Auburn, CA 95603-9075
Telephone: (916)-885-7591 Fax: (916)-885-8404
Contact: Francis Rodriguez - Clinical Nursing Supervisor
Case support for HIV patients

Roseville Hospital Home Health/Hospice Care
333 Sunrise Avenue
Roseville, CA 95661
Telephone: (916)-781-3355 Fax: (916)-781-3581
Contact: Ruth Dunmore - Director of Hospice Services
Home health/hospice care

Medical Services

Placer-Nevada County Medical Society
1230 High Street
Room 211
Auburn, CA 95603
Telephone: (916)-885-3951
Medical Referrals

Roseville Hospital
333 Sunrise Avenue
Roseville, CA 95661
Telephone: (916)-784-7266
HIV patient care

Testing Sites

Planned Parenthood of Sacramento Valley, Roseville
151 North Sunrise
Suite # 815
Roseville, CA 95661
Telephone: (916)-781-3310 Fax: (916)-781-2338
Contact: Linda Allenby - Area Director
HIV testing

Riverside County

Community Services

Community Counseling and Consultation Center, Inc.
750 Vella Road
Palm Springs, CA 92264-1452
Telephone: (619)-323-2118 Fax: (619)-323-9865
Contact: Marc Haupert - Project Director
HIV health center, Primary care, social services, counseling, bereavement,home care

Desert AIDS Project - Community Counseling/Consortium
750 Vella Road
Palm Springs, CA 92264
Telephone: (619)-323-2118 Fax: (619)-323-9865
Contact: Richard See
HIV anonymous testing, counseling, referrals, support groups for PWA's andfamilies, home care, case management, benefits counseling, legal clinic

Inland AIDS Project
1240 Palmyrita Avenue
Suite E
Riverside, CA 92507-1704
Telephone: (909)-784-2437 Fax: (909)-784-5416
Contact: Mr. John Salley
HIV testing (anonymous), pre/post counseling, case management, foodbaskets, legal clinic, shelter, hospice care, education, outreach referrals

County Health Depts

Riverside County Department of Public Health
4065 County Circle Drive
PO Box 7600
Riverside, CA 92513-7600
Telephone: (909)-358-6400 Fax: (909)-358-6414
Contact: Dr. Bradley Gilbert
HIV testing (anonymous & confidential), pre/post counseling, casemanagement, referral, education, outreach

Medical Services

El Progresso Del Desierto, Inc.
51-800 Harrison
PO Box 245
Coachella, CA 92236-0245
Telephone: (619)-398-7277 Fax: (619)-398-8905
Contact: Cally Ramos
Medical and dental clinic, education, counseling, referrals

Sacramento County

Community Services

C.A.R.E.S. - Sacramento
2710 Capitol Avenue
Sacramento, CA 95816-6005
Telephone: (916)-443-3299 Fax: (916)-443-6629
Contact: Susan Strong - Executive Director
Health care, health education, HIV education, counseling, relatives &fashions & monitoring, health services

Legal Services of Northern California
515 12th Street
Sacramento, CA 95814-1418
Telephone: (916)-444-6760 Fax: (916)-444-6700
HIV/AIDS panel

Home Health Care

Country Home Health
10535 East Stockton Boulevard
Suites A and B
Elk Grove, CA 95624
Telephone: (916)-685-9815 Fax: (916)-686-8845
Contact: Barbara Case - Administrator
Skilled nursing, physical & occupational therapy

Critical Care America
1515 Sports Drive, #2
Sacramento, CA 95834
Telephone: (916)-928-0200 Fax: (916)-928-0420
Contact: Don Lewis
Infusion, equipment, medical services, etc.

Homedco Infusion
4244 A South Market Court
Sacramento, CA 95815
Telephone: (916)-927-5500 Fax: (916)-927-5533
Contact: Chris Jackson - Manager
Antibiotics, chemo, hydration, TPN, enternal

O.P.T.I.O.N. Care of Sacramento
3671 Business Drive
Sacramento, CA 95820-2165
Telephone: (916)-454-0444 Fax: (916)-454-3586
Contact: Ramona Moenter
Antibiotics, pain control, TPN, IV & aerosolized pentamidine, HIV supportgroups

Olsten Kimberly Quality Care
2020 Hurley Way
Suite # 485
Sacramento, CA 95825-3214
Telephone: (916)-929-2229 Fax: (916)-929-5431
Contact: Chris Stetner
Home care, home health aides

Medical Services

California Children Services, HIV Children Program
Sacramento County
10161 Croydon Way
Sacramento, CA 95827
Telephone: (916)-366-4000 Fax: (916)-369-0639
Contact: Alice Baber-Banks - Program Coordinator
Diagnostic Testing, Medical Treatment, Medical Support Services, Counseling

Sacramento Blood Center
1625 Stockton Boulevard
Sacramento, CA 95816-7089
Telephone: (916)-456-1500 Fax: (916)-452-9232
Donor center

Testing Sites

Bi-Valley Medical Clinic, Inc.
2100 Capitol Avenue
Sacramento, CA 95816-5721
Telephone: (916)-442-4985 Fax: (916)-442-1029
Contact: Daniel Steinhartator - AIDS Education Coordinator
AIDS education and prevention projects, HIV testing

Planned Parenthood of Sacramento Valley, AIDS Education
3510 Auburn Avenue
Suite 8
Sacramento, CA 95821
Telephone: (916)-482-8300 Fax: (916)-482-2149
Contact: Paula Adams
HIV testing (anonymous & confidental), counseling, training, outreach

San Benito County

County Health Depts

San Benito County Health Department
439 Fourth Street
Hollister, CA 95023
Telephone: (408)-637-5367 Fax: (408)-637-9073
Contact: Claudia Arnold, RN
HIV testing (confidential), counseling (pre & post), referrals, education

San Bernardino County

Community Services

Family Service of San Bernardino
1669 North E Street
San Bernardino, CA 92405-4498
Telephone: (909)-886-6737 Fax: (909)-881-3871
Contact: Mr. Woodward McHarg - Executive
Counseling, referral

Foothills AIDS Project
8880 Benson Avenue
Suite 114
Mont Clair, CA 91763
Telephone: (909)-920-9265 Fax: (909)-920-4139
Contact: Paul Miailovich - Administrative Assistant
Case management, buddy program, speakers bureau, support groups, foodpantry, care givers

West End Family Counseling Service
855 N. Euclid Avenue
Suite 3
Ontario, CA 91762
Telephone: (909)-983-2020 Fax: (909)-983-6847
HIV/AIDS counseling

Home Health Care

Caremark Connection Network
10431 Commerce Street
Redlands, CA 92374-4529
Telephone: (909)-796-0422
Contact: Operations Manager - Bonnie Kenneford;
Clinical support & infusion therapies: nutrition, antimicrobials, chemo.,Hematopoe

Modern Home Care
24711 Redlands Blvd.
Suite J
San Bernadino, CA 92408
Telephone: (909)-796-5306 Fax: (909)-799-9637
Contact: Robin Mendoza, RN
Home care, case management, referrals, infusion, nutritional advice, socialservice, extended care, IV medication

O.P.T.I.O.N. Care of the High Desert
15367-B Tamarack Road
Victorville, CA 92392-2443
Telephone: (619)-241-0424 Fax: (619)-241-3083
Home IV and Nutritional Services

Medical Services

California Children Services, HIV Children Program
San Bernardino County
351 Mountain View Avenue
San Bernardino, CA 92415-0001
Telephone: (909)-387-6200 Fax: (909)-387-6241
Contact: Ms. Tressa Hayes, PhN
Diagnostic testing, medical treatment, case management, counseling

Testing Sites

San Bernardino County Medical Center, Infectious Disease Unit
780 East Gilbert Street
San Bernardino, CA 92415-0001
Telephone: (909)-387-8111 Fax: (909)-387-0412
Contact: Dr. Steven Beutler
HIV testing (confidental), pre/post counseling, referrals

San Diego County

Community Services

Armed Services YMCA
500 West Broadway
San Diego, CA 92101-3506
Telephone: (619)-232-1133 Fax: (619)-237-0330
HIV Crisis Intervention Counseling & Referral for Military Personnel/Families.

Center for Social Services, Lesbian/Gay Community Center
P.O. Box 3357
San Diego, CA 92163-3357
Telephone: (619)-692-2077 Fax: (619)-260-3092
Contact: Dr. Jeff Leiphart - RHD
Massage, acupuncture, HIV testing, counseling, referrals

Navy Family Service Center, Miramar Naval Air Station
Building M-273
Code 320
Mirimar N.A.S., CA 92145
Telephone: (619)-537-4099 Fax: (619)-537-6447
Counseling, information, referrals, benefits and employment assistance

San Diego Council of Community Clinics, SANE
4646 Mission Gorge Pl.
San Diego, CA 92120
Telephone: (619)-265-2100 Fax: (619)-265-1414
Contact: Rick Siordian - Executive Director
AIDS Education and Prevention Projects

County Health Depts

San Diego County Department of Health Services
Office of AIDS Coordinator
P.O. Box 85524
San Diego, CA 92138-0524
Telephone: (619)-236-2254 Fax: (619)-236-2660
Contact: Bonnie Calender
Applies for federal grants and funds, referrals, housing coordinator forpeople with HIV

San Diego County Department of Health Services
1700 Pacific Hwy.
San Diego, CA 92138-5222
Telephone: (619)-236-2237 Fax: (619)-692-8448
Contact: Jane Young
AIDS Education and Prevention Projects, Training of Resource Personnel, Testing

Home Health Care

Caremark Health Care
5754 Pacific Center Blvd.
Suite 201
San Diego, CA 92121-4208
Telephone: (619)-597-0123
Contact: Branch Manager
Clinical support and infusion therapies: nutrition, antimicrobials, chemo.,hematopoeti

Critical Care America
5490 Complex St, #605
San Diego, CA 92123
Telephone: (619)-576-6969 Fax: (619)-974-6606
Contact: Scott Sales
Coordinate & integrate all clinical & psychosocial services for HIV+

Home Intensive Care, Inc.
6199 Cornerstone Court E
Suite 106
San Diego, CA 92121
Telephone: (619)-535-1547 Fax: (619)-455-1811
Contact: Director of Nursing
Home dialysis care

VCSD Home Care
6711 Convoy Court
San Diego, CA 92111
Telephone: (619)-744-7710 Fax: (619)-495-0382
Home Health Care

Medical Services

AIDS Ocular Treatment Center
UCSD Treatment Center Eye Clinic
2760 5th Ave, Ste 200
San Diego, CA 92103
Telephone: (619)-543-5099 Fax: (619)-543-1235
Contact: Dr. William Freeman - Director

Apogee Medical Group
3415 6th Avenue
San Diego, CA 92103
Telephone: (619)-295-4448 Fax: (619)-295-4499
Contact: Steve Anderson - Office Operations
HIV services for men & women

Beach Area Community Clinic
3705 Mission Boulevard
San Diego, CA 92109-7104
Telephone: (619)-488-0644 Fax: (619)-539-0517
Contact: Iris Payne
Primary care, health education, psychiatric and nutrition services

California Children Services, HIV Children Program
San Diego
6255 Mission Gorge Road
San Diego, CA 92120
Telephone: (619)-560-3400
Contact: Robyn Phelps
Diagnostic Testing, Medical Treatment, Medical Support Services, Counseling

North County Health Services
348 Rancheros Drive
San Marcos, CA 92069-2995
Telephone: (619)-471-2100 Fax: (619)-471-4694
Contact: Rick Duffer - AIDS Project Director
HIV testing, AIDS case management, dental care, mental health; Spanish &English

San Diego American Indian Health Center
2561 First Avenue
San Diego, CA 92103-6588
Telephone: (619)-234-2158 Fax: (619)-234-0206
Contact: William Poff - Executive Director
Medical & mental services; HIV counseling & testing; alcohol & substanceabuse counseling

Sharp Cabrillo Hospital
3475 Kenyon Street
San Diego, CA 92110-5066
Telephone: (619)-221-3400 Fax: (619)-221-3509
Contact: James Schibanoff, MD
Comprehensive HIV/AIDS medical services, testing

Sharp Memorial Hospital
7901 Frost Street
San Diego, CA 92123-2786
Telephone: (619)-541-3400 Fax: (619)-541-3514
Comprehensive HIV/AIDS medical services

University of California San Diego, Medical Center
UCSD Med. Ctr., H-672A
200 West Barbara Drive
San Diego, CA 92103-8681
Telephone: (619)-294-6255 Fax: (619)-297-8858
Contact: Willian C. Matthews - Medical Director;
HIV/AIDS testing, Comprehensive HIV/AIDS medical care.

Testing Sites

Linda Vista Health Care Center, San Diego County Health Dept
6973 Linda Vista Road
San Diego, CA 92111-6339
Telephone: (619)-279-0925 Fax: (619)-279-6471
Contact: Susan Cary
HIV Antibody Test Site, Counseling, Medical Services

San Diego Department of Health Services
104 South Barnes Street
Oceanside, CA 92054-3406
Telephone: (619)-967-4401 Fax: (619)-967-4644
Contact: Celis Gordon
HIV Antibody Test Site, Counseling, Medical Services

San Francisco County

Community Services

18th Street Services
217 Church Street
San Francisco, CA 94114-1319
Telephone: (415)-861-4898
Outpatient substance abuse counseling for gay & bisexual men

African American Men's Health Project
74 New Montgomery Street
600
San Francisco, CA 94105-3411
Telephone: (415)-597-9137 Fax: (415)-597-9213
Contact: Thomas J. Coates, PhD
Information, Education, Referrals

AIDS Benefit Counselors
470 Castro Street, #202
San Francisco, CA 94114-2061
Telephone: (415)-558-9845
Contact: Matthew Landis
Social Services; Information on Health Care, Social Security, Disability, etc.

AIDS Emergency Fund
1540 Market Street
#320
San Francisco, CA 94109-4708
Telephone: (415)-558-6999
Contact: Mark Tomaszweski
Funds for food, housing & other life emergencies for qualified.

AIDS Health Project
PO Box 0884
San Francisco, CA 94143
Telephone: (415)-476-6430 Fax: (415)-476-3655
Support groups for women who are sero-positive and worried well.

AIDS Legal Referral Panel
114 Sansome St, #31103
Suite 1129
San Francisco, CA 94104-3803
Telephone: (415)-291-5454 Fax: (415)-291-5833
Contact: Christine Chamber
Samples of wills and powers of attorney to persons with AIDS/ARC.

American Civil Liberties Union
1663 Mission Street, #460
San Francisco, CA 94103-2492
Telephone: (415)-621-2493
Contact: Dorothy Ehrlich
Legal Services

Baker New Place
3350 24th Street
San Francisco, CA 94110
Telephone: (415)-826-9574
Provides living space for people who have been sober for one month

Black and White Men Together/Men of All Colors Together
2261 Market Street
Box 506
San Francisco, CA 94114
Telephone: (415)-261-7922
Contact: Lee Woo
Information, Education, Referrals, Social Activities

The Bridge for Kids
1101 O'Farrell
San Francisco, CA 94117
Telephone: (415)-552-2437 Fax: (415)-567-7465
Childcare for families living with AIDS

California Department of Fair Employment and Housing
30 Van Ness, 3rd Floor
San Francisco, CA 94102-6020
Telephone: (415)-557-2006
Toll-Free: (800)-884-1684
Legal/Advocacy Services

Catholic Charities Hearing Impaired Program (Voice)
2891 Bush Street
San Francisco, CA 94115-2904
Telephone: (415)-749-3812 Fax: (415)-567-0916
Contact: Millie Stansfield - 415-567-0540
Counseling and Social Work for Hearing Impaired

Center for Southeast Asian Refugee Resettlement
875 O'Farrell
San Francisco, CA 94109-7005
Telephone: (415)-885-2743 Fax: (415)-885-3253
Contact: Kyle Moroe-Spencer
Information, education, referrals; Cant., Mand., Laotian, Viet., Cambodian

Commodity Supplemental Food Program
70 10th Street, 3rd Fl
San Francisco, CA 94103
Telephone: (415)-243-3100 Fax: (415)-243-3198
For pregnant women or children under 6 years of age.

Dept of Soc Services/Aid to Families with Dependent Children
170 Otis Street
San Francisco, CA 94103
Telephone: (415)-557-5723 Fax: (415)-557-5724
Financial aid

Employment Law Center/Legal Aid Society of San Francisco
1663 Mission Street #400
San Francisco, CA 94103-2449
Telephone: (415)-864-8848 Fax: (415)-864-8194
Contact: Joan Graff
Assistance for people with AIDS/ARC who have experienced employmentdiscrimination

Episcopal Sanctuary
201 8th Street
(at Howard Street)
San Francisco, CA 94103-3901
Telephone: (415)-863-3893 Fax: (415)-252-1743
Contact: Barbara Solomon
Emergency shelter only; no medical or nursing, wheelchair accessible,clinic two days a week for shelter residents

Family Link
400 Baker Street
Apt 102
San Francisco, CA 94117-2007
Telephone: (415)-346-0770
Contact: Ray Cope
Low cost accomodations for relatives/friends of people with-life-threatening illness.

Forensic AIDS Project-San Francisco Dept. of Public Health
798 Brannan Street
San Francisco, CA 94103-4919
Telephone: (415)-863-8237 Fax: (415)-863-3975
Contact: Ralle Greensburg
Information, Education, Counseling, Crisis Intervention, Referrals

Gay Legal Referral Service
114 Sansome Street
Suite 1129
San Francisco, CA 94104
Telephone: (415)-621-3900
Legal/Advocacy Services

Glide Memorial Church
330 Ellis Street
San Francisco, CA 94102-2793
Telephone: (415)-771-6300 Fax: (415)-921-6951
Contact: Leon Bacchues
Daily breakfast, lunch, & dinners for seniors and families with children;HIV clinic

Godfather Service Fund
584 Castro Street, #225
San Francisco, CA 94114-2588
Telephone: (415)-565-4433
Contact: Robert Docca - Co-Chairman
Social Services; Care Packages for Persons Hospitalized with AIDS/ARC

Haight Ashbury Alcohol Treatment Services
1698 Haight Street
San Francisco, CA 94117-2113
Telephone: (415)-552-7230 Fax: (415)-552-1645
Outpatient Alcohol Abuse Treatment

Haight Street Soup Kitchen
1525 Waller Street
off Belvedere Street
San Francisco, CA 94117-2817
Telephone: (415)-566-0366
Tu-Fri:Noon-1:00/Women with children at 11:30. Vegetarian alternative each day.

Japanese Community Youth Council
1596 Post Street
San Francisco, CA 94109-6511
Telephone: (415)-202-7905 Fax: (415)-563-1345
Contact: Jimmy Naritomi
Information, Education, Referrals, Support Services

Jewish Family and Child Services, AIDS Fund and Project
1600 Scott Street
San Francisco, CA 94115-3912
Telephone: (415)-567-8860 Fax: (415)-922-5938
Contact: Jody Reese - AIDS Project Coordinator
Counseling, Emergency Financial Assistance, Outreach

Larkin Street Youth Services (Street Youth)
1044 Larkin Street
San Francisco, CA 94109-5707
Telephone: (415)-673-0911 Fax: (415)-923-1378
Contact: Roxanne White
Referral services, awareness group, support group, housing for HIV, testing

Mano a Mano Project
2639 24th Street
San Francisco, CA 94110-3510
Telephone: (415)-647-5450 Fax: (415)-647-0740
Contact: Juanita Quintaro - Team Leader
Counseling and Support Groups; Latino/Spanish Speaking

Martin de Porres
225 Potrero Street
between 15th & 16th St.
San Francisco, CA 94103-4814
Telephone: (415)-552-0240
Contact: Barbra Collier
Soup kitchen

Most Holy Redeemer AIDS Support Group
100 Diamond Street
San Francisco, CA 94114-2414
Telephone: (415)-863-1581 Fax: (415)-863-2189
Contact: Louis Coloia, PhD.
Homecare buddy system, support for AIDS patients

Most Holy Redeemer Support Group
22 Henry Street
San Francisco, CA 94114-1215
Telephone: (415)-861-2329
Contact: William Reese
Home care, transportation to doctors &/or hospital

Narcotics Anonymous
205 13th Street
San Francisco, CA 94103-7365
Telephone: (415)-621-8600
Contact: ; ; - 1
Referrals to 12-step meetings in San Francisco. Also AIDS/ARC meetings.

Permanent Housing
3350 24th Street
San Francisco, Ca 94110
Telephone: (415)-826-9574
Terminally ill patients that are sober

Peter Clavor Community
1340 Golden Gate
San Francisco, CA 94115-4707
Telephone: (415)-749-3800 Fax: (415)-563-3153
Contact: Barbara Collins
Long-term Residential Care for PWAs/PWARCs with History of Substance Abuse

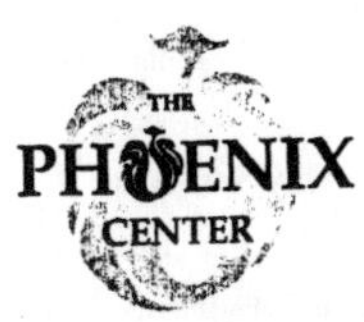

The Phoenix Center
2707 Pine Street
San Francisco, CA 94115
Telephone: (415)-563-7600
Fax: (415)-563-1544
Contact: Kenneth M. Abrams MD. - Medical Director; Pamela Brown - Coordinator
Provides 24-hr skilled Nursing Care and supervision. A full service 20 bed unit includes; Case Management, counseling, Family Support Services, complete nutritional program and activities, and hospice care.

Planned Parenthood - Alameda/San Francisco
815 Eddy Street, #300
San Francisco, CA 94109-7701
Telephone: (415)-441-7858 Fax: (415)-776-1449
Contact: Amanda Newsletter
Free anonymous HIV testing, education, medical services

Project Open Hand
2720 17th Street
San Francisco, CA 94110-1405
Telephone: (415)-558-0600 Fax: (415)-621-0755
Contact: Steve Burns - Director, Client Services
Services: prepare and deliver meals to PWA'S; AIDS food bank

Project Open Hand Food Bank
401 Duboce Abe
San Francisco, CA 94117
Telephone: (415)-252-1931 Fax: (415)-621-0755
Food assistance for HIV positive individuals

Richmond Area Multi-Services, MAXI Center
3626 Balboa Street
San Francisco, CA 94121-2604
Telephone: (415)-668-5955 Fax: (415)-668-0246
Counseling and Support Groups; Cantonese, Vietnamese, Cambodian, Korean

Salvation Army - Center for Social Services
445 9th Street
San Francisco, CA 94103-4410
Telephone: (415)-861-0755
Contact: Harry DeRuyter
Food or vouchers given on a case-by-case basis; call for appointment.

San Francisco AIDS Foundation's Emergency Housing Program
Baker Places, Inc.
310 Townsend
San Francisco, CA 94107
Telephone: (415)-546-9446 Fax: (415)-546-9947
Halfway houses, specialized residential treatment for gays/lesbians in recovery

San Francisco City, Dept. of Public Health, AIDS Office
25 Van Ness Avenue
4th Floor
San Francisco, CA 94102
Telephone: (415)-554-9173 Fax: (415)-431-9547
Contact: Coordinator - Jeff Amory;
Information, Education, Referrals

San Francisco Suicide Prevention
3940 Geary Boulevard
San Francisco, CA 94118-3219
Telephone: (415)-221-1423
Variety of support and referral services.

Shanti Project
525 Howard Street
San Francisco, CA 94105-3080
Telephone: (415)-777-2273 Fax: (415)-777-5152
Contact: Gloria Anadabo
Referrals, emotional & pratical support

Shanti Project (TTY)
525 Howard Street
San Francisco, CA 94105-3080
Telephone: (415)-495-7495 Fax: (415)-777-5152
Contact: Arlene Gonolez - Operations Manager
Information, referrals, support program, counseling

Audrey L. Smith Developmental Center/Childcare
1101 Masonic Avenue
San Francisco, CA 94117-2914
Telephone: (415)-863-0909 Fax: (415)-346-7931
Contact: 346-3268
Childcare, emergency services to families in crisis.

The National Center for Lesbian Rights
1663 Mission Street
5th Floor
San Francisco, CA 94103-2449
Telephone: (415)-621-0674 Fax: (415)-621-6744
Contact: Liz Hendrickson
Legal Assistance Services

United Way of the Bay Area, San Francisco
50 California Street
#200
San Francisco, CA 94111-4696
Telephone: (415)-772-4312 Fax: (415)-291-8352
Contact: Jackie Ruggles

Westside AIDS/ARC Project/Community Mental Health Center
1153 Oak Street
San Francisco, CA 94117
Telephone: (415)-431-9000 Fax: (415)-431-8351
Will coordinate housing, employment, income, and other maintenance services.

Home Health Care

Caremark Connection Network
1635 Divisadero Street
Suite 625
San Francisco, CA 94115
Telephone: (415)-202-9950 Fax: (415)-202-9950
Contact: Don Lawhorn - HIV Program Manager
Clinical Support and Infusion Therapies: Nutrition, Antimicrobials,Chemotherapy, Hematopoeti

CHS Home Health Agency
399 Buena Vista East
San Francisco, CA 94117-4170
Telephone: (415)-621-4562 Fax: (415)-431-1388
Private insurance & Medicare services: visiting RN, physical therapy, aidesetc

Coming Home Hospice/Visiting Nurses & Hospice of SF
Hospice Programs
1390 Market, Ste 510
San Francisco, CA 94102
Telephone: (415)-861-8705 Fax: (415)-431-4071
Contact: Director
Residential facility providing 24-hr care & supervision. Sliding scale fees.

Public Health Nurses
3850 17th St
near Noe Street
San Francisco, CA 94114-2031
Telephone: (415)-554-9770
Contact: Carol Suto
Monitor general physical condition, assess ability to manage at home. No fee.

Zen Center Hospice - Volunteer Program
273 Page Street
San Francisco, CA 94102-5699
Telephone: (415)-863-2910 Fax: (415)-863-1768
Training of Volunteers to Assist Outpatients

Medical Services

Acceptance Place
673 San Jose Avenue
San Francisco, CA 94110-4914
Telephone: (415)-695-1708 Fax: (415)-695-0829
Comprehensive 90-day resident alcohol and drug treatment program for gay males.

Alcoholism Evaluation and Treatment Center
San Francisco General Hosp./Ward 23
1001 Potrero Ave, Bldg 20
San Francisco, CA 94110
Telephone: (415)-206-8091 Fax: (415)-206-4232
42-day inpatient alcohol treatment program. Sliding scale.HIV support and HIV housing

Bay Area Addiction Research and Treatment (BAART)
1040 Geary Street
San Francisco, CA 94109-6908
Telephone: (415)-928-7800 Fax: (415)-928-7641
Methadone maintenance program for opiate addicts, counseling

California Detoxification Programs, Inc.
1040 Geary Street
San Francisco, CA 94109-6908
Telephone: (415)-928-7800
Short-term detoxification with counseling, medical services, and referral.

California Pacific Medical Center
2333 Buchanan St. at Clay
San Francisco, CA 94115
Telephone: (415)-563-4321
HIV testing, counseling & treatment, homecare, hospice, research

Chinatown-North Beach Clinic
1548 Stockton Street
San Francisco, CA 94133-3306
Telephone: (415)-398-0981 Fax: (415)-398-2305
Mental health counseling; Cantonese, Cambodian, Mandarin, Vietnamese,Italian/English

Continuum
10 United Nations Plaza
Suite 200
San Francisco, CA 94102
Telephone: (415)-241-5500 Fax: (415)-241-5511
Contact: Executive Director
Licensed day health care for people with AIDS

Continuum: HIV Day Services
10 United Nations Plaza
Suite 200
San Francisco, CA 94102-4910
Telephone: (415)-241-5507 Fax: (415)-241-5511
Contact: William D. Glenn - Director
Health care services

Department of Social Services/Medi-Cal
150 Otis Street
San Francisco, CA 94120-1221
Telephone: (415)-557-6188 Fax: (415)-557-5730
Medical office visits, nursing home care, lab, prescriptions, medicalsupplies

District Health Center No. 3/City of San Francisco Health
1525 Silver Avenue
(near San Bruno Avenue)
San Francisco, CA 94134-1221
Telephone: (415)-468-3664 Fax: (415)-467-3320
Screening for people without health care coverage. By appointment only.

Family Addiction Center for Education and Treatment
1040 Geary Street
San Francisco, CA 94109-6908
Telephone: (415)-928-7800
Comprehensive medical & psychological treatment for pregnant & postpartumaddicts

Financial District Women's Health Center
222 Front Street, 6th FL
San Francisco, CA 94111-4403
Telephone: (415)-982-0707 Fax: (415)-982-6304
Education, Medical Services, Free Anonymous HIV Testing

Independent Living
1326 4th Avenue
San Francisco, CA 94117-1419
Telephone: (415)-664-1868
Substance abuse residential treatment for AIDS/ARC/HIV positive men & women.

Letterman Army Medical Center/Screening & Education
Presidio of San Francisco
San Francisco, CA 94129-5000
Telephone: (415)-561-3929 Fax: (415)-561-6459
Screening, education, & medical for active duty military personnel & families.

Lyon-Martin Clinic
1748 Market, Suite 201
San Francisco, CA 94102
Telephone: (415)-565-7667 Fax: (415)-252-7490
Medical Services for Women, AIDS Prevention and Education

Medical Center Building
1726 Fillmore Street
Suite 201
San Francisco, CA 94115-3130
Telephone: (415)-346-1380
Contact: Hank Bermanpy/Consultant
Psychotherapy & counseling for HIV patients & families

Mt. Zion Hospital and Medical Center
1600 Divisadero Street
San Francisco, CA 94115-3010
Telephone: (415)-476-6356 Fax: (415)-885-7751
Contact: Laurance Drew
Outpatient services, HIV testing, research

Quan Yin Healing Project Center
1748 Market
San Francisco, CA 94102-5806
Telephone: (415)-861-4964 Fax: (415)-861-0579
Contact: Joe Browning - Administrator
Alternative treatment options, HIV education

Rape Treatment Center, San Francisco General Hospital
995 Potrero
Bldg. 80, Ward 87
San Francisco, CA 94110-2859
Telephone: (415)-821-3222 Fax: (415)-206-6859
Contact: Marilyn Lewis
Medical services, HIV testing, counseling, information and referrals

Richard A. Cazen, M.D.
45 Castro Street Annex
Suite 100
San Francisco, CA 94114-1010
Telephone: (415)-565-6288
Contact: Jeff Pound
Gastroenterology, Internal Medicine

San Francisco City, CMH - Team #2
298 Montery
San Francisco, CA 94131
Telephone: (415)-337-4795 Fax: (415)-337-4816
Mental health services only, no physical support provided

San Francisco City, CMH - Team #2
298 Monterey Blvd.
San Francisco, CA 94131
Telephone: (415)-337-4795 Fax: (415)-337-4816
Contact: BJ Douglass
Mental Health Services

San Francisco City, CMH - Team #2
298 Monterey Blvd
San Francisco, CA 94131-3140
Telephone: (415)-337-4795 Fax: (415)-337-4816
Mental Health Services

San Francisco General Hospital
Ward 86, Building 80
995 Potrero Avenue
San Francisco, CA 94110
Telephone: (415)-206-8830
Screening for people with AIDS/ARC symptoms. Appointment only/Thursday a.m.

St. Francis Memorial Hospital
900 Hyde Street
San Francisco, CA 94109-4899
Telephone: (415)-775-4321 Fax: (415)-353-6692
Contact: Joan Mazleyxt

Tenderloin Outpatient Clinic
251 Hyde Street
San Francisco, CA 94102-4008
Telephone: (415)-673-5700 Fax: (415)-292-7140
Contact: Cindy Gyori
AIDS/HIV counseling, crisis intervention & medical evaluation.

University of California Center on Deafness (Voice)
333 California Street
#10
San Francisco, CA 94143-1208
Telephone: (415)-476-4980 Fax: (415)-476-7113

Mental Health Services, Consultation, Inservice Training

Westside Methadone Treatment Program
1301 Pierce Street
San Francisco, CA 94115-4005
Telephone: (415)-563-8200 Fax: (415)-563-5985
Contact: JoAnn Newman
Long term & short term programs, counseling, medical services & referrals.

Testing Sites

Children's Hospital of San Francisco
3698 California Street
Suite 324
San Francisco, CA 94118-1697
Telephone: (415)-387-8700
Contact: 750-6160 - Emergency; 750-6031 - General Information; 750-6041
AIDS testing, social services

City Clinic
356 7th Street
San Francisco, CA 94103-4029
Telephone: (415)-864-8100 Fax: (415)-495-6463
Contact: Paul Mark Gibson
Call for appointments for testing early AIDS, HIV care program referrals

Health Center 1
3850 17th Street
San Francisco, CA 94114-2031
Telephone: (415)-554-9750
Contact: Carol Suto, RN
HIV testing and counseling, referral

South of Market Health Center
551 Minna Street
San Francisco, CA 94103-2831
Telephone: (415)-626-2951 Fax: (415)-626-1096
Contact: Anand Chaudhary
HIV testing

San Joaquin County

Community Services

San Joaquin AIDS Foundation, Community Education/Prevention
4410 North Pershing
Suite C-5
Stockton, CA 95207-6928
Telephone: (209)-476-8533 Fax: (209)-476-8142
Contact: Ronn Stockman
Legal referrals

San Joaquin Local Health District, AIDS Info. and Educ. Proj
1601 E Hazelton Avenue
Stockton, CA 95202
Telephone: (209)-468-3495
Contact: Project Coordinator - William Dorn; Substance Abuse Educator - Hipolita Villa; Latino Outreach Educator
Case management, benefits counseling, children's services, education andprevention

Home Health Care

Lodi Memorial Hospital Home Health Agency
975 South Fairmont
Lodi, CA 95240
Telephone: (209)-339-7581 Fax: (209)-368-7813
Contact: Marilyn Maki - Director
Nursing services

San Luis Obispo County

Community Services

AIDS Support Network
P.O. Box 12158
San Luis Obispo, CA 93406
Telephone: (805)-781-3660 Fax: (805)-781-3660
Contact: Susan Hughes
Counseling

Home Health Care

Home Health Care
P.O. Box 1489
San Luis Obispo, CA 93401
Telephone: (805)-781-4141 Fax: (805)-781-1236
Contact: Michele Groff
Home health, hospice, & AIDS case management program

Medical Services

California Children Services, HIV Children Program
2156 Sierra Way
San Luis Obispo, CA 93406
Telephone: (805)-781-5529 Fax: (805)-781-5541
Contact: Program Coordinator
Diagnostic Testing, Medical Treatment, Medical Support Services, Counseling

San Luis Obispo County Drug & Alcohol Services
1102 Laurel Lane
San Luis Obispo, CA 93408
Telephone: (805)-781-4753 Fax: (805)-781-1227
Contact: Paul Hyman
Mental health, social services

Testing Sites

San Luis Obispo County Health Services
12191 Johnson Avenue
San Luis Obispo, CA 93406
Telephone: (805)-781-5500 Fax: (805)-781-1235
Contact: Marsha Bollinger
Medical services; HIV testing & counseling

San Mateo County

Community Services

AIDS Project of San Mateo County
3700 Edison Street
San Mateo, CA 94403
Telephone: (415)-573-2588 Fax: (415)-573-2895
Full range of services

Don Mariacher
1779 Woodside Road
Suite #201
Redwood City, CA 94061
Telephone: (415)-776-0778
Psychotherapy (individual, families, couples) and crisis intervention

Home Health Care

Caremark Consortium
1048 El Camino Real
Redwood City, CA 94062
Telephone: (415)-364-6563 Fax: (415)-364-9001
Contact: Michael Edell
IV infusion treatments, participates in Clinical Drug Trials

Healthdyne Home Infusion Therapy, Inc.
884 Dubuque
San Francisco, CA 94080
Telephone: (415)-589-8962 Fax: (415)-589-2905
Contact: Craig Sheffer
Home infusion therapy, In-home Nursing and Attendant Care, P.T. Services,Pentamidine

Healthdyne Home Infusion Therapy, Inc.
884 Dubuque Ave.
S San Francisco, CA 94080
Telephone: (415)-589-8962
Home/Infusion/Therapy

nmc HOMECARE
200 Saginaw Drive
Redwood City, CA 94063
Telephone: (415)-366-1901
Fax: (415)-366-2760
Contact: Bill Zimmerman
National JCAHO-Accredited company providing a full range of Infusion and Respiratory therapies and specializing in the care of HIV/AIDS patients. National Case Manager is also available at 800-445-1188

West Bay Home Care Service
1900 Sullivan Avenue
Daly City, CA 94015
Telephone: (415)-991-6680 Fax: (415)-991-6368
Homemaking tasks, personal care

Medical Services

Central County Mental Health Center
3080 La Selva
San Mateo, CA 94403
Telephone: (415)-573-2544 Fax: (415)-573-2841
Outpatient mental health clinic

San Mateo General Hospital
3700 Edison
San Mateo, CA 94403-4364
Telephone: (415)-573-2222 Fax: (415)-573-2474
HIV counseling

Testing Sites

Ellipse - Peninsula AIDS Services
173 S. Blvd
San Mateo, CA 94402
Telephone: (415)-572-9702 Fax: (415)-572-1788
AIDS testing, food pantry for eligible patients

Santa Barbara County

Community Services

AIDS: Counseling & Assistance Program
126 E. Haley Street
Suite A17
Santa Barbara, CA 93101
Telephone: (805)-963-3636 Fax: (805)-963-9086
Contact: Nancy Self
Case management, support services/No fee.

Gay & Lesbian Resource Center
126 East Haley Street
Suite A17
Santa Barbara, CA 93101
Telephone: (805)-963-3636 Fax: (805)-963-9086
Contact: Derek Gordon
AIDS counseling & assistance programs; support groups, food pantry,volunteers, social work, management, HIV testing

Home Health Care

Critical Care America
1933 Cliff Dr, Ste 10
Santa Barbara, CA 93109
Telephone: (805)-965-6333
Contact: Jayne Johann
Coordinate & integrate all clinical & psychosocial services for HIV+

Integrated Care Systems
1933 Cliff Drive, #10
Santa Barbara, CA 93109
Telephone: (805)-965-6333
Contact: Jayne Johann
Superior, quality traditional and innovative infusion therapies in home

Santa Barbara Visiting Nurse Association
222 E Canon Perdido St
Santa Barbara, CA 93101-2263
Telephone: (805)-963-6794
Contact: Barbara Franzen - Nursing service/Hospice
Home Health Care and Hospice Services

Medical Services

California Children Services, HIV Children Program
Santa Barbara County
315 Camino Del Remedio
Santa Barbara, CA 93110
Telephone: (805)-681-5360
Contact: Elizabeth Kasehagen
Diagnostic Testing, Medical Treatment, Medical Support Services, Counseling

Calle Real Mental Health Service Center
4444 Calle Real
Santa Barbara, CA 93110
Telephone: (805)-681-5190 Fax: (805)-681-5239
Psychiatric Assessment, Eval., Crisis Intervention, Therapy, Case Management

Testing Sites

Planned Parenthood
518 Garden Street
Santa Barbara, CA 93101
Telephone: (805)-963-5801 Fax: (805)-965-2292
Contact: Wendy Raffetto
Anonymous and confidential testing.

Planned Parenthood
415 E. Chapel St
Santa Maria, CA 93454
Telephone: (805)-922-8317 Fax: (805)-928-7671
Contact: Ray Flemings - Director
HIV testing & counseling; community education; referrals

Santa Barbara Health Care Services/Public Health Clinic
315 Camino del Remedio
Santa Barbara, CA 93110
Telephone: (805)-681-5488 Fax: (805)-681-5424
Contact: Dr. Scott
Social, Medical, Education & Support/Testing by Appointment/Anonymous

Santa Clara County

Community Services

Adult Independence Development Center
1601 Clinic Center
Suite 100
Santa Clara, CA 95050
Telephone: (408)-985-1243 Fax: (408)-985-0671
Contact: Attendant Care Specialist
Support services for physically disabled persons toward independence in living.

American Cancer Society
535 Race Street
PO Box 26007
San Jose, CA 95159-3452
Telephone: (408)-287-5973 Fax: (408)-298-0112
Contact: Georgia Porter
Referrals, counseling

American Civil Liberties Union of Northern California
Santa Clara Valley Chapter
P.O. Box 215
Los Gatos, CA 95030-0215
Telephone: (408)-293-2584
Legal Aid

Aris Project
595 Millich Drive
104
Campbell, CA 95008
Telephone: (408)-370-3272
Contact: Executive Director - Julian di Ciurcio; Director,Volunteer Serv. -
Support services, education, housing for AIDS/ARC

Combined Addicts and Professional Services, Inc.
135 E Gish Road
Suite 200
San Jose, CA 95112
Telephone: (408)-441-7707
Contact: Outpatient Director - Jacqueline Novads
Outpatient Counseling/Groups for Drug Abusers not Requiring Residential Care

Community Services Agency of Mountain View and Los Altos
204 Stierlin Road
Mountain View, CA 94043
Telephone: (415)-968-0836 Fax: (415)-968-2164
Contact: Tom Pamilla
Homeless shelter, food, clothes closet, emergency rental assistance, foodkitchen

Deaf Counseling, Advocacy and Referral Agency
25 Dana Avenue
San Jose, CA 95126-2806
Telephone: (408)-298-6770 Fax: (408)-298-7971
Contact: Tony Papalia
Information & Referral for Deaf, Living Skills Training, Counseling, Job Help

Diocese of San Jose, Saint Julie Parish
366 Saint Julie Drive
San Jose, CA 95119
Telephone: (408)-629-3030
Contact: Parochial Vicar
Personal counseling for individual with AIDS/ARC or HIV positive, family.

Downtown Fellowship II & III, Inc.
561 South Almaden Avenue
San Jose, CA 95110
Telephone: (408)-998-4170
Contact: John Kerr - Executive Director
Male Only Alcohol Recovery Services, Room/Board, Recovery Classes, AA Oriented

Downtown Multi-Service Center
1075 East Santa Clara St.
San Jose, CA 95116
Telephone: (408)-299-6175
Counseling, individual, groups & family/Crisis services/Medication evaluation.

Emergency Housing Consortium
P.O. Box 2346
San Jose, CA 95109-2346
Telephone: (408)-993-0833
Contact: Rite Kemic - Assistant Director
Homelessness resource and learning center, transitional housing program

Hispanic AIDS Project
650 South Bascom
San Jose, CA 95128
Telephone: (408)-299-4734 Fax: (408)-299-8751
Contact: Juanita Pena Franco
Emotional and practical support, community outreach and counseling,suppport groups

Jewish Family Service
14855 Oka Road
Suite 3
Los Gatos, CA 95030
Telephone: (408)-356-7576 Fax: (408)-356-8736
Contact: Dr. Raymond Stovich - Executive Director
Counseling, Referral, Education to Community (Jewish Target Population)

Legal Aid of Santa Clara County
PO Box 103
San Jose, CA 95103-0103
Telephone: (408)-998-5200 Fax: (408)-298-3782
Contact: Harry Ramos
Advocacy, emergencies

Lima Family Mortuaries
710 Willow Street
San Jose, CA 95125
Telephone: (408)-295-5160
Funeral Services

Los Altos/Mountain View Ministers Association
1347 Richardson Avenue
Los Altos, CA 94022
Telephone: (415)-968-5778
Contact: Dr. Don Grant
Emotional/Spiritual Support to PWAs/Families, Referral to Ministers & Churches

Narvaez Hispanic AIDS Project - Josefa Narvaez MHC
Santa Clara County Health Dept.
650 S. Bascam Street
San Jose, CA 95128
Telephone: (408)-299-8751 Fax: (408)-275-6716
Contact: Project Coordinator
Community education, support, case management, counseling

Santa Clara County Bureau of Alcoholism Services/North County Center
270 Grant Avenue
Room 150
Palo Alto, CA 94306
Telephone: (415)-328-1441 Fax: (415)-329-8728
Contact: Cathleen Sheil

Santa Clara County Bureau of Alcoholism Services/West Valley
375 Knowles Drive
Los Gatos, CA 95030
Telephone: (408)-379-7020 Fax: (408)-379-6337
Contact: Kim Flatmo

Santa Clara County Outpatient Drug-Free Counseling Program
1675 Burdette Drive
Suite B
San Jose, CA 95121
Telephone: (408)-270-2587
Contact: Ernie Ortiz
Outpatient program for drug & alcohol abuses

SCC Bureau of Alcoholism Services/STEPS
1445-47 Oakland Rd
San Jose, CA 95112
Telephone: (408)-289-1070
Alcoholism services, AIDS education & services

South Valley Counseling Center
8475 Forrest Street, Suite A-2
P.O. Box 534
Gilroy, CA 95020
Telephone: (408)-842-7138
Contact: Beverly Nelson
Non-Residential Individual/Group/Family Therapy, Community Outreach, Referrals

County Health Depts

Santa Clara County Health Department
Hillview Clinic
1675 Burdette Dr., Ste A
San Jose, CA 95121
Telephone: (408)-274-7520
Outpatient Heroin Detox, Methadone Maintenance; Counseling, Medical Referrals

Santa Clara County Health Department AIDS Program
976 Lenzen Avenue
San Jose, CA 95126
Telephone: (408)-299-6245 Fax: (408)-275-9667
Contact: Marc Madsen - Clinic Coordinator
Free anonymous HIV antibody testing, early intervention project

Santa Clara County Health Department, Drug Abuse Bureau
South County Office
80 Highland Avenue
San Martin, CA 95046
Telephone: (408)-683-4053
Outpatient Heroin Detox, Methadone Maintenance; Counseling, Medical Referrals

Santa Clara County Health Department, Women's Health
976 Lienzen Avenue
San Martin, CA 95126
Telephone: (408)-683-4570 Fax: (408)-299-6245
Contact: Mark Madsen
AIDS education, administration, clinic, anonymous HIV testing by appt.only, early intervention program

Santa Clara County Health Dept, Mental Health Svcs. Bureau
Narvaez Mental Health
614 Tully Road
San Jose, CA 95111
Telephone: (408)-299-4734
Contact: Peter Digiulio, LMFCC
Mental Health Services: Individual/Group Counseling, Referral, Crisis Services

Santa Clara County HIV/AIDS Program
976 Lenzen Avenue
San Jose, CA 95126
Telephone: (408)-299-4151 Fax: (408)-275-9667
Contact: Mark Madsen - Coordinator
Clinical, alternative test site, early intervention, education, prevention

Home Health Care

Beverly Home Care
2875 Moorpark Avenue, #10
San Jose, CA 95128-1807
Telephone: (408)-247-5880 Fax: (408)-247-3426
Contact: Yvette Dudote
Licensed or Non-Licensed Help: RNs, LVNs, Live-Ins, CNAs

Beverly Home Health Center
2875 Moorpark Ave
Suite 100
San Jose, CA 95128
Telephone: (408)-326-3530 Fax: (408)-247-3426
Contact: Staffing Coordinator - Bobbi or Glenyce; 408-247-5880 (San Jose) -
Will provide licensed or non-licensed help as needed. Fees.

East Valley Public Health Nursing/Milpitas PHN
1989 McKee Road
San Jose, CA 95116
Telephone: (408)-251-2760 Fax: (408)-259-2308
Contact: Sonya Meissner
Comprehensive in-home support for AIDS/ARC patients.

Fair Oaks Public Health Nursing
660 S. Fair Oaks Avenue
Sunnyvale, CA 94086
Telephone: (408)-732-3720 Fax: (408)-245-3838
Contact: Sonya Meisner; Jeanette Richards -
Comprehensive in-home support for AIDS/ARC patients.

Homemaker Services, Inc.
2025 Gateway Place
Suite 234
San Jose, CA 95110
Telephone: (408)-452-1134 Fax: (408)-453-1222
In-home, non-medical supportive services for homebound; AIDS attendant care.

Hospice of the Valley
1150 S. Bascom Avenue
Suite 7A
San Jose, CA 95128
Telephone: (408)-947-1233 Fax: (408)-288-4172
Contact: Barbara Noggle
In-home medical & hospice care for terminally ill patients.

HSSI Home Care
1361 South Winchester Blvd
Suite 109
San Jose, CA 95128
Telephone: (408)-376-3522 Fax: (408)-376-3590
Contact: Connie Anderson - Supervisor
Services to homebound patients; Spanish, Japanese.

Narvaez Public Health Nursing
614 Tully Road
San Jose, CA 95111-1033
Telephone: (408)-299-4305
Contact: SPHN - Sandy Couser; SPHN - Shirley Garcie; PHN
In-Home Support for AIDS/ARC Patients, Referral, Nutritional Screening,TB and pregnancy testing

O'Connor Home Health Care Agency
455 O'Connor Drive
San Jose, CA 95128-1694
Telephone: (408)-947-2724 Fax: (408)-947-2572
Contact: Doris Miles
Nursing, home infusion therapy, womb care specialist, physical, socialwork, occupational, speech therapist, dietary

Olsten Health Care
1101 S Winchester Blvd
Suite L239
San Jose, CA 95128
Telephone: (408)-261-2801 Fax: (408)-261-9202
Contact: Susan Meyer - Director of Nurses
Private nursing care

Santa Clara Health Department, PHN Administration
2220 Moorpark Avenue
San Jose, CA 95128-2613
Telephone: (408)-299-5971 Fax: (408)-292-3750
Contact: Dena Dickinson
Comprehensive in-home support for AIDS/ARC patients; PHN Case Management

Visiting Nurse Association
2025 Gateway Place
Suite 205
San Jose, CA 95110
Telephone: (408)-452-1380 Fax: (408)-453-1222
Contact: Sharon Miller
Case Management, Home Care, In-Home Hospice, Attendant Care

Medical Services

Alexian Brothers Hospital
225 North Jackson Avenue
San Jose, CA 95116-1691
Telephone: (408)-259-5000
Contact: Mary Ann Palmieri, RN - Social Worker/Discharge
Acute Care Hospital

Armstrong Infectious Disease Clinic
340 Dardanelli Ln, Ste 26
Los Gatos, CA 95030-1418
Telephone: (408)-374-5340
Infectious disease. Initial evaluation and consultation

Avenues to Mental Health
86 S 14th St
San Jose, CA 95112
Telephone: (408)-293-6141
Contact: Director of Development
24-hour residential treatement, housing and case management

Combined Addicts and Professional Services, Inc.
398 12th Street
San Jose, CA 95112
Telephone: (408)-294-5425
Contact: Jacqueline Novads - Executive Director
6-Month Residential Drug Treatment Prog. for Total Abstinence and Self-Support

Dr. Greg Loitz, DDS, MD
150 North Jackson Avenue
Suite 108
San Jose, CA 95116
Telephone: (408)-254-0500 Fax: (408)-254-9536
Contact: Heather Hickerson
Oral & manillofacial surgeon

East Valley Clinic
1993 McKee Road
San Jose, CA 95116
Telephone: (408)-259-9160 Fax: (408)-258-2812
Contact: Jean Middaugh, RN - Clinical Nurse
Outpatient Clinic Services for East Side Residents, Multilingual

Evergreen Valley College, Student Health Center
3095 Yerba Buena Road
San Jose, CA 95135
Telephone: (408)-270-6480 Fax: (408)-238-3179
Contact: Doris DeCecco
Student Primary Health Clinic, Family Planning Services, Health Education,anonymous HIV testing, pre/post counseling, students olny

George I. Deabill
PO Box 60365
Palo Alto, CA 94306
Telephone: (415)-494-3363
General psychotherapy, clinical sexology, marriage and family counseling.

Good Samaritan Hospital
2425 Samaritan Drive
San Jose, CA 95124
Telephone: (408)-559-2276
Contact: Nancy Ricossa, MSW - Infection Control Nurse
Acute Care Hospital, Psychosocial Counseling, Referrals, Home Care Planning

Interaction Psychotherapy and Counseling Center
925 West Hedding Street
San Jose, CA 95126
Telephone: (408)-246-4422
Psychological Assessment; Brief, Long-Term Individual, Family, CoupleCounseling

Kaiser Foundation Hospital Milpitas
770 East Calaveras Blvd.
Milpitas, CA 95035
Telephone: (408)-945-2933
Contact: Donna DeClue
Full Service Medical Center

Kaiser Foundation Hospital Santa Clara
900 Kiely Boulevard
Santa Clara, CA 95051-5386
Telephone: (408)-236-4170 Fax: (408)-236-6981
Contact: HIV Service Coordinator
Medical Services, Hemophilia Services, Counseling, Discharge Planning,Referrals

Kaiser Mountainview Clinic
555 Castro Street
Mountain View, CA 94041
Telephone: (415)-903-3000
Contact: Catherine Collins, MD - Internal Medicine; Roger Newton, MD - Internal Medicine
General service, pediatrics, OB-GYN

Mission Oaks Hospital
15891 Los Gatos Almaden Rd
Los Gatos, CA 95030
Telephone: (408)-356-4111 Fax: (408)-358-5633
Contact: Maureen Texeira - Infection Control
Acute care hospital

Mountain View Community Health Center, Inc.
P.O. Box 447
101 Stierlin Road
Mountain View, CA 94043
Telephone: (415)-965-3323 Fax: (415)-965-0706
Contact: Belinda Montes
General medical services, diagnosis/treatment of STDs, referrals

San Jose Medical Center
675 East Santa Clara ST.
San Jose, CA 95112-1982
Telephone: (408)-998-3212
Contact: Director Patient - Nenna Kirschner; Infection Control;
Acute Care hospital with specialty units.

Santa Clara County California Children Services, HIV Children Program
720 Empey Way
San Jose, CA 95128-2613
Telephone: (408)-299-5891 Fax: (408)-971-3538
Contact: Rosita Saw - Program Coordinator
Diagnostic Testing, Medical Treatment, Medical Support Services, Counseling

Santa Clara County Health Department AIDS Program
Medical Services Division
2220 Moorpark Avenue
San Jose, CA 95128
Telephone: (408)-299-4151
Contact: David Burgess - Director; Millicent Kellogg - Administrative Coordinator
Provides community education, clinical services and consultation.

Santa Clara County Health Dept, Mental Health Svcs. Bureau
Downtown Multiservice Ctr
1075 East Santa Clara St.
San Jose, CA 95116
Telephone: (408)-299-6175 Fax: (408)-298-0182
Contact: Rich Galvan
Mental Health Services: Individual/Group Counseling, Referral, Crisis Services

Santa Clara County Health Dept, Mental Health Svcs. Bureau
East Valley Mental Svcs
1991 McKee Road
San Jose, CA 95116
Telephone: (408)-926-2900 Fax: (408)-258-5528
Contact: Shirley Miller
Mental Health Services: Individual/Group Counseling, Referral, Crisis Services

Santa Clara County Health Dept, Mental Health Svcs. Bureau
Access Center
2221 Enborg Lane
San Jose, CA 95128
Telephone: (408)-299-5800
Contact: Louis Pollard
Mental health services, referrals, grief access program

Santa Clara Valley Medical Center, AIDS Program
751 South Bascom Avenue
San Jose, CA 95128-2699
Telephone: (408)-299-5523 Fax: (408)-299-8806
Contact: Onnie Lang - RN; Dr. Stanley Dereskinski - Chief Infectious Disease
Emergency and Inpatient Acute Care, Outpatient AIDS Followup, Research Protocol

Santa Clara Valley Medical Ctr.
751 South Bascom
Annex Bldg
San Jose, CA 95128-2699
Telephone: (408)-299-5746 Fax: (408)-299-8806
Contact: Onnie Lang - AIDS Program Coordinator
Education, primary treatment, research, testing

Santa Teresa Community Hospital
250 Hospital Parkway
San Jose, CA 95119-1199
Telephone: (408)-972-3000
Acute Care Hospital

SCC Bureau of Alcoholism Services/Proyecto Primavera
614 Tully Road
San Jose, CA 95111-1033
Telephone: (408)-977-1591
Alcoholism services, knowledge of AIDS-related issues.

South Valley Hospital
9400 No Name Uno
Gilroy, CA 95020
Telephone: (408)-842-5621
Acute care hospital, HIV testing, counseling

South Valley Medical Clinic
90 Highland Avenue
San Martin, CA 95046
Telephone: (408)-683-0310 Fax: (408)-683-4393
Contact: Louise Deal
Primary care

West Valley Mental Services
375 Knowles Drive
Los Gatos, CA 95030
Telephone: (408)-379-7020
Individual/group counseling, referral, crisis service & HIV referrals

Testing Sites

Family Planning Alternatives, Inc.
505 West Olive Avenue
#210
Sunnyvale, CA 94086
Telephone: (408)-739-5151 Fax: (408)-739-5258
Anonymous HIV Testing, Pre and Post Test Counseling by American Red Cross

Planned Parenthood
1691 The Alameda
San Jose, CA 95126-2203
Telephone: (408)-287-7532 Fax: (408)-971-6935
Contact: Lynn Fielder - AIDS Counselor
HIV testing, anonymous and confidential. Pre and post-test counseling.

Santa Cruz County

Community Services

Santa Cruz AIDS Project
911 A Central Street
Santa Cruz, CA 95060
Telephone: (408)-427-3900 Fax: (408)-427-0398
Contact: John Laird - Director
Home care, outreach, HIV testing (anonymous), pre/post counseling,referrals

Shasta County

County Health Depts

Shasta County Health Department
2650 Breslawer Way
Redding, CA 96001
Telephone: (916)-225-5591 Fax: (916)-225-5074
Contact: Steven Plank, MD
Testing, counseling, educational services

Home Health Care

Owens Pharmacy - O.P.T.I.O.N Care
2021 Court Street
P.O. Box 90550
Redding, CA 96099
Telephone: (916)-241-2273 Fax: (916)-241-1563
Home IV and Nutritional Services

Sierra County

County Health Depts

Sierra County Health Department
202 Front Street
PO Box 7
Loyalton, CA 96118
Telephone: (916)-993-6700
Contact: Donna Hall, PHN - AIDS Coordinator

Siskiyou County

Home Health Care

Siskiyou Home Health Services
1217 South Main, Suite B
Eureka, CA 96097
Telephone: (916)-842-7325
Home health care, intravenous on call

Solano County

Community Services

Solano AIDS Task Force
355 Tuolumne Street
Vallejo, CA 94590
Telephone: (707)-553-5033 Fax: (707)-553-5071
Contact: Curt Smith
Case management, support groups, benefits, counseling

Solano County AIDS Task Force
PO Box 749
Fairfield, CA 94533
Telephone: (707)-553-5033 Fax: (707)-553-5071
Contact: Lisa Swehla
Case management, referrals, housing, support groups, benefits, counseling

Home Health Care

Northbay Health at Home and Hospice
1101 B Gale Wilson Blvd
#301
Fairfield, CA 94533
Telephone: (707)-429-7756 Fax: (707)-429-6846
Contact: Barbara Walters
Home Health Care, Hospice

Solano County Home Health Services
355 Tuolumne Street
Vallejo, CA 94590
Telephone: (707)-553-5571 Fax: (707)-553-5649
Contact: Sharon Blake
Home Health Care

Medical Services

Genesis House
1149 Warren Street
Vallejo, CA 94590
Telephone: (707)-552-5295 Fax: (707)-552-5295
Contact: Lloyd Gieg
Long-term residential alcohol and drug treatment, hotline 707-557-3165

Primary Care Clinic
2100 West Texas
Fairfield, CA 94533
Telephone: (707)-421-6650 Fax: (707)-421-6659
Contact: Dr. Maus
Family clinic, HIV testing & counseling, STD, prenatal

Vacaville Community Clinic
40 Eldridge Avenue
Suite E-10
Vacaville, CA 95688
Telephone: (707)-446-0196 Fax: (707)-446-4024
Contact: Executive Director
Medical Services, AIDS-Related Projects

Testing Sites

Planned Parenthood, Fairfield Center
1325 Travis Boulevard
Suite C
Fairfield, CA 94533
Telephone: (707)-429-8855 Fax: (707)-429-0285
HIV testing and counseling

State of California - Dept of Corrections
Calif. Medical Facility
P.O. Box 2000
Vacaville, CA 95696-2000
Telephone: (707)-448-6841 Fax: (707)-453-7010
Contact: Dr. Bick
HIV testing and counseling

Sonoma County

Community Services

Face to Face/Sonoma City AIDS Network
P.O. Box 1599
Guerneville, CA 95446
Telephone: (707)-887-1581 Fax: (707)-869-1461
Contact: Terry Scott - MSW
Case management, benefits counseling, education, housing assistance,support groups, emergency funding

Sonoma County AIDS Project
3313 Chanate Road
Santa Rosa, CA 95404
Telephone: (707)-576-4363 Fax: (707)-576-4694
Contact: Pat Kuta
Schedules HIV testing at 5 different sites, prevention education, outreach,training hotline

Home Health Care

Homedco Infusion
960 Hopper Avenue
Santa Rosa, CA 95403
Telephone: (707)-579-3020 Fax: (707)-579-5408
Contact: Nicola Dempsey
Experienced in providing quality home infusion therapy to HIV/AIDS patients

Medical Services

Scott Cozza - Professional Counseling
159 Kentucky Street
Room 10
Petaluma, CA 94952
Telephone: (707)-762-1557
Contact: Scott Cozza
HIV education, literature, outreach, counseling

Stanislaus County

County Health Depts

Stanislaus County Department of Public Health
820 Scenic Drive
Modesto, CA 95350-6194
Telephone: (209)-525-7301 Fax: (209)-525-5337
Contact: Kris Owens, MPH - Director, Public Health
AIDS education and prevention projects, training, phoneline

Stanislaus County Public Health Department
820 Scenic Drive
Modesto, CA 95350
Telephone: (209)-525-7339 Fax: (209)-525-5337
Contact: Jean Yokotobi - Chaiman
Testing, case management, nutritional service, surveillance, education

Home Health Care

Community Hospice
601 McHenry Avenue
Suite C
Modesto, CA 95350
Telephone: (209)-577-0615
Contact: Ann Bonfiglio
Hospice, case management

Home Care of Memorial
1800 Coffee Road
Suite 50
Modesto, CA 95355
Telephone: (209)-572-7104 Fax: (209)-572-7058
Home Health Care

Home Health Care and Hospice of Emanuel
P.O. Box 2120
825 Delbon Avenue
Turlock, CA 95381-2120
Telephone: (209)-667-4663 Fax: (209)-667-4689
Contact: Renette Bronkin - RN
Home health care, hospice, case management

Home Health Services of Doctor's Medical Center
P.O. Box 4921
1700 McHenry Ave. Ste 27B
Modesto, CA 95350
Telephone: (209)-578-0507 Fax: (209)-522-9887
Contact: Barbara Norquist
Skilled nursing care

Homedco Infusion
4230 Kiernan Ave
Modesto, CA 95356
Telephone: (209)-545-8540 Fax: (209)-545-6072
Infusion therapy to home HIV/AIDS patients

Sutter County

County Health Depts

Sutter County Health Department
1445 Circle Drive
P.O. Box 1510
Yuba City, CA 95993
Telephone: (916)-741-7215 Fax: (916)-741-7223
Contact: Allen L. Leavitt - Health Officer
Free confidential HIV antibody testing, referral services.

Tehama County

County Health Depts

Tehama County Health Department
1860 Walnut Street
Red Bluff, CA 96080-3698
Telephone: (916)-527-6824 Fax: (916)-527-0249
Contact: Cathy Crocecer; Valerie Lucero - AIDS Coordinator; Jeanette Smith, PHN - Chairman, AIDS Task Force
AIDS services, AIDS task force, community education and preventionprojects, HIV testing & counseling

Home Health Care

St. Elizabeth Hospital Home Health Agency and Hospice
2550 St. Mary Columbia Dr
Red Bluff, CA 96080-4397
Telephone: (916)-527-4880 Fax: (916)-527-3368
Contact: Bobbie Krup
Home Health Care, Hospice

Medical Services

Tehama County Medical Society
P.O. Box 1212
Red Bluff, CA 96080-1212
Telephone: (916)-527-7082 Fax: (916)-527-2972
Medical Referrals

Tehama County Mental Health Services
1860 Walnut Street
Red Bluff, CA 96080-3698
Telephone: (916)-527-5631 Fax: (916)-527-0249
Contact: Carl Havener
Drug Treatment, Community Services

Trinity County

Community Services

Trinity County Counseling Center
P.O. Box 1640
Weaverville, CA 96093-1640
Telephone: (916)-623-1362 Fax: (916)-623-5830
Contact: Dr. Donald Williams
Drug Treatment, Community Services, Counseling

County Health Depts

Trinity County Health Department
P.O. Box 1257
Weaverville, CA 96093
Telephone: (916)-623-1358 Fax: (916)-623-3480
Contact: Donald Krouse - Helath Officer
AIDS Services, AZT Drug Program

Home Health Care

Trinity Home Health Agency
P.O. Box 1229
410 North Taylor Street
Weaverville, CA 96093-1229
Telephone: (916)-623-5541 Fax: (916)-623-3073
Contact: Patty Olives-Matz
Home Health Care

Tulare County

Community Services

Woodlake Family Health Centers
180 East Antelope
Woodlake, CA 93286
Telephone: (209)-564-8067 Fax: (209)-564-8420
AIDS-Related Projects

Home Health Care

Critical Care America
430 W Caldwell Avenue
Suite A
Visalia, CA 93227
Telephone: (209)-734-2896 Fax: (209)-734-6451
Contact: Barbara Beaty
Coordinate & integrate all clinical & psychosocial services for HIV+

Tuolumne County

Community Services

Sierra AIDS Council
P.O. Box 1062
Sonora, CA 95370-1602
Telephone: (209)-533-2873
Contact: Mr. Gail Brabec
Client care, support groups, education, prevention & outreach

Medical Services

Tuolumne County Medical Society
1 Forest Road
PO Box 3234
Sonora, CA 95370
Telephone: (209)-532-4843
Contact: Mary Ellinger
Medical Referrals

Tuolumne County Mental Health Svcs, Alcohol & Drug Services
P.O. Box 4255
Sonora, CA 95370-4255
Telephone: (209)-533-5775 Fax: (209)-536-1948
Contact: Bea Readel - Substance Control Coordinator
Drug treatment education, prevention & outreach, referrals

Tuolumne Medical Clinic
P.O. Box 1386
Tuolumne, CA 95379-1386
Telephone: (209)-928-4225 Fax: (209)-928-1598
Contact: Jerry Boyajian - Director
HIV referrals

Ventura County

Community Services

Alcoholics Anonymous
321 N Aviador St, #115
Camarillo, CA 93010-8333
Telephone: (805)-389-1444
Contact: Shirley McCormack

All Saints Episcopal Church Oxnard
144 South "C" Street
Oxnard, CA 93030
Telephone: (805)-483-2347
Church and Spiritual Support

Buena Ventura Legal Clinic
1239 E. Main Street
Ventura, CA 93001-3180
Telephone: (805)-653-7642 Fax: (805)-653-5976
Legal Services

Catholic Social Services
402 North A Street
Oxnard, CA 93030
Telephone: (805)-486-2900
Nutrition Resources, Limited Emergency Food, Temporary Emergency Housing

Church of the Oaks
United Church of Christ
950 Warwick Avenue
Thousand Oaks, CA 91360
Telephone: (805)-495-4587
Contact: Frank Johnson - Pastor
Church and Spiritual Support

Crystal Lodge
1787 Thompson
Ventura, CA 93001
Telephone: (805)-648-2272
Accommodations, Accepts Vouchers from General Relief

Meals on Wheels, Conejo Valley/Thousand Oaks
401 Hoden Camp Road
Thousand Oaks, CA 91360
Telephone: (805)-496-2009
Contact: Judy Brown
Nutrition, Meals for Homebound Persons

Meals on Wheels, Santa Paula
P.O. Box 569
Santa Paula, CA 93061
Telephone: (805)-525-8277
Nutrition, Meals for Homebound Persons

Meals on Wheels, Ventura and Oxnard
234 Vince
Ventura, CA 93001
Telephone: (805)-643-5653
Nutrition, Meals for Homebound Persons

Ocean View
1690 East Thompson
Ventura, CA 93001
Telephone: (805)-648-2494
Accommodations

Salvation Army
138 West Hill Street
Oxnard, CA 93030
Telephone: (805)-483-9235
Contact: Lt. Fred Morasky
Limited Emergency Food for People in Need, Temporary Emergency Housing

Simi Valley Council on Aging, Meals on Wheels
3900 Avenida Sim
Simi Valley, CA 93065
Telephone: (805)-526-9237 Fax: (805)-583-6300
Contact: Kathryn B. Oliver
Nutrition, Meals for Homebound Persons, noon time meals

Ventura Alcoholics Anonymous
739 East Main Street
Ventura, CA 93001
Telephone: (805)-652-7823
Drug and Alcohol Abuse Program

Ventura County Public Social Services Agency
Ventura District Office
4651 Telephone Road
Ventura, CA 93003
Telephone: (805)-658-4100 Fax: (805)-658-4116
Contact: Maria Older
Social Services, General Relief, Medi-Cal, food stamps

Ventura County Public Social Services Agency
Santa Paula Dist. Office
1320 East Main Street
Santa Paula, CA 93060
Telephone: (805)-525-1505 Fax: (805)-933-8447
Contact: Teresa Eleness
Social Services, General Relief, Medi-Cal, food stamps

Ventura County Public Social Services Agency
Oxnard District Office
1400 Vangard Avenue
Oxnard, CA 93030
Telephone: (805)-385-8519 Fax: (805)-385-1894
Contact: Cynthia Bengston
Social services, general relief, medi-cal, food stamps

Ventura County Public Social Services Agency
Simi Valley Dist. Office
2003 East Royal Avenue
Simi Valley, CA 93065
Telephone: (805)-584-4840 Fax: (805)-548-4814
Contact: Kathi Strahl
Social Services, General Relief, Medi-Cal, food stamps

Ventura County Rescue Mission
234 East Sixth Street
Oxnard, CA 93030
Telephone: (805)-487-8252 Fax: (805)-487-2427
Contact: David Shaw
Limited Emergency Food, Temporary Emergency Housing for Men Only

County Health Depts

Ventura County Health Department
3147 Loma Vista Road
Ventura, CA 93009
Telephone: (805)-652-5918 Fax: (805)-652-5784
Contact: Martina Rippey, PHN - AIDS Coordinator, Diane Seyl - Testing Coordinator
Medical Services, HIV Antibody Testing, Alternative (Anonymous) Test Site

Home Health Care

American Cancer Society
1363 Del Norte Road
Camarillo, CA 93010
Telephone: (805)-497-0114 Fax: (805)-983-3751
Contact: Nancy Shook
Home health care and hospice services

Camarillo Hospice
2309 Antonio Avenue
Camarillo, CA 93010
Telephone: (805)-484-2831 Fax: (805)-389-5631
Home Health Care and Hospice Services

Help Unlimited
402 W. Ojai Avenue, #202
Ojai, CA 93023
Telephone: (805)-656-4000 Fax: (805)-640-0612
Contact: Gayle Bertsch
Nursing/home health services

Hospice Caring Neighbors, Help of Ojai
P.O. Box 621
111 West Santa Ana Street
Ojai, CA 93023
Telephone: (805)-646-9752
Hospice services and support counseling

Meditech
4562 Westinghouse Street
Suite A
Ventura, CA 93003
Telephone: (805)-963-8949 Fax: (805)-658-2195
Contact: Sharon Bick
Nursing/Home Health Services

Olsten Kimberly Quality Care
1901 N Solar Drive
Suite 175
Oxnard, CA 93030
Telephone: (805)-485-8585 Fax: (805)-485-4313
Contact: Barbara Bucher
Nursing/Home Health Services

Ombudsman Program
1841 Knoll Drive
Ventura, CA 93003
Telephone: (805)-656-1986
Skilled nursing care, residential care, pre-placement, support group

Santa Clara Valley Hospice
P.O. Box 365
121 Davis Street
Santa Paula, CA 93060
Telephone: (805)-525-1333
Contact: Kathryn Anderson - Executive Director
Hospice services

Medical Services

Buena Ventura Medical Clinic, Inc.
2705 Loma Vista Road
Ventura, CA 93003
Telephone: (805)-652-5200 Fax: (805)-652-5178
Medical Services, Immediate care 24 hours a day

Community Health Projects, Methadone Clinic, Oxnard
2055 Saviers Road
Suite 10
Oxnard, CA 93030
Telephone: (805)-483-2253 Fax: (805)-483-2255
Drug and Alcohol Abuse Program

Dental Society of Santa Barbara/Ventura County
1607 East Thompson Blvd.
Ventura, CA 93001
Telephone: (805)-656-3166 Fax: (805)-648-5154
Dental Referrals

Oxnard Mental Health
1400 Vangard Avenue
Oxnard, CA 93033
Telephone: (805)-385-8665 Fax: (805)-385-9105
Contact: Robert Soliz
Counseling and Mental Health Services

Sierra Vista Family Clinic
4531 Alamo Avenue
Simi Valley, CA 93065
Telephone: (805)-584-4885
Medical services, primary care referrals to Ventura County Clinic

Simi Mental Health
3150 Los Angeles Avenue
Simi Valley, CA 93065
Telephone: (805)-584-4881
Contact: Hector Trevino
Counseling

Ventura Clinic Special Projects
95 East Thompson Blvd.
Suite 250
Ventura, CA 93001
Telephone: (805)-648-9522 Fax: (805)-658-4188
Contact: Lynn Evans-Reister
Drug and alcohol abuse, HIV testing, counseling

Ventura County Medical Center
3291 Loma Vista Road
Ventura, CA 93003
Telephone: (805)-652-6236
Contact: Waldi Holloway
Drug & Alcohol Abuse Program, Counseling, Referral, Antabuse and Detox Services

Ventura County Medical Society
625 East Santa Clara
Ventura, CA 93001
Telephone: (805)-656-3407 Fax: (805)-643-5337
Medical Referrals to Private Physicians

Ventura County Mental Health Outpatient Services
1400 Bandguard Avenue
Oxnard, CA 93030
Telephone: (805)-385-8665 Fax: (805)-385-9105
Contact: Robert Soliz
Mental Health, Counseling, Therapy

Ventura County Mental Health Services
300 Hillmont Avenue
Ventura, CA 93003
Telephone: (805)-652-6768
Counseling and mental health services; crisis -- 805-652-6727

Westside Family Practice
400 E. Santa Barbara Street
Suite A
Santa Paula, CA 93060
Telephone: (805)-525-2121
Ventura County Clinic, Medical Services

Testing Sites

Oxnard Multi-Service Center
2500 South "C" Street
Suite D
Oxnard, CA 93030
Telephone: (805)-385-8647 Fax: (805)-385-9134
Contact: Sally Malisky
Medical Services, HIV Antibody Testing, Alternative (Anonymous) Test Site

Yolo County

County Health Depts

Yolo County Health Department
10 Cottonwood Street
Woodland, CA 95695
Telephone: (916)-666-8649 Fax: (916)-666-8674
Contact: Cris Cipperly
AIDS services, AZT drug program, AIDS task force, AIDS-related projects

Home Health Care

Woodland Memorial Hospital Home Health Care
1325 Cottonwood Street
Woodland, CA 95695
Telephone: (916)-662-3961 Fax: (916)-662-3961
Contact: Sue Rollansbee
Home health care

Medical Services

Yolo County Department of Alcohol and Drug Programs
201 West Beamer Street
Woodland, CA 95695
Telephone: (916)-666-8650
Contact: Joan Parnas - Administrator
Drug treatment, community services, HIV testing, support

Testing Sites

Davis Community Clinic
620 G Street
Davis, CA 95616
Telephone: (916)-758-2060 Fax: (916)-758-8490
Contact: Cheryl Lathan - HIV Coordinator
HIV testing

Esparto Family Practice
P.O. Box 134
Esparto, CA 95627
Telephone: (209)-948-5410
Contact: Deanna Rangel - HIV Coordinator
HIV testing program (Mon & Wed)

Yuba County

County Health Depts

Marysville County Health Department
6000 Lindhurst Avenue
Suite 601-B
Marysville, CA 95901-0429
Telephone: (916)-741-6259 Fax: (916)-741-6397
Contact: Val Spooner, RN
HIV testing anonymous confidential, pre-post counseling, referrals,education

Yuba City County Health Department
P.O. Box 429
938 14th Street
Marysville, CA 95901
Telephone: (916)-741-6366 Fax: (916)-741-6397
Contact: Jackie Travis - Public Health Admin
HIV testing (anonymous & confidential), referrals, education, communityoutreach

Home Health Care

Fremont Rideout Home Health
P.O. Box 303
16911 Willow Glen Road
Brownsville, CA 95919
Telephone: (916)-692-1410
Contact: Cindy White RN
Intermittent nursing, home health aides, physical therapy, counseling

Fremont Rideout Home Health
P.O. Box 2128
319 G Street
Marysville, CA 95901
Telephone: (916)-741-8688 Fax: (916)-749-4386
Contact: Mary Ann Anderson RN
Intermittent nursing, home health aides, physical therapy, counseling

Fremont Rideout Home Health
P.O. Box 303
16911 Willow Glen Road
Brownsville, CA 95919
Telephone: (916)-692-1410
Contact: Cindy White
Home Health Care

Medical Services

Norte Clinic Inc.
4941 Olivehurst Avenue
Olivehurst, CA 95961
Telephone: (916)-743-6638 Fax: (916)-743-2613
Contact: Nursing Director
HIV testing, education, dental clinic

COLORADO

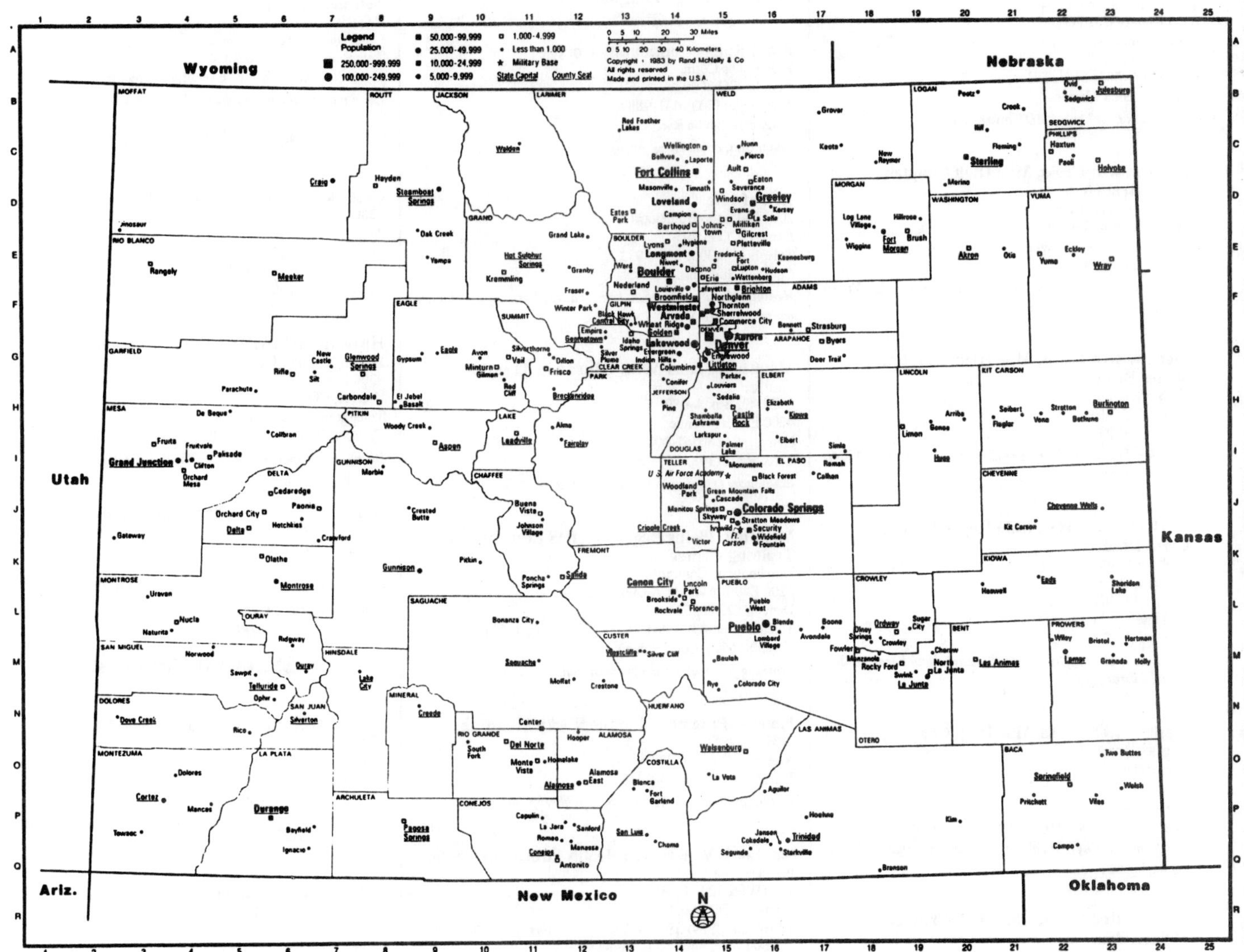

From City/County Planning Atlas Copyright 1989 by Reed McNally & Company, R.L. 90-S-28

Colorado

General Services

Education

American Red Cross
Weld County Chapter
804 23rd Avenue
Greeley, CO 80631
Telephone: (303)-352-7212
Contact: Leona Martens
Information brochures, AIDS awareness

American Red Cross, Mile High Chapter, Aurora Branch
10450 E. 1st Avenue
Aurora, CO 80010-4309
Telephone: (303)-343-1249
Contact: Jim Chesnut
Education/Training, Speakers Bureau, Brochures, Video Lending Library

American Red Cross, Mile High Chapter, Boulder Branch
5378 Sterling Dr.
Boulder, CO 80301-2351
Telephone: (303)-442-0577
Education/Training, Speakers Bureau, Brochures, Video Lending Library

American Red Cross, Mile High Chapter, Denver Branch
444 Sherman St.
170 Steele Street
Denver, CO 80203-3521
Telephone: (303)-399-0550
Contact: Judi Dunn
Education/Training, Speakers Bureau, Brochures, Video Lending Library

American Red Cross, Mile High Chapter, Douglas Branch
444 Sherman Street
Denver, CO 80203
Telephone: (303)-688-1551
Contact: Judy Dunn - HIV Statewide Coordinator
Education/Training, Speakers Bureau, Brochures, Video Lending Library

American Red Cross, Mile High Chapter, Jefferson Branch
10030 W. 27th Avenue
Lakewood, CO 80215-6601
Telephone: (303)-237-7785
Education/Training, Speakers Bureau, Brochures, Video Lending Library

American Red Cross, Mountain West Region
444 Sherman Street
Denver, CO 80203-3521
Telephone: (303)-722-7474 Fax: (303)-722-9588
Contact: Dallis J. Pierson - REO; Kathryn A. Forbes - Chairman
AIDS information & classes

American Red Cross, Pikes Peak Chapter
P.O. Box 7640
1600 N. Cascade
Colorado Springs, CO 80907-7640
Telephone: (719)-632-3563
Contact: Marry Rettner; Larry Decker
Education/Training, Speakers, Video Lending Library, Brochures, Referral

Centennial Area Health Education Center (CAHEC)
1024 9th Avenue
Suite B
Greeley, CO 80631
Telephone: (303)-351-0755 Fax: (303)-351-0786
Contact: Bob Guthman
Health education for rural health care providers.

Front Range Community College
7639 Owns Court
Arvada, CO 80005
Telephone: (303)-431-9887
Contact: Claudia Riel
Education, counseling, prevention

Hall of Life
2001 Colorado Boulevard
Denver, CO 80205
Telephone: (303)-329-5933
Contact: Sue Palmer
Health Education for 5th-12th grades, businesses, teacher training in AIDS

Mountain Plains AIDS Education Training Center
UCHSC, Box A-089
4200 E. 9th Avenue
Denver, CO 80262-0001
Telephone: (303)-355-1301
Education/Training, Speakers Bureau

Mountain Plains Regional AIDS Education and Training Center
University of Colorado
4200 E. 9th Ave, Bx A-096
Denver, CO 80262
Telephone: (303)-355-1301 Fax: (303)-355-1448
Contact: Mary Lou Johnson
Training for health care professionals

Planned Parenthood of the Rocky Mountains
1537 Alton Street
Aurora, CO 80010-1716
Telephone: (303)-321-2458
Education/Training, Advocacy, Speakers, Counseling

San Louis Valley Area Health Education Center
Box 4
1560 West 12th Street
Alamosa, CO 81101
Telephone: (719)-589-4977 Fax: (719)-589-4978
Contact: Al Kelly - Executive Director
Regional AIDS Training Center workshops

Southeastern Colorado Area Health Education Center
1225 Grand Avenue
Suite 103
Pueblo, CO 81003
Telephone: (719)-544-7833
Contact: Judy Weaver, RN - Special Projects Coord.
Regional health education center

University of Colorado Health Sciences Center
4200 E. Ninth Avenue
Box A-021
Denver, CO 80262-0001
Telephone: (303)-270-8875 Fax: (303)-270-8886
Counseling, Education/Training, Speakers, Referral

Hotlines

Colorado Dept of Health AIDS Info Line
1210 East Colfax
Suite 307
Denver, CO 80218
Telephone: (303)-333-4741
Contact: Jim Smith - Executive Director

Southern Colorado AIDS Project
P.O. Box 311
Colorado Springs, CO 80901
Telephone: (719)-540-8894
Contact: Richard Blair - Executive Director
Case management, educational outreach

State Health Departments

Colorado Department of Health
4300 Cherry Creek Drive S
A-3
Denver, CO 80222-1530
Telephone: (303)-399-0550
Contact: Ellen Mangione, M.P.

Hispanic HIV/AIDS Group, Colorado Department of Health
4300 Cherry Creek Street
Denver, CO 80220
Telephone: (303)-331-8706
Contact: Linda Lucero - Minority AIDS Coordinator
Bilingual Support Group for PWAs and HIV+

Northeast Colorado Health Department
700 Columbine Street
Sterling, CO 80751-3728
Telephone: (303)-522-3741
Contact: Loreen Miller - Health Education, RN
STD Clinic, Free Confidential HIV Testing/Counseling, referral, education,literature

Statewide Services

Black AIDS Project at Large (B-A-PAL)
1525 Josephine St.
Denver, CO 80206-1406
Telephone: (303)-388-9780
Contact: Steve Arrington
Education and training, advocacy, speakers bureau, information and referral.

Colorado Department of Social Services
1575 Sherman Street
Denver, CO 80203-1714
Telephone: (303)-866-5815 Fax: (303)-866-2704
Education, Medicaid, home health care, drug coverage

Colorado Department of Social Services, Medical Services
1575 Sherman Street
Denver, CO 80203
Telephone: (303)-866-3176
Contact: Janet Campbell
AZT therapy assistance & other assistance

Mount Evans Home Health Care, Inc.
P.O. Box 2770
Evergreen, CO 80439
Telephone: (303)-674-6400
Home and hospice program network, advocacy, education and training

U.S. Public Health Service
1961 Stout Street
4th Floor

Denver, CO 80294
Telephone: (303)-844-6163 Fax: (303)-844-2019
Contact: Jane Wilson - Regional AIDS Coordinator
Education/Training Information, Referrals, Federal Grant Assistance

Adams County

County Health Depts

Tri-County Health Department
10190 Bannock St. #100
North Glen, CO 80221
Telephone: (303)-341-9370
Contact: Pam Moores
Free Confidential HIV Testing/Counseling

Tri-County Health Department
15400 E. 14th Place
Aurora, CO 80011
Telephone: (303)-341-9370
Free Confidential HIV Testing/Counseling

Arapahoe County

County Health Depts

Tri-County Health Department
4857 South Broadway
Englewood, CO 80110
Telephone: (303)-761-1340 Fax: (303)-761-1528
Contact: Hugh H. Rohrer, MD - Director
Free Confidential HIV referrals/Counseling

Tri-County Health Department
4857 South Broadway
Englewood, CO 80110-6865
Telephone: (303)-761-1340
Contact: Betty Schmidt RND - Director
Free confidential HIV testing/pre & post counseling, referrals , and home health care

Caremark Connection Network
7042 South Revere PW
Englewood, CO 80112
Telephone: (303)-863-0102
Contact: Andrea Woodell - HIV Program Manager
Clinical Support and Infusion Therapies: Nutrition, Antimicrobials, Chemo.,Hematopoe, AIDS education

Homedco Infusion
300 East Mineral Ave
Littleton, CO 80122
Telephone: (303)-795-6000 Fax: (303)-347-1361
Experienced in providing quality infusion therapy to home HIV/AIDS patients

Homedco Infusion
300 East Mineral Avenue
Suite 10
Littleton, CO 80121-2627
Telephone: (303)-795-6000 Fax: (303)-795-1280
Contact: Richard Iriye
Nationwide experience in providing home infusion therapy to AIDS patients

nmc HOMECARE
7032 So. Revere Pkwy, Bldg D
Englewood, CO 80112
Telephone: (303)-790-0271
Fax: (303)-790-0284
Contact: Danette Stephens
National JCAHO-Accredited company providing a full range of Infusion and Respiratory therapies and specializing in the care of HIV/AIDS patients. National Case Manager is also available at 800-445-1188

Boulder County

Community Services

Hispanic Support Group, Boulder County Health Department
3470 Broadway
Boulder, CO 80304
Telephone: (303)-776-5925
Contact: Jerry Frazier
Bilingual Support Group for PWAs, HIV+, and Families

Home Health Care

Home Care
2825 Marine Street
Boulder, CO 80303-1027
Telephone: (303)-449-7740 Fax: (303)-449-6961
Contact: Llona Steur
Home health care

Medical Services

Belle Bonfils Memorial Blood Center
3113 28th Street
Tebo Plaza
Boulder, CO 80301
Telephone: (303)-442-8270
Patient transfusions, referrals

Wardenbury Student Health Service
University of Colorado
Campus Box 119
Boulder, CO 80309-0119
Telephone: (303)-492-5101 Fax: (303)-492-1747
Contact: Sue Husler - Director of Nursing
HIV free clinic

Clear Creek County

Community Services

Clear Creek County Department of Social Services
P.O. Box 2000
Georgetown, CO 80444
Telephone: (303)-534-5777
Contact: Susie A. Lala - Director
Counseling, social services, family planning, home health care, education.

Delta County

County Health Depts

Delta County Health Department
255 West 6th Street
Delta, CO 81416
Telephone: (303)-874-2165 Fax: (303)-874-0222
Contact: Debbie Tittle RN
Sexually Transmitted Disease Clinic, HIV testing

Denver County

Community Services

Belle Bonfils Memorial Blood Center
4200 East 9th Avenue
Box B-128
Denver, CO 80262-4318
Telephone: (303)-355-7366 Fax: (303)-322-5159
Education and training, speakers bureau.

Catholic Hispanic AIDS Education (CHALE)
1209 West 36th Avenue
Denver, CO 80211
Telephone: (303)-477-6958
Contact: Richard Velasqez
Latino support group for HIV infected persons, family, and friends.

Colorado AIDS Project
P.O. Box 18529
1576 Sherman Street
Denver, CO 80218-0529
Telephone: (303)-837-0166
Contact: Julian Rush - Executive Director
Support groups for PWAs, HIV infected, and care providers, food bank

Colorado AIDS Project
1576 Sherman Street
Denver, CO 80218-0529
Telephone: (800)-333-2437
Contact: Julian Rush
Food bank, financial aid, clothing

Denver Department of Social Services, AIDS Program
2200 W. Alameda Avenue
Denver, CO 80223-1996
Telephone: (303)-727-2437
Counseling, Financial/Food Assistance, Information, Referral

Human Services, Inc., Counseling Services
899 Logan Street, #500
Denver, CO 80203-3156
Telephone: (303)-830-2714
AIDS prevention education, family counseling

Human Services, Inc., Traveler's Aide
1245 East Colfax
Suite 408
Denver, CO 80218
Telephone: (303)-832-8194
Material Assistance, Food, Transportation, Referrals to New/Displaced Residents

Jewish Community AIDS Task Force
Allied Jewish Federation
300 South Dahlia Street
Denver, CO 80222
Telephone: (303)-321-3399
Contact: Shelly Watters - Planning Director
Social services, counseling, education.

Legal Aid Center
455 Sherman Street
Denver, CO 80203
Telephone: (303)-722-0300

Legal information and Assistance for disabled, elderly, AIDS patients

Mile High Council on Alcoholism and Drug abuse
1444 Wazee, Suite 125
Denver, CO 80202
Telephone: (303)-825-8113
Information and Referrals on Substance Abuse Treatment Centers

Parents and Friends of Lesbians and Gays
AIDS Family Support Group
P.O. Box 18901
Denver, CO 80218-0901
Telephone: (303)-333-0286
Contact: Nancy Keene - President
Referral, counseling, bereavement, support, education, speakers, financail food assistance

The Empowerment Program
1245 E. Colfax Avenue
#404
Denver, CO 80218-2216
Telephone: (303)-863-7817
AIDS support group for women

Home Health Care

HNS, Inc.
700 West Mississippi
Suite C-3
Denver, CO 80223
Telephone: (303)-733-0808
Contact: Beth Smith
Home Infusion Therapy, In-home Nursing and Attendant Care, PhysicalTherapy, Pentamidine

Hospice of Metro Denver
3955 East Exposition Ave.
Denver, CO 80209
Telephone: (303)-778-1010 Fax: (303)-722-4524
Contact: Richard Bear
Hospice Care, Home Health Care, Bereavement Counseling, Education/Training

Hospice of Peace
1620 Meade
Denver, CO 80204
Telephone: (303)-575-8357 Fax: (303)-575-8390
Contact: Ann F. Luke - Director
Hospice home care/ home health agency

Medical Services

Belle Bonfils Memorial Blood Center
4200 East 9th Avenue
Box B-128
Denver, CO 80262-4318
Telephone: (303)-355-7366

Denver Community Program for Clinical Research on AIDS
605 Bannock Street
Denver, CO 80204-4507
Telephone: (303)-436-7200
AIDS/STD prevention clinic

Testing Sites

Colorado Department of Health - Lab
4210 East 11th Avenue
Denver, CO 80220
Telephone: (303)-331-8471
Contact: Larry Briggs
HIV testing

Mountain States Regional Hemophilia Center, UCHSC/MSRHC
4200 E. Ninth Avenue
Box C-220
Denver, CO 80262-0001
Telephone: (303)-372-1750
Medical Care, Counseling, HIV Testing, Referral

El Paso County

Community Services

El Paso County Medical Society
Task Force on AIDS
2760 N. Academy Blvd.#207
Colorado Springs, CO 80917
Telephone: (303)-591-2424
Contact: Carol Walker

Lambda House
P.O. Box 10069
512 W. Colorado
Colorado Sprngs, CO 80905-1069
Telephone: (719)-635-7671
Contact: Joe Brady
Housing for HIV+/AIDS individuals. No medical services provided.

Southern Colorado AIDS Project
P.O. Box 311
Colorado Springs, CO 80901-0311
Telephone: (719)-578-9092 Fax: (719)-578-8690
Contact: Marvin Harrison - President
Home meals, peer support, food service, HIV testing, counseling, medicalassistance

County Health Depts

El Paso County Department of Health
301 South Union Blvd
Colorado Springs, CO 80910
Telephone: (719)-578-3148
Contact: John Potterat; Lynn Drzewiczewski - Coordinator
Medical referral, education, HIV testing, follow-up, counseling, notification.

El Paso County Health Department
301 S Union
Colorado Springs, CO 80910
Telephone: (719)-578-3199 Fax: (719)-578-3192
Contact: John B. Muth, MD - Director; Lynn Phillips; John Potterat

Home Health Care

nmc HOMECARE
1506 N. Hancock Ave.
Colorado Springs, CO 80903
Telephone: (719)-633-8803
Fax: (719)-633-9175
Contact: Karen Popham
National JCAHO-Accredited company providing a full range of Infusion and Respiratory therapies and specializing in the care of HIV/AIDS patients. National Case Manager is also available at 800-445-1188

Pikes Peak Hospice
3630 Sinton Rd. Ste 302
Colorado Sprngs, CO 80907-5098
Telephone: (719)-633-3400 Fax: (719)-633-1150
Home health care, hospice care

Gunnison County

Community Services

Gunnison/Hinsdale County Department of Social Services
200 East Virginia Avenue
Gunnison, CO 81230
Telephone: (303)-641-3244
Counseling, Financial and Social Services, Family Planning, Physician Referral

Huerfano County

Community Services

Huerfano County Department of Social Services
121 West Sixth Avenue
Walsenburg, CO 81089
Telephone: (719)-738-2810
Contact: Roberta F. Vallejos - Social Services Supervisor
Counseling, Financial and Social Services, Case Management.

County Health Depts

Huerfano County Health Department
119 E. 5th Street
Walsenburg, CO 81089-2094
Telephone: (719)-738-2650
Contact: Amy Bevsek - RN
Free Confidential HIV Testing/Counseling, education

Jefferson County

Community Services

Belle Bonfils Memorial Blood Center
1050 South Wadsworth Blv.
Lakewood, CO 80226-4318
Telephone: (303)-936-7174
Referrals

Gilpin County Department of Social Services
280 Janjowski Drive
Black Hawk, CO 80403
Telephone: (303)-443-1210
Social services including home health care, hospice care, physician referral

County Health Depts

Jefferson County Department of Health and Environment
260 S. Kipling
Lakewood, CO 80226-1099
Telephone: (303)-232-6301
Contact: Mark B. Johnson, MD - Director
Counseling

Home Health Care

Hospice of St. John
1320 Everett Court
Lakewood, CO 80215
Telephone: (303)-232-7900 Fax: (303)-232-3614
Contact: Bernard Heese - Admissions Coordinator; Janelle M. Betley, RN - Director of Nursing
Hospice Care, Home Health Care, Bereavement Counseling, Social services

Hospice of St. John, Inc.
1320 Everett Court
Lakewood, CO 80215
Telephone: (303)-232-7900 Fax: (303)-232-3614
Contact: Bernard Heese; Janelle M. Betley, RN - Director of Nursing
Hospice Care, Home Health Care, Bereavement Counseling, social work, AIDS support group

Mount Evans Home Health / Hospice Care Inc.
P.O. Box 2770
Evergreen, CO 80439
Telephone: (303)-674-6400 Fax: (303)-674-8813
Contact: Louisa B. Walthers - Executive Director
Home health care, counseling, support groups.

Mount Evans Home Health / Hospice Care Inc.
P.O. Box 2770
3709 Evergreen Parkway
Evergreen, CO 80439
Telephone: (303)-674-6400 Fax: (303)-674-8813
Contact: Louisa B. Walthers - Executive Director; 303-674-6400 answered 24 hrs. -
Home health care, counseling, support groups.

Kit Carson County

Community Services

Kit Carson County Department of Social Services
Courthouse 251 Sixteenth Street
Suite 101
Burlington, CO 80807
Telephone: (719)-346-8732
Contact: Norma H. Pankratz - Director
Social Services

La Plata County

Medical Services

Southern Colorado Ute Service Unit
P.O. Box 899
Ignacio, CO 81137
Telephone: (303)-563-4581 Fax: (303)-563-0206
Contact: George Maxted, MD - Clinical Director
Indian Health Service

Testing Sites

San Juan Basin Health Unit
San Juan Basin Health Department
3803 North Main
Durango, CO 81301-0140
Telephone: (303)-247-5702
Contact: Lynne Westberg, RN - Director
Confidential HIV Testing/Counseling

Larimer County

County Health Depts

Larimer County Health Department
Municipal Building, #201
P.O. Box 1137
Estes Park, CO 80517-1137
Telephone: (303)-586-2077
STD Clinic, HIV Testing, Counseling, Education/Training, Information/Referral

Larimer County Health Department
205 E. 6th Street
Loveland, CO 80537-5606
Telephone: (303)-532-4401 Fax: (303)-679-4580
Contact: Gene Berger RN - HIV Testing
STD Clinic, HIV Testing, Counseling, Education/Training, Information/Referral

Larimer County Health Department
1525 Blue Spruce Street
Fort Collins, CO 80524
Telephone: (303)-221-7460
Contact: Ann Watson - Health Education Sup.
Education & training services, family planning, HIV and STD testing & counseling

Las Animas County

County Health Depts

Las Animas County Health Department
412 Benedicta Avenue
Trinidad, CO 81081-2005
Telephone: (719)-846-2213
Contact: Lora Melnicoe, MD - Director
Free Confidential HIV Testing/Counseling

Logan County

County Health Depts

Northeast Colorado Health Department
700 Columbine Street
PO Box 3300
Sterling, CO 80751
Telephone: (303)-522-3741 Fax: (303)-522-1412
Contact: Loreen Miller
STD Clinic, Free Confidential HIV Testing/Counseling

Medical Services

Centennial Mental Health Center
211 West Main
Sterling, CO 80751
Telephone: (303)-522-4392 Fax: (303)-522-4211
Counseling. Community mental health center.

Mesa County

County Health Depts

Western Colorado Health Network, Colorado Dept. of Health
1003 Main Street
Grand Junction, CO 81501-2758
Telephone: (303)-243-2437 Fax: (303)-248-7198
Contact: Shelly Nelson
Case managementm support for PWAs and HIV+, wellness group

Montezuma County

County Health Depts

Montezuma County Health Department
106 West North
Cortez, CO 81321-3119
Telephone: (303)-565-3056
Free Confidential HIV Testing/Counseling, Home Health Care

Otero County

County Health Depts

Otero County Health Department
Courthouse Bldg, Rm 111
La Junta, CO 81050-1591
Telephone: (719)-384-2584
Contact: Rodger Stasiak - MD
Testing center, counseling, referrals

Park County

Community Services

Park County Department of Social Services
P.O. Box 156
Fairplay, CO 80440
Telephone: (719)-836-2771 Fax: (719)-836-2771
Contact: Victoria McCullough-Matt - Director
Social Services and Community Resource

Phillips County

Community Services

Phillips County Department of Social Services
246 South Interocean
Holyoke, CO 80734
Telephone: (303)-854-2280
Contact: Shirley Thompson - Director
Social Services, referrals

Pitkin County

Community Services

Aspen AIDS Project
P.O. Box 4807
Aspen, CO 81612
Telephone: (303)-925-2752
Contact: Bernard Welage - Chairperson
Counseling, Education, Training, Financial and Social Services, Testing Center

Testing Sites

Community Health Services VNA
405 Castle Creek Rd.#6
Aspen, CO 81611-1557
Telephone: (303)-920-5420 Fax: (303)-920-5558
Contact: Sarah Oliver
Free Confidential HIV Testing/Counseling

Pueblo County

County Health Depts

Pueblo City/County Health Department, Pueblo AIDS Coalition
151 Central Main Street
Pueblo, CO 81003-4212
Telephone: (719)-544-8376 Fax: (719)-545-9800
Contact: Dan Otoupalik - Health Educator
Counseling, Education, HIV Testing, Referral, STD Clinic, south corridorAIDS project

Home Health Care

nmc HOMECARE
2648 Santa Fe Dr, Suite 15
Pueblo, CO 81006
Telephone: (719)-542-0202
Fax: (719)-542-2419
Contact: Karen Popham
National JCAHO-Accredited company providing a full range of Infusion and Respiratory therapies and specializing in the care of HIV/AIDS patients. National Case Manager is also available at 800-445-1188

Testing Sites

Colorado Department of Health - Field Office
720 North Main Street
Pueblo, CO 81003-3028
Telephone: (719)-545-4050
Contact: Perry Bethea
Medical referral, education, HIV testing, follow-up, counseling, notification.

Teller County

Community Services

Teller County Department of Social Services
P.O. Box 9033
Woodland Park, CO 80866
Telephone: (719)-687-3335 Fax: (719)-687-0429
Contact: Debbie Layden - Family Therapist
Social Services

Weld County

County Health Depts

Weld County Health Department
1517 16th Ave Ct
Greeley, CO 80631-4597
Telephone: (303)-353-0639
Contact: Jill Burch - Weld County AIDS Coalitio
STD Clinic, Free Confidential HIV Testing/Counseling

Yuma County

Community Services

Yuma County Social Services
310 Ash Street
Wray, CO 80758
Telephone: (303)-332-4877 Fax: (303)-332-3411
Contact: Tom Westfall - Director
Food stamps, general assistance

CONNECTICUT

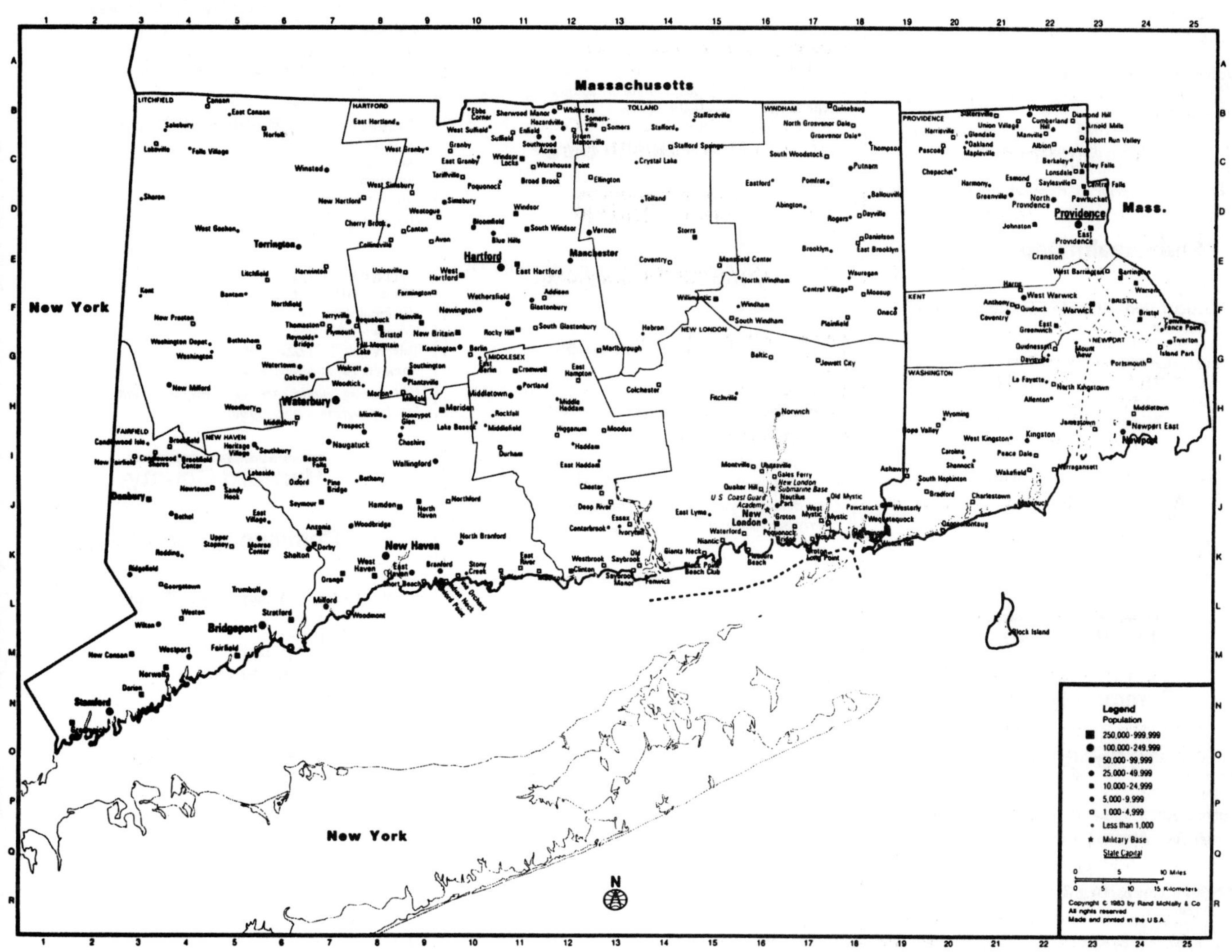

From City/County Planning Atlas Copyright 1989 by Reed McNally & Company, R.L. 90-S-28

Connecticut

General Services

Education

Hospice Education Institute
190 Westbrooke Road
Essex, CT 06426-1113
Telephone: (203)-767-1620 Fax: (203)-767-2746
Contact: J.M. Galazka - Executive Director; Ellen J. Laskarin - Administrator
HOSPICELINK Directory of Hospices, Education, Speakers Bureau, Training

State Health Departments

Connecticut Department of Health Services AIDS Section
Bureau of Health Promotion
150 Washington Street
Hartford, CT 06106
Telephone: (203)-566-1157
Contact: Beth Wienstein - Chief of AIDS Section

Connecticut Department of Health Services AIDS Section
150 Washington Street
Hartford, CT 06106
Telephone: (203)-566-1157
Contact: Susan Murray - AIDS Public Information

Fairfield County

Community Services

AIDS Project of Greater Danbury
PO Box 91
Bethel, CT 06801
Telephone: (203)-778-2437 Fax: (203)-743-1439
Case mgt: food, financial, counseling & support services

AIDS/HIV Counseling & Test Site
137 E Avenue
Norwalk, CT 06851
Telephone: (203)-854-7979 Fax: (203)-854-7934
Contact: Karen Gorman - Counselor
HIV counseling & testing (confidential)

American Red Cross
986 Bedford Street
Stamford, CT 06905
Telephone: (203)-324-6182 Fax: (203)-363-1041
Contact: Phillis Berry Weinstein
Case mgt, financial, social services & educational program

Norwalk Health Department
137 East Avenue
Norwalk, CT 06851
Telephone: (203)-854-7776 Fax: (203)-854-7934
Contact: Jan Boardman
Counseling, testing, referrals, STD & Tuberculosis clinic

Stamford Health Dept. AIDS Program
888 Washington Blvd
PO Box 10152
Stamford, CT 06904-2152
Telephone: (203)-977-4387 Fax: (203)-977-5460
Contact: Debra Katz - Coordinator
HIV testing (anonymous & confidential), pre/post counseling, HIV/AIDS education, case management, community outreach, referrals

County Health Depts

Danbury Dept of Health
20 West Street
Danbury, CT 06810
Telephone: (203)-797-7900
Contact: Susan Durgy - AIDS/HIV Coordinator
HIV testing; pre & post-individual counseling; follow-up visits for HIV+, community outreach

Home Health Care

O.P.T.I.O.N. Care of Connecticut
87 Sand Pit Road
Danbury, CT 06810-4044
Telephone: (203)-744-0466 Fax: (203)-797-1104
Contact: Bob Tendler, RPh; 800-422-9229 (NY)
Home IV and Nutritional Services

Medical Services

Bridgeport Community Health Center
471 Barnum Avenue
Bridgeport, CT 06608
Telephone: (203)-333-6864 Fax: (203)-332-0376
Contact: Darlene Delagdo - Case Manager
Case management, counseling testing, pediatrics, medical-referrals, prescriptions

Bridgeport Community Health Center
471 Barnum Ave
Bridgeport, CT 06608
Telephone: (203)-333-6864
Contact: Rafael Muniz - Coordinator
Medical assistance for adults & children

Southwest Community Health Center
361 Bird Street
Bridgeport, CT 06605
Telephone: (203)-576-8446 Fax: (203)-576-8444
Contact: Susan M. Hanewisz, RN
Primary care, substance abuse counseling, family counseling, dental OB GYN, pediatrics

Zane K. Saul, MD
Brick Walk, Suite 301
Fairfield, CT 06430
Telephone: (203)-259-8087
Internal Medicine, Infectious Diseases

Testing Sites

AIDS/HIV Counseling & Test Site
229 North Street
Stamford, CT 06904-2152
Telephone: (203)-967-2437 Fax: (203)-977-5460
Contact: Debbie Katz; Victoria Valdez -
HIV counseling & testing, confidential and anonymous

AIDS/HIV Counseling & Test Site
Public Health Program
20 West Street
Danbury, CT 06810
Telephone: (203)-797-7900 Fax: (203)-796-1596
Contact: Susan Durgy
Confidential counseling & testing, AIDS educators, bilingual

AIDS/HIV Counseling & Test Site
Town Hall/101 Field Pt
Greenwich, CT 06830
Telephone: (203)-622-6460 Fax: (203)-622-7770
Contact: Thomas Mahoney - Health Educator
Confidential counseling & testing

Bridgeport Dept of Health
752 E Main Street
Bridgeport, CT 06608
Telephone: (203)-576-7469 Fax: (203)-576-8311
Contact: Robin Clark-Smith - AIDS/HIV Counseling Coordinato
AIDS/HIV testing; pre & post counseling; follow-up; referrals, intervention& needle exchange program

Danbury County Health AIDS Program
20 West Street
Danbury, CT 06810
Telephone: (203)-778-2437
Contact: Susan Durgy
HIV testing & counseling

Greenwich Dept of Health
Office of HIV info/svc
101 Field Point Rd
Greenwich, CT 06836
Telephone: (203)-622-6496
Contact: Thomas Mahoney
HIV testing, home care, referrals, individual counseling; buddy program, support groups

Hartford County

Community Services

AIDS Ministries Program of CT, Inc.
1335 Asylum Ave
Hartford, CT 06105
Telephone: (203)-233-4481
Contact: John Murzeus Bennett
Home care, referrals & education

AIDS Program Hotline (Weekdays)
150 Washington Street
Hartford, CT 06106
Telephone: (203)-566-1157
Contact: Beth Weinstein
Counseling, testing, education, legal help, referral

AIDS Project Hartford
30 Arbour Street
Hartford, CT 06106
Telephone: (203)-247-2437 Fax: (203)-231-1996
Contact: Judith A. Fox
Outreach education, hotline; buddy, group & hospital support; casemanagement, peer counseling

American Red Cross, Northeast Region
100 Corporate Drive
Suite 110
Windsor, CT 06095
Telephone: (203)-298-7202
Contact: Bonnie J. Wright - REO; Martha Dunn-Strohecker - Chairman

Community Health Service
5020 Albony Ave
Hartford, CT 06120
Telephone: (203)-249-9625
Contact: Angela Sysom
Testing, counseling & referral

Hispanic Health Council
96-98 Cedar Street
Hartford, CT 06120
Telephone: (203)-724-0437

Contact: Todd Nusome
Project Cope, Project Orgullo (gay outreach)

Latinos/as Contra SIDA
331 Weatherfield Avenue
Hartford, CT 06114
Telephone: (203)-724-1169
Contact: Manuel S. Magaz
Referrals, counseling, case management, prevention

Home Health Care

HNS, Inc.
152 Rockwell Road
Unit B-3
Newington, CT 06111
Telephone: (203)-665-1331 Fax: (203)-665-1521
Toll-Free: (800)-872-4467
Contact: John Leonard
Home infusion therapy, in-home nursing

Homedco
141 South Street
West Hartford, CT 06110
Telephone: (203)-493-6200 Fax: (203)-493-6212
Contact: Judy Jennings - Customer Service Super.
Respiratory, HME, Infusion Therapy

Homedco Pharmacy
85 Holmes Road
Newington, CT 06111
Telephone: (203)-666-6199 Fax: (203)-667-8112
Contact: Rick Eleck - Pharmacist
Services for CT, RI, Westchester, NY, Northern NJ, home infusion

Visiting Nurse & Home Care Inc
103 Woodland Street
Hartford, CT 06105
Telephone: (203)-249-4862 Fax: (203)-246-8734
Contact: Sue Keefe, RN, MS
Case mgt/health care, skilled nursing, physical therapy, homemaker, IV therapy, social workers, meals on wheels

Medical Services

Hartford Hospital/AIDS Program
80 Seymour St
P.O. Box 5037
Hartford, CT 06102-5037
Telephone: (203)-545-5555
Contact: Lynn Bryant
Health care, HIV Counseling & Test Site/Confidential anonymous

Testing Sites

AIDS/HIV Counseling & Test Site
31 High Street
New Britain, CT 06051
Telephone: (203)-224-2420 Fax: (203)-826-3475
Contact: Gail Ide - Coordinator
AIDS/HIV counseling & test site/confidential

Hartford Health Department
Burgdorff Health Center
80 Coventry St
Hartford, CT 06112
Telephone: (203)-722-6742 Fax: (203)-722-6719
Contact: Daniel Barrone ; Migdalia Belliveau
HIV Counseling & Test Site/Confidential

Middlesex County

Testing Sites

Community Health Center
635 Main Street
Middletown, CT 06457
Telephone: (203)-347-6971 Fax: (203)-347-2043
Contact: Sally Baumer - HIV Program Coordinator
Testing & counseling

New Haven County

Community Services

Hispanos Unidos
263 Grand Ave
New Haven, CT 06513
Telephone: (203)-772-1777 Fax: (203)-772-1773
Contact: Luz Z. Gonzalez - Executive Director
Case management group for women, HIV testing

Waterbury Dept of Health/AIDS Services
402 E Main Street
Waterbury, CT 06702
Telephone: (203)-574-6883 Fax: (203)-597-3481
Contact: Thomas Butcher - AIDS Coordinator
Preventive education & outreach, HIV testing & counseling; case managementservices, bi-lingual, Spanish service

County Health Depts

New Haven Dept of Health
1 State Street
New Haven, CT 06511
Telephone: (203)-787-6453
Contact: Pam Foster (C/FP)

Home Health Care

Caremark Connection Network
7 Barnes Industrial Park
Wallingford, CT 06492
Telephone: (203)-284-8558 Fax: (203)-284-8580
Toll-Free: (800)-458-3431
Contact: Polly Bader - Branch Manager
Clinical Support and Infusion Therapies: Nutrition, Antimicrobials, Chemo.,Hematopoe

Homedco
5 Hamden Park Drive
Hamden, CT 06517-3150
Telephone: (203)-288-7938 Fax: (203)-230-0202
Contact: Tim Johns - Distribution Supervisor
Respiratory, HME, Infusion Therapy

nmc HOMECARE
900 Northrop Road
Wallingford, CT 06405
Telephone: (203)-294-9744
Fax: (203)-294-9754
Contact: John Fogarty
National JCAHO-Accredited company providing a full range of Infusion and Respiratory therapies and specializing in the care of HIV/AIDS patients. National Case Manager is also available at 800-445-1188

Medical Services

Hill Health Center
428 Columbus Ave
New Haven, CT 06519
Telephone: (203)-776-9594
Contact: Robert Killpatric
Counseling, testing, education, free services, case managers, referrals fordetox & housing, mental health specialist.

Hospital of St. Raphael
Infectious Disease Clinic
1450 Chapel Street
New Haven, CT 06511
Telephone: (203)-789-4135 Fax: (203)-784-3222
In-patient and Out-patient, Social services, Nutrition services, MedicalDoctors

Planned Parenthood of Connecticut
129 Whitney Ave
New Haven, CT 06510
Telephone: (203)-865-5158
Contact: Jean Larson - Program Director
Clinic/walk-in, referrals, social services, STD testing/treatment

Yale New Haven Hospital
AIDS Care Program
135 College Street
New Haven, CT 06510
Telephone: (203)-785-3184
Contact: June Holmesis
Medical services, in-patient & out-patient care; counseling & testing;HIV/AIDS education, out reach, clinical trials

Testing Sites

AIDS/HIV Counseling & Test Site
STD Clinic
1 State Street
New Haven, CT 06511
Telephone: (203)-787-6453 Fax: (203)-772-7234
Contact: Jesus Gomez - 203-787-8181
HIV Counseling & Test confidential & anonymous

AIDS/HIV Counseling & Test Site
Public Health Nursing
402 E Main/N Elm St
Waterbury, CT 06702
Telephone: (203)-574-6883 Fax: (203)-597-3481
Contact: Thomas Butcher, Debbie Becking -
HIV counseling & test confidential & anonymous, case management

New Haven Health Dept.
South Central CT
One State Street
New Haven, CT 06511
Telephone: (203)-787-6453 Fax: (203)-772-7234
Contact: Suzanne Jasper
Pre & post counseling & testing

New London County

Home Health Care

Homedco
159 Sachem Street
Norwich, CT 06360
Telephone: (203)-886-2486 Fax: (203)-885-1505

Contact: Cheryl Jolly - Customer Service
Respiratory, HME, Infusion Therapy

Testing Sites

AIDS/HIV Counseling & Test Site
120 Broad Street
New London, CT 06320
Telephone: (203)-447-2437
Contact: Betsy Ryan - Coordinator
HIV counseling & test confidential & anonymous

William W. Backus Hospital
326 Washington St
Norwich, CT 06360
Telephone: (203)-823-6343 Fax: (203)-823-6329
AIDS counseling & testing, STD clinic, infectious disease

New London AIDS Counseling & Testing Services
120 Broad Street
New London, CT 06320
Telephone: (203)-447-2437 Fax: (203)-447-5260
Contact: Betsy Ryan, RN
Testing & counseling, educational presentations

Windham County

Community Services

Windham AIDS Program
112 Mansfield Ave
Williamantic, CT 06226
Telephone: (203)-423-4447
Counseling, testing, post counseling case management, buddy program, hosthome program, support group

DELAWARE

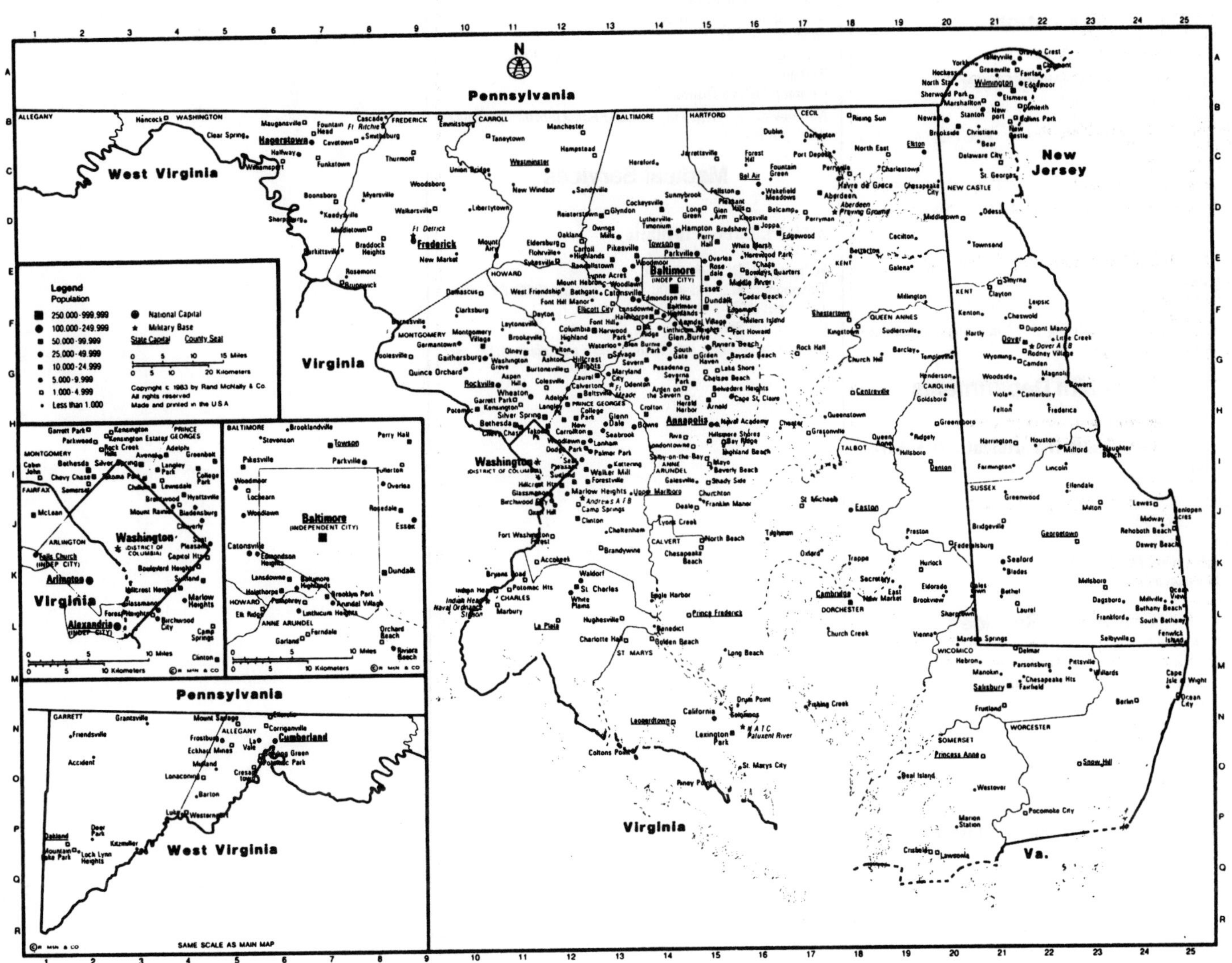

From City/County Planning Atlas Copyright 1989 by Reed McNally & Company, R.L. 90-S-28

Delaware

General Services

Education

Latin American Community Center
403 North Van Buren Street
Wilmington, DE 19805-3606
Telephone: (302)-655-7338 Fax: (302)-655-7334
Contact: Emperatriz Alaix
HIV education

University of Delaware
Student Health Services
University of Delaware
Newark, DE 19716
Telephone: (302)-451-8806
Health education, counseling for University of Delaware students.

State Health Departments

Delaware State Health Departments., HIV/AIDS Epidemiology
300 Newport Gap Pike
Building G
Wilmington, DE 19808
Telephone: (302)-995-8422
Contact: Mary Herr
AIDS surveillance

Statewide Services

Children's Bureau of Delaware
2005 Baynard Boulevard
Wilmington, DE 19802-3999
Telephone: (302)-658-5177
Contact: Alvin Snyder
Foster care for HIV infected children.

Delaware Council on Crime and Justice
501 Shipley Street
Wilmington, DE 19801-2226
Telephone: (302)-658-7174
Contact: Lisa Carr
Health education to prison population/includes peer education program.

Delaware Division of Libraries
43 S Dupont Highway
Dover, DE 19901
Telephone: (302)-739-4748
AIDS educational resources

Kent County

County Health Depts

Kent Court Health Unit
805 River Road
PO Box 1401
Dover, DE 19901-3753
Telephone: (302)-739-5305 Fax: (302)-739-6264
Contact: Lorraine Ryan Jones - Clinical Manager
Family planning, STD program, pre-natal clinic, dental services forchildren,

New Castle County

Home Health Care

Homedco Infusion
4637 Stanton Ogletown Rd
Newark, DE 19713
Telephone: (302)-737-7979 Fax: (302)-737-6719
Toll-Free: (800)-762-7991
Contact: Debbie Home
Nationwide experience in providing home infusion therapy to AIDS patients

Medical Services

Alfred I. DuPont Institute
1600 Rockland Road
Wilmington, DE 19803-3616
Telephone: (302)-651-4000 Fax: (302)-651-4055
Toll-Free: (800)-344-5437
Contact: Dr. Steven C. Eppes
Children's services: infectious disease treatment, AIDS care

DISTRICT OF COLUMBIA

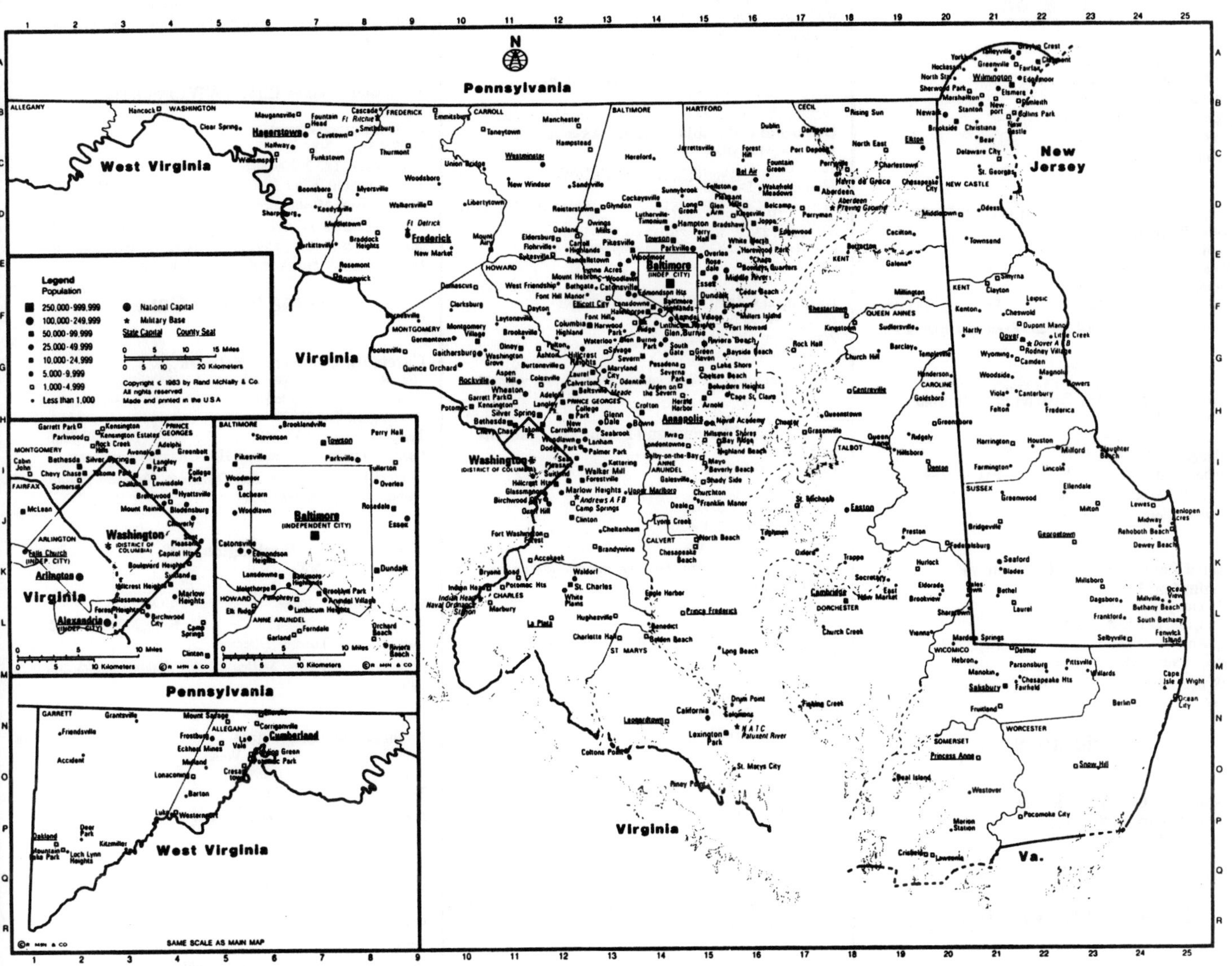

From City/County Planning Atlas Copyright 1989 by Reed McNally & Company, R.L. 90-S-28

District of Columbia

General Services

Education

American Red Cross
1750 K Street
Washington, DC 20036-3078
Telephone: (202)-737-8300
Contact: L.F. Barker
Educational services

George Washington Univ., Intergovt. Health Policy Project
2021 K. Street NW
Suite 800
Washington, DC 20006-1808
Telephone: (202)-872-1445 Fax: (202)-785-0114
Publisher of Brochure on AIDS and Prescription Drug Therapy

Medical Society of the District of Columbia
Pub Info and Educ Comm.
1707 L Street NW, Ste 400
Washington, DC 20036-5402
Telephone: (202)-466-1800 Fax: (202)-452-1542
Contact: P. Douglas Torrence
Professional organization for doctors

Planned Parenthood of Metropolitan Washington, Inc.
2811 Pennsylvania Ave. SE
Washington, DC 20020-3865
Telephone: (202)-581-5710 Fax: (202)-581-5714
Contact: Lauren Molloy - Manager
AIDS information and specified training inservices, HIV testing.

Hotlines

Washington DC AIDS Hotline
1407 South Street Northwest
Washington, DC 20009
Telephone: (202)-332-2437
Contact: Brian Glover

State Health Departments

District of Columbia Commission of Public Health
Office of AIDS Activities
1660 L Street, N.W., Suite 700
Washington, DC 20036
Telephone: (202)-673-6888 Fax: (202)-727-2386
Long term care, preventive health services, agency for HIV/AIDS referralsto services in DC

Washington County

Community Services

American Red Cross National Headquarters
1709 New York Ave. N.W.
Suite 208
Washington, DC 20006
Telephone: (202)-434-4084
Contact: Carol Kaufman - Executive Director, Allen P. Born - Associate, Mktg. & Distr.

Church of the Disciples
1638 R Street NW
Washington, DC 20009-6446
Telephone: (202)-387-5230
Support programs for gay/lesbians PWAs/PWARCs and their significant others.

Damien Ministries
P.O. Box 10202
Washington, DC 20018-0202
Telephone: (202)-387-2926
Housing program, counseling, speakers bureau.

District of Columbia Hospital Association
Task Force on AIDS
Suite 700
Washington, DC 20005
Telephone: (202)-682-1581 Fax: (202)-371-8151
Contact: Joan Lewis
Coordination of DC hospitals' response to AIDS

Episcopal Caring Response to AIDS
733 15th Street NW, #315
Washington, DC 20005-2112
Telephone: (202)-347-8077
AIDS chaplaincy, speakers bureau for parishes, volunteers

Federation of Parents and Friends of Lesbians and Gays
Family AIDS Project
P.O. Box 27605
Washington, DC 20038
Telephone: (202)-638-4200
Contact: Laurie Coburn
Support groups, referral services, information packets for families of PWA's

Interfaith Conference of Metropolitan Washington
AIDS Task Force
1419 V Street, NW
Washington, DC 20009
Telephone: (202)-234-6300
Emergency food & shelter

Parents of Gays
8020 Eastern Avenue, NW
Washington, DC 20012-1311
Telephone: (202)-726-3223
Contact: Eugene Baker - Coord. of Programs & Services
Parents' counseling and support groups for helping PWAs, educationalmaterials, referrals to AIDS/HIV sources

Rap
3451 Holmead Place, NW
Washington, DC 20010-3407
Telephone: (202)-462-7500 Fax: (202)-462-7507
Contact: Kokayi Patterson - AIDS/HIV Office
Individual group counseling, 5-7 bed residential facility for men

Salud
2701 Ontario Road Northwest
Suite 2
Washington, DC 20009-0734
Telephone: (202)-483-6806 Fax: (202)-387-5239
Toll-Free: (800)-322-7432
Contact: Miriam Murillo - Case Mgmt Coordinator
AIDS/HIV testing; individual counseling; case management; Spanish speakingcounselors

Society of Friends
Friends Meeting House
2111 Florida Avenue, NW
Washington, DC 20008
Telephone: (202)-283-3310
Support for PWAs/PWARCs and their significant others.

St. Francis Center
5417 Sherrier Place, NW
Washington, DC 20016-2561
Telephone: (202)-363-8500 Fax: (202)-363-4989
Contact: Elizabeth Haase - Dir of Clinical Services
Provide counseling to AIDS/HIV patients; counseling for family & friends ingrief, in-home visitation, trained counselors for children

Whitman-Walker Clinic (WWC)-Sunnye Sherman
AIDS Education Project
1407 S Street, NW
Washington, DC 20009-3840
Telephone: (202)-797-3560 Fax: (202)-797-3504
Contact: Rick Musher - Media Coordinator
Comprehensive services: testing, counseling, AIDS/HIV care, nineresidential facilities, speakers bureau, street outreach, Latinooutreach, professional training

Home Health Care

Caremark Connection Network
1623 R Connecticut Ave NW
PO Box 53091, Temple Hts.
Washington, DC 20009
Telephone: (202)-387-7411 Fax: (202)-387-7565
Contact: Debbie LaFontaine - HIV Clinical Coordinator
Clinical Support and Infusion Therapies: Nutrition, Antimicrobials,Chemo.,Hematopoe

Hospice Care of Washington, D.C.
1325 Mass Ave NW
Suite 606
Washington, DC 20066
Telephone: (202)-347-1700 Fax: (202)-347-4285
Contact: Anne Towne - Director
In-home hospice care, Skilled nursing & home health aide care, Counseling.

Lutheran Social Services
4406 Georgia Avenue North West
Washington, DC 20011-3895
Telephone: (202)-829-5283
Pediatric AIDS hospice respite care.

Visiting Nurse Association
5151 Wisconsin Ave NW
#400
Washington, DC 20016-4154
Telephone: (202)-686-8702
Nursing care, IV therapy, home health aides, counseling by social workers.

Medical Services

Children's Hospital, National Medical Center
Hemophilia Center
111 Michigan Avenue, NW
Washington, DC 20010
Telephone: (202)-884-2140 Fax: (202)-884-5685
Contact: Gordon L. Bray - MD
Medical Services for Hemophiliacs, Children with AIDS, Hemophiliacs with AIDS

Testing Sites

Planned Parenthood of Metropolitan Washington, Inc.
1108 16th Street, NW
Washington, DC 20036-4890
Telephone: (202)-347-8500 Fax: (202)-783-1007
Contact: Clinical Services

AIDS information and specified training inservices, HIV testing.

Whitman-Walker Clinic
1407 South Street NW
Washington, DC 20009
Telephone: (202)-797-3534 Fax: (202)-797-3504
HIV testing, AIDS research

FLORIDA

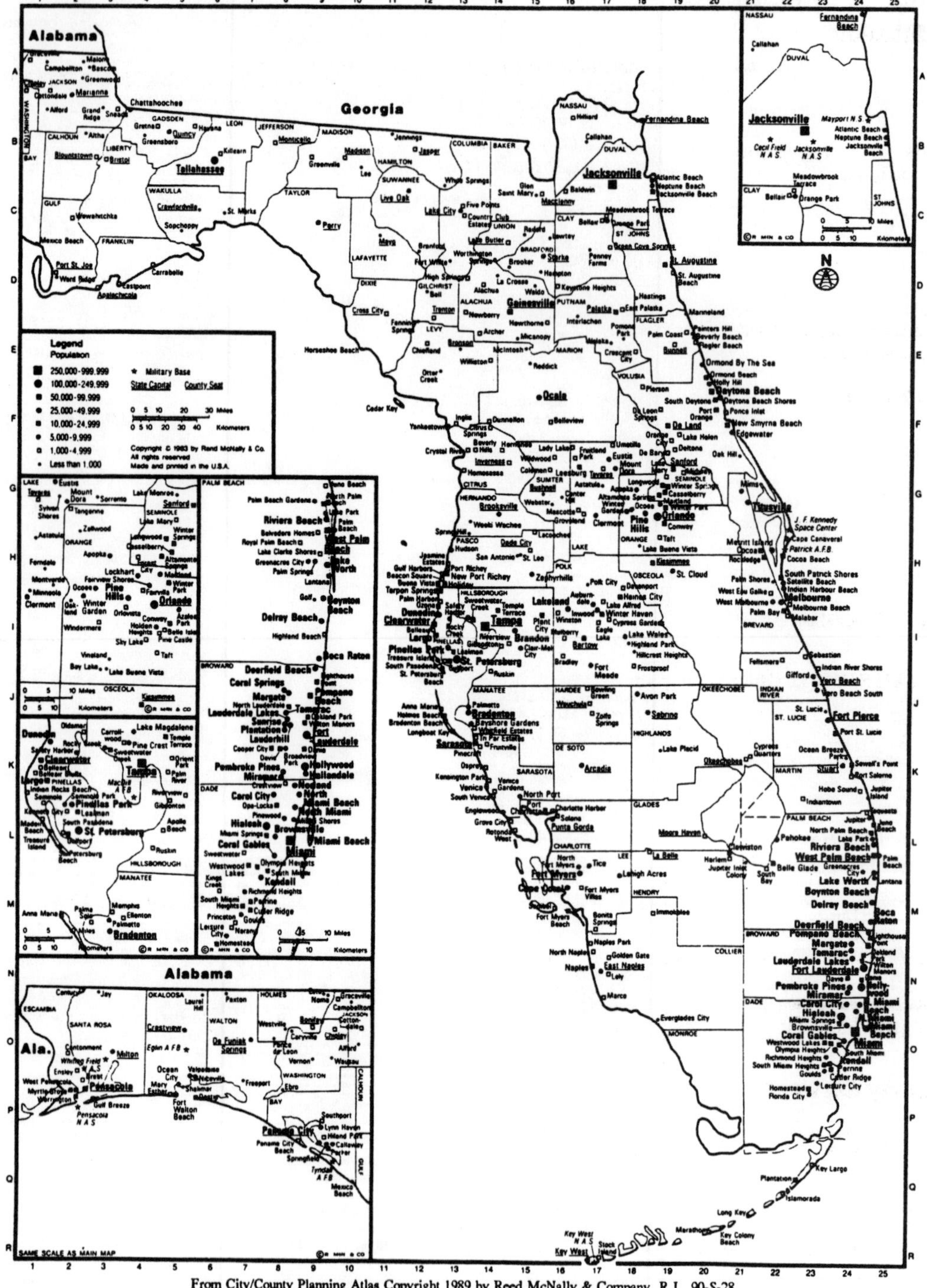

From City/County Planning Atlas Copyright 1989 by Reed McNally & Company, R.L. 90-S-28

Florida

General Services

Education

American Red Cross
1675 N.W. 9th Ave
Miami, FL 33136
Telephone: (305)-326-8888 Fax: (305)-326-6648
Education, training for health care workers

District 3 Office
1000 Northeast 16th Ave
Building G, Room 107
Gainesville, FL 32601
Telephone: (904)-336-5217
Contact: Robert Davis - Administrator of AIDS Program
General AIDS/HIV educational materials

Hotlines

Health Crisis Network
5050 Biscayne Blvd
P.O. Box 42-1280
Miami, FL 33137
Telephone: (305)-326-8833 Fax: (305)-751-7775
Contact: Francis Penka
AIDS hotline 305/751-7751

State Health Departments

Florida Health Office AIDS/STD/TB Office
1317 Winewood Blvd.
Tallahassee, FL 32399-0700
Telephone: (904)-922-6675
Contact: Gill Silva - Dept. of Human Resources Mgr.
Resources and referrals

State of Florida Health Dept. (HRS)
5100 West College Road
Key West, FL 33040
Telephone: (305)-294-4641
Contact: Mark Sureck - Program Director
AIDS/HIV testing, pre & post counseling, AIDS/HIV prevention clinic,outreach program on Marathon Tabernier.

Alachua County

Community Services

Alachua County Social Services
730 NE Waldo Road
Suite # 200
Gainesville, FL 32601-5398
Telephone: (904)-336-2471
Entitlement benefits for eligible clients with no resources.

American Red Cross
821 Northwest 13th Street
Gainesville, FL 32601
Telephone: (904)-376-4669 Fax: (904)-376-4267
Contact: Darlene Burlingame - Health & Safety Coordinator
AIDS/HIV workplace program; offer course on preventing transmissiondiseases

Catholic Charities Bureau, Inc.
1717 NE 9th Street
Suite 126
Gainesville, FL 32609
Telephone: (904)-372-0294
Contact: Leonard Spikane - Director
Emergency assistance with rent, food, utilities & transportation

Community Action Agency - North Central Florida
1204 NW 8th Avenue
Gainesville, FL 32602
Telephone: (904)-373-7667
Self-help loans (repayable).Serves Alachua, Levy, & Marion Counties.

Coordinated Transportation System
2711 NW 6th Street
Suite B
Gainesville, FL 32602
Telephone: (904)-373-8747 Fax: (904)-334-1600
Transportation for the disadvantaged.

Corner Drug Store/Transitions
1300 NW 6th Street
Gainesville, FL 32601
Telephone: (904)-378-1588
Contact: Shirley Walker - Out-patient Coordinator
Therapy for substance abuse problems.

Gainesville Housing Authority
1900 S.E. 4th Street
Gainesville, FL 32602
Telephone: (904)-377-8851
Housing

Goodwill Industries
716 North Main Street
Gainesville, FL 32601
Telephone: (904)-376-9041
Low-cost clothing, household goods and furniture.

Housing Authority - Gainesville
1900 SE 4 Street
Gainesville, FL 32602
Telephone: (904)-377-8853
Public housing program. (Rental subsidies call: 377-3099.)

Legal Services
11 SW 1 Street
Gainesville, FL 32601
Telephone: (904)-372-0519
Court & administrative representation in civil actions for indigents

Medicaid Program
1000 NE 16th Avenue
Bldg NSC
Gainesville, FL 32609
Telephone: (904)-336-5176 Fax: (904)-336-3317
Services for Medicaid recipients.

Metamorphosis
306 NE 7th Street
Gainesville, FL 32601
Telephone: (904)-377-8787
24-hour residential drug rehabilitation program.

North Central Florida AIDS Network (NCFAN)
P.O. Box 5755
Gainesville, FL 32602-5755
Telephone: (904)-372-4370
Toll-Free: (800)-824-6745
Contact: Jesse Smith
Support, buddy groups, speakers, newsletter, public awarenessprojects,education

Salvation Army
639 E University Avenue
Gainesville, FL 32602
Telephone: (904)-376-1743 Fax: (904)-375-3235
Services to homeless, indigent and veterans.

Samaritan Counseling Center of North Central Florida
606 SW 3rd Avenue
Gainesville, FL 32601
Telephone: (904)-371-2797
Contact: Dr. Richard Horn
Professional counseling-spiritual,emotional,& personal relationships,individual, couple & family therapy

St. Francis House
PO Box 12491
Gainesville, FL 32604
Telephone: (904)-378-9079
Contact: Bib Tanzic - Executive Director
Emergency housing and daily lunches, (no fees).

County Health Depts

Alachua County Public Health Unit
Dental Care
730 N Waldo Road
Gainesville, FL 32602
Telephone: (904)-336-2415
Dental care for children and adults

Alachua County Public Health Unit
P.O. Box 1327
730 NE Waldo, 500, Bldg B
Gainesville, FL 32601-1327
Telephone: (904)-336-2356
Contact: Bobby Davisuore - Administrator AIDS Program
Health department, education, HIV pre/post testing, medical follow-up,referral, social service

Home Health Care

Hospice of North Central Florida, Inc.
3615 Southwest 13th Street
Gainesville, FL 32608
Telephone: (904)-378-2121 Fax: (904)-378-4111
Serves terminally patients and their families.

Kimberly Quality Care Homecare Services
5200 Newberry Road
Suite A-1
Gainesville, FL 32607
Telephone: (904)-375-8199
Provides care in hospitals and at home.

Olsten HealthCare
327 N.W. 23rd Ave.
Gainesville, FL 32069
Telephone: (904)-373-7539 Fax: (904)-372-9127
Home health services incl: infusion therapy, nutritional support

Project AIDS Care Florida-Medicaid
Alachua Cty Health Unit
730 NE Waldo Road, Suite 600
Gainesville, FL 32602
Telephone: (904)-336-2364 Fax: (904)-336-2376
Case management, private-duty nursing, home-delivered meals,etc.

Santa Fe Home Care
801 SW 2nd Avenue
Gainesville, FL 32602
Telephone: (904)-338-2189 Fax: (904)-338-6709
Certified home health care, home infusion

Upjohn Health Care Services
327 NW 23rd Avenue
Gainesville, FL 32609
Telephone: (904)-373-7539 Fax: (904)-374-9127
Certified and licensed home health care, case management

Medical Services

Alachua County Mental Health
4300 SW 13th St
Gainesville, FL 32608
Telephone: (904)-374-5600
Detox program

Alachua General Hospital
801 SW 2nd Avenue
Gainesville, FL 32601
Telephone: (904)-372-4321

Family Practice Medical Group
625 SW 4th Avenue
Gainesville, FL 32601
Telephone: (904)-373-6771
Provides basic medical, psychiatric, nurtritional and nursing services.

Pediatric Immunology Clinic
Shands Teaching Hospital
1600 SW Archer Road
Gainesville, FL 32611
Telephone: (904)-392-2961 Fax: (904)-392-0481
Accepts referrals from doctors & health departments.

Shand's Teaching Hospital
1600 SW Archer Road
Gainesville, FL 32610
Telephone: (904)-395-0110
904-395-0050 emergency.

Shand's Teaching Hospital - Psychology Clinic
1600 SW Archer Road
Ground Flr, Rm A-73
Gainesville, FL 32611
Telephone: (904)-395-0294 Fax: (904)-392-7060
Contact: Dr. Nathan Perry - Clinical & Health Psychology
Group, family, marital therapy; pain & stress mgmt-in & out-patient.

Shands Teaching Hospital, Immunology (Pediatric)
1600 South West Archer Road 1st Floor
Gainesville, FL 32610
Telephone: (904)-392-8491
Care for asymptomatic & symptomatic HIV infection.

Student Health Care Center
University of Florida
P.O. Box 117500
Gainesville, FL 32611-7500
Telephone: (904)-392-1161
Medical care, preventative medicine, counseling and health education

Veterans Affairs Medical Center
1601 SW Archer Road
Gainesville, FL 32608
Telephone: (904)-376-1611
HIV/AIDS treatment for veterans

Vista Pavilion
8900 NW 39th Avenue
Gaineville, FL 32606
Telephone: (904)-338-0097
Medically supervised in & out-patient treatment programs for recovery.

Testing Sites

Alachua Clinic
310 North Main Street
P.O. Box 1060
Alachua, FL 32615
Telephone: (904)-462-2542 Fax: (904)-462-4381
Anonymous HIV Test Site

Gainesville Health Center
720 NW 23rd Street
Gainesville, FL 32609
Telephone: (904)-377-5055
Comprehensive services for men & women; anonymous HIV screening.

Hawthorne Clinic
107 NW 3rd Street
P.O. Box 1481
Hawthorne, FL 32640-1481
Telephone: (904)-481-2388 Fax: (904)-481-2699
Anonymous HIV Test Site

Herpes Support Group
914 NOrthwest 13th Street
Gainesville, FL 32601
Telephone: (904)-376-9000 Fax: (904)-374-6823
STD/AIDS testing, gynecological

Planned Parenthood of North Central Florida
914 Northwest 13th Street
Gainesville, FL 32601
Telephone: (904)-377-0881 Fax: (904)-374-6823
Gynecological, AIDS testing, pregnancy tests

Baker County

County Health Depts

Baker County Public Health Unit
657 South 6th Street
Macclenny, FL 32063-2607
Telephone: (904)-259-6291 Fax: (904)-259-4761
Contact: Kerry Dunleavy - Director of Nursing
Confidential HIV testing, treatment for HIV/AIDS, STD-pre-natal, pediatrics,educational information.

Bay County

County Health Depts

Bay County Public Health Unit
605 MacArthur Avenue
Panama City, FL 32401-3680
Telephone: (904)-872-4455 Fax: (904)-872-7779
Contact: Nancy Nichols - Nurse Supervisor
HIV anonymous test site, confidential testing, information referrals

Bradford County

County Health Depts

Bradford County Public Health Unit
329 North Church Street
Starke, FL 32091-3415
Telephone: (904)-964-7732
Contact: Wanda Norman - CPHU Director; Audrey Michael - Business Manager; Kenneth Pabst - Environmental Health
Health services, education, HIV pre-post testing, medical follow up,referrals

Home Health Care

Olsten HealthCare
221 S. Orange St.
Starke, FL 32091
Telephone: (904)-964-8772
Home health services incl: infusion therapy, nutritional support,pediatric care.

Medical Services

Acorn Dental Clinic
Route 1 Box 59
Hwy #231
Brooker, FL 32622
Telephone: (904)-485-1133
Primary medical & dental care

Brevard County

County Health Depts

Brevard County Public Health Unit
P.O. Box 560-474
1744 South Cedar Street
Rockledge, FL 32956-0747
Telephone: (407)-632-6010
Contact: Manuel J. Garcia, MD - CPHU Director; Renick 'Nick' Brandt - Business Manager; Willie Humphrey, DDS
Pretesting, post testing, counseling, education

Home Health Care

Olsten Kimberly Quality Care
1571 Robert J Conlan Blvd. NE
Suite 118
Palm Bay, FL 32905
Telephone: (407)-723-9600 Fax: (407)-723-0306
Home health services incl: infusion therapy, nutritional support,pediatric care.

Broward County

County Health Depts

Broward County Public Health Unit
2421 Southwest Sixth Ave
Ft. Lauderdale, FL 33315-2613
Telephone: (305)-467-4811
Contact: Lisa Aqatte
Education, pre & post testing, medical follow-up, referrals

District 10 Office
201 West Broward Blvd
Ft. Lauderdale, FL 33301-1846
Telephone: (305)-467-4298 Fax: (305)-467-4623
Contact: Lisa Agatte - District Administrator; Myra Bomba - Deputy District Admin.; Theresa Coleman - District AIDS Coordinator
Public services

Home Health Care

Caremark Connection Network
100 E. Commercial Blvd.
Fort Lauderdale, FL 33334
Telephone: (305)-938-9944 Fax: (305)-938-9010
Clinical Support and Infusion Therapies: Nutrition, Antimicrobials,Chemo.,Hematopoe

Critical Care America
10102 USA Today Way
Miramar, FL 33025
Telephone: (305)-436-0400 Fax: (305)-436-0405
Toll-Free: (800)-765-9614
Coordinate & integrate all clinical & psychosocial services for HIV+

Curaflex Infusion Services
3330 NW 53rd St. #301
Ft Lauderdale, FL 33309-6352
Telephone: (305)-771-4208
Contact: Lisa Kasten
Home IV therapy: TPN, Enteral, IV Antibiotics, Aerosolized/IV, pentamidine,chemotherapy

HNS, Inc.
5249 NW 33rd Ave, Bldg 6
Ft. Lauderdale, FL 33309
Telephone: (305)-735-5080
Home infusion therapy

Infusion Care of Fort Lauderdale
315 Southeast 14th Street
Ft. Lauderdale, FL 33316
Telephone: (305)-524-2250 Fax: (305)-524-4555
Contact: Verne Appleby
Comprehensive HIV services

nmc HOMECARE
1350 East Newport Center Drive, Suite 100
Deerfield, FL 33442
Telephone: (305)-427-7200
Fax: (305)-427-7263
Contact: Karen Kaczmarek
National JCAHO-Accredited company providing a full range of Infusion and Respiratory therapies and specializing in the care of HIV/AIDS patients. National Case Manager is also available at 800-445-1188

Olsten HealthCare
3600 W. Commercial Blvd.
Ft. Lauderdale, FL 33309
Telephone: (305)-486-2257 Fax: (305)-731-2861
Home health services incl: infusion therapy, nutritional support, pediatriccare

Olsten HealthCare
3860 Sheriden St.
Hollywood, FL 33021
Telephone: (305)-962-5507 Fax: (305)-962-5710
Home health services incl: infusion therapy, nutritional support

Resource Opportunities, Inc.
800 Cypress Creek Road W
Suite 340
Ft. Lauderdale, FL 33309
Telephone: (305)-776-5189 Fax: (305)-776-5792
Contact: Patrica Hubrig, RN
Catastrophic case management, vocational rehab., life care plans, experttestimonies

Medical Services

INFUSIONCARE of FT. LAUDERDALE
315 SE 14th St
Ft. Lauderdale, FL 33316
Telephone: (305)-524-4555
Fax: (305)-524-5833
Full service ambulatory HIV/AIDS clinic with primary care physicians providing aerosolized infusion therapies and other comprehensive care for the HIV/AIDS patient.

Northwest Health Center
624 Northwest 15 Way
Ft. Lauderdale, FL 33311
Telephone: (305)-467-4532 Fax: (305)-467-4676
Contact: Jasmin Shirley Moore
Medical, dental, social, case management, counseling, home health care,hospice

Calhoun County

County Health Depts

Calhoun County Public Health Unit
1507 West Central Street
Blountstown, FL 32424-0239
Telephone: (904)-674-5645 Fax: (904)-674-5420
Contact: Claudette Pratt - R.N.
AIDS testing, counseling, education, minimal services.

Charlotte County

County Health Depts

Charlotte County Public Health Unit
514 East Grace Street
Punta Gorda, FL 33950
Telephone: (813)-639-1181 Fax: (813)-639-3350
Contact: John Piacitelli, MD - CPHU Director
Testing, counseling, education

Citrus County

County Health Depts

HRS Citrus County Public Health Unit
3700 West Souerign Path
Lecanto, FL 34461-8071
Telephone: (904)-726-1731
Contact: Marybeth Nayfield
Health services, education, HIV pre & post testing, medical followup, referrals

Clay County

County Health Depts

Clay County Public Health Unit
P.O. Box 566
1305 Idlewild Avenue
Green Cove Springs, FL 32043-0566
Telephone: (904)-284-6340
Contact: Lynette Smith - CPHU Administrator

Home Health Care

Olsten HealthCare
2020 Kingsley Ave.
Letter F
Orange Park, FL 32073
Telephone: (904)-272-8367
Home health services incl: infusion therapy, nutritional support, pediatriccare; 2-hour AIDS class

Collier County

Community Services

Collier AIDS Resources & Education Service Inc. (CARES)
3080 Miami Trail North
Naples, FL 33940
Telephone: (813)-263-2273 Fax: (813)-263-2303
Contact: Rob McMurrough - Peer Educator; Michael Kaiser - Executive Director
Education, case management, testing, outreach, support groups,medical/dental referrals

County Health Depts

HRS Collier County Public Health Unit
3301 E Tamiami Trail
P.O. Box 428
Naples, FL 33939-0428
Telephone: (813)-774-8200 Fax: (813)-774-5653
Contact: Roger Evans
HIV Anonymous Test Site, Infectious disease clinic, community healtheducation, AIDS & epidemilogy services.

Home Health Care

Olsten HealthCare
660 9th St. N
Suite 5
Naples, FL 33940
Telephone: (813)-263-7787
Home health services incl: infusion therapy, nutritional support,pediatric care.

Columbia County

County Health Depts

Columbia County Public Health Unit
249 E. Franklin Street
Lake City, FL 32055-2915
Telephone: (904)-755-4100 Fax: (904)-755-4326
Contact: Michael Tow
Anonymous HIV Test Site

Home Health Care

Olsten HealthCare
Rte 10
Box 971
Lake City, FL 32055
Telephone: (904)-755-9500
Home health services incl: infusion therapy, nutritional support, pediatric care, Ryan White case management

Dade County

Community Services

Camilius House
726 Northeast First Avenue
Miami, FL 33132
Telephone: (305)-374-1065 Fax: (305)-372-1402
Homeless shelter

Children's Home Society: Project SMILE (AIDS)
800 Northwest 15th Street
Miami, FL 33136
Telephone: (305)-324-1262 Fax: (305)-326-7430
Contact: Issa Cuadra
Adoptions, shelters, teenage shelters

Dade County Government - Alcohol & Drug Abuse
2500 Northwest 22nd Avenue
Miami, FL 33142
Telephone: (305)-638-6540
Referrals, detox unit

Dade County Government - Emergency Housing Services
2301 Northwest 54th Street
Miami, FL 33142
Telephone: (305)-638-6001 Fax: (305)-638-5608
Contact: Shesha Tarber
AIDS hotline 305-795-1562

Dade County Government - Metro DHR
140 West Flagler Street
902 Suite
Miami, FL 33139
Telephone: (305)-375-5656
Contact: Claudia Thompson
General Information (Emergency Assistance)

Douglas Gardens Community Mental Health Center
701 Lincoln Road
2nd Floor
Miami Beach, FL 33139-3813
Telephone: (305)-531-5341 Fax: (305)-532-5322
Mental health services

Genesis House 1
3675 South Miami Avenue
Miami, FL 33133
Telephone: (305)-856-1043 Fax: (305)-856-1633
Contact: Anna Marie Martin
Residential services for AIDS patients

League Against AIDS, Inc.
2699 Biscayne Blvd
Suite 4
Miami, FL 33137
Counseling, therapy

Legal Services of Greater Miami
225 NE 34th Street
Miami, FL 33137
Telephone: (305)-576-0080
Contact: Clint Hurst - Legal Aid
Legal aid for AIDS/HIV patients

Narcotics-Anonymous (South)
4705 Southwest 75th Avenue
Miami, FL 33155
Telephone: (305)-662-0280
Referral service for recovering addicts

Paratransit Operations
2775 Southwest 74th Avenue
Miami, FL 33155
Telephone: (305)-263-5400 Fax: (305)-269-6325
Medicaid eligible, transportation service

Refugee Assistance Program
1621 Southwest 107 Avenue
Miami, FL 33165
Telephone: (305)-227-5021
Food stamps, emergency assistance

She Center
12550 Biscayne Blvd.
North Miami, FL 33181
Telephone: (305)-895-5555 Fax: (305)-899-9402
AIDS support group, counseling

United Way
1 Southeast 3rd Avenue
Suite #1950
Miami, FL 33131
Telephone: (305)-579-2200 Fax: (305)-579-2212
Fund raising

Youth and Family Development
1701 NW 30th Avenue
Miami, FL 33125
Telephone: (305)-633-6481
Psychological counseling

County Health Depts

Dade County Health Department (Pre-Natal)
1350 Northwest 14th Street
Miami, FL 33125
Telephone: (305)-324-2452 Fax: (305)-324-5959
Contact: Joan Davis
Prenatal care, infant care, STD., WIC.

Dade County Public Health Unit
1444 Biscayne Blvd.
Miami, FL 33125-1609
Telephone: (305)-377-5022 Fax: (305)-377-7238
Contact: George Mettelus, MD, MPH - CPHU Director
HIV testing, confidential and anonymous; counseling; patient care and referrals

Dade County Public Health Unit
615 Collins Avenue
Miami Beach, FL 33139-6213
Telephone: (305)-538-0525
HIV Anonymous Test Site, Primary care to HIV clients

Home Health Care

Hospice
4770 Biscaine Blvd.
Suite 250
Miami, FL 33137
Telephone: (305)-576-9333
In home patient care units of terminally ill, AIDS care

nmc HOMECARE
2628 NE 191st St
No. Miami Beach, FL 33180
Telephone: (305)-933-1307
Fax: (305)-935-9846
National JCAHO-Accredited company providing a full range of Infusion and Respiratory therapies and specializing in the care of HIV/AIDS patients. National Case Manager is also available at 800-445-1188

nmc HOMECARE
8405 N.W. 53rd St, Suite C 106
Miami, FL 33166
Telephone: (305)-477-7777
Fax: (305)-477-6730
National JCAHO-Accredited company providing a full range of Infusion and Respiratory therapies and specializing in the care of HIV/AIDS patients. National Case Manager is also available at 800-445-1188

Olsten HealthCare
6303 Blue Lagoon Drive
Suite 195
Miami, FL 33126
Telephone: (305)-262-5333 Fax: (305)-262-5397
Home health services incl: infusion therapy, nutritional support

Olsten HealthCare
16853 NE 2nd Ave.
Miami, FL 33162
Telephone: (305)-652-6611 Fax: (305)-651-1154
Home health services incl: infusion therapy, nutritional support

Medical Services

Bayview Center for Mental Health
12550 Biscayne Blvd.
Miami, FL 33181-2024
Telephone: (305)-892-4600 Fax: (305)-893-1224
Therapy group, Pharmacy, Counseling, Testing, Social workers

Borinquen Health Care Center
5700 NE 4 Court
Miami, FL 33137-2689
Telephone: (305)-751-5322 Fax: (305)-751-5051
Contact: Helene Augustin - Aids Coordinator
Evaluation, testing, medical & dental care

Coconut Grove Family Health Center
3230 Hibiscus Street
Miami, FL 33133-4906
Telephone: (305)-447-4950 Fax: (305)-447-9740
Early intervention: labs, pharmacy, medical visits & social services

Community Health of South Dade, Inc.
10300 SW 216 Street
Miami, FL 33190-1003
Telephone: (305)-253-5100 Fax: (305)-254-2011
Testing, Medical care, Social and Counseling Services, Referrals

Community Health of South Dade, Inc.
10300 SW 216 Street
Miami, FL 33190
Telephone: (305)-252-4877 Fax: (305)-254-2011
Contact: Amber Wallace - AIDS Coordinator
General practice, specialists, mental health pharmacy, testing, counseling

Dade County Public Care Department
1350 Northwest 14th Street
Miami, FL 33125-1609
Telephone: (305)-324-2441 Fax: (305)-324-5959
Basic dental services

Douglas Gardens Community Mental Health Center
701 Lincoln Road
2nd Floor
Miami, FL 33139
Telephone: (305)-531-5341
Contact: Jeanne Adams - Dir of Outpatients Services
Therapy, psychotherapy, medication

Hialeah Family Health Center
490 East Hialeah Drive
Hialeah, FL 33010-5347
Telephone: (305)-887-0004 Fax: (305)-887-8466
Contact: Carmen Tejada - HIV Counselor
Medical care, testing, counseling

Jackson Memorial Hospital
1611 NW 12th Ave
Miami, FL 33136
Telephone: (305)-325-7429
Contact: Barbara K. Lloyd
Case management

James E. Scott Center
7200 NW 22nd Avenue
Miami, FL 33147-6222
Telephone: (305)-835-8122 Fax: (305)-835-6906
Primary Health Care

Liberty City Health Services Center
1320 NW 62nd Street
Miami, FL 33147-8016
Telephone: (305)-835-2200 Fax: (305)-696-6910
Full primary care, group counseling, psychosocial counseling, casemanagement, referrals, outreach, transportation

Martin Luther King Jr., Clinica Campesina
810 West Mowry Street
Homestead, FL 33030-574
Telephone: (305)-248-4334 Fax: (305)-245-1161
Contact: Amber Wallace - AIDS Coordinator
Comprehensive medical care, pharmacy, dentist, mental health counseling

Miami Mental Health Center
2141 SW 1st Street
Miami, FL 33135-1699
Telephone: (305)-643-1660 Fax: (305)-642-7010
AIDS testing

New Horizons Community Mental Health
1469 NW 36th Street
Miami, FL 33142-5583
Telephone: (305)-635-0366

North Dade Health Center
16555 NW 25th Avenue
Miami, FL 33054-6598
Telephone: (305)-621-8888 Fax: (305)-624-5296
Primary care, Dental, Case management, Relaxation classes, Pharmacy, X-ray

Spectrum
11033 Northeast 6th Avenue
Miami, FL 33161
Telephone: (305)-754-1683
Contact: Carolyn Boyett
Out-patient Drug & Alcohol, inpatient & outpatient AIDS treatment

Stanley Myers Community Health Center
710 Alton Road
Miami Beach, FL 33139
Telephone: (305)-538-8835 Fax: (305)-532-5766
General and special medical care, pharmacy, testing, social services

University of Miami School of Medicine
Dept. of OB/GYNU
P.O. Box 016960 (D-136)
Miami, FL 33101
Telephone: (305)-585-6950 Fax: (305)-325-1282
Contact: Dr. Mary O'Sullivan

Westchester Mental Health
2700 SW 87th Avenue
Suite 209
Miami, FL 33165
Telephone: (305)-553-4322
Psychological and psychiatric services

Westchester Mental Health Center
2468 S.W. 87th Avenue
Suite 208
Miami, FL 33165-2031
Telephone: (305)-553-4322
Outpatient therapy, Testing, Evaluation counseling

Dixie County

County Health Depts

Dixie County Public Health Unit
P.O. Drawer 2099
Cross City, FL 32628-9999
Telephone: (904)-498-1360
HIV testing

Duval County

County Health Depts

Duval County Public Health Unit
962 N.Main St.
Jacksonville, FL 32202
Telephone: (904)-358-8386
Contact: Sharron Stanton - Deputy Director
STD treatment, HIV clinic, counseling & testing (anonymous), medical care

Home Health Care

Caremark, Inc.
9143 Phillips Hwy
Suite 300
Jacksonville, FL 32256
Telephone: (904)-363-3089 Fax: (904)-363-2159
Contact: Mike Young - General Manager
Clinical Support and Infusion Therapies: Nutrition, Antimicrobials,Chemotherapy Hematopoe

Critical Care America
8301 Cypress Plaza Dr
Suite 123
Jacksonville, FL 32256
Telephone: (904)-281-9727
Contact: 800-331-6856
Hone care; coordinate & integrate all clinical & psychosocial services forHIV+

HNS, Inc.
8031 Phillips Highway
Suite 1
Jacksonville, FL 32256
Telephone: (904)-737-9843 Fax: (904)-737-9871
Contact: Janet Stock Palmer
Home Infusion Therapy, In-home Nursing and Attendant Care, PhysicalTherapy, Pentamidine

nmc HOMECARE
2700 University Blvd West, Suite 81
Jacksonville, FL 32217
Telephone: (904)-296-8700
Fax: (904)-733-1626
Contact: Joanne Ryan
National JCAHO-Accredited company providing a full range of Infusion and Respiratory therapies and specializing in the care of HIV/AIDS patients. National Case Manager is also available at 800-445-1188

O.P.T.I.O.N Care of North Florida
88 W. 63rd Street
Jacksonville, FL 32208-4124
Telephone: (904)-766-9608 Fax: (904)-766-2849
Contact: Rudolf Elliott
Home IV, nutritional services, chemotherapy, pharmacy, on call nurses

Olsten HealthCare
8101 Southside Blvd.
Suite 1
Jacksonville, FL 32256
Telephone: (904)-641-2700 Fax: (904)-641-2702
Toll-Free: (800)-852-4381
Home health services incl: infusion therapy, nutritional support

Testing Sites

Main St Clinic (AIDS Program)
962 N. Main Street
Jacksonville, FL 32202-3081
Telephone: (904)-358-8386
Contact: Sharon Stanton
Anonymous HIV testing clinic

Escambia County

Home Health Care

Caremark Connection Network
5401 Corporate Woods Dr.
Suite 150
Pensacola, FL 32504
Telephone: (904)-494-1121 Fax: (904)-494-0240
Contact: ; Joanne Peoples - Nurse Manager; Angela Kelly - Clinical Sales Rep.
Clinical Support and Infusion Therapies: Nutrition, Antimicrobials, Chemo.,Hematopoe

Olsten HealthCare
4400 Bayou Blvd
Suite 14 B
Pensacola, FL 32503
Telephone: (904)-479-0885 Fax: (904)-484-6847
Home health services incl: infusion therapy, nutritional support, pedes care.

Testing Sites

Escambia AIDS Services and Education (EASE)
P.O. Box 13584
Pensacola, FL 32591-3584
Telephone: (904)-456-7079 Fax: (904)-457-0902
Contact: Phil Cudahy; Fred Chappa -
HIV Anonymous Test Site

Flagler County

County Health Depts

Flagler County Public Health Unit
P.O. Box 847
301 South Lemon St.
Bunnell, FL 32110-0847
Telephone: (904)-437-3113
Contact: Debbie Panchella - Medical Executive Dir.; Steve McClintock, DDS - Dental

Gadsden County

County Health Depts

Gadsden County Public Health Unit
P.O. Box 1000
Quincy, FL 32353-1000
Telephone: (904)-487-3952
Contact: Edward J. Wynn - CPHU Director
Testing, counseling, referrals

Gilchrist County

County Health Depts

Gilchrist County Public Health Unit
P.O. Box 368
Trenton, FL 32693
Telephone: (904)-463-2312 Fax: (904)-463-6320
Contact: Jana Land
Confidential HIV Test Site

Home Health Care

Olsten HealthCare
Box 1032, RR 1 Hwy. 26
Trenton, FL 32693
Telephone: (904)-463-6510 Fax: (904)-463-6520
Toll-Free: (800)-228-4236
Home health services incl: infusion therapy, nutritional support

Glades County

County Health Depts

Glades County Public Health Unit
P.O. Box 489
Building 998, Hwy 27 N.
Moore Haven, FL 33471-0489
Telephone: (813)-946-0707 Fax: (813)-946-3097
Contact: Martha Valiant - MD
Primary care, counseling, testing, education, home-visiting nurse, speakers

Gulf County

County Health Depts

Gulf County Public Health Unit
502 Fourth Street
Port St. Joe, FL 32456
Telephone: (904)-227-1276
Contact: Verna Mathis - CPHU Director
Screening for AIDS, education

Hamilton County

County Health Depts

Hamilton County Public Health Unit
209 SE Central Avenue
P.O. Box 267
Jasper, FL 32052
Telephone: (904)-792-1414
Contact: Nancy Wiegand
Anonymous HIV test site, education, referrals

Hardee County

County Health Depts

Hardee County Public Health Unit
P.O. Box 788
316 North 7th Avenue
Wauchula, FL 33873-0788
Telephone: (813)-773-4161
Contact: Jane Counts - CPHU Director
Testing, referral, education

Hendry County

County Health Depts

Hendry County Public Health Unit
P.O. Box 70
133 Bridge Street
LaBelle, FL 33935-0070
Telephone: (813)-675-0313
Contact: George Roberson - Coordinator
Medical care, case management, rental assistance, HIV testing, education,drug abuse referral

Hernando County

County Health Depts

Hernando County Public Health Unit
300 South Main Street
Brooksville, FL 34601
Telephone: (904)-754-4067
Contact: Jackie Carol - CPHU Director
HIV testing, referrals, education

Hernando County Public Health Unit
7465 Forest Oaks Blvd.
Spring Hill, FL 34606-2449
Telephone: (904)-688-5067
Contact: Liz Jennings
Confidential testing, referral, counseling

Highlands County

County Health Depts

Highlands County Public Health Unit
7205 South George Blvd
Sebring, FL 33872-5847
Telephone: (813)-382-1193
Contact: Juva Fassler, MD - CPHU Director
HIV testing, patient care follow-up, home visits, financial counseling,education

Home Health Care

Olsten Kimberly Quality Care
259 US 27 North
Sebring, FL 33870
Telephone: (801)-382-8855
Contact: Lynne Stacy
Home health services incl: infusion therapy, nutritional support,pediatric care.

Hillsborough County

Community Services

District 6 Office
P.O. Box 5135
Tampa, FL 33614
Telephone: (813)-871-7520 Fax: (813)-873-4751
Contact: Lisle House - District Administrator
Case management financing, education, counseling; confidential referral fortesting

Tampa Bay Area AIDS Network
11215 North Nebraska Avenue
Suite B
Tampa, FL 33612
Telephone: (813)-978-8683 Fax: (813)-878-3515

County Health Depts

HRS Hillsborough County Public Health Unit
P.O. Box 5135
1105 East Kennedy Blvd
Tampa, FL 33675-5135
Telephone: (813)-272-6300
Contact: Luis Miranda, MD - CPHU Director
HIV testing & counseling (confidential) & medical services; education, STDclinic

Home Health Care

Critical Care America
8509-A Benjamin Road
Clearwater, FL 33634-1224
Telephone: (813)-573-0336
Home infusion therapy

Critical Care America
8509A Benjamin Road
Tampa, FL 33634
Telephone: (813)-888-7545 Fax: (813)-887-3198
Clinical pharmacy, IV infusion

HNS, Inc.
5402 Beaumont Center Blvd
Suite 114
Tampa, FL 33634
Telephone: (813)-882-0083
Contact: Bob McChesney
Home Infusion Therapy, In-home Nursing and Attendant Care, PhysicalTherapy, Pentamidine

nmc HOMECARE
6308 Benjamin Rd
Tampa, FL 33634
Telephone: (813)-576-7070
Fax: (813)-579-0259
Contact: Daniel Sweeney
National JCAHO-Accredited company providing a full range of Infusion and Respiratory therapies and specializing in the care of HIV/AIDS patients. National Case Manager is also available at 800-445-1188

Olsten Kimberly Quality Care
5802 Breckenridge Pkwy #1
Suite 103
Tampa, FL 33610
Telephone: (813)-620-3368
Home health services incl: infusion therapy, nutritional support,pediatric care.

Medical Services

BAY COMPREHENSIVE HEALTHCARE
3217A S MacDill Ave
Tampa, FL 33629
Telephone: (813)-651-2238
Fax: (813)-831-3516
Contact: Cyndie Smith
Full service ambulatory HIV/AIDS clinic with primary care physicians providing aerosolized infusion therapies and other comprehensive care for the HIV/AIDS patient.

Testing Sites

Hillsborough County Public Health Unit
1105 East Kennedy Blvd.
Tampa, FL 33602-3512
Telephone: (813)-272-6200 Fax: (813)-272-6039
Contact: Mr. George Hughes - STD Programming Manager
HIV confidental & anonymous test site, pre & post counseling, referrals,case management

Holmes County

County Health Depts

Holmes County Public Health Unit
P.O. Box 337
603 Scenic Circle Drive
Bonifay, FL 32425-0337
Telephone: (904)-547-3691
Contact: Margie Barefield
HIV testing & counseling

Jackson County

County Health Depts

Jackson County Public Health Unit
P.O. Box 310
3045 Fourth Street
Marianna, FL 32446-0310
Telephone: (904)-526-2412
Contact: Jimmy Rigsby - CPHU Administrator, Rosemary Everitt - Administrative Assistant; Sara Schulz, MD - Medical Director
HIV testing, counseling, evaluation

Jefferson County

County Health Depts

Jefferson County Public Health Unit
1255 W. Washington St.
Monticello, FL 32344-1128
Telephone: (904)-997-5422
Contact: Dr. Anna Vazguez - CPHU Administrator
HIV testing, counseling & evaluation

Lafayette County

County Health Depts

HRS Lafayette County Public Health Unit
Route 3, Box 8
Highway 27
Mayo, FL 32066-9429
Telephone: (904)-294-1321
Contact: Nancy McCullers - CPHU Administrator
HIV testing & counseling

Lake County

County Health Depts

Lake County Public Health Unit
249 Collins Street
Umatilla, FL 32784-0523
Telephone: (904)-669-2432 Fax: (904)-669-1228
Primary care, Project AIDS care

Lee County

County Health Depts

District 8 Office
P.O. Box 06085
12381 South Cleveland
Ft. Myers, FL 33906-6085
Telephone: (813)-936-2211
Contact: Gail Counts - AIDS/HIV Coord.
Regional office of state HRS dept., educational materials on prevention &treatment, referrals to county health offices and private agencies; serves7-county area

Lee County Public Health Unit
3920 Michigan Avenue
Ft. Myers, FL 33916-2298
Telephone: (813)-332-9510
Contact: Judith A. Hartner - Medical Director
HIV testing; pre & post test, counseling, education & awareness program forAIDS/HIV; make referrals to Lee county AIDS/HIV task force

Lee County Public Health Unit
3920 Michigan Avenue
Ft. Myers, FL 33916
Telephone: (813)-332-9501 Fax: (813)-332-9609
Contact: Terry Ogilbey
HIV Anonymous Test Site

Home Health Care

Olsten HealthCare
1620 Medical Lane
Suite 135
Fort Myers, FL 33907
Telephone: (813)-275-5505 Fax: (813)-275-5995
Home health services incl: infusion therapy, nutritional support,pediatric care.

Testing Sites

Cape Coral Hospital
Del Prado Boulevard
Cape Coral, FL 33990-2695
Telephone: (813)-574-2323
Contact: Lynda Nugteren
HIV Anonymous Test Site

Leon County

County Health Depts

District 2 Health Program Office
2639 North Monroe Street
Tallahassee, FL 32303-4051
Telephone: (904)-487-2546
Contact: Philip E. Reichert - AIDS/HIV Coord.
Regional administrative office of state HRS dept., educational materials onprevention & treatment, referrals to county health offices and privateagencies

Leon County Public Health Unit
2965 Municipal Way
Tallahassee, FL 32304-3822
Telephone: (904)-487-3186 Fax: (904)-487-3162
Toll-Free: (904)-487-7954
Contact: Paul Mazzotta; Gloria Guimaraes
HIV Anonymous Test Site, HIV/AIDS Education

Home Health Care

Olsten Kimberly Quality Care
1861 Capital Cir NE
Tallahassee, FL 32308
Telephone: (904)-878-2191 Fax: (904)-942-2147
Home health services incl: infusion therapy, nutritional support, pedes care.

Levy County

County Health Depts

Levy County Public Health Unit
P.O. Box 40
66 South Main Street
Bronson, FL 32621-0040
Telephone: (904)-486-2101
Contact: Jeffrey Rubin, MD - CPHU Director; Barbara Locke, RN - Nursing
Testing & counseling for HIV

Liberty County

County Health Depts

Liberty County Public Health Unit
P.O. Box 489
North Central Street
Bristol, FL 32321-0489
Telephone: (904)-643-2415
Contact: Julian Giraldo; June Glass, Nursing -
HIV testing, counseling

Madison County

County Health Depts

Madison County Public Health Unit
801 SW Smith Street
Madison, FL 32340-1245
Telephone: (904)-973-6651
Contact: Roger McCollum - CPHU Administrator; Diane Webb - Staff Assistant
Confidential HIV testing/ counseling, education & limited referral services

Manatee County

County Health Depts

HRS Manatee County Public Health Unit
410 Sixth Avenue East
Bradenton, FL 34208
Telephone: (813)-748-0666 Fax: (813)-747-7347
Contact: John Ambrusko, MD - CPHU Director; C. Wolford - Assistant Director
Case management, anonymous testing & counseling

Home Health Care

Olsten Kimberly Quality Care
1999 Lincoln Drive
Suite 101
Sarasota, FL 34205
Telephone: (813)-366-4320 Fax: (813)-955-9597
Home health services incl: infusion therapy, nutritional support,pediatric care.

Marion County

Community Services

AIDS Network
3820 East Silver Springs Blvd.
Suite 8
Ocala, FL 34470
Telephone: (904)-629-5124
24 hour support

Home Health Care

Olsten Kimberly Quality Care
3304 SW 34th Cir #104
Ocala, FL 34474
Telephone: (904)-237-6111 Fax: (904)-237-6836
Contact: Maryann Wilhelm
Home health services incl: infusion therapy, nutritional support,pediatric care.

Medical Services

Charter Hospital
3130 South West 27th Avenue
Ocala, FL 34474
Telephone: (904)-331-8559
Psychiatric counseling, chemical dependency programs

Martin County

County Health Depts

Martin County Public Health Unit
620 S. Dixie Hwy
Stuart, FL 34994-3407
Telephone: (407)-221-4000
Contact: Betty Kroesen, RN - CPHU Administrator
General care

Monroe County

Medical Services

Immunecare of Key West
520 Southard St.
Key West, FL 33040
Telephone: (305)-296-4990 Fax: (305)-296-4866
Contact: Chuck Kessler
HIV care, financial counseling

Nassau County

County Health Depts

Nassau County Public Health Unit
P.O. Box 517
4th and Ash Street
Fernandina Bch, FL 32034-0517
Telephone: (904)-277-7280 Fax: (904)-277-7286
Contact: Maries Riley, RN - AID/HIV Coordinator
Testing; pre & post counseling, referrals for medical services

Okaloosa County

County Health Depts

Okaloosa County Public Health Unit
221 Hospital Drive NE
Ft. Walton, FL 32548-5066
Telephone: (904)-244-5175
Contact: Dr. Mathew Kinzelman
HIV testing, counseling

Okeechobee County

County Health Depts

Okeechobee County Public Health Unit
1728 Northwest 9th Avenue
Okeechobee, FL 34972-2586
Telephone: (813)-763-3419
Contact: Richard Katz, MD - CPHU Director
HIV counseling & testing

Orange County

County Health Depts

District 7 Office
400 West Robinson Street
Suite F-1014
Orlando, FL 32801-1736
Telephone: (407)-423-6245
Contact: Ed Carson - AIDS/HIV Coord.
Regional administrative office of state HRS dept.; educational materials onprevention & treatment; referrals to county health offices and privateagencies

Orange County Public Health Unit
832 West Central Blvd
Orlando, FL 32805-1851
Telephone: (407)-836-2680 Fax: (407)-836-2522
Contact: Victor Harris, PhD - CPHU Director; Stan Wagy - AIDS Manager
Anonymous testing & counseling, medical care, educational advisor,social worker

Home Health Care

Critical Care America
6355 Metrowest Blvd #220
Orlando, FL 32835-6206
Telephone: (407)-831-1224
Coordinate & integrate all clinical & psychosocial services for HIV+

Testing Sites

Orange County Public Health Unit
PO Box 3187
Orlando, FL 32805-1851
Telephone: (407)-836-2680 Fax: (407)-836-2522
Contact: Stan Wagy
HIV Anonymous Test Site, AIDS Patient Care Program,Outpatient SurveillanceProgram

Osceola County

County Health Depts

Osceola County Public Health Unit
1875 Boggy Creek Road
Kissimmee, FL 34745
Telephone: (407)-870-1400 Fax: (407)-870-1488
Contact: George Grant, MD - CPHU Director, Nancy Amhrein - Nursing Director
HIV counseling & testing

Palm Beach County

Community Services

Compass, Inc.
2670 Forest Hill Blvd.
Suite 106
West Palm Beach, FL 33406
Telephone: (407)-966-3050 Fax: (407)-966-0039
Contact: Lisa McWhorter - Executive Director
Gay & lesiban organization, support group, acupuncture clinic, outreachprogram for adults, teen awareness

District 9 Office Health Program Office
705 North Olive Street
West Palm Beach, FL 33401-5214
Telephone: (407)-837-5187
Contact: Nancy L. Heinrich - AIDS Coordinator
Total AIDS Care

County Health Depts

Palm Beach County Public Health Unit
P.O. Box 29
826 Evernia Street
West Palm Beach, FL 33402-5709
Telephone: (407)-355-3119
Contact: Jean Marie Malecki, MD
Public Health: medical services

Palm Beach County Public Health Unit
225 South Congress
Delray Beach, FL 33445
Telephone: (407)-274-3100 Fax: (407)-274-3144
Contact: Dorothy Gruber
HIV Anonymous Test Site

Home Health Care

Caremark Connection Network
3345 Burns Road
Suite 302
Palm Beach Gardens, FL 33410
Telephone: (407)-775-7544 Fax: (407)-775-8711
Contact: Bob Phelan - Branch Manager
Clinical Support and Infusion Therapies: Nutrition, Antimicrobials, Chemo.,Hematopoe

nmc HOMECARE
1315 53rd Street Unit #1
W. Palm Beach, FL 33407
Telephone: (407)-840-1500
Fax: (407)-840-1591
Contact: Gary McFadden
National JCAHO-Accredited company providing a full range of Infusion and Respiratory therapies and specializing in the care of HIV/AIDS patients. National Case Manager is also available at 800-445-1188

Testing Sites

Palm Beach County Public Health Unit
701 North Olive
West Palm Beach, FL 33407-4318
Telephone: (407)-355-4664 Fax: (407)-840-4564
Contact: Michelle Thomas
HIV Anonymous Test Site

Pasco County

County Health Depts

Pasco County Public Health Unit
10841 Little Road
New Port Richey, FL 34654
Telephone: (813)-862-0782 Fax: (813)-869-3900
Contact: Marc Yacht, MD - CPHU Director

Home Health Care

Olsten Kimberly Quality Care
6014 US 19, Suite 100
New Port Richey, FL 34652
Telephone: (813)-842-9579 Fax: (813)-849-9256
Home health services incl: infusion therapy, nutritional support,pediatric care

Pinellas County

County Health Depts

Pinellas County Public Health Unit
500 7th Avenue South
St. Petersburg, FL 33701-4820
Telephone: (813)-823-0401
Contact: Preston Goodale
HIV Anonymous Test Site, AIDS Patient Care Clinic, Medicaid Waiver Program

Home Health Care

nmc HOMECARE
10901 D Roosevelt Blvd, Suite 300
St. Petersburg, FL 33716
Telephone: (813)-576-7070
Fax: (813)-579-0259
Contact: Daniel Sweeney
National JCAHO-Accredited company providing a full range of Infusion and Respiratory therapies and specializing in the care of HIV/AIDS patients. National Case Manager is also available at 800-445-1188

Olsten HealthCare
2 Corporate Dr.
Suite 170
Clearwater, FL 34622
Telephone: (813)-572-6600 Fax: (813)-572-1317
Contact: Ruth Sanovich
Home health services incl: infusion therapy, nutritional support,pediatric care

Polk County

County Health Depts

Polk County Public Health Unit
1290 Golfview Ave., 4th Floor
Bartow, FL 33830
Telephone: (813)-533-4276 Fax: (813)-534-7046
Contact: Julia Hemelbracht - Health Information
Patient care clinic; administration for AIDS education, counseling, testing

Home Health Care

Olsten HealthCare
706 Jones Ave.
Haines City, FL 33844
Telephone: (813)-422-3422 Fax: (813)-422-8801
Toll-Free: (800)-292-9331
Home health services incl: infusion therapy, nutritional support

Olsten HealthCare
1257 Lakeland Hills Blvd.
Lakeland, FL 33805
Telephone: (813)-683-6431 Fax: (813)-687-2788
Contact: Joanne Weiss
Home health services incl: infusion therapy, nutritional support,pediatric care

Putnam County

County Health Depts

Putnam County Public Health Unit
2801 Kennedy Street
Palatka, FL 32177
Telephone: (904)-329-0420
Contact: Helen Morgan
Anonymous test site, confidential testing, speakers

Home Health Care

Olsten HealthCare
800 Zeagler Dr. #420
Palatka, FL 32178
Telephone: (904)-325-2771 Fax: (904)-325-5679
Toll-Free: (800)-562-0114
Home health services incl: infusion therapy, nutritional support,pediatric care

Medical Services

Family Medical & Dental Center
P.O. Drawer 817
Palatka, FL 32178-0817
Telephone: (904)-328-8371
Federally subsidized Community Health Center

Saint Johns County

County Health Depts

St. Johns County Public Health Unit
180 Marine Street
St. Augustine, FL 32084-5153
Telephone: (904)-825-5055
Contact: Colleen Buxinie - Nurse Specialist
Case management, precare, confidential testing, follow-up

Saint Lucie County

County Health Depts

St. Lucie County Public Health Unit
P.O. Box 580
714 Avenue C
Ft. Pierce, FL 34950
Telephone: (407)-468-3945 Fax: (407)-468-3954
Contact: Mary V. Mitchell - Health Education Coordinator

Education, prevention outreach, social worker assistance.Santa Rosa County

County Health Depts

Santa Rosa County Public Health Unit
503 Stewart Street, North
Milton, FL 32570-4375
Telephone: (904)-623-4604
Contact: Sherilyn KulasMD - HIV/AIDS Nurse
HIV/AIDS testing

Sarasota County

County Health Depts

Sarasota County Public Health Unit
P.O. Box 2658
Sarasota, FL 34230-2658
Telephone: (813)-954-2950
Contact: Mark Magenheim, MD - CPHU Director; Chander Malik, DDS
Clinical services, nutrition, educational facilities, & anonymous testing

Home Health Care

Olsten HealthCare
1999 Lincoln Dr.
Sarasota, FL 34236
Telephone: (813)-366-4320
Home health services incl: infusion therapy, nutritional support,pediatric care, AIDS in-services education

Seminole County

Home Health Care

nmc HOMECARE
976 Florida Ctrl Prkwy
Longwood, FL 32750
Telephone: (407)-339-8648
Fax: (407)-332-8229
Contact: William Bolgar
National JCAHO-Accredited company providing a full range of Infusion and Respiratory therapies and specializing in the care of HIV/AIDS patients. National Case Manager is also available at 800-445-1188

HNS, Inc.
715 West State Road 434
Suite Q
Longwood, FL 32750
Telephone: (407)-830-5354 Fax: (407)-830-5503
Contact: Mark Curran
Home Infusion Therapy, In-home Nursing and Attendant Care, PhysicalTherapy, Pentamidine

Olsten HealthCare
250 Intnl Pkwy
Heathrow, FL 32746
Telephone: (407)-333-0043 Fax: (407)-333-2320
Home health services incl: infusion therapy, nutritional support

Sumter County

County Health Depts

Sumter County Public Health Unit
Highway 301 North
P.O. Box 98
Bushnel, FL 33513
Telephone: (904)-793-2701 Fax: (904)-793-1506
Contact: Alann Knight
HIV testing & screening, primary care, drug assistance program, STDcounseling, educational information

Suwannee County

County Health Depts

Suwannee County Public Health Unit
P.O. Drawer 268
Branford, FL 32008-0368
Telephone: (904)-935-1133
Contact: Wanda Crowe
HIV/AIDS testing & counseling

Suwannee County Public Health Unit
1001 Nobles Ferry Road
P.O. Drawer 6030
Live Oak, FL 32060-0327
Telephone: (904)-362-2708
Contact: Wanda Crowe
HIV counseling, screening, referral

Taylor County

County Health Depts

Taylor County Public Health Unit
P.O. Box 425
1215 Peacock Street
Perry, FL 32347-0425
Telephone: (904)-584-5087
Contact: Jerry Boland, M.D. - Director
HIV counseling, screening, referral

Union County

County Health Depts

Union County Public Health Unit
495 East Main Street
Lake Butler, FL 32054-1701
Telephone: (904)-496-3211
Contact: Sally Keller
HIV testing referral, screening, basic HIV care, limited case management

Volusia County

County Health Depts

HRS Volusia County Public Health Unit, Pierson Clinic
216 North Frederick Street
Pierson, FL 32180
Telephone: (904)-749-2193 Fax: (904)-749-2482
Contact: Chris Culver
HIV Anonymous Test Site

Volusia County Public Health Unit
501 S. Clyde Morris Blvd
Daytona Beach, FL 32114-3929
Telephone: (904)-257-1700
Contact: Bill Drahos
HIV Anonymous Test Site; patient care, counseling

Wakulla County

County Health Depts

Wakulla County Public Health Unit
P.O. Box 368
Highway 319
Crawfordville, FL 32326-0368
Telephone: (904)-926-3591
Contact: David Keen, M.D. - Director
Primary care, medication program, confidential testing

Walton County

County Health Depts

Walton County Public Health Unit
Route 8, Box 10
605 North 9th Street
DeFuniak Sprngs, FL 32433-9401
Telephone: (904)-892-8015 Fax: (904)-892-8024
Contact: JunEllen Ray, RN - CHN Supervisor; Genny Crocker, ARNP - CHN Director
HIV testing (confidential), pre/post counseling, HIV education

Washington County

County Health Depts

Washington County Public Health Unit
404 South Boulevard, West
Chipley, FL 32428-2218
Telephone: (904)-638-6240 Fax: (904)-638-6244

Contact: Cookie Anderson RN - CPHU Director, Jim Parmer - Administrative Assistant

HIV testing (confidential), pre/post counseling, HIV/AIDS education,referrals

GEORGIA

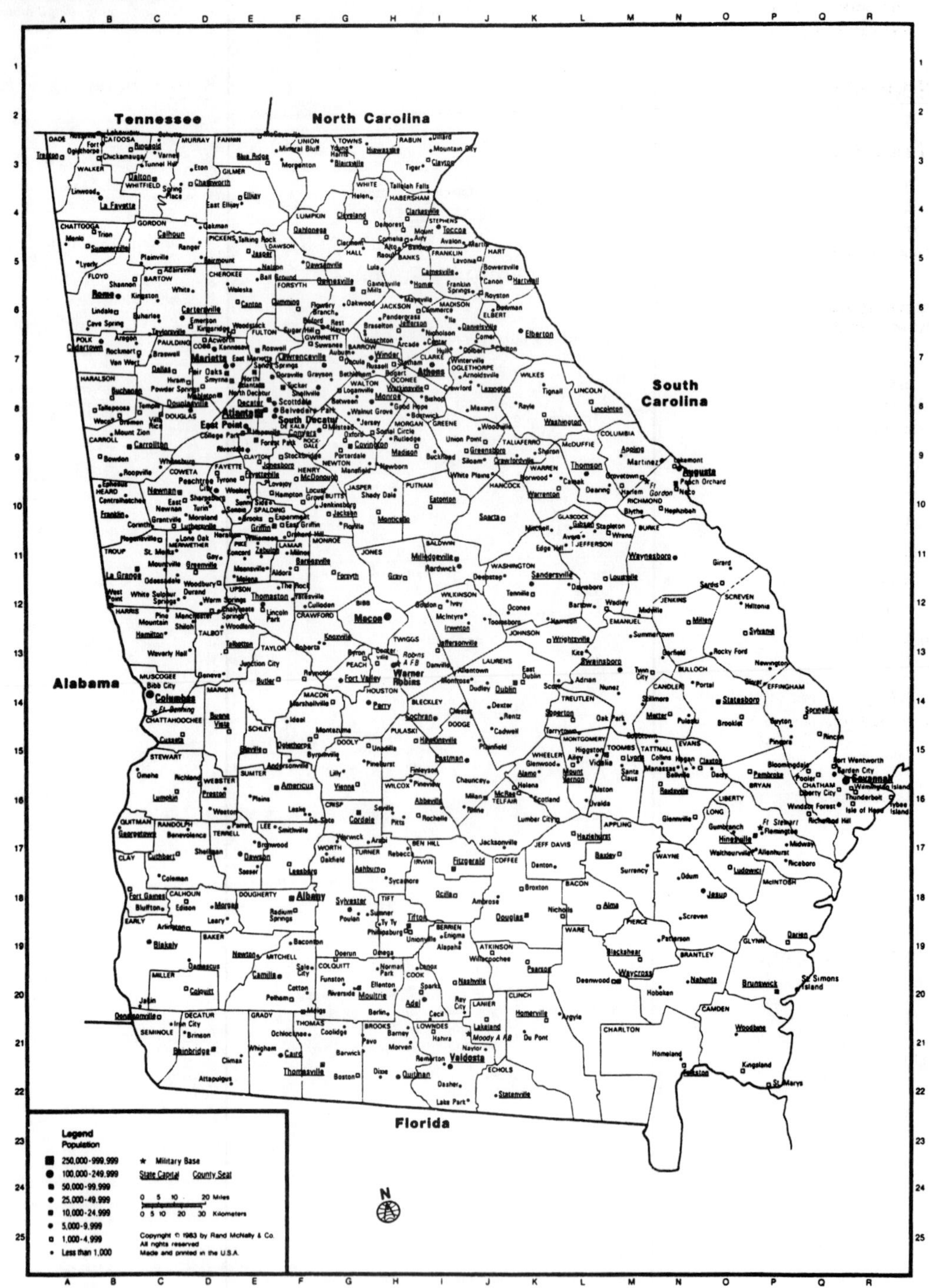

From City/County Planning Atlas Copyright 1989 by Reed McNally & Company, R.L. 90-S-28

Georgia

General Services

Education

American Red Cross of Atlanta
1955 Monroe Dr NE
Atlanta, GA 30324
Telephone: (404)-881-9800
Contact: Diane Hamilton
Community Education and Outreach

Georgia Dept of Human Resources, Epidemiology & Prevention Branch
2 Peach Tree Street NW
Atlanta, GA 30303
Telephone: (404)-894-5304
Contact: Dr. Katheen Tooney
AIDS education for community worksites, schools and professional groups

Outreach, Inc.
3030 Camp Bellton Road
Atlanta, GA 30311
Telephone: (404)-873-5992
AIDS education in minority community

Rehabilitation-Exposure, Inc.
756 West Peachtree Street
Atlanta, GA 30308
Telephone: (404)-880-8767 Fax: (404)-880-8886
Aids education for Korean, Haitians, Vietnamese, communities

SCLC-Women's National AIDS Program
334 Auburn Avenue
Atlanta, GA 30303
Telephone: (404)-351-7105
Contact: Margie Shannon
Community outreach and education, training for the church community

State Health Departments

Georgia Div. Public Health - Office of Infectious Disease
#2 Peachtree Street Northwest
Suite 400
Altanta, GA 30303
Telephone: (404)-657-3100
Main office for community based AIDS organizations

Statewide Services

Georgia Legal Services Program
161 String Street
5th Floor
Atlanta, GA 30303
Telephone: (404)-656-6021
Contact: Phyllis J. Holman
Legal Services

Insurance Commissioner of Georgia
2 Martin Luther King Jr. Drive
West Tower Room 716
Atlanta, GA 30334
Telephone: (404)-656-2056 Fax: (404)-656-7628
Consumer services insurance claims

Clarke County

Home Health Care

St. Mary's Hospice
PO Box 6588
Athens, GA 30604-6588
Telephone: (404)-548-8923
Hospice Programs

Clayton County

Community Services

Community Center Services Authority, Inc.
667 S Avenue
Forrest Park, GA 30051-1808
Telephone: (404)-366-0517
Clothing, food, rent, utilities, transportation, legal aid, weatherization,day care

Salvation Army of Riverdale
Box 757
Joansberg, GA 30237
Telephone: (404)-603-6258
Rent, utilities, food, prescription drugs, appointment system

Home Health Care

Nurses Around the Clock
6338 Riverdale Rd
Riverdale, GA 30274
Telephone: (404)-991-2515 Fax: (404)-991-1557
Situational staffing

Cobb County

Community Services

Cobb County Legal Aid
159 Dobbs Street, Norteast
Marietta, GA 30060
Telephone: (404)-528-2565
Legal services, special funding for AIDS/HIV

Cobb Family Resources
377 Henry Drive
Marietta, GA 30064
Telephone: (404)-428-2601
Clothing, food, rent, utilities, transportation, prescriptions,employment,emergency housing

Department of Family and Children Services
25 Fairground
Marietta, GA 30060
Telephone: (404)-528-5000
Financial, Clothing, Energy and Food Assistance (food stamps, Medicaid,rent)

Home Health Care

Caremark Home Care
2150 New Market Parkway
Suite 108
Marietta, GA 30067
Telephone: (404)-952-3021 Fax: (404)-952-6840
Contact: Jan Jordan
IV home care

Critical Care America
805 Franklin Ct. Ste A
Marietta, GA 30067-8942
Telephone: (404)-933-8624
Coordinate & integrate all clinical & psychosocial services for HIV+

Home Nutrition Support (HNS)
425 Franklin
Suite 545
Marietta, GA 30067
Telephone: (404)-426-4933 Fax: (404)-426-7488
Home health care, home infusion therapy, social workers

Kennestone Regional Hospice
PO Box 1208
Marietta, GA 30061-1208
Telephone: (404)-426-3131 Fax: (404)-793-7370
Hospice Programs-Home care & support for terminally ill patients & family

De Kalb County

Community Services

Decatur Cooperative Ministry
PO Box 457
Decatur, GA 30031
Telephone: (404)-377-5365
Spiritual Support

DeKalb County Legal AID
340 West Ponce DeLeon Avenue
Decatur, GA 30030
Telephone: (404)-377-0701 Fax: (704)-377-2349
Legal Services

Home Health Care

VA Medical Center Atlanta
1670 Clairmont Road
Decatur, GA 30033
Telephone: (404)-728-7680
Hospice programs in development

Medical Services

Dekalb Medical Center
2701 N Decatur Rd
Decatur, GA 30033
Telephone: (404)-501-5400 Fax: (404)-501-1761
HIV/AIDS Support Groups -- PWA/PWARCs; Family/Friends

Dougherty County

Home Health Care

Albany Community Hospice
P.O. Box 1828
Albany, GA 31703
Telephone: (912)-883-4484
Contact: Tricia Helms
Hospice Programs

Douglas County

Community Services

Department of Family and Children Services
6218 Hospital Way
PO Box 1135
Douglasville, GA 30133
Telephone: (404)-489-3000 Fax: (404)-489-3035
Financial, Clothing, Energy, and Food Assistance (food stamps, Medicaid,rent)

Fulton County

Community Services

AID ATLANTA (main)
1438 W Peachtree St NW
#100
Atlanta, GA 30309-2955
Telephone: (404)-872-0600 Fax: (404)-885-6799
Toll-Free: (800)-551-2728
Contact: Todd Lambert
Blood tests, therapy, minor treatments, education, case management

American Lung Association
2452 Spring Road
Smyrna, GA 30380
Telephone: (404)-434-5864
Contact: Sandra Colt
Financial help for people with lung disease, e.g. PCP

Atlanta Chapter of NAPWA
44 12th Street
Atlanta, GA 30303
Telephone: (404)-874-7926 Fax: (404)-872-1192
HIV/AIDS Support Groups:

Cathedral of Faith Church of God in Christ (S.W. Atlanta)
30003 Howell Mill Road
Atlanta, GA 30327
Telephone: (404)-237-6491 Fax: (404)-264-0470
Contact: Dr. Bill Carr - Grief Counselor
Spiritual Support

Central Presbyterian Church
201 Washington
Atlanta, GA 30303
Telephone: (404)-659-7119
Contact: Jewl Louis
Assistance with prescription drugs, rent, food, utilities

Drug Abuse Service Section
3201 Atlanta Industrial Park
Bldg 100, Suite 101
Atlanta, GA 30331
Telephone: (404)-699-4300 Fax: (404)-699-4328
Substance Abuse Counseling, Education, Support

Ebenezer Baptist Church
407 Auburn Avenue NE
Atlanta, GA 30312-1599
Telephone: (404)-688-7263
Contact: Rev Sharon G. Alston
Assistance with prescription drugs, rent, food, utilities

Episcopal Church
453 Peachtree Street
Atlanta, GA 30365
Telephone: (404)-885-1386
Contact: Father Isaias Rodriguez
Spiritual support, Spanish speaking

Fulton County Indigent Funerals
501 Pulliam Street
Southwest Atlanta, GA 30312
Telephone: (404)-656-6089
Contact: John Flemming
For funeral planning, cremation & reduced fees

Fulton County Legal Aid
151 Spring Street
Atlanta, GA 30335
Telephone: (404)-524-5811
Contact: Chip Rowan
Legal Services

Jerusalem House, Inc.
100 Edgewood Ave
Suite 1228
Atlanta, GA 30303
Telephone: (404)-527-7665 Fax: (404)-527-7629
Contact: Sue Thompson - Program Director
Housing

Metro Community Church
1379 Tull Road
Atlanta, GA 30329
Telephone: (404)-325-4143 Fax: (404)-325-1372
Spiritual support, AIDS/HIV counseling

Operation Blessing
PO Box 450008
Atlanta, GA 30345
Telephone: (404)-633-4700 Fax: (404)-636-0700
Rent, utilities, food, prescription drugs, on matching funds basis

Outreach, Inc.
3030 Campbellton Rd, S.W.
Atlanta, GA 30311
Telephone: (404)-346-3922 Fax: (404)-346-3036
Contact: Sandra McDonald - President; Alfred White - Vice President
HIV testing, alcohol abuse programs

Salvation Army of Atlanta (Luckie Street)
400 Luckie Street Northwest
Atlanta, GA 30313
Telephone: (404)-688-2884
Contact: Hope Smyly - Director
Rent, utilities, food, prescription drugs, job counseling

The Bridge
1559 Johnson Road, Northwest
Atlanta, GA 30318
Telephone: (404)-792-0070 Fax: (404)-794-0444
Substance Abuse Counseling/Education/Support

Home Health Care

Alliance Against AIDS
3525 Piedmont Rd NE
Atlanta, GA 30305
Telephone: (404)-261-6210 Fax: (404)-233-8603
Home Health Care

Community Care
2600 Skyland Drive NE
Atlanta, GA 30319
Telephone: (404)-679-4799 Fax: (404)-679-4913
Home Health Care, including Medicaid

Curaflex Infusion Services
120 Interstate N. Parkway
#440
Atlanta, GA 30339-2158
Telephone: (800)-825-2735 Fax: (404)-952-6889
Contact: Kirk Jones
Home IV therapy: TPN, Enteral, IV Antibiotics, Aerosolized/IV Pentamidine

Health Force
2601 Flowers Rd S, #160
Koger Management Ctr
Atlanta, GA 30341
Telephone: (404)-458-8500 Fax: (404)-458-9050
Home Health Care

Homecare Equipment Services
199 Hildebrand Dr NE
Atlanta, GA 30328
Telephone: (404)-252-4663 Fax: (404)-256-9076
Home Health Care

Hospice Atlanta
133 Luckie Street Northwest
Atlanta, GA 30303
Telephone: (404)-527-8070 Fax: (404)-527-0757
Hospice Programs

nmc HOMECARE
120 Interstate North Parkway, Suite 158
Atlanta, GA 30339
Telephone: (404)-953-0899
Fax: (404)-933-0224
Contact: Jeff Hill
National JCAHO-Accredited company providing a full range of Infusion and Respiratory therapies and specializing in the care of HIV/AIDS patients. National Case Manager is also available at 800-445-1188

Northside Hospice
5825 Glenridger Drive
Building 4
Atlanta, GA 30328
Telephone: (404)-851-6300 Fax: (404)-252-7708
Hospice care, RN's, social workers, health technicians, pharmacy

Omni Home Medical
4025 Pleasantdale Rd
Suite 565
Atlanta, GA 30340
Telephone: (404)-447-8680
Home Health Care, medical supplies, T.P.N., enteral therapy

Medical Services

AID ATLANTA, Social Services
1438 W Peachtree St NW
#100
Atlanta, GA 30309-2955
Telephone: (404)-874-6517
HIV/AIDS Support Groups

Dunwoody Medical Center
4575 N Shallowford Road
Atlanta, GA 30338
Telephone: (404)-454-2000 Fax: (404)-454-4279
Acute care facility, Diagnostics evaluation

Feminist Woman's Health Center
580 14th Street N.W.
Atlanta, GA 30318
Telephone: (404)-874-3028
Toll-Free: (800)-877-6013
Contact: Sherry Sutton
HIV/STD testing, referrals

Infectious Disease Program
341 Ponce De Leon Avenue
Atlanta, GA 30308
Telephone: (404)-616-2440 Fax: (404)-898-1442
Outpatient clinic and treatment, education, counseling, dispensingmedication, dental services, social services

Veterans Positive
Veterans Administration Medical Center
1670 Clairmont Road
Atlanta, GA 30329
Telephone: (404)-321-6111
Outpatient medical care, testing, counseling, family support, socialworkers

Testing Sites

Charter Oak/Rice Heights
2452 Spring Road
Smyrna, GA 30380
Telephone: (404)-952-1096
Contact: Lona Pointeka
HIV/AIDS counseling, testing pre & post, (confidential), outreach,casemanagement

Glynn County

Community Services

Coastal Area Support Team (CAST)
2917 Sifer Mill Road
Brunswick, GA 31521
Telephone: (912)-264-2111
Contact: Loretta Sams - Director
HIV/AIDS Support Groups: PWA, ARC (Th.7:30-9 P.M.), HIV+ (Tu 7:30-9 P.M)

Home Health Care

Hospice of the Golden Isles
2228 Starling
Brunswick, GA 31520
Telephone: (912)-265-4735 Fax: (912)-265-6100
Hospice Programs

O.P.T.I.O.N Care
3029 Altama Avenue
Brunswick, GA 31520-4608
Telephone: (912)-267-6192 Fax: (912)-267-0042
Contact: Pat Patel, RPh; K. Jackson, RN
Home IV and Nutritional Services

Gwinnett County

Community Services

Salvation Army of Lawrenceville
PO Box 1613
Lawrenceville, GA 30246-1613
Telephone: (404)-962-2988
Rent, utilities, food, prescription drugs

Lowndes County

Home Health Care

Barnes O.P.T.I.O.N Care
101 Northside Drive
Valdosta, GA 31602
Telephone: (912)-244-4248
Contact: Casey Moye - Director of Nursing
Home IV and Nutritional Services

Muscogee County

Home Health Care

Columbus Hospice
Physicians Bldg, Ste 104
Columbus, GA 31901
Telephone: (706)-327-5153
Hospice Programs, home care services for terminally ill patients

Pickens County

Home Health Care

Northwest Home Health Agency, Inc.
1425 Church Street
Jasper, GA 30143
Telephone: (706)-692-3491 Fax: (706)-692-5767
Contact: Marguerite Cammerta - Director
Hospice Programs; IV therapy, lab, medical care, home health aides,physical therapy, social workers

Richmond County

Home Health Care

St. Joseph's Hospice
2260 Wrightsboro Rd
Augusta, GA 30910
Telephone: (706)-481-7000 Fax: (706)-481-7852
Hospice Programs

Troup County

Home Health Care

LaGrange Hospice
1514 Vernon Road
LaGrange, GA 30240
Telephone: (404)-882-1411
Hospice Programs

Ware County

County Health Depts

Ware County Board of Health
Southeast Health Unit
1101 Church Street
Waycross, GA 31501
Telephone: (912)-285-6002 Fax: (912)-285-6004
Contact: John Holloway, M.D.; Helen Wildes - Program Coordinator; Melissa Alpern - Evaluator
AIDS/HIV testing, education

HAWAII

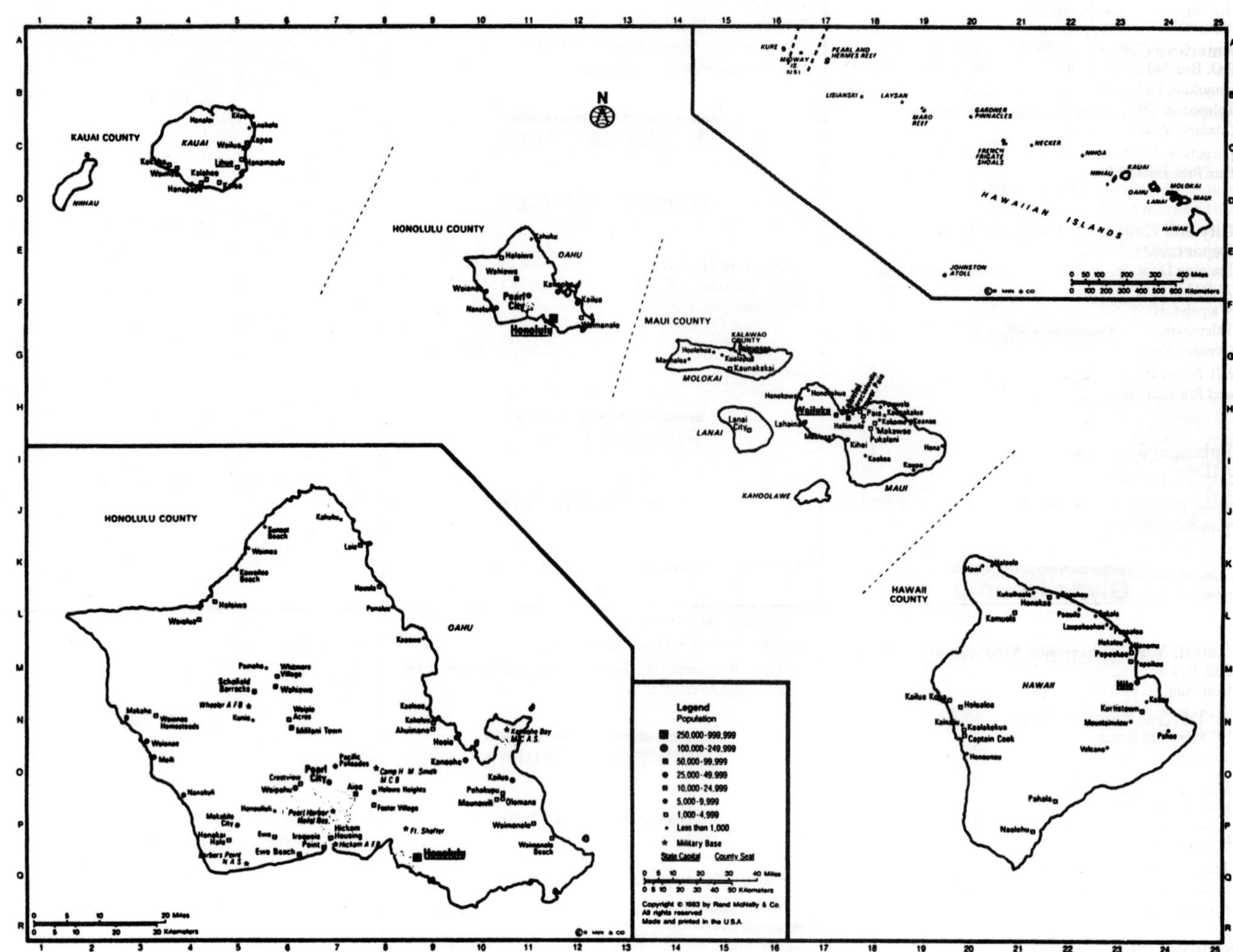

From City/County Planning Atlas Copyright 1989 by Reed McNally & Company, R.L. 90-S-28

Hawaii

General Services

Education

American Civil Liberties Union of Hawaii
P.O. Box 3410
Honolulu, HI 96801-3410
Telephone: (808)-545-1722 Fax: (808)-545-2993
Contact: Vanessa Chong
Litigation, Education & Lobbying for AIDS Discrimination, Due Process & Privacy

City and County of Honolulu, Honolulu Police Department
Training Division
93-093 Waipahu Depot Road
Waipahu, HI 96797
Telephone: (808)-677-1474
Contact: Fabian Loo
HIV Education and Training Sessions for Police, Information and Precautions

Episcopal Diocesan Advisory Committee on AIDS
P.O. Box 813
Kihei, HI 96753-0813
Telephone: (808)-879-0161
Contact: The Rev. Morley E. Frech, Jr.
Educational Resource for Episcopal Congregations, Institutions and Schools;monthly meetings

Hawaii Medical Services Association (HMSA)
P.O. Box 860
Honolulu, HI 96808
Telephone: (808)-944-2414
Contact: Karen Sugai - Community Relations

Hawaii Planned Parenthood
1441 Kapiolani Blvd.
Suite 1400
Honolulu, HI 96814
Telephone: (808)-941-0516
Contact: Cheryl Vasconcellos
Education materials

Kalihi-Palama Immigrant Service Center, HIV Education Proj.
720 North King Street
Honolulu, HI 96817-4511
Telephone: (808)-848-0936 Fax: (808)-842-1962
Contact: Richard Chabot
HIV Training for Bilingual Service Providers: SE Asians, Chinese, Koreans,education with a focus on immigrant teenagers

Womens Health Center, - Molokai General Hospital
204 2nd Street East
Kaunakakai, HI 96748-0408
Telephone: (808)-553-5331
Free Confidential STD and Anonymous HIV Antibody Counseling and Testing

State Health Departments

Hawaii State Dept. of Health, AIDS Research & Seroprevalence
Leahi Hospital
3675 Kilauea Avenue
Honolulu, HI 96816
Telephone: (808)-735-0440
Contact: Lanette Shizuru - PhD
Coordinates CDC & State prevalence and incidence for State planningcoordination

Hawaii State Dept. of Health, Seropositivity
3627 Kilauea Avenue
Suite 306
Honolulu, HI 96816-2317
Telephone: (808)-732-0026
Contact: Suzanne Richmond-Crum
Subsidized Confidential Medical Care, HIV+ Volunteers for Medical Follow-up

State Department of Health, AIDS Surveillance Program
3627 Kilauea Avenue
Suite 306
Honolulu, HI 96816-2317
Telephone: (808)-733-9010
Contact: Dave Sohmen
Maintains AIDS Registry, Contact with Medical Facilities, Validation Studies

State Dept. of Health, HIV Counseling/Testing Site, Kauai
3040 Umi Street
Lihue, HI 96766-1356
Telephone: (808)-241-3495
Contact: Tom Jones
Free Confidential STD and Anonymous HIV Antibody Counseling and Testing

State Dept. of Health, HIV Counseling/Testing Site, Lanai
Lanai Community Hospital
Lanai City, HI 96763-0763
Telephone: (808)-565-6622
Contact: Jan Squirres
Free Confidential STD and Anonymous HIV Antibody Counseling and Testing

Honolulu County

Community Services

American Cancer Society, Hawaii Pacific Division
200 North Vineyard Blvd.
Honolulu, HI 96817-3998
Telephone: (808)-531-1662 Fax: (808)-526-9729
Toll-Free: (800)-227-2545
Contact: Grace Y. Iwahashi - Medical Affairs Director
AIDS Cancer Svcs: Referral, Home Care Items, Transport, Support Groups, Rehab.

City and County of Honolulu, Department of Housing
Rental Assist Branch, S-8
842 Bethel Street, 1st Fl
Honolulu, HI 96813
Telephone: (808)-523-4266 Fax: (808)-527-5545
Contact: Sandra Toma - Administrator
Rental Assistance for Low Income Families, Elderly, Disabled, and Handicapped

Hawaii AIDS Task Group
1951 East-West Road
Honolulu, HI 96822
Telephone: (808)-956-7400 Fax: (808)-956-9481
Contact: Milton Diamond, PhD - Chairman
Provide forum for agency/individuals - Gov't & Private, STD HIV related

Hawaii Centers for Independent Living (Offices on 4 Islands)
677 Ala Moana Boulevard
Suite 118
Honolulu, HI 96813-5419
Telephone: (808)-537-1941 Fax: (808)-599-4851
Contact: Erica C. Jones - Executive Director
Referrals; Benefits, Housing, Care & Job Assistance; Advocacy; Peer Counseling

Hawaii Long Term Care Association
1948 St. Louis Drive
Honolulu, HI 96816-1935
Telephone: (808)-732-6463 Fax: (808)-734-1760
Contact: Lynda Johnson
Association of Nursing Homes, Legislative Advocacy, Care Enhancement

Hemophilia Foundation of Hawaii
1164 Bishop St.
Suite 1501
Honolulu, HI 96813-2829
Telephone: (808)-521-5483 Fax: (808)-528-7430
Contact: Marion Poirier, MA, RN - Executive Director
Hemophilia Services: Treatment Cost Help, Rehab., Summer Camp; Public Education

HIV Community Care Program, Dept. of Human Services
33 S. King St. #223
Honolulu, HI 96813
Telephone: (808)-586-5545 Fax: (808)-586-5606
Contact: Lori Treschuk - RN, Program Specialist
Services for Medicaid PWAs: Case Mgmt, Counseling, Subst Abuse, Respite Care

Ho'omana'olana (AIDS Housing Project, Gregory House)
770 Kapiolani Blvd
Suite 515
Honolulu, HI 96813-2424
Telephone: (808)-522-9022 Fax: (808)-522-9049
Contact: Michael Burnett - Director
Flexible Housing to Homeless HIV+; Fosters Holistic Life, Independence, Dignity

Life Foundation
P.O. Box 88980
Honolulu, HI 96830-8980
Telephone: (808)-971-2437 Fax: (808)-971-7850
Contact: Paul S. Groesbeck - Executive Director
Case management, education, newsletter, advocacy, counseling, supportgroup, buddies, legal aid

Home Health Care

Hospice Hawaii, Inc.
445 Seaside Avenue
Suite 604
Honolulu, HI 96815-3738
Telephone: (808)-924-9255
Contact: Robert W. Luck - Executive Director
Home Care, Hospice, Pallative Care, Respite Care, Therapy, Counseling

Kuakini-at-Home
347 North Kuakini Street
Honolulu, HI 96817-2377
Telephone: (808)-547-9478
Contact: Barbara Idela - Acting Director
Home Care: Nursing, Therapy, Social Services, Aides, Counseling, Equipment

Medical Personnel Pool
1441 Kapiolani Boulevard
Suite 1320

Honolulu, HI 96814-4441
Telephone: (808)-955-1102
Contact: Carol Kikkawa-Ward - President
Provides Home Health, Companion and Chore Aides; Nurses; Medical Social Workers

Saint Francis Hospice, The Sister Maureen Keleher Center
24 Puiwa Road
Honolulu, HI 96817-1127
Telephone: (808)-595-7566
Contact: Sister Francine Gries - RN, MS
Hospice Care

Medical Services

Blood Bank of Hawaii
2043 Dillingham Boulevard
Honolulu, HI 96819
Telephone: (808)-845-9966 Fax: (808)-848-4737
Contact: Kirk Hazeltt - Communications Director
State Blood Center, Provides Safe and Adequate Blood

Castle Medical Center
640 Ulukahiki Street
Kailua, HI 96734-4498
Telephone: (808)-263-5500 Fax: (808)-263-5393
Contact: Collen Assavapisitkul - Infection Control Coord.
General Hospital, Speakers Bureau, Education Center, Substance Abuse ServiceMental Health

Drug Addictions Services of Hawaii (DASH)
1031 Auahi Street
Honolulu, HI 96814-4918
Telephone: (808)-523-0704 Fax: (808)-591-8304
Contact: Lisa Cook - Executive Director
Outpatient Methadone, Advocacy, Education, Referrals, Case Management,Support

Kokua Kalihi Valley Health Center
1846 Gulick Avenue
Honolulu, HI 96819
Telephone: (808)-848-0976
Contact: Merina Sapolu
Multilingual Primary Care Clinic, Staff Training, Group Education

Salvation Army Treatment Services
3624 Waokanaka Street
Honolulu, HI 96817-5224
Telephone: (808)-595-6371 Fax: (808)-595-8250
Contact: Martin Matthews - HIV Counseling
Residential/outpatient substance abuse services, AIDS education, counseling

Waikiki Health Center
277 Ohua Avenue
Honolulu, HI 96815-3695
Telephone: (808)-922-4787 Fax: (808)-922-4794
Contact: Rev. Frank Chong - Executive Director
Low-Cost Outpatient Medical Care, Testing/Counseling, Outreach to High-Risk

Testing Sites

Waianae Coast Comprehensive Health Center
86-260 Farrington Highway
Waianae, HI 96792-3199
Telephone: (808)-696-5561 Fax: (808)-696-7093
Contact: Joyce O'Brien
Outpatient Medical, Testing/Counseling, Home Care, Minorities, Prevention Educ.

Kauai County

Community Services

Malama Pono (Kauai AIDS Project)
P.O. Box 1500
Kapaa, HI 96746-7500
Telephone: (808)-822-0878 Fax: (808)-822-0644
Contact: Don Gershberg
Case management, community, education, outreach

Maui County

Community Services

Maui AIDS Foundation
PO Box 1538
55 Kaahumanu Avenue
Kahului, HI 96732-1538
Telephone: (808)-871-2437 Fax: (808)-877-6363
Contact: Greg Lamb
Volunteer in home support, food assistance, hospital visits, support &groups

IDAHO

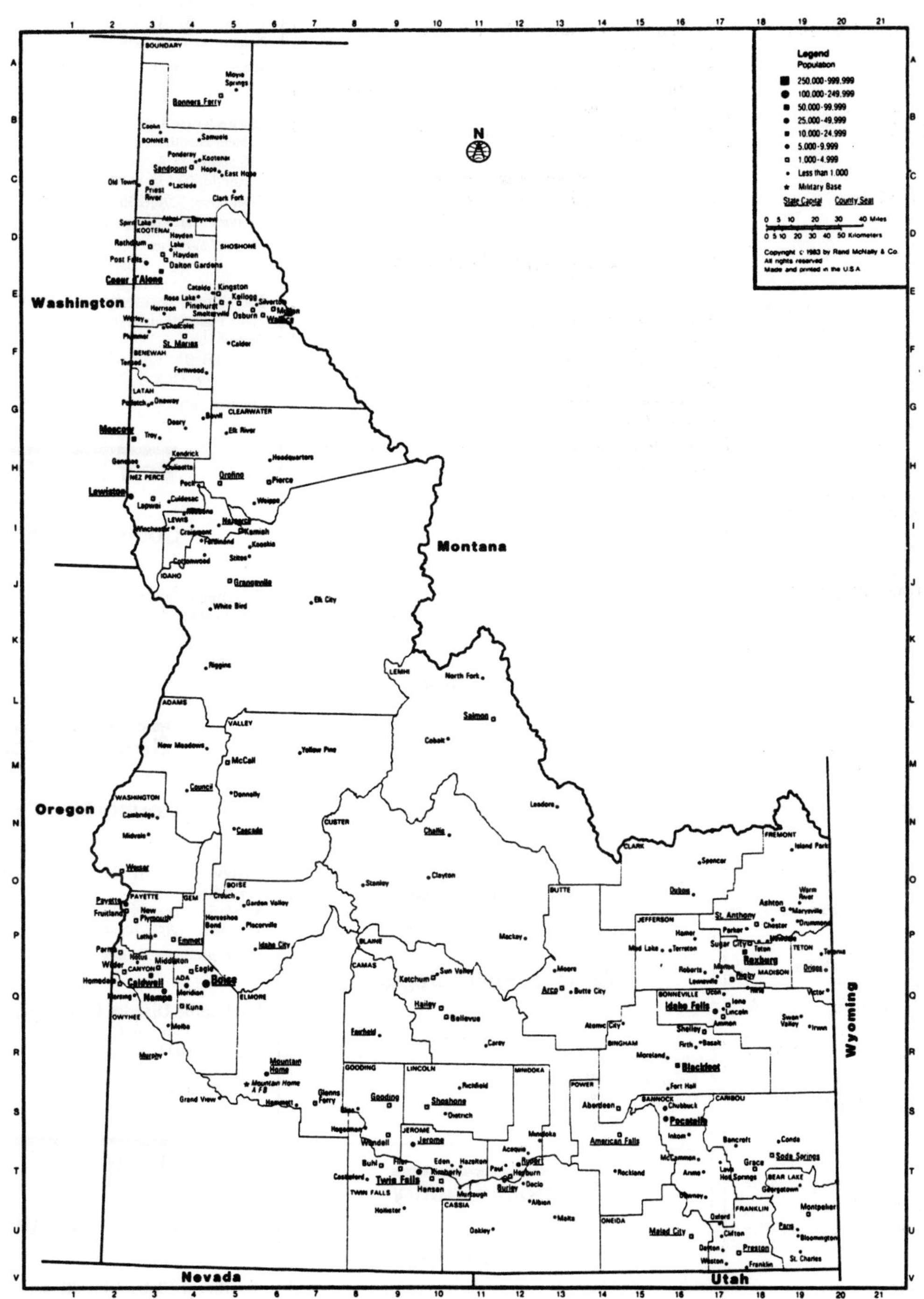

From City/County Planning Atlas Copyright 1989 by Reed McNally & Company, R.L. 90-S-28

Idaho

General Services

Education

North Idaho College
1000 West Garden Avenue
Coeur d'Arlene, ID 83814
Telephone: (208)-769-3300
Contact: Linda Michael
Counseling, Education

North Idaho Indian Health Service
P.O. Drawer 367
Lapwai, ID 83540
Telephone: (208)-843-2271
Contact: Leroy Seth
Education, Counseling

Planned Parenthood
4301 Franklin Road
Boise, ID 83705
Telephone: (208)-345-0839 Fax: (208)-336-5504
Contact: Sabrina Shalz
Counseling, General AIDS Information

State Health Departments

District 7 Health Department
P.O. Box 1855
Idaho Falls, ID 83403-1855
Telephone: (208)-522-0310
Education, Social Workers, Counseling, HIV Counseling/Testing, Health Care

District Seven Health Department
245 E Street
Idaho Falls, ID 83403
Telephone: (208)-522-0310 Fax: (208)-522-0310
Contact: Melda Hines, R.N.; Lyla Stanger -
Case Mgt, Dental, HIV/STD testing & counseling, home care

Idaho Department of Health and Welfare
Bureau of Communicable Disease Prevention
STD/AIDS Program, 450 West State Street
Boise, ID 83720
Telephone: (208)-334-5932 Fax: (208)-334-6581
Contact: John Glaza - Supervisor

Statewide Services

Idaho AIDS Foundation
2933 Woodside Blvd.
Hailey, ID 83333
Telephone: (208)-788-4372
Contact: Polly Street
Counseling

Ada County

Community Services

Idaho AIDS Foundation
PO Box 421
Boise, ID 83702-0421
Telephone: (208)-345-2277
Contact: Bill Lorenzo

Medical Services

Physicians Immediate Care
1625 West State Street
Boise, ID 83702
Telephone: (208)-336-8800
Medical Services

Physicians Immediate Care
1525 South Owyhee
Boise, ID 83705
Telephone: (208)-344-8621 Fax: (208)-344-8728
Medical Services

St. Alphonsus Hospital
Emergency Room
1055 North Curtis Road
Boise, ID 83706
Telephone: (208)-378-3221 Fax: (208)-378-3564
Medical Services

St. Luke's Hospital
Emergency Room
190 E. Bannock Street
Boise, ID 83702
Telephone: (208)-386-2344 Fax: (208)-384-4556
Medical Services

Veterans Administration
500 West Fort Street
Boise, ID 83702
Telephone: (208)-336-5100 Fax: (208)-338-7257
Health Care

Testing Sites

Central District Health Department
707 N. Armstrong Place
Boise, ID 83704-2277
Telephone: (208)-375-5211
Contact: Ann Davis
Testing, Counseling, Education Services, Referral Services

Adams County

County Health Depts

Adams County Health Department
104 Illinois Avenue
Council, ID 83612
Telephone: (208)-253-4300
HIV Counseling/Testing

Bannock County

County Health Depts

Southeast District Health Department
465 Memorial Drive
Pocatello, ID 83201-4008
Telephone: (208)-322-9080
Contact: Jack Bennett
Educational, Counseling, HIV Counseling, Testing, Health Care

Medical Services

Bannock Regional Medical Center Emergency Room
651 Memorial Drive
Pocatello, ID 83201-4004
Telephone: (208)-239-1800 Fax: (208)-239-1935
Medical Services

Idaho State University
Student Health Center
990 South 8th Avenue
Pocatello, ID 83209-0001
Telephone: (208)-236-2330 Fax: (208)-236-4696
Contact: Carol Morgan, R.N.P.
Medical Services

Physicians Immedicate Care Center
1246 Yellowstone Avenue
Suite E1
Pocatello, ID 83201-4374
Telephone: (208)-237-1122 Fax: (208)-237-0830
Medical Services

Bear Lake County

County Health Depts

Southeast District Health Department
455 Washington Street #2
Montpelier, ID 83254-1544
Telephone: (208)-847-3000
Social Services

Benewah County

County Health Depts

Benewah County Health Department
711 Jefferson
St. Maries, ID 83861
Telephone: (208)-245-4556
HIV Counseling/Testing

Panhandle District Health Department
711 W. Jefferson Ave.
St. Maries, ID 83861-1831
Telephone: (208)-245-4556
Social Services

Bingham County

County Health Depts

Southeast District Health Dept.
412 West Pacific
Blackfoot, ID 83221
Telephone: (208)-785-2160
Contact: Alice Taylor, R.N.
Referral for STD services; HIV counseling & testing

Medical Services

Aberdeen Area Health Clinic
306 North Main, Box 419
Aberdeen, ID 83210
Telephone: (208)-397-4126
Medical Services

Fort Hall Indian Health Center
P.O. Box 717
Fort Hall, ID 83203
Telephone: (208)-238-2400 Fax: (208)-238-6272
Contact: Bernadine Ricker - Administrative Officer
Medical Services

Blaine County

County Health Depts

Blaine County Health Department
513 North Main Street
Hailey, ID 83333
Telephone: (208)-788-4335
Contact: Linda Johnson
HIV Counseling/Testing

Bonner County

Testing Sites

Panhandle District Health Department
1020 Michigan
Sandpoint, ID 83864
Telephone: (208)-263-5159 Fax: (208)-263-6963
HIV testing, counseling.

Bonneville County

Medical Services

Family Emergency Center-East
1995 East 17th
Idaho Falls, ID 83404
Telephone: (208)-529-5252 Fax: (208)-529-4434
Medical Services

Family Emergency Center-West
250 South Skyline
Idaho Falls, ID 83402
Telephone: (208)-525-2600 Fax: (208)-525-2611
Medical Services

U.S. Navy Base Dispensary
550 First Street
Idaho Falls, ID 83401
Telephone: (208)-522-1288 Fax: (208)-526-0454
Medical Services

Testing Sites

Eastern Idaho Regional Hospital
3100 Channing Way
P.O. Box 2077
Idaho Falls, ID 83403-2077
Telephone: (208)-529-6111 Fax: (208)-529-7007
Medical Services-HIV testing

Boundary County

County Health Depts

Boundary County Health Department
440 Kaniksu Street
Bonners Ferry, ID 83805
Telephone: (208)-267-5558 Fax: (208)-267-3795
Contact: Kathy Harden
HIV Counseling/Testing

Butte County

County Health Depts

Southeast District Health Dept.
178 Sunset
Arco, ID 83213
Telephone: (208)-527-3463
Referral for STD services

Canyon County

County Health Depts

Southwest District Health Department
920 Main Street
Caldwell, ID 83605-3700
Telephone: (208)-459-0744
Contact: Barbara Hyde, RN
Educational, Counseling, Social Workers, HIV Counseling/Testing, Health Care

Medical Services

Mercy Hospital
Emergency Room
1512 12th Avenue Road
Nampa, ID 83651
Telephone: (208)-467-1171 Fax: (208)-463-5144
Medical Services

Cassia County

County Health Depts

Cassia County Health Department
129 East 14th Street
Burley, ID 83318
Telephone: (208)-678-8221
HIV Counseling/Testing

Clark County

Testing Sites

Clark County Courthouse
120 West Main Street
DuBoise, ID 83423
Telephone: (208)-374-5216
Contact: Elaine Hoggan
HIV Counseling/Testing

Clearwater County

County Health Depts

Clearwater County Health Department
25 Hospital Drive
Orofino, ID 83544
Telephone: (208)-476-7850
Contact: Margaret Hoglan, R.N.
HIV Counseling/Testing

Medical Services

Clearwater Valley Hospital
Emergency Room
Cedar Street
Orofino, ID 83544
Telephone: (208)-476-4555
Medical Services

Medical Park Associates
P.O. Box 2079
Orofino, ID 83544
Telephone: (208)-476-5777 Fax: (208)-476-7192
Medical Services

Pioneer Medical Clinic
Community Center Building
Pierce, ID 83546
Telephone: (208)-464-2578
Contact: Susan Aleida
Medical Services

Custer County

County Health Depts

District 7 Health Department
1025 Valley-P.O. Box 508
Challis, ID 83226-0385
Telephone: (208)-879-2504
HIV Counseling/Testing

Elmore County

County Health Depts

Elmore County Health Department
520 East 8th Street North
Mountain Home, ID 83647
Telephone: (208)-587-4407
HIV Counseling/Testing

Medical Services

Glenns Ferry Health Center
516 West First
Glenns Ferry, ID 83623
Telephone: (208)-366-7416
Contact: Seanak Daly, M.D.
Medical Services

Franklin County

County Health Depts

Southeast District Health Department
42 West 1st South
Preston, ID 83263
Telephone: (208)-852-0479
Social Services

Fremont County

County Health Depts

District 7 Health Department
Fremont County Courthouse
PO Box 490
St. Anthony, ID 83445
Telephone: (208)-624-7585
Social Services

Gem County

County Health Depts

Southwest District Health Department
1008 E Locust
Emmett, ID 83617
Telephone: (208)-365-6371
Contact: Jeanine Gardner, RN
HIV Counseling/Testing

Gooding County

County Health Depts

Gooding County Health Department
1120 Montana
Gooding, ID 83330
Telephone: (208)-934-4522
HIV Counseling/Testing

Idaho County

County Health Depts

Idaho County Health Department
320 W. Main
Grangeville, ID 83530
Telephone: (208)-983-2842
Contact: Linda Blair, R.N.
HIV Counseling/Testing

Jefferson County

County Health Depts

Jefferson County Health Department
365 Farnsworth Way
P.O. Box 508
Rigby, ID 83442
Telephone: (208)-745-7297
HIV Counseling/Testing

Jerome County

County Health Depts

Jerome County Health Department
602 S. Lincoln
Jerome, ID 83338
Telephone: (208)-324-7565 Fax: (208)-324-8838
Contact: Mary Detienne - RN
HIV Counseling/Testing

Kootenai County

Medical Services

Kootenai Medical Center
2003 Lincoln Way
Coeur d'Arlene, ID 83814
Telephone: (208)-667-6441
Health Care

Testing Sites

Panhandle District Health Department
2195 Ironwood Court
Coeur d'Arlene, ID 83814-2620
Telephone: (208)-667-3481
Contact: Jan Palmer
Counseling, Educational, Social Workers, HIV Counseling, Testing, DrugAbuse

Latah County

County Health Depts

North Central District Health Department
333 E. Palouse River Dr
Moscow, ID 83843
Telephone: (208)-882-7506
Social Services; counseling & testing for AIDS

Medical Services

University of Idaho
Student Health Center
831 Ash
Moscow, ID 83843
Telephone: (208)-885-6511 Fax: (208)-885-6693
Medical Services

Lemhi County

County Health Depts

Lemhi County Health Department
P.O. Box 280
Salmon, ID 83467-0280
Telephone: (208)-756-2123
HIV Counseling/Testing

Lewis County

County Health Depts

North Central District Health Department
611 4th Street
Kamiah, ID 83536
Telephone: (208)-935-2124
Social services

Lincoln County

County Health Depts

Lincoln County Health Department
P.O. Box 429
Shoshone, ID 83352
Telephone: (208)-886-7663
HIV Counseling/Testing

Madison County

County Health Depts

Madison County Health Department
314 North Third East
Box 2
Rexburg, ID 83440
Telephone: (208)-356-3239
Contact: Myrdean Smith, RN
HIV Counseling/Testing

Minidoka County

County Health Depts

South Central Health District
Minidoka County Courthous
PO Box 474
Rupert, ID 83350-0474
Telephone: (208)-436-7185
Contact: Sandra Stoller, R.N.
Social services, counseling & testing

Nez Perce County

County Health Depts

North Central District Health Department
215 10th St.
Lewiston, ID 83501
Telephone: (208)-799-3100
Contact: Alice Vollerecht
Educational, Counseling, HIV Counseling/Testing, Health Care, Support, Referral

Medical Services

St. Joseph's Regional Medical Center
415 6th Street
Lewiston, ID 83501
Telephone: (208)-743-2511 Fax: (208)-799-5528
Contact: Doris Ziegeldorf, RN
Acute health care

Oneida County

County Health Depts

Southeast District Health Department
220 Bannock
Malad City, ID 83252-1256
Telephone: (208)-766-4764
Contact: Jackie Pfeiffer
Social services; counseling & testing

Owyhee County

Medical Services

Marsing Clinic
201 Main Street
Box 516
Marsing, ID 83639
Telephone: (208)-896-4159
Medical Services

Payette County

County Health Depts

Payette County Health Department
16 South 9th Street
Payette, ID 83661
Telephone: (208)-642-9321
Contact: Mary Beaver, R.N.
HIV Counseling/Testing

Medical Services

Valley Family Health Care
1441 Northeast 10th Avenue
HC 80, Box 45
Payette, ID 83661
Telephone: (208)-642-9314 Fax: (208)-642-5598
Contact: Jennie Rodiguez
Medial Services

Power County

County Health Depts

Southeast District Health
Department (Power County)
590 1/2 Gifford
American Falls, ID 83211
Telephone: (208)-226-5096
Contact: Cindy Holt
Referral for STD services

Teton County

County Health Depts

Teton County Health Department
30 West Depot Street
Driggs, ID 83422
Telephone: (208)-354-2220
HIV Counseling/Testing

Twin Falls County

County Health Depts

South Central District Health Department
324 2nd Street East
Box 547
Twin Falls, ID 83301
Telephone: (208)-734-5900
Contact: Cheryl Becker
Educational, Social Workers, Counseling, HIV Counseling/Testing, Health Care

Valley County

County Health Depts

Central District Health Department
703 North 1st Street
McCall, ID 83638
Telephone: (208)-634-7194
Social Services

Washington County

County Health Depts

Washington County Health Department
Main Street
Cambridge, ID 83610
Telephone: (208)-257-3355
HIV Counseling/Testing

Home Health Care

South West District Health Dept.
H6 West Court Street
Weiser, ID 83672
Telephone: (208)-549-2370
HIV Counseling/Testing

Testing Sites

Southwest District Health Dept
46 West Court
Weiser, ID 83672
Telephone: (208)-549-2370
Contact: Ms. Clare Howland, R.N.
HIV testing/counseling, STD testing/treatment

ILLINOIS

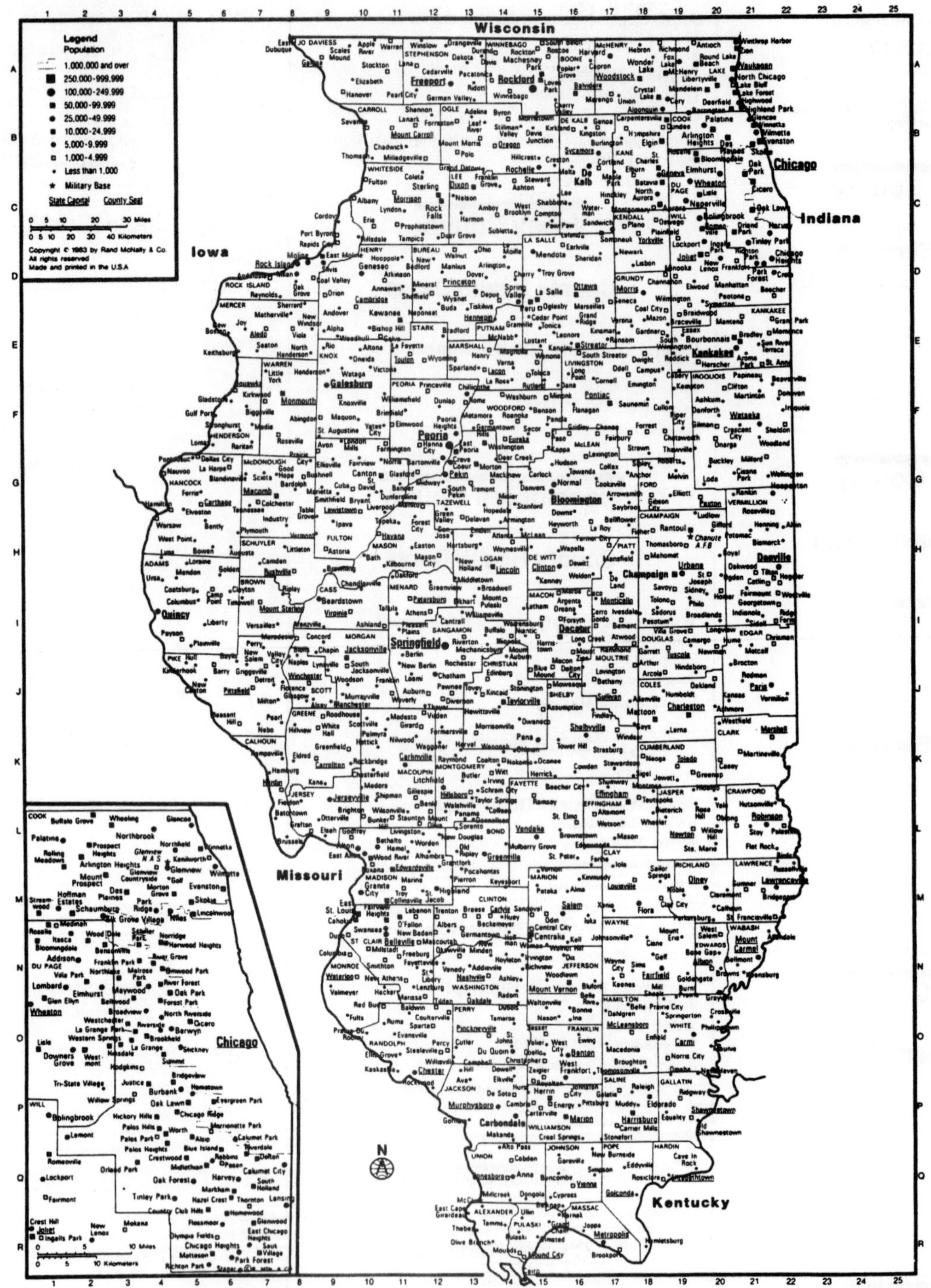

From City/County Planning Atlas Copyright 1989 by Reed McNally & Company, R.L. 90-S-28

Illinois

General Services

Education

Midwest AIDS Education and Training Center
Univ. of Illinois/Chicago Room 173
808 South Wood Street MC 779
Chicago, IL 60612
Telephone: (312)-996-1426 Fax: (312)-413-4184
Contact: Dr. Nathan L. Linsk, PhD - ;
Provide Professional Education

Midwest AIDS Training and Education Center
Univ of IL at Chicago
M/C 779, 808 S. Wood St.
Chicago, IL 60612-4325
Telephone: (312)-996-5574
Contact: Dr. Nathan L. Linsk - Director, Barbara Schechtman - Admin. Director, Caryn Berman - Program Director
AIDS education for health care professionals; assist schools in developingAIDS educational materials

Northwest Suburban Alcoholism/Drug Dependency Program
4811 Emerson
Palatine, IL 60067-7416
Telephone: (708)-397-0095 Fax: (708)-397-4192
HIV education

Reimer Foundation
3023 North Clark
1000
Chicago, IL 60657
Telephone: (312)-935-7233
Contact: Del Barrett
Educational resources

South Side Help Center
10420 South Halsted
Chicago, IL 60628
Telephone: (312)-264-6610
Contact: Betty Smith
Education and risk reduction for high risk youth, Black Male Mentor Program

Southside Help Center
10420 South Halsted
Chicago, IL 60609
Telephone: (312)-264-6610
Contact: Betty Smith
AIDS Education/Outreach, HIV prevention, Referrals

Stop AIDS Chicago
909 West Belmont Ave.
Chicago, IL 60657
Telephone: (312)-871-3300 Fax: (312)-871-2528
Contact: Matt Denckla
Referrals and informal, at-home AIDS awareness discussion groups

State Health Departments

Illinois Department of Public Health AIDS Activity Section
160 N. La Salle, 7th Floor
Chicago, IL 60601-3103
Telephone: (312)-814-4846 Fax: (312)-814-4844
Contact: Chet Kelly
Education, seroprevalance

Statewide Services

ACLU/Roger Baldwin Foundation
203 North LaSalle
Suite 1405
Chicago, IL 60601
Telephone: (312)-201-9740
Contact: John Hammel; Matt Nosanchuck
Legal assistance for HIV discrimination in housing, health care and other areas

Illinois Department of Health and Human Services
1900 Hassell Road
Hoffman Estates, IL 60195-2308
Telephone: (708)-882-4445
counseling

Illinois Department of Human Rights
100 West Randolph Street
Suite 10-100
Chicago, IL 60601
Telephone: (312)-917-6200
Investigate discrimination

Illinois Department of Public Aid
Central Office
624 South Michigan Ave
Chicago, IL 60605
Telephone: (312)-793-4706
Toll-Free: (800)-252-8635
Financial assistance, food stamps, medical card

Illinois Dept. of Children & Family AIDS Project Service
750 West Montrose
Chicago, IL 60613
Telephone: (312)-989-5884
Contact: Maria Ayala
Training for parents on care to children with AIDS, case management, referrals

Public Health Service
105 West Adams Street
17th Floor
Chicago, IL 60603
Telephone: (312)-353-3832 Fax: (312)-353-0718
Contact: John Krzemien, PhD
Referrals

The Kupona Network
4611 South Ellis Avenue
Chicago, IL 60653-3624
Telephone: (312)-536-3000
Contact: Susan Watts
Support groups, counseling, education, outreach programs, speakers,referrals

Adams County

County Health Depts

Adams County Health Department
333 North Sixth Street
Quincy, IL 62301-2796
Telephone: (217)-222-8440 Fax: (217)-222-8508
Contact: Carleen Orton

Alexander County

Testing Sites

HIV Counseling/Testing Site
3104 Elm Street
Cairo, IL 62914
Telephone: (618)-734-4167
Contact: Theresa Lasley

Bond County

County Health Depts

Bond County Health Department
503 South Prairie
Greenville, IL 62246-1897
Telephone: (618)-664-1442

Boone County

County Health Depts

Boone County Health Department
601 North Main Street
Belvidere, IL 61008-2600
Telephone: (815)-544-2951 Fax: (815)-547-8701
Contact: Dale Sterud

Brown County

County Health Depts

Brown County Health Department
111 West Washington St.
Mt. Sterling, IL 62353-1287
Telephone: (217)-773-2714

Calhoun County

County Health Depts

Calhoun County Health Department
P.O. Box 158
Hardin, IL 62047-0158
Telephone: (618)-576-2428
Contact: Judy Zahrli, RN

Cass County

County Health Depts

Cass County Health Department
331 South Main
Virginia, IL 62691-1524
Telephone: (217)-452-3057
Contact: Connie Sebetti
Home health care

Champaign County

County Health Depts

Champaign-Urbana Public Health District
710 North Neil Street
Box 1847
Champaign, IL 61820-3013
Telephone: (217)-352-7961
Contact: Gale Fella - MPH, RS

Christian County

County Health Depts

Christian County Health Department
902 West Spring Field
Taylorville, IL 62568
Telephone: (217)-824-4113
Contact: Cornelia Colonius
Home health care, communicable disease counseling, family counseling

Clay County

County Health Depts

Clay County Health Department
201 East North Avenue
P.O. Box 579
Flora, IL 62839-2029
Telephone: (618)-662-4406
Contact: Jeff Workman - Director
Counseling

Coles County

County Health Depts

Coles County Health Department
825 18th Street
Charleston, IL 61920-2996
Telephone: (217)-348-0530
Contact: Fred Edgar - Public Health Admin.
HIV/AIDS testing & counseling

Cook County

Community Services

Actor's Fund
203 North Wabash
Suite 1308
Chicago, IL 60601
Telephone: (312)-372-0989
Contact: Sheila Sheehan
Financial assistance & case mgt. for actors and entertainers, AIDSinitiative, referrals, counseling

Ascension Respite Care
1133 North LaSalle
Chicago, IL 60610
Telephone: (312)-751-8887
Contact: Kathy Thill
Respite child care, meals, case management, family support group, counseling

B.R.O.T.H.E.R.S.
6540 South Woodlawn Ave.
Chicago, IL 60637
Telephone: (312)-667-8313
Contact: Elliot Matthews - Director
Support groups for black, gay substance abusers; HIV/AIDS information

CAMEO (Chicago Area Mens Enrichment Organization)
P.O. Box 791
Hillside, IL 60163
Telephone: (708)-449-3478
Contact: James Wolfe
Food delivery for men with AIDS

Catholic Charities, Archdiocese of Chicago
126 North Des Plaines
Chicago, IL 60661
Telephone: (312)-236-5172 Fax: (312)-655-7000
Contact: Loretta Norton
Advocacy, education, counseling, necessity assistance

Chicago House and Social Service Agency
913 West Belmont
Chicago, IL 60657
Telephone: (312)-248-5200 Fax: (312)-248-5019
Contact: Mary Ellen Krems
Residential services for HIV

Chicago Urban League
4510 South Michigan Ave.
Chicago, IL 60653
Telephone: (312)-285-5800
Contact: David Wok
Case management, referrals, information

Community Family Services & Mental Health Center
1023 Burlington Ave
Western Springs, IL 60558
Telephone: (708)-354-0826 Fax: (708)-354-0867
Individual & family counseling

Comprehensive Counseling Associates
151 North Michigan Avenue
#2905
Chicago, IL 60601
Telephone: (312)-883-1643
Contact: Chuck Stemberg
Individual, couples & family counseling, and support groups for people withHIV

Counseling Center of Lakeview
3225 North Sheffield
Chicago, IL 60657-2210
Telephone: (312)-549-5886 Fax: (312)-549-3265
Contact: Norman Groetzinger - Executive Director
Counseling, case management

Counseling Centers of Chicago
4740 North Clark Street
Suite 208
Chicago, IL 60640
Telephone: (312)-326-0601
Contact: Rebecca Reusch
HIV case management

DePaul Legal Clinic
23 East Jackson
#950
Chicago, IL 60604
Telephone: (312)-341-8294 Fax: (312)-362-6918
Contact: Howard Rubin
General legal assistance for people with low income; family law

Family Service of Wilmette, Glenview, Northbrock, Kenilworth
1167 Wilmette Avenue
Wilmette, IL 60091-2603
Telephone: (708)-251-7350 Fax: (708)-446-5606
Contact: Dr. Robert Noone
Drug abuse counseling, HIV counseling

Great Lakes Psychological Services
111 North Wabash Avenue
Suite 1400
Chicago, IL 60602-1901
Telephone: (312)-443-1400 Fax: (312)-443-1307
Contact: Dr. John Fusco
counseling, testing

Health Care Financing Administration
15th Floor
Chicago, IL 60603
Telephone: (312)-353-1670 Fax: (312)-353-5927
Contact: Jan Cekan
Health care financing administration

Hispanic Health Alliance
1579 North Milwaukee
Suite 203
Chicago, IL 60622
Telephone: (312)-276-2185
Contact: Cecil Romano; Marta Munoz -
Referrals, counseling

Horizons Community Services, Inc.
961 W. Montana Street
Chicago, IL 60614-2408
Telephone: (312)-472-6469
Contact: Elizabeth Huesemann - Coordinator of Programs
Support groups for gay PWA/HIVs; free 24-hour anti-violence program 871-CARE

Kaleidoscope
1279 North Milwaukee
Suite 250
Chicago, IL 60622
Telephone: (312)-278-7200
Contact: Star Program
Child welfare agency providing services to HIV affected/infected families

Lifeline, Inc.
4746 North Marine Drive
Chicago, IL 60640
Telephone: (312)-275-9393 Fax: (312)-275-6690
Toll-Free: (800)-827-4898
Contact: Sheryl Smith
Substance abuse treatment and referrals

Marillac House
2822 West Jackson
Chicago, IL 60612
Telephone: (312)-772-7440
Contact: Sister Antoinette
Emergency food pantry and clothing, with supplemental for low income or SSI

Oak Park Family Services
120 S. Marion St
Oak Park, IL 60302-2809
Telephone: (708)-383-7500 Fax: (708)-383-7780
Contact: Pamela Robbins - Social Worker & Therapist
Mental health & substance abuse counseling

Planned Parenthood Association - Chicago Area
14 East Jackson Blvd.
10
Chicago, IL 60604-2204
Telephone: (312)-781-9550

Referrals

Safer Foundation
571 West Jackson
Chicago, IL 60661
Telephone: (312)-922-2200 Fax: (312)-922-7640
Contact: Ewing Foulks
AIDS information and referrals for former offenders

Skokie Health Department
5127 Oakton Street
Skokie, IL 60077-3633
Telephone: (708)-673-0500
Contact: Frieda Kagan
AIDS referrals

Social Security Administration
600 W. Madison St.,10th Fl
P.O. Box 8280
Chicago, IL 60680
Telephone: (312)-353-1733 Fax: (312)-353-0781
Contact: Mary Mahler
Social Security, Supplemental Security Income benefits, low income

St. Catherine Catholic Worker
P.O. Box 377585
Chicago, IL 60637
Telephone: (312)-288-3688
Contact: Tom Heuser
Temporary housing for men and women with HIV

Tinley Park Mental Health
7400 West 183rd Street
Tinley Park, IL 60477
Telephone: (708)-614-4014
Contact: Central Admission
Group counseling and information, referral for mentally ill

Travelers and Immigrants Aid
208 South La Salle
Suite 1818
Chicago, IL 60604
Telephone: (312)-404-1113
Primary care, case management, hospital discharge planning, emergency shelter

Village of Mt. Prospect - Human Services Division
50 South Emerson St.
Mt. Prospect, IL 60056-3218
Telephone: (708)-870-5680 Fax: (708)-392-6022
Home delivered meals, home nursing services

Village of Schaumburg Family Counseling Center
217 South Civic Drive
Schaumburg, IL 60193-1257
Telephone: (708)-529-1505 Fax: (708)-529-2201
Contact: Du Ree Brynant
Family and Counseling for HIV

Westside Association for Community Action
3600 West Ogden Avenue
Chicago, IL 60623
Telephone: (312)-762-4022
Contact: Gloria Jenkins
Food baskets, toys, financial help, AIDS outreach education, case management

Woodlawn Organization
1447 East 65th Street
Chicago, IL 60637
Telephone: (312)-493-6116
In-house treatment program, counseling, job training, AA/CA/NA meetings,HIV counseling

County Health Depts

Cook County Bureau of Health Services
HIV Primary Care Center
1900 West Polk Street-CCSN Floor 12
Chicago, IL 60612
Telephone: (312)-633-5182
HIV-antibody testing, counseling, primary care, case management, pharmacy

Cook County Department of Public Health
16501 South Kedzie Pkwy.
Markham, IL 60426
Telephone: (708)-210-4500 Fax: (708)-210-4619
Counseling & referral, HIV testing, (HIV testing phone 708-445-2437)

Cook County Department of Public Health
1015 Lake Street
Suite 300
Oak Park, IL 60301
Telephone: (708)-445-2437
Contact: Karen Scott - MD, MPH
HIV counseling, testing

Evanston Health Department
2100 Ridge Avenue
Evanston, IL 60204-2796
Telephone: (708)-866-2952 Fax: (708)-475-7259
Contact: Helen Sethuraman
HIV testing, counseling

Oak Park Department of Health
One Village Hall Plaza
Oak Park, IL 60301
Telephone: (708)-383-6400
Contact: Nancy Haggerty - Public Health Admin.

Stickney Township Public Health District
5635 State Road
Burbank, IL 60459-2097
Telephone: (708)-424-9200
Contact: Robert Peters - Public Health Admin.

Home Health Care

Alternate Site Infusion Technologies Inc.
5695 W. Howard Street
Niles, IL 60714
Telephone: (708)-647-8896 Fax: (708)-647-8898
Contact: Tom Abbott - Manager Client Relations
Clinical support, inhalation therapy, infusion, enteral and parenteralnutrition, antibiotics, chemotherapy, hematopoetics, transfusions andinvestigational agents

Ancilla Home Help
1350 Remington Road
Schaumburg, IL 60173-4822
Telephone: (708)-882-9595 Fax: (708)-882-9640
Contact: Ralph Eaton
Home care, nursing services

Caremark Connection Network
1125 W 175th Street
Homewood, IL 60430-4604
Telephone: (708)-957-9572 Fax: (708)-957-8531
Contact: Margaret Frued - Branch Manager
Clinical support and infusion therapies: Nutrition, Antimicrobials, Chemo.,Hematopoeti

Caremark Connection Network
c/o Seton Medical Center
711 W North Ave, Ste. 205
Chicago, IL 60610
Telephone: (312)-664-2037
Contact: Ronald Ohlsen - Branch Manager
Clinical support and infusion therapies: nutrition, & social-services, aerosolized pentamidine service, blood tranfusions & otherintraven therapies

Caremark Corp.
1471 Business Center Dr.
Suite 500
Mt Prospect, IL 60056-6041
Telephone: (708)-803-9600 Fax: (708)-803-8635
Contact: Ronald Ohlsen - Branch Manager, Patricia Conklin - Operations Manager
Clinical Support and Infusion Therapies: Nutrition, Antimicrobials, Chemo.,Hematopoeti

Community Nursing Service - West
1041 West Madison
Oak Park, IL 60302
Telephone: (708)-386-4443 Fax: (708)-386-7453
Contact: Kathie Nash
Visiting nurse, certified nursing aides for support care, homemaker support

Concerned Care, Inc.
8950 Gross Point Road
Suite E
Skokie, IL 60077
Telephone: (708)-966-8700 Fax: (708)-966-8566
Toll-Free: (800)-241-2666
Contact: Mora Raith - Intake Worker
Homemaker Service

Critical Care America
945 Busse Road
Elk Grove Village, IL 60007-2400
Telephone: (708)-437-2273 Fax: (702)-437-2719
Toll-Free: (800)-876-3399
Infusion therapies in home

Department of Rehabilitative Services
6200 North Hiawatha
Suite 300
Chicago, IL 60646
Telephone: (312)-794-4803
Contact: Linda Cianfrani
Home Health Services

El Dorado Home Health
2405 West North Avenue
Chicago, IL 60647
Telephone: (312)-227-2520
Contact: Janet Lapidos
Nursing services, home health aid, physical/occupational/speech therapy

Extended Health Services
7434 Skokie Blvd.
Skokie, IL 60077
Telephone: (708)-679-6565 Fax: (708)-674-4677
Contact: Diane Muench - Administrator
Intermittent and private duty nursing, therapy, homemakers and companions

Five Hospital Program
600 West Diversey
Chicago, IL 60614
Telephone: (312)-549-5822
Contact: Intake Nurse
Home health care specializing in infusion therapies

Harbor Home Support Services
1010 Lake Street
Suite 100
Oak Park, IL 60301
Telephone: (708)-386-1100 Fax: (708)-386-1108
Contact: Marc Krupowicz - Supervisor
Comprehensive care to home-bound individuals with HIV or AIDS

Hardy Associates Home Health Service
8053 South Stony Island
Chicago, IL 60617
Telephone: (312)-731-6574
Contact: Brenda Adams, R.N.
Comprehensive home health services with RNs, LPNs, home health aides,certified nurses aides

Haymarket House
120 North Sangamon Ave.
Chicago, IL 60607
Telephone: (312)-226-7984
Contact: Debra Carter
Residential recovery home for those with a history of substance abuse

Horizon Hospice
2800 North Sheridan Road
Chicago, IL 60657-6156
Telephone: (312)-871-3658
Contact: Intake Mgr.
Home Health Care Services

Hospice of North Shore
2821 Central Street
Evanston, IL 60201-1221
Telephone: (708)-467-7423 Fax: (708)-866-6023
Contact: Pat Huesing - Coordinator of Patient Care
Home and Hospice Services, Bereavement Support

Hospice Suburban South
2609 Flossmoor Road
PO Box 258
Flossmoor, IL 604220258
Telephone: (708)-957-7177
Contact: Susie Zanuodnyik
Home Health Care Services

Hospital & Medicare Center
2929 South Ellis Street
Chicago, IL 60616
Telephone: (312)-791-2050 Fax: (312)-791-3577
Contact: Patricia Moss, R.N. - HIV Clinical Specialist
HIV support group, HIV clinic, impatient care, nutritional counseling,mental health care, social work support

Howard Brown Health Center
945 West George Street
Chicago, IL 60657-5007
Telephone: (312)-871-5777
Contact: Client Service Representative
Home Health Care Services

Illinois Masonic Hospice
836 West Wellington Ave.
Chicago, IL 60657
Telephone: (312)-296-7048
Contact: Oscar Bemard
Full range of in-home hospice services

Interim Health Care
10735 S Cicero Avenue
Oak Lawn, IL 60453-6205
Telephone: (708)-422-2934 Fax: (708)-422-2934
Contact: JoAnne McGovern - Director
Home Health Services

LaGrange Memorial Home Care Hospice
6406 Joliet Road
Countryside, IL 60525-4642
Telephone: (708)-352-6696 Fax: (708)-352-9459
Contact: Mary Jo Long - Patient Care Coordinator
Home care; nursing, social work, home health aides, bereavement care

Little Company of Mary Hospital
2800 West 95th
Evergreen Park, IL 60642-2795
Telephone: (708)-422-6200
Home Health Care Services

Medical Personnel Pool
990 Grove Road
Evanston, IL 60201
Telephone: (708)-869-7601 Fax: (708)-869-7836
Contact: Nancy Williams
Medical Services

Meridian Hospice
9204 S. Commercial Ave.
Suite 212
Chicago, IL 60617
Telephone: (312)-768-2500 Fax: (312)-768-5786
Contact: Maria Van Gemert - Executive Director
Home care, hospice

nmc HOMECARE
8120 Lehigh, Suite 104
Morton Grove, IL 60053
Telephone: (312)-792-1821
Fax: (312)-966-2863
Contact: Raj King
National JCAHO-Accredited company providing a full range of Infusion and Respiratory therapies and specializing in the care of HIV/AIDS patients. National Case Manager is also available at 800-445-1188

Northwestern Memorial Hospice Program
303 East Superior Street
9th Floor East
Chicago, IL 60611-3053
Telephone: (312)-908-7476 Fax: (312)-908-4020
Contact: Jeanne Martinez - Clinical Manager
Full service hospice (hospital based), home care social services, nursesaides, volunteers, interdisciplinary service, acute care, inpatientfacility

Nursefinders
5301 West Pempster Street
Skokie, IL 60077-1835
Telephone: (708)-470-8550
Contact: Terri Peri
Health care services for HIV patients

Nursefinders
1512 Fremont Street
#203
Chicago, IL 60622
Telephone: (312)-654-2050 Fax: (312)-654-2059
Health care agency: nurses, LPN, home health aides

Park Forest Health Department
Nine Centre
Park Forest, IL 60466
Telephone: (708)-748-1118
Contact: Lois Coxworth - Director of Public Health
Home health and education/information

Rainbow Hospice
460 South NW Highway
Suite 103
Parkridge, IL 60068-4986
Telephone: (708)-292-0550 Fax: (708)-292-0556
Home Health Care Services

Rush Home Care - North Shore
8700 Waukegan Road
Suite 136
Morton Grove, IL 60053-2103
Telephone: (708)-965-8250 Fax: (708)-965-5161
Care for all ages

Rush Home Care Network
1201 West Harrison
Chicago, IL 60607-3319
Telephone: (312)-850-7500 Fax: (312)-850-7501
Contact: Marilyn O'Rourke - Agency Director
Certified home care agency: skilled nursing, physical therapy, occupationaltherapy, speech pathology, social work, psychiatric nursing, home healthaides, life line program

Senior's Home Health Care, Ltd.
10716 South Ewing Avenue
Chicago, IL 60617-6619
Telephone: (312)-768-8100
Contact: Susan Orlando - Office Manager
Nurses, nurses aides, physical therapy, occupational therapy, speechtherapy

Staff Builders Home Visits Plus
1459 Ring Road
Calumet, IL 60409
Telephone: (708)-730-3624
Contact: Geri Griffie
Skilled nursing visits, home health aides, homemakers, respite care services

Visiting Nurse Association North
2008 Dempster Avenue
Evanston, IL 60202-1017
Telephone: (708)-328-1900 Fax: (708)-328-9253
Home health care-takes care of AIDS patients

Visiting Nurse Association of Chicago
322 South Greene Street
Suite 500
Chicago, IL 60607-3599
Telephone: (312)-738-8622
Contact: Elaine Sampson - Corporate VP
Home health aides, speech therapist, social services, hospice pgm., volunteers

West Towns Visiting Nursing Service
6438 W. 34th Street
Berwyn, IL 60402-1258
Telephone: (708)-749-7171
Contact: Sue Svec, M.S.W. - Development Director
Home health & hospice services, counseling

Medical Services

AIDS Alternative Health Project
4753 North Broadway
Suite 1110
Chicago, IL 60640
Telephone: (312)-561-2800 Fax: (312)-561-8225
Contact: Sal Iacopelli
Alternative therapy

Alden-Lakeland
820 West Lawrence
Chicago, IL 60640
Telephone: (312)-769-2570 Fax: (312)-769-0607
Contact: Rose Guptierrez

Long-term care, skilled nursing

Alivio Medical Center
2355 South Western
Chicago, IL 60608
Telephone: (312)-650-1200 Fax: (312)-650-1226
Contact: Carmen Velasquez
HIV-antibody testing, counseling, primary care, case management

American Indian Health Services
838 West Irving Park Rd.
Chicago, IL 60613
Telephone: (312)-883-9100 Fax: (312)-883-0005
Contact: Tim Vermillion
Community health center services for American Indians, HIV counseling

Cermak Health Services
2800 S. California Ave.
Chicago, IL 60608
Telephone: (312)-890-9300 Fax: (312)-890-7177
Contact: Delia Rozier-Johnson
HIV-antibody testing, counseling, case mgt., HIV education, support groups

Children's Memorial Comprehensive Hemophilia Center
2300 Children's Plaza
Chicago, IL 60614
Telephone: (312)-880-4620 Fax: (312)-880-3053
Contact: Susan Garnermann - Hemophilia Clinican Nurse
Primary care, dental, orthopedic, social svcs., support groups, financial aid

Children's Memorial Hospital
2300 Children's Plaza
Chicago, IL 60614-3394
Telephone: (312)-880-3718 Fax: (312)-880-3208
Contact: Judy Swanson
HIV-antibody testing, inpatient/outpatient medical care, counseling

Erie Family Health Center
1656 West Chicago Avenue
Chicago, IL 60622
Telephone: (312)-666-3488 Fax: (312)-666-5867
Contact: Irma Gerena; David Ley -
HIV-antibody testing, counseling, pharmacological treatment, medical support

Garfield Counseling Center
4132 West Madison
Chicago, IL 60624
Telephone: (312)-533-0433 Fax: (312)-533-6288
Contact: Richard Shelton
Case management, residential treatment and rehabilitation for IDUs

Glen Oaks Nursing Center
270 Skokie Blvd.
Northbrook, IL 60062
Telephone: (708)-498-9320 Fax: (708)-498-2990
Contact: Carol Lisy - Director of Admissions
Long-term care with services for PWA/HIV

Humana HMO
2545 South King Drive
Chicago, IL 60616
Telephone: (312)-842-7117 Fax: (312)-842-7595
Contact: Dr. Arthur Moswin
Primary care, nursing care, social services & case management for hemophiliacs

Illinois Masonic Medical Center
836 W. Wellington Ave.
Chicago, IL 60657-5147
Telephone: (312)-975-1600 Fax: (312)-296-5372
Contact: Dr. David Moore & David Blatt - Unit 371
In-patient medical care with special HIV/AIDS unit

Lawnside Christian Health Center
3860 West Ogden
Chicago, IL 60623
Telephone: (312)-521-5006 Fax: (312)-762-5772
Contact: Alice Pizzano
Primary outpatient care, case management, HIV-antibody testing, counseling

Leyden Family Services & Mental Health Center
10001 West Grand Avenue
Franklin Park, IL 60131-2564
Telephone: (708)-451-0330 Fax: (708)-451-1652

Loyola Medical Center HIV/AIDS Clinic
Mulcahy Outpatient Center
2nd Floor
Maywood, IL 60153
Telephone: (708)-216-5024 Fax: (708)-216-8198
Contact: Scott Chinburg, R.N.
HIV screening, counseling, primary medical care, social services, referrals, nutritional counseling

Lutheran General Hospital
1775 Dempster
Park Ridge, IL 60068-1174
Telephone: (708)-696-2210 Fax: (708)-318-2332
Primary medical care, HIV testing, social & counseling services, pharmacy, speakers, education

Mt. Sinai Hospital
15th at California
Chicago, IL 60608
Telephone: (312)-542-2000 Fax: (312)-257-6548
Contact: Dr. Mark Levin
Primary and inpatient medical care, and home health services

Near North Health Service
1276 North Clybourn
Chicago, IL 60610
Telephone: (312)-337-1073 Fax: (312)-337-7616
Contact: Linda Murray, M.D.
Outpatient services, HIV-antibody testing, counseling, AZT & pentamidine

Northside HIV Treatment Center
4753 North Broadway
Suite 518
Chicago, IL 60640
Telephone: (312)-271-6335
Contact: Arthur Shattuck
Alternative healthcare for PWA/HIVs incl. acupuncture, massage, Chinese herbs

Northwest Community Hospital and Hospice
800 West Central Road
Arlington Hgts., IL 60005-2392
Telephone: (708)-259-1000
Contact: Marcia Beckerdite
Basic inpatient medical services, hospice services, long-term care, supportgroups

Oak Forest Hospital
15900 South Cicero Ave.
Oak Forest, IL 60452
Telephone: (708)-687-7200 Fax: (708)-687-7979
Contact: Admissions Office
Long term care

Olympia Fields Osteopathic Hospital & Medical Center
20201 South Crawford
Olympia Fields, IL 60461-1080
Telephone: (708)-747-4000 Fax: (708)-503-3299
Contact: Dr. Basil Williams
Counseling, testing, medical services, referrals, lab

Rush North Shore Medical Center
9600 Gross Point Road
Skokie, IL 60076-1257
Telephone: (708)-677-9600 Fax: (708)-933-6756
Inpatient care, counseling, labs, pharmacy, referrals

Rush Presbyterian St. Luke's Medical Center
Infectious Disease Dept
600 South Paulina, #143
Chicago, IL 60612
Telephone: (312)-942-5865 Fax: (312)-942-2184
Contact: Harold Kessler
Studies, private practice, referrals

Rush-Prebyterian-St. Luke's Medical Center
1653 West Congress Parkway
Chicago, IL 60612-3833
Telephone: (312)-942-5000 Fax: (312)-942-2184
Contact: Dr. Trenholme
In-patient medical care and clinical trials

St. Bernard Hospital
326 West 64th Street
Chicago, IL 60621
Telephone: (312)-962-4075
Contact: Ron Campbell
Basic inpatient medical care, and HIV-antibody testing with counseling

St. Francis Hospital of Evanston
355 Ridge Ave.
Evanston, IL 60202-3399
Telephone: (708)-866-2775 Fax: (708)-492-3307
Contact: Dr. Fred Zar
Basic inpatient medical care

St. Joseph Hospital
2900 N. Lake Shore Drive
Chicago, IL 60657-6274
Telephone: (312)-975-3000 Fax: (312)-665-3601
Contact: Debbie Septofki
AIDS unit provides care for PWA/HIVs

University of Illinois College of Medicine
Mail Code 856
840 South Wood St
Chicago, IL 60612
Telephone: (312)-996-6714 Fax: (312)-413-1526
Contact: Kenneth Rich
Counseling, HIV testing, research

West Suburban Hospital
Erie at Austin
Oak Park, IL 60302-2599
Telephone: (708)-383-6200
HIV testing, medical treatment, counseling, referrals, family counseling

West Suburban Hospital
Erie A7 Austin
Oak Park, IL 60302
Telephone: (708)-383-6200
HIV testing, medical treatment, counseling, referrals, pharmacy family counseling

Western Clinic Health Services
63 East Adams Street
Suite 201
Chicago, IL 60603
Telephone: (312)-939-7047 Fax: (312)-939-7905
Contact: Nel Stokes
Group/individual counseling, outpatient methadone treatment, case management

Daniel Hale Williams Center
5044 South State Street
Chicago, IL 60609
Telephone: (312)-538-6700 Fax: (312)-538-4325
Contact: Bernice Wilson
Primary medical care, case management, HIV-antibody testing, and counseling

Winfield Moody Community Health Center
1276 North Clybourn
Chicago, IL 60610
Telephone: (312)-337-1073 Fax: (312)-337-7616
Contact: Linda Murray - MD
Primary care, case management, anonymous HIV-antibody testing, counseling, etc.

Testing Sites

Chicago Department of Health
333 South State Street
2nd Floor
Chicago, IL 60604
Telephone: (312)-744-4312
Contact: Judith Johns
Free, anonymous and confidential HIV-antibody testing; counseling; referrals

Crossroads Health Center
512 N Plum Grove Rd, #100
Palatine, IL 60067-3522
Telephone: (708)-359-7575
HIV testing & counseling

El Rincon Supportive Services
1874 North Milwaukee Ave.
Chicago, IL 60647
Telephone: (312)-276-0200 Fax: (312)-276-4226
Contact: Efrain Valentin; Pedro Garcia
Bilingual; HIV testing and support groups

Health Services at University of Chicago
5841 South Maryland Ave.
Chicago, IL 60637
Telephone: (312)-702-1572 Fax: (312)-702-2468
HIV-antibody testing, STD testing, counseling, referrals

Komed Health Center
501 East 43rd
Chicago, IL 60653
Telephone: (312)-268-7600 Fax: (312)-268-9088
Contact: Jenny Donner
Primary care, HIV-antibody testing with pre- and post-test counseling

New City Healthcare Center
5500 South Damen
Chicago, IL 60636
Telephone: (312)-737-5400 Fax: (312)-737-5567
Contact: Della Jones
Primary care, HIV-antibody testing, counseling, case management

Westside Clinic CDC
1306 South Michigan Avenue
Chicago, IL 60605
Telephone: (312)-747-0103 Fax: (312)-747-0160
Contact: Bill Erwin
Counseling, testing, referral & partner notification program

Crawford County

County Health Depts

Crawford County Health Dept.
301 South Cross
Commercium Bldg., Suite 284
Robinson, IL 62454
Telephone: (618)-544-8798
Contact: Michael P. Henry - MA

Cumberland County

County Health Depts

Cumberland County Health Department
Box 130
Toledo, IL 62468-0130
Telephone: (217)-849-3211
Contact: Nancy Nees
Education & counseling services

De Kalb County

County Health Depts

DeKalb County Health Department
2337 Sycamore Road
DeKalb, IL 60115-2088
Telephone: (815)-758-6673
Contact: LaDonne McShannon
HIV testing and counseling

De Witt County

County Health Depts

Dewitt-Piatt Bi-County Health Department
910 Route 54 East
P.O. Box 518
Clinton, IL 61727
Telephone: (217)-935-3427
Contact: Richard J. Bennett - Public Health Admin.

Douglas County

County Health Depts

Douglas County Health Department
209 E. Van Allen Street
Tuscola, IL 61953-1841
Telephone: (217)-253-4137
Contact: Kimberly Bassett - RN
Referral services

Du Page County

Community Services

Addison Township
Human Services Dept.
401 North Addison Road
Addison, IL 60101
Telephone: (708)-530-8161 Fax: (708)-530-1952
Financial assistance and food pantry for persons with low income in AddisonTwp

AIDS Pastoral Care Network
Edward Hospital
801 South Washington
Naperville, IL 60566
Telephone: (708)-527-3560
Contact: Rev. Robert Hansen
Support groups, pastoral counseling, referrals, and speakers

Downers Grove Health & Human Resources
842 Curtis Street
Downers Grove, IL 60515
Telephone: (708)-719-4595
Contact: Barbara Lieber
Individual and group counseling on grief surrounding HIV/AIDS

DuPage County Department of Public Aid
146 West Roosevelt Road
Villa Park, IL 60181
Telephone: (708)-530-1120
Contact: Marsha Wojcik
Financial assistance, food stamps, referrals to home health care, homemakersvc general referrals for all services

DuPage County Para-Transit
421 North County Farm Rd.
Wheaton, IL 60187
Telephone: (708)-682-7400
Contact: Margo Schreiber
Financial assistance for rent and utilities, transportation, housing& referral

Hope Fair Housing Center
154 South Main Street
Lombard, IL 60148
Telephone: (708)-495-4844 Fax: (708)-495-4845
Contact: Bernard Kleina - Executive Director
Housing discrimination, financial assistance, referrals, advocacy, andcounseling

County Health Depts

DuPage County Health Department
111 North County Farm Rd.
Wheaton, IL 60187-3988
Telephone: (708)-682-7979
Contact: Kevin M. Sherin - MD

Home Health Care

Curaflex Infusion Services
1360 North Wood Dale Rd
Suite K
Wood Dale, IL 60191-1038
Telephone: (800)-333-8710 Fax: (708)-766-8387
Toll-Free: (800)-333-8710
Contact: Michael Lattrell - General Manager
Home IV therapy: TPN, Enteral, IV Antibiotics, Aerosolized/IV Pentamidine

EHS Homecare
2311 W. 22nd Street
Suite 300
Oak Brook, IL 60521
Telephone: (708)-572-1232 Fax: (708)-572-9797
Visiting nurse, physical, respiratory, psychological therapy, socialworkers

Evangelical Health Systems, Inc.
2025 Windsor Drive
Oak Brook, IL 60521-1586
Telephone: (708)-572-1232 Fax: (708)-572-9797
Contact: Kate O'Neil
Hi-tech nursing care, maternal-child care, pediatrics, physical therapy,respiratory therapy, occupational therapy, home health aides

HNS, Inc.
342 Carol Lane
Elmhurst, IL 60126
Telephone: (708)-941-3008 Fax: (708)-941-3276
Toll-Free: (800)-872-4467
Contact: Dave Anderson
Home Infusion Therapy, In-home Nursing and Attendant Care, PhysicalTherapy, Pentamidine

Homedco Infusion
655 West Grand Avenue
Unit 100
Elmhurst, IL 60126-1060
Telephone: (708)-832-5800
Toll-Free: (800)-466-4363
Contact: Denise McGuire
Nationwide experience inproviding home infusion therapy to AIDS patients

Hospice of Du Page
690 East North Avenue
Carol Stream, IL 60188
Telephone: (708)-690-9000 Fax: (708)-690-9064
Contact: Kathy Schwartz, R.N. - Nursing Manager
Pain and symptom support, case management, emotional and spiritual support

Hospitals Home Health
4255 Westbrook Drive
Aurora, IL 60504
Telephone: (708)-898-0122
Contact: Mary Rausch
Home healthcare and HIV-antibody testing with pre- and post-test counseling

St. Thomas Hospice
7 Salt Creek Lane
Suite 204
Hinsdale, IL 60521
Telephone: (708)-920-8300 Fax: (708)-850-3969
Contact: Patricia Morrissey
Home Health Care Services

Vitas Corp.
100 West 22nd Street
Suite 101
Lombard, IL 60148-4877
Telephone: (708)-495-8484 Fax: (708)-495-1598
Contact: - Director of Admissions
Hospices Care Services

Medical Services

Edward Hospital
801 South Washington St.
Naperville, IL 60566
Telephone: (708)-527-3562
Contact: Sheri Flum - Social Worker
Weekly support group for PWHIV/PWAs, and basic hospital medical care

Elmhurst Memorial Hospital
200 Bertreau Avenue
Elmhurst, IL 60126
Telephone: (708)-833-1400 Fax: (708)-782-7892
Contact: Charles Ross
Inpatient care, HIV-antibody testing, counseling, hospice care, home health

Effingham County

County Health Depts

Effingham County Health Department
901 West Virginia
P.O. Box 685
Effingham, IL 62401-2012
Telephone: (217)-342-9237 Fax: (217)-342-9324
Contact: Ted Crump - Public Health Admin.
Anonymous testing/counseling

Fayette County

County Health Depts

Fayette County Health Department
509 West Edwards
P.O. Box 340
Vandalia, IL 62471-2707
Telephone: (618)-283-1044 Fax: (618)-283-5038
Contact: Cara Kelly - RN
Anonymous HIV testing

Franklin County

County Health Depts

Franklin William Bican County Health Dept
Franklin Heights Plaza
Benton, IL 62812
Telephone: (618)-439-0951
Contact: Robin Rice
HIV Counseling/Testing Site

Fulton County

County Health Depts

Fulton County Health Department
700 East Oak Street
Canton, IL 61520-3168
Telephone: (309)-647-1134
Contact: Fred Fiebenmann - Public Health Admin.
Education

Greene County

County Health Depts

Greene County Health Department
310 Fifth Street
Carrollton, IL 62016-1393
Telephone: (217)-942-6961
Contact: Darlene Ridings - Public Health Admin.
AIDS education, home health

Grundy County

County Health Depts

Grundy County Health Department
1320 Union Street
Morris, IL 60450-2426
Telephone: (815)-941-3112 Fax: (815)-941-3400
Contact: Polly Daly - Public Health Admin.
Counseling

Hamilton County

County Health Depts

Hamilton County Health Dept.
County Courthouse, Room 5
McLeansboro, IL 62859
Telephone: (618)-643-3522
Contact: Martha Heflin - RN, Public Health Admin.

Hancock County

County Health Depts

Hancock County Health Department
Box 357
73 South Adams Street
Carthage, IL 62321-0357
Telephone: (217)-357-2171
Contact: Lee Ourth - Public Health Admin.
Information, counseling, testing, home health

Henderson County

County Health Depts

Henderson County Health Department
P.O. Box 268
Gladstone, IL 61437
Telephone: (309)-627-2812
Contact: Louise Webb
Case management

Henry County

County Health Depts

Henry County Health Department
4424 U.S. Highway 34
Kewanee, IL 61443
Telephone: (309)-852-0197
Contact: Louise Tharp - Public Health Admin.
Home health services

Stark County Health Dept.
4424 US Hwy 34
Kewanee, IL 61443
Telephone: (309)-852-3115
Contact: Louise Tharp - Public Health Admin.

Iroquois County

County Health Depts

Ford-Iroquois Public Health Department
114 North 3rd Street
P.O. Box 427
Watseka, IL 60970
Telephone: (815)-432-2483
Contact: John A. Pickering - Public Health Admin.

Jackson County

County Health Depts

Jackson County Health Department
Route 13 at Country Club Road
P.O. Box 307
Murphysboro, IL 62966
Telephone: (618)-684-3143
Contact: Virginia Scott - Public Health Admin.
Anonymous testing, counseling, STD clinic

Jasper County

County Health Depts

Jasper County Health Department
106 East Edwards Street
Newton, IL 62448-1736
Telephone: (618)-783-4436
Contact: Christine Hampton - Public Health Admin.
Testing, home visits, counseling

Jersey County

County Health Depts

Jersey County Health Department
208 South Lafayette St.
Jerseyville, IL 62052-1657
Telephone: (618)-498-9565
Contact: Therese Macias - Public Health Admin.

Jo Daviess County

County Health Depts

Jo Daviess County Health Department
9483 U.S. Rt. 20 West
P.O. Box 318
Galena, IL 61036-9102
Telephone: (815)-777-0263 Fax: (815)-777-2977
Contact: Peggy Murphy - Public Health Admin.
Call for information about specific services

Johnson County

Testing Sites

HIV Counseling/Testing Site
PO Box 603
Vienna, IL 62995
Telephone: (618)-658-5011
Contact: Mary Trovillion, RN
Counseling and Testing for HIV and AIDS

Kane County

County Health Depts

Kane County Health Department
1330 North Highland Ave.
Aurora, IL 60506-1441
Telephone: (708)-897-1124
Contact: Robert S. Pietrusiak - Public Health Admin.
HIV testing & counseling

Home Health Care

Fox Valley Hospice
113 East Wilson
Batavia, IL 60510
Telephone: (708)-879-6064 Fax: (708)-879-6639
Contact: Vivian Nimmo
For patients with life expectancy of days, weeks, or months

Medical Services

Copley Memorial Hospital
502 South Lincoln Avenue
Aurora, IL 60505
Telephone: (708)-844-1030 Fax: (708)-892-5058
Inpatient care, AIDS education, and pastoral care

Sherman Hospital
934 Center Street
Elgin, IL 60120
Telephone: (708)-742-9800
Contact: Infectious Disease Unit
Basic inpatient medical services, HIV-antibody testing, counseling, referrals

Testing Sites

HIV Counseling/Testing Site
164 Division St
Elgin, IL 60120
Telephone: (708)-695-1093
Contact: Hugh Epping
HIV testing, Counseling, Case Management, Medical Care

Kankakee County

County Health Depts

Kankakee County Health Department
1115 Riverlane Drive
Bradley, IL 60915
Telephone: (815)-937-7888
Contact: Clayton Pape - Public Health Admin.
HIV testing, pre & post individual counseling, referrals

Kendall County

County Health Depts

Kendall County Health Department
111 West Fox Street
Yorkville, IL 60560
Telephone: (708)-553-4132 Fax: (708)-553-4214
Contact: Ruth Ann Little - Public Health Admin.

Knox County

County Health Depts

Woodford County Health Dept.
106 South Darst
Eureka, IL 61430
Telephone: (309)-467-3064
Contact: Nancy Allen - Public Health Admin.

La Salle County

County Health Depts

Lasalle County Health Department
717 Etna Road
Ottawa, IL 61350-1097
Telephone: (815)-433-3366
Contact: Margo Schmitz Myers - Public Health Admin.
Information, referrals, educational videos, risk-prevention-materials

Lake County

Community Services

Bethany Ministry
Deerfield - Wilmont Roads
Deerfield, IL 60015
Telephone: (708)-945-1678
Support group for family and friends of persons living with HIV/AIDS

County Health Depts

Lake County Health Department
2400 Belvedere Road
Waukegan, IL 60085
Telephone: (708)-360-6892
Contact: Ann Jensen - RN, HIV/STD, Coordinator
HIV pre & post testing, referral, support counseling, early interventionclinic

Home Health Care

Hospice of Highland Park
718 Glenview Avenue
Highland Park, IL 60035
Telephone: (708)-480-3858
Contact: Karen Holub
Full hospice services, nurse visits, social workers, volunteers

Hospice of Northeastern Illinois, Inc.
410 South Hagen Avenue
Barrington, IL 60010
Telephone: (708)-381-5599
Services for terminally ill and families

Hospital Home Health
660 North Westmoreland
Lake Forest, IL 60045
Telephone: (708)-234-6118
Physician ordered home care with nurse or trained aide, referrals tohospice, meals on wheels & telecare, physical, speech & occupationaltherapy

S.T.A.R. Hospice
2615 W. Washington Blvd.
Waukegan, IL 60085
Telephone: (708)-240-5897
Contact: Pam Boyd
Home care and holistic services (psycho/social/spirit)

Lawrence County

County Health Depts

Lawrence County Health Department
R.R. #3, Box 414
Lawrenceville, IL 62439-9499
Telephone: (618)-943-3302 Fax: (618)-943-3657
Contact: Sylvia Pulleyblank - Public Health Admin.
Home health, outpatient counseling, psychiatric counsultation

Lee County

County Health Depts

Lee County Health Department
1315 Franklin Grove Rd.
Suite 110
Dixon, IL 61021-9185
Telephone: (815)-284-3371
Contact: Richard Innis - Public Health Admin.

Livingston County

County Health Depts

Livingston County Health Department
Livingston Health/Ed Bldg
R.R. #4
Pontiac, IL 61764
Telephone: (815)-844-7174
Contact: Merylin Elliott - AIDS Administrator
Home health, TB testing

Logan County

County Health Depts

Logan County Health Department
2120 West 5th Street Road
Lincoln, IL 62656-9149
Telephone: (217)-735-2317
Contact: Mary Anderson - AIDS Coordinator
Anonymous HIV screening & counseling

Macon County

County Health Depts

Macon County Health Department
1221 East Condit Street
Decatur, IL 62521-1405
Telephone: (217)-423-6988
Contact: Jerry Andrews - Public Health Admin.
Free, confidential counseling, AIDS education

Macoupin County

County Health Depts

Macoupin County Health Department
805 North Broad
Carlinville, IL 62626-1075
Telephone: (217)-854-3223
Contact: Karen Hazzard - Director of Nursing

Madison County

County Health Depts

Madison County Health Department, Branch Office
WIC Building
Market Square Mall
Huntsville, IL 35804
Telephone: (205)-534-1651
Contact: Susan Zlotnick-Hale
HIV testing, counseling, home care services, referrals, education,speakers & medical services

Testing Sites

AIDS Madison County
2016 Madison Avenue
Granite City, IL 62040
Telephone: (618)-877-5110 Fax: (618)-877-0772
Contact: Sandra Stokka - Director
HIV testing, counseling, outreach, case management, home services

HIV Counseling/Testing Site
2016 Madison Avenue
Granite City, IL 62040
Telephone: (618)-877-5110
Contact: Sandra Stokka - Director
HIV counseling and testing, Case management, Home service and Educationaloutreach

Mason County

County Health Depts

Mason County Health Department
Route 136 East
P.O. Box 557
Havana, IL 62644
Telephone: (309)-543-2201
Contact: Beth Irwin, R.N.
Referrals, educational seminars

Massac County

Testing Sites

HIV Counseling/Testing Site
PO Box 133
Metropolis, IL 62960
Telephone: (618)-524-2212
Contact: Mary Trovillion
Confidential & anonymous testing

Mc Donough County

County Health Depts

McDonough County Health Department
505 East Jackson Street
Macomb, IL 61455-2390
Telephone: (309)-837-9951
Contact: Linda Delgado - Nurse
HIV/TB testing, counseling

Mc Henry County

Community Services

AIDS Support Coalition
PO Box 141
Crystal Lake, IL 60039-0141
Telephone: (815)-459-1985
HIV support groups

County Health Depts

McHenry County Health Department
2200 North Seminary Ave.
Woodstock, IL 60098-2600
Telephone: (815)-338-2040
Contact: J. Bacon - Public Health Admin.
Testing & counseling

Home Health Care

Northern Illinois Medical Center Home Health Care
4201 Medical Center Drive
McHenry, IL 60050
Telephone: (815)-344-6602
Contact: Ann Mattson
Skilled therapist or medical aide upon doctor's order (no homemaker service)

Medical Services

Northern Illinois Medical Center
4201 Medical Center Drive
McHenry, IL 60050
Telephone: (815)-344-5000 Fax: (815)-344-9848
Basic inpatient medical services

Mc Lean County

County Health Depts

McLean County Health Department
905 North Main Street
Normal, IL 61761-1598
Telephone: (309)-888-5450
Contact: Robert Keller - Public Health Admin.
HIV testing & counseling, TB testing, STD program

Menard County

County Health Depts

Menard County Health Department
809 Old Salem Road
Petersburg, IL 62675-1798
Telephone: (217)-632-7864 Fax: (217)-632-7873
Contact: James Diekroeger - Public Health Admin.
Counseling, referrals, education, literature.

Mercer County

County Health Depts

Mercer County Health Dept.
409 Northwest 9th Avenue
Aledo, IL 61231
Telephone: (309)-582-5301
Contact: Bruce Peterson - Public Health Admin.

Montgomery County

County Health Depts

Montgomery County Health Department
Route 185, P.O. Box 128
Hillsboro, IL 62049
Telephone: (217)-532-2001 Fax: (217)-532-2089
Contact: C. Tom Larson - Public Health Admin.
Partner notification, referrals, counseling, education, mental health.

Morgan County

County Health Depts

Morgan County Health Department
345 West State Street
Jacksonville, IL 62650-2062
Telephone: (217)-245-5111 Fax: (217)-243-5354
Contact: Dan Williams - Coordinator
Anonymous HIV testing, counseling, referrals.

Ogle County

County Health Depts

Ogle County Health Department
104 South Fifth Street
Oregon, IL 61061-1624
Telephone: (815)-732-3201
Contact: Michael Williams - Public Health Admin.

Peoria County

County Health Depts

Marshall County Health Department
c/o Peoria Health Dept.
2116 North Sheridan Road
Peoria, IL 61604
Telephone: (309)-685-6181
Contact: Robert L. Murray - Public Health Admin.
Testing, counseling, home visits

Peoria City/County Health Department
2116 North Sheridan Road
Peoria, IL 61604-3492
Telephone: (309)-685-6181 Fax: (309)-679-6030
Contact: Robert Murray - Public health Admin.
STD clinic, HIV testing, counseling, referrals, education.

Putnam County Health Department
c/o Peoria Health Dept.
2116 North Sheridan Rd.
Peoria, IL 61604
Telephone: (309)-679-6000 Fax: (309)-685-3312
Contact: Robert Murray - Public Health Admin.
Anonymous HIV testing, counseling, referrals, education.

Perry County

County Health Depts

Perry County Health Department
907 South Main Street
Pinckneyville, IL 62274-1700
Telephone: (618)-357-5371 Fax: (618)-357-3190
Contact: Bonita Griffin, R.N. - Administrator
Anonymous HIV testing, counseling, referrals, education, literature.

Pike County

County Health Depts

Pike County Health Department
113 East Jefferson Street
Pittsfield, IL 62363-1420
Telephone: (217)-285-4407 Fax: (217)-285-4639
Contact: Judith Schlieper - R.N., Public Health
Anonymous HIV testing, counseling, education, referrals.

Pulaski County

County Health Depts

Southern Seven Health Department
PO Box 78
Jonesboro, IL 62992
Telephone: (618)-833-8561
Contact: Carolyn Kissair
HIV testing & counseling

Testing Sites

Southern Seven Health Department
R.R. #1
Ullin, IL 62992-9801
Telephone: (618)-634-2297 Fax: (618)-634-9394
Contact: Carolyn Kissair - R.N.
Anonymous HIV testing, counseling, education, referrals.

Randolph County

County Health Depts

Monroe-Randolph Bi-County Health Department
1227 State Street
Chester, IL 62233-1649
Telephone: (618)-826-5007 Fax: (618)-826-5223
Contact: Thomas Smith - Public Health Admin.
Education, home health care

Home Health Care

O.P.T.I.O.N Care of Sparta
110 S Market Street
Sparta, IL 62286-2062
Telephone: (618)-443-4524
Contact: James V. Hayes
Home IV and Nutritional Services

Rock Island County

County Health Depts

Rock Island County Health Department
2112 25th Avenue
Rock Island, IL 61201-5317
Telephone: (309)-794-7050
Contact: Virginia Riener - Coordinator
Anonymous HIV testing, counseling, referrals, education.

Rock Island County Health Department
2112 25th Avenue
Rock Island, IL 61201-5317
Telephone: (309)-794-7050
Contact: Ginny Reiner
HIV Alternate Test Sites

Saint Clair County

Community Services

Bethany Place
224 West Washington St.
Belleville, IL 62220
Telephone: (618)-234-0291 Fax: (618)-234-4391
Contact: Carol Baltosiewich - Director
Social services

County Health Depts

St. Clair County Health Department
19 Public Square
Suite 150
Belleville, IL 62221
Telephone: (618)-233-7703 Fax: (618)-233-7713
Contact: Kevin Hutchinson - Public Health Admin.
Anonymous testing & counseling

Testing Sites

East Side Health District
638 North 20th Street
East St. Louis, IL 62205
Telephone: (618)-874-4713
Contact: Robert E. Klutts - Public Health Admin.
Testing, counseling, case management

Saline County

County Health Depts

Egyptian Health Department
1412 US 45 North
Eldorado, IL 62930-9324
Telephone: (618)-273-3326
Contact: Edith Frederica Garnett - Public Health Admin.

Sangamon County

Community Services

AZT Assistance
IL Dept. of Public Health
525 W. Jefferson, 1st fl.
Springfield, IL 62761
Telephone: (217)-524-5983   Fax: (217)-524-6090
Contact: Terry Dobbs
Federally-funded program to assist with AZT cost

County Health Depts

Sangamon County Department of Public Health
200 South 9th Street
Room 301
Springfield, IL 62701-1629
Telephone: (217)-535-3100   Fax: (217)-535-3104
Contact: Pat Howard, R.N.
Referrals

Testing Sites

Springfield Department of Public Health
1415 East Jefferson St.
Springfield, IL 62703-1098
Telephone: (217)-789-2182
Contact: Gail Danner
Testing

Schuyler County

County Health Depts

Schuyler County Health Department
127 South Liberty
P.O. Box 320
Rushville, IL 62681-1419
Telephone: (217)-322-4373
Contact: Francis Wilson - Public Health Admin.
Referrals

Shelby County

County Health Depts

Shelby County Health Department
R.R. #2, Box 54
1810 West South Third St.
Shelbyville, IL 62565-9510
Telephone: (217)-774-9555   Fax: (217)-774-2355
Contact: Joel Clark - Public Health Admin.
Health education to groups, some counseling

Stephenson County

County Health Depts

Stephenson County Health Department
15 North Galena Avenue
Freeport, IL 61032-4390
Telephone: (815)-235-8271
Contact: Clayton Pate - Public Health Admin.
Referrals

Tazewell County

County Health Depts

Tazewell County Health Department
21306 IL Route #9
Tremont, IL 61568
Telephone: (309)-925-5511
Contact: Sarah Fenton - Clinic Coordinator
Testing & counseling.

Vermilion County

County Health Depts

Vermilion County Health Department
R.R. #1, Box 12-B
Tilton Road
Danville, IL 61832-9754
Telephone: (217)-431-2662
Contact: Stephen Laker - Public Health Admin.

Wabash County

County Health Depts

Wabash County Health Department
130 West 7th Street
Mt. Carmel, IL 62863
Telephone: (618)-263-3873
Contact: Michael Henry - Public Health Admin.
Counseling, education

Washington County

County Health Depts

Washington County Health dept.
711 West Adams
Nashville, IL 62263
Telephone: (618)-327-3644
Contact: Bonita Griffin - Public Health Admin.

Wayne County

County Health Depts

Wayne County Health Department
P.O. Box 445,RR 45 South
Fairfield, IL 62837-0445
Telephone: (618)-842-5166
Contact: Martha Heflin - Public Health Admin.

Whiteside County

County Health Depts

Whiteside County Health Department/AIDS Network
18929 Lincoln Road
Morrison, IL 61270-9500
Telephone: (815)-772-7411
Contact: Michael Zurn - Public Health Admin.
Counseling & testing

Will County

County Health Depts

Will County Health Department
501 Ella Avenue
Joliet, IL 60433-2799
Telephone: (815)-727-8480
Contact: James Zelko - Public Health Admin.
Testing, referrals, support groups

Williamson County

County Health Depts

Franklin-Williamson Bi-County Health Department
Williamson County Airport
Marion, IL 62959
Telephone: (618)-993-8111
Contact: Larry Castrale - Public Health Admin.
Testing

Winnebago County

County Health Depts

Winnebago County Health Department
401 Division Street
Rockford, IL 61104-2096
Telephone: (815)-962-5092

Contact: Joseph Orthoefer - Public Health Admin.
Testing & counseling

Home Health Care

Caremark Connection Network
1953 Harlem Road
Suite 9
Loves Park, IL 61111
Telephone: (815)-636-2100
Contact: Ronald Ohlsen - Branch Manager
Clinical support and infusion therapies: nutrition, antimicrobials,chemotherapy, hematopoetics, infusion therapies

INDIANA

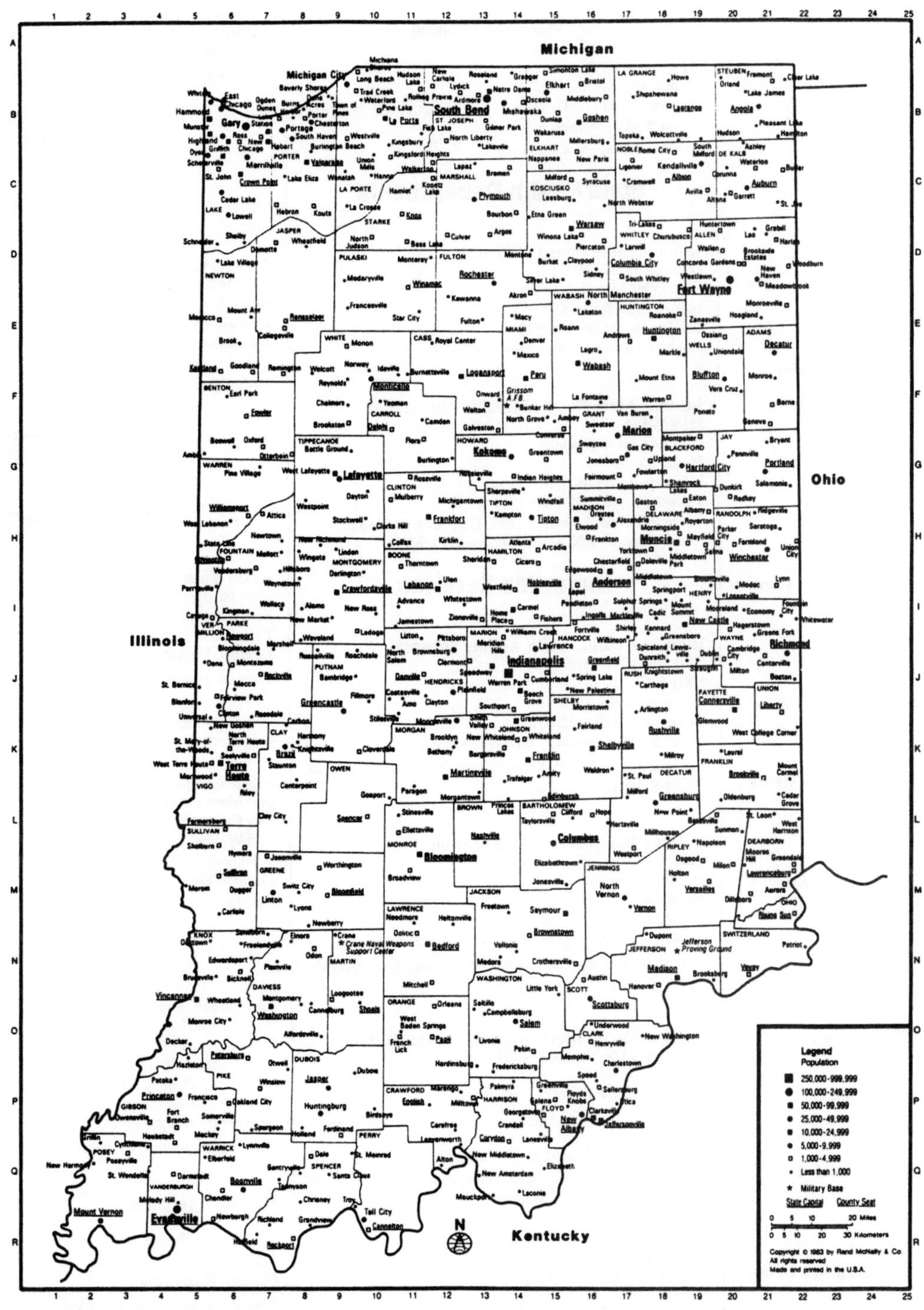

From City/County Planning Atlas Copyright 1989 by Reed McNally & Company, R.L. 90-S-28

Indiana

General Services

Education

American Red Cross
Indianapolis Area Chapter
441 East Tenth Street
Indianapolis, IN 46202-
Telephone: (317)-634-1441
Contact: Donna Plummer
AIDS education

American Red Cross
791 E. 83rd Ave.
Merryville, IN 46410-6204
Telephone: (219)-756-5360
Contact: Beth Ann Wisch
Prevention education, community outreach, literature

American Red Cross
501 North Lake
Warsaw, IN 46580-2654
Telephone: (219)-267-5244
Contact: Becky Notestine
HIV/AIDS Education materials

Clinical Training Associates, Inc./ Marott Center
342 Massachusetts Ave.
Suite 403
Indianapolis, IN 46204
Telephone: (317)-631-5535
Contact: Kathryn M. Connell,MPH
HIV/AIDS Education Materials and Programs, Information/Referral Services

Elkhart County Chapter - American Red Cross
306 West High Street
Elkhart, IN 46516-2826
Telephone: (219)-293-6519
Contact: Duane E. Cook
HIV/AIDS Education materials, presentations, referral

Hancock County American Red Cross
114 W. South St.
Greenfield, IN 46140-2336
Telephone: (317)-462-4343
Contact: Myra Bleill
HIV/AIDS Educational Materials, Transportation

Kosciusko County Health Department
100 West Center Street
3rd Floor, Room 2
Warsaw, IN 46580-2846
Telephone: (219)-372-2349 Fax: (215)-269-2023
Contact: Jon Cupp - Chief Administrator
HIV/AIDS education materials

LaPorte County Chapter - American Red Cross
905 Maple Avenue
LaPorte, IN 46350-3427
Telephone: (219)-362-6208
Contact: Lamar Koontz
HIV/AIDS education materials, educational programs

Madison County Red Cross
914 Chase
Anderson, IN 46016-1335
Telephone: (317)-643-6621
Contact: Lorri Branch - Director of Health & Safety
AIDS educational materials and referrals

Marshall County AIDS Task Force
9726 Sunnyside Drive
Plymouth, IN 46563-2115
Telephone: (219)-936-2726
Contact: Harriet Wilson
HIV/AIDS education materials

Morgan County Memorial Hospital
2209 J.R. Wooden Drive
Education Department
Martinsville, IN 46151
Telephone: (317)-342-8441 Fax: (317)-349-5411
Contact: Jan Swinney, RN
HIV/AIDS education materials

State Health Departments

Indiana State Board of Health
Division of HIV/AIDS
1330 West Michigan Street
Indianapolis, IN 46202
Telephone: (317)-633-0893
Contact: Dennis Stover - Director

Indiana State Dept. of Health, Division of HIV/STD
Office of AIDS Activity
PO Box 1964
Indianapolis, IN 46206-1964
Telephone: (317)-633-0100
Contact: Dennis L. Stover - MS, Dir., Barbara Kempf, Family Health - RN, Judith Ganser, MD, MPH,

Statewide Services

Indiana Comm. AIDS Action Network
3951 North Meridian Street
Suite 200
Indianapolis, IN 46208
Telephone: (317)-632-0123
Contact: Dennis Stover - Project Coordinator
Educational, Legal, Political Action, Volunteer Programs, Referral Services

Indiana Department of Education
Statehouse Rm 229
251 East Ohio Street
Indianapolis, IN 46204-2798
Telephone: (317)-232-6875
Contact: Leah M. Ingraham - HIV/AIDS Ed. Cons
Education, minority outreach, speakers bureau, referrals, reports

Indiana Early Intervention Program/ ICAAN
3951 North Meridian Street
Suite 200
Indianapolis, IN 46208
Telephone: (317)-920-3190 Fax: (317)-920-3199
Toll-Free: (800)-659-7580
Contact: Mary M. Coudret - Assistant Director
Statewide services, early intervention, drug assistance, advocacy program,outreach program

Indiana State Board of Health
1330 WEst Michigan Street
PO Box 1964
Indianapolis, IN 46206-1964
Telephone: (317)-633-0893
Contact: Mr. Dennis Stover - Division Director; Ms. Rosemary Igney - Asst.Division Director
Hot line; fund facilities for HIV programs

Indiana State Welfare Department
State Office Building
Indiana Government Center South P.O. Box 7083
Indianapolis, IN 46207
Telephone: (317)-232-4324
Contact: James Hmurovich - Director
Financial Services, Social Workers, Information/Referral Services

Mental Health Association of Indiana
55 Mounument Circle
Suite 700
Indianapolis, IN 46204
Telephone: (317)-269-1569
Statewide advocacy & public policy agency

Adams County

County Health Depts

Adams County Health Department
804 Mercer Avenue
Room 5
Decatur, IN 46733
Telephone: (219)-724-8215
Contact: Louise Busse
HIV/STD testing

Allen County

Community Services

AIDS Task Force, Inc.
2124 Fairfield Ave.
Fort Wayne, IN 46802-5158
Telephone: (219)-424-0844
Contact: John Roach - Executive Director
Care coordination site, residential facility for HIV+

County Health Depts

Allen County Health Dept.
One Main Street
City County Bldg - R505
Fort Wayne, IN 46802-1810
Telephone: (219)-428-7504 Fax: (219)-427-1391
Contact: Dwight James; Jeff Markley
HIV Testing/counseling, STD testing/counseling.

Home Health Care

Caremark Branch Network.
431 Femhill Ave
Fort Wayne, IN 45805
Telephone: (219)-484-4442 Fax: (219)-484-4637
Contact: J. Thomas Edsall - Pharmacy Manager; Evelyn Ladd - Nurse Manager
CLINICAL SUPPORT AND INFUSION THERAPY: Nutrition, Antimicrobials, Chemo., Hematopoeti

Homedco Infusion
7515 Westfield Drive
Fort Wayne, IN 46825
Telephone: (219)-484-8696
Contact: Rick Clapp
Nationwide experience in providing home infusion therapy to AIDS patients

O.P.T.I.O.N Care
3722 Lake Ave.
Ft Wayne, IN 46805
Telephone: (219)-420-2050 Fax: (219)-423-6101
Contact: Sandra Patterson - Nursing Director
Home IV and Nutritional Services

Testing Sites

American Red Cross - Allen/Wells Chapter
P.O. Box 5025
Fort Wayne, IN 46895-5025
Telephone: (219)-480-8100
Contact: Marita Marquardt
HIV Counseling/Testing

Bartholomew County

County Health Depts

Bartholomew County Health Department
1971 State Street
Columbus, IN 47201-6965
Telephone: (812)-379-1555
Contact: Debbie Overfelt - RN
HIV/AIDS counseling, testing, educational materials, referrals

Boone County

County Health Depts

Boone County Health Department
416 West Camp Street
Lebanon, IN 46052-1796
Telephone: (317)-482-3942
Contact: Millie Barry
HIV/AIDS educational materials & information

Brown County

County Health Depts

Brown County Health Department
County Office Bldg.
P.O. Box 281
Nashville, IN 47448
Telephone: (812)-988-2255 Fax: (812)-988-5520
Contact: Donna Browning
HIV/AIDS educational materials, housing assistance

Carroll County

County Health Depts

Carroll County Health Department
Courthouse
Delphi, IN 46923
Telephone: (317)-564-3420 Fax: (317)-465-4851
Contact: Alicia Wright, RN
HIV/AIDS Educational Materials

Cass County

Medical Services

Logansport State Hospital
R.R. 2 Box 38
Logansport, IN 46947-9802
Telephone: (219)-722-4141 Fax: (219)-735-3414
Contact: Mike Leonard

Clark County

Community Services

SE Indiana AIDS Program
207 Sparks Avenue
Medical Arts Building Room 303
Jeffersonville, IN 47130-3725
Telephone: (812)-282-7521
Contact: Kent Wells
Community Action Group, HIV testing & counseling; case management,education programs

Testing Sites

Clark County Health Dept., SE Indiana Counseling/Testing Site
207 Sparks Avenue
Medical Arts Building Room 303
Jeffersonville, IN 47131
Telephone: (812)-288-2706 Fax: (812)-288-2711
Contact: Kent Wells - DIS
HIV/AIDS counseling, testing, educational materials & programs, carecoordination, partner notification, STD clinic

Delaware County

County Health Depts

Delaware County Health Department
100 West Main Street
Muncie, IN 47305-2879
Telephone: (317)-747-7721
Contact: Robert Jones - Administrator
HIV Counseling/Testing/Education materials

Medical Services

Ball Memorial Hospital
2401 W University Avenue
Muncie, IN 47303-3499
Telephone: (317)-747-3111 Fax: (317)-747-0137
Contact: Mike Langona
HIV Counseling/Testing, Health Care

Testing Sites

Planned Parenthood
110 North Cherry
Muncie, IN 47305-1599
Telephone: (317)-282-8011
Contact: Carol Suro
HIV counseling, testing, educational materials

Elkhart County

Community Services

Association for Disabled of Elkhart County
P.O. Box 398
Bristol, IN 46507-0398
Telephone: (219)-848-7451 Fax: (219)-848-5917
Contact: Karen Powell, R.N.

Elkhart General Hospital
600 East Blvd
P.O. Box 1329
Elkhart, IN 46515-2499
Telephone: (219)-294-2621 Fax: (219)-523-3389
Contact: Joan Adams
Support gropus

Rosewood Terrace
1001 West Hively
Elkhart, IN 46517
Telephone: (219)-294-7641 Fax: (219)-522-3071
AIDS action group

County Health Depts

Elkhart County Health Department
315 South Second Street
Elkhart, IN 46516-3188
Telephone: (219)-523-2328
Contact: Joyce Bontrager, RN
HIV/AIDS Counseling/Testing/Education materials, Health Care, Housing

Home Health Care

O.P.T.I.O.N. Care of Northern Indiana
25416 County Road 6th East
Elkhart, IN 46514-3968
Telephone: (219)-264-4488 Fax: (219)-262-8452
Contact: Delisa Purchase
Health Care

Fulton County

County Health Depts

Fulton County Health Department
175 South 50 East
Rochester, IN 46975-1536
Telephone: (219)-223-5152
Contact: Diane Jones, RN
HIV/AIDS Education materials, referrals

Grant County

Home Health Care

Olsten Kimberly Quality Care
2020 Southwestern Ave.
Marion, IN 46953
Telephone: (317)-664-4073 Fax: (317)-664-6157
Contact: Pat Lau
Home care for AIDS patients, elderly

Hendricks County

County Health Depts

Hendricks County Health Department
Courthouse Annex
P.O. Box 310
Danville, IN 46122
Telephone: (317)-745-9217
Contact: Linda Hibner
Refers Patients to Bell Flower Clinic

Howard County

County Health Depts

Howard County Health Department
120 East Mulberry
Room 206
Kokomo, IN 46901-4632
Telephone: (317)-456-2408
Contact: Jeri Malone
HIV testing site, AIDS educator, support group, helpline, counseling &referrals

Home Health Care

Homedco Infusion
711 South Reed Road
Kokomo, IN 46901-5628
Telephone: (317)-457-6613 Fax: (317)-457-6639
Contact: Peggy Beck
Nationwide experience in providing home infusion therapy to AIDS patients

Testing Sites

Planned Parenthood, Kokomo
404 B Arnold Ct.
P.O. Box 2943
Kokomo, IN 46904-2943
Telephone: (317)-455-2400
STD testing, AIDS information

Huntington County

County Health Depts

Huntington County Health Department
Room 205, Courthouse
Huntington, IN 46750
Telephone: (219)-356-5227
Contact: Tracie Walker
HIV/AIDS Education materials

Jasper County

County Health Depts

Jasper County Health Department
105 West Kellner Blvd.
Rensselaer, IN 47978-2629
Telephone: (219)-866-4918
Contact: Nancy Bailey, RN
HIV/AIDS educational materials

Kosciusko County

Home Health Care

Warsaw O.P.T.I.O.N Care
519 E Center Street
Warsaw, IN 46580-3319
Telephone: (219)-267-6767 Fax: (219)-267-4389
Contact: Nancy Highley
Home IV and Nutritional Services

Testing Sites

Kosciusko Community Hospital
2101 East Dubois Drive
Warsaw, IN 46580-3288
Telephone: (219)-267-3200
Contact: Judy Slone
HIV testing, educational materials, health care

Planned Parenthood
630 South Buffalo Street
Warsaw, IN 46580-4372
Telephone: (219)-267-3889
STD testing, birth control, pregnancy tests

Lagrange County

County Health Depts

LaGrange County Health Department
County Office Bldg
114 West Michigan Street
LaGrange, IN 46761
Telephone: (219)-463-2183 Fax: (219)-463-7563
Contact: Ann Jack, RN; Allen Martin, MD -
HIV counseling, health care

Lake County

Home Health Care

Hospice of the Calumet Area, Inc.
600 Superior Avenue
Munster, IN 46321-3198
Telephone: (219)-922-2732 Fax: (219)-922-1947
Contact: Walter Knishk
Counseling, health care, in home care for terminally ill patients

Medical Services

Tri City Community Mental Health
4522 Indianapolis Blvd.
East Chicago, IN 46312-2555
Telephone: (219)-392-6061 Fax: (219)-392-6003
Contact: Michael White, ACSW
HIV/AIDS educational materials, counseling, housing

Testing Sites

Gary AIDS Counseling/Testing Site
1145 West Fifth Avenue
Gary, IN 46402-1744
Telephone: (219)-882-5565
Contact: Aleicia James
HIV Counseling/Testing

Hammond City Health Department
649 Conkey Street
Hammond, IN 46324
Telephone: (219)-853-6358 Fax: (219)-853-6403
Contact: George Stahura
HIV/AIDS education materials, housing, HIV testing, counseling

Planned Parenthood of NW/NE Indiana
8645 Connecticut
Merrillville, IN 46410-6222
Telephone: (219)-769-3500 Fax: (219)-736-0938
HIV/AIDS Education Services, HIV Counseling/Testing

Madison County

Community Services

Community Hospital
1515 North Madison
Anderson, IN 46012-3454
Telephone: (317)-646-5145 Fax: (317)-646-5207
Contact: Calire Lee
Financial services, referrals & counseling, treatment

Social Security Administration
1304 Main Street
Anderson, IN 46016-1541
Telephone: (800)-234-5772
Contact: Claims Rep
Financial services, referrals, disability

County Health Depts

Madison County Health Department
STD Clinic
16 East 9th Street
Anderson, IN 46016
Telephone: (317)-641-9688
HIV/AIDS educational materials, HIV testing & counseling, STD treatment & testing

Home Health Care

St. John's Medical Center
Hospice Care
2015 Jackson Street
Anderson, IN 46016
Telephone: (317)-646-8334
Health Care

Visiting Nurse Association of North Central Indiana
1354 South B
P.O. Box 7
Elwood, IN 46036-
Telephone: (317)-552-3393 Fax: (317)-552-3994
Toll-Free: (800)-404-4852
Contact: Carole Baer
Health Care

Visiting Nurse Health Care
P.O. Box 30
Anderson, IN 46015-0030
Telephone: (317)-643-7371 Fax: (317)-643-1289
Contact: Glenda Shirley
Home health aides, speech therapy

Medical Services

Community Hospital of Anderson & Madison County
1515 North Madison
Anderson, IN 46011
Telephone: (317)-646-5172 Fax: (317)-646-5209
Contact: Jane McCarthy
Health Care, Physician Referral

Mercy Hospital
1331 South A Street
Elwood, IN 46036-1942
Telephone: (317)-552-3336
Contact: Candy Robinson
Health Care, Physician Referral

Marion County

Community Services

Flanner House Multi-Service Center
2424 Dr. Martin Luther
King Jr.
Indianapolis, IN 46208-5598
Telephone: (317)-925-4231
Counseling, Financial Services, Housing, Social Workers, Info/Referral Service

Indianapolis Bar Association
Lawyers Referral Service
10 West Market, Ste 440
Indianapolis, IN 46204
Telephone: (317)-632-8240
Contact: Rosie Felton - Director
HIV/AIDS assistance & referral services

Marion County Department of Public Welfare
1125 Brookside Avenue
Suite 1
Indianapolis, IN 46202
Telephone: (317)-924-7608
Financial assistance, Medicaid, social workers, information and referralservices

Near Eastside Multi-Service Center
2236 East 10th Street
Indianapolis, IN 46201
Telephone: (317)-633-8330
Counseling,financial services, housing, information/referral services

County Health Depts

Family Home Health Center
1500 North Ritter
Room 1501
Indianapolis, IN 46219-3027
Telephone: (317)-541-2000 Fax: (317)-541-2130
Health Care, Information/Referral Services

Marion County Health Department
3838 North Rural
First Floor
Indianapolis, IN 462050
Telephone: (317)-541-2000 Fax: (317)-541-2130
Counseling, drug abuse and AIDS information, educational materials,referrals, testing

Marion County Health Department
3838 N. Rural St.
Indianapolis, IN 46205-2930
Telephone: (317)-633-9752
Drug Abuse & AIDS Info, Educational Materials, Health Care, Referrals, Testing

Marion County Health Dept.
38 North Rural
Indianapolis, IN 46205
Telephone: (317)-630-7221
Contact: Deborah Long
HIV testing & counseling

Home Health Care

Critical Care America
8770 Guion Road, #F
Indianapolis, IN 46268
Telephone: (317)-875-6770 Fax: (317)-875-7018
Toll-Free: (800)-537-5356
Contact: Chuck Spraas
Coordinate & integrate all clinical & psychosocial services for HIV+

HNS, Inc.
6330 East 75th Street
Suite 122
Indianapolis, IN 46250
Telephone: (219)-478-4822 Fax: (317)-576-5953
Contact: Steve Burleson
Home infusion therapy

HNS, Inc.
The Metro Centre
6330 East 75th St, #122
Indianapolis, IN 46250
Telephone: (317)-576-5950 Fax: (317)-576-5953
Contact: Doug Gruene
Home infusion therapy, in-home nursing, attendant care, physicaltherapy, pentamidine

Homedco Infusion
1604 South Franklin Road
Indianapolis, IN 46239-9596
Telephone: (317)-352-1646 Fax: (317)-357-8131
Contact: Melody Renjhan - CS Rep
Nationwide experience in providing home infusion therapy to AIDS patients

Indiana Home Health Services
2039 North Capitol Avenue
Indianapolis, IN 46202
Telephone: (317)-923-4663 Fax: (317)-927-3815
Health Care, Information/Referral Services

nmc HOMECARE
7112 Zionsville Rd.
Indianapolis, IN 46268
Telephone: (317)-297-9616
Fax: (317)-297-9684
Contact: Kathy Hammontree
National JCAHO-Accredited company providing a full range of Infusion and Respiratory therapies and specializing in the care of HIV/AIDS patients. National Case Manager is also available at 800-445-1188

Nurses House Call
9302 N. Merridean
Suite 155
Indianapolis, IN 46260
Telephone: (317)-581-2600 Fax: (317)-581-2612
Toll-Free: (800)-852-1970
Contact: Carole Woods
Home care agency

Nurses Professional Registry, Inc.
2915 North High School Rd
Indianapolis, IN 46224-2915
Telephone: (317)-299-4222
Contact: Mabel Andrews, RN
Registry of private duty nurses: RN's, LPN's, general duty

R.N. Registry, Inc.
5670 Caito Drive
Suite 125
Indianapolis, IN 46226-1347
Telephone: (317)-547-2411 Fax: (317)-547-4202
Toll-Free: (800)-945-2411
Contact: Dolly Green, RN
Information/Referral Services

Visiting Nurse Affiliates of Indiana
950 North Illinois
Indianapolis, IN 46204-1059
Telephone: (317)-236-0445 Fax: (317)-236-8201
Toll-Free: (800)-248-6540
Contact: Laine Franklin
Home Health Care covering state of Indiana

Medical Services

Adult Amb. Care Center Methodist Hospital
1633 North Capital Avenue
Indianapolis, IN 46202-1261
Telephone: (317)-929-8851
Primary care

Barrington Health Center
3118 Bethel Avenue
Indianapolis, IN 46203-3336
Telephone: (317)-788-4716
Contact: Teresa Tyree - HIV Clinical Manager
Health Care

Bell Flower Clinic
1101 West Tenth Street
Indianapolis, IN 46202-4800
Telephone: (317)-630-7192 Fax: (317)-687-8132
HIV/AIDS Educational Materials, Health Care, Counseling/Testing, Referrals

Indiana University Hospital (Adult)
550 North University Boulevard
Indianapolis, IN 46202
Telephone: (317)-274-3746 Fax: (317)-274-8132
Health Care, Social Workers

Indiana University School of Dentistry
1121 West Michigan Street
Indianapolis, IN 46202-5211
Telephone: (317)-274-7474 Fax: (317)-274-2419
Contact: Dr. John Valentine
Health Care, Dental Referral

Methodist Hospital of Indianapolis
1701 North Senate Blvd.
Indianapolis, IN 46202-1299
Telephone: (317)-929-2915 Fax: (317)-929-2499
Contact: Terry Ridge - Lifecare Program Coord.
Health Care, Physician/Dental Referral, Social Workers, HIV Lifecare Program

People's Health Center
2340 East 10th Street
Indianapolis, IN 46201
Telephone: (317)-633-7360 Fax: (317)-633-7302
Contact: Robin Davis-Reed, MSW - Care Coordinator
Confidential HIV testing, pharmacy, dental services, social services,counseling

Regenstrief Health Center (Wishard)
1001 W. 10th Street
Indianapolis, IN 46202-2859
Telephone: (317)-630-7400 Fax: (317)-630-6962
Health Care, HIV Counseling/Testing

Riley Hospital For Children
I.U. Medical Center
Indianapolis, IN 46202
Telephone: (317)-274-8312 Fax: (317)-274-8712
Health Care, Social Workers

Southwest Health Center
2202 West Morris Street
Indianapolis, IN 46221-1499
Telephone: (317)-488-2020 Fax: (317)-488-2031

Health Care; HIV testing & counseling, patient care

Veterans Administration
1481 West 10th Street
Indianapolis, IN 46202-2803
Telephone: (317)-635-7401 Fax: (317)-267-8763
Health Care

Testing Sites

Methodist Hospital of Indiana-Life Care Program
1701 N. Senate Blvd.
Rm. B-127, PO Box 1367
Indianapolis, IN 46206-1367
Telephone: (317)-929-2915 Fax: (317)-929-2499
Contact: Terry Ridle - Lifecare Program Coord.
HIV testing

Southeast Health Center
901 South Shelby Street
Indianapolis, IN 46203-1151
Telephone: (317)-488-2040 Fax: (317)-488-2051
Contact: Shannon Merrill
Health Care; HIV testing & counseling

Miami County

County Health Depts

Miami County Health Department
Courthouse, Room 110
Peru, IN 46970
Telephone: (317)-472-3901 Fax: (317)-472-1412
Contact: Aletha Hartleroad, RN
HIV/AIDS education materials, information

Montgomery County

County Health Depts

Montgomery County Health Department
Benford Street
Crawfordsville, IN 47933-1709
Telephone: (317)-364-6440
Community Services

Morgan County

Community Services

South Central Community Action, Inc.
Morgan County Branch Offc
70 West Washington Street
Martinsville, IN 46151
Telephone: (317)-342-1518
Contact: Luanne Swan
Housing, HIV/AIDS Information

Noble County

County Health Depts

Noble County Health Department
2090 North State Rd 9
Suite C
Albion, IN 46701
Telephone: (219)-636-2191 Fax: (219)-636-2192
Contact: Nancy Huffman, RN
HIV/AIDS education materials

Parke County

County Health Depts

Parke County Health Dept.
116 W. High Street
Rockville, IN 47872-1785
Telephone: (317)-569-4008
Contact: Marvel Waldridge - RN

Medical Services

Family Health & Help Clinic
109 Jefferson Street
Rockville, IN 47872
Telephone: (317)-569-6665
Adult clinic, referrals, videos, home care

Porter County

County Health Depts

Porter County Health Department
1401 North Calumet
Valparaiso, IN 46383-3198
Telephone: (219)-465-3525 Fax: (219)-465-3531
Contact: Jan Garvey - RN
HIV/AIDS counseling, testing, educational materials

Pulaski County

Community Services

Parkview Haven
Constitution Drive
P.O. Box 797
Francesville, IN 47946
Telephone: (219)-567-9149
Contact: Amy Jo Schmicker - Director of Nursing
Health care, counseling, nursing home

Pulaski Memorial
616 East 13th Street
Winamac, IN 46996-1117
Telephone: (219)-946-6131
Contact: Richard Mynark
General health care & medical services (no HIV)

County Health Depts

Pulaski County Health Department
County Bldg Suite 205
125 South Riverside Drive
Winamac, IN 46996
Telephone: (219)-946-6080
Contact: Gene Widup
HIV/AIDS education materials

Medical Services

Pulaski Health Care Center
624 East 13th Street
Winamac, IN 46996-1100
Telephone: (219)-946-3394
Contact: Dan Dolezal
Nursing Home

Randolph County

County Health Depts

Randolph County Health Department
211 South Main Street
Winchester, IN 47394
Telephone: (317)-584-7070
Contact: Myma Peacock - RN

Saint Joseph County

Community Services

Michiana Friends/Family/Lovers
P.O. Box 1521
South Bend, IN 46634-1521
Telephone: (219)-232-6930
Contact: John Roxy
Support group

Michiana HIV Positive Support Groups
County-City Building
9th Floor
South Bend, IN 46601
Telephone: (219)-284-9725
Contact: Christine Veal
Pre & post test counseling

County Health Depts

St. Joseph County Health Department
County-City Building
Room 825
South Bend, IN 46601
Telephone: (219)-235-9750 Fax: (219)-235-9960
Contact: John Frybort - AIDS Coordinator
HIV/AIDS education materials, HIV counseling, testing, housing

Home Health Care

Hospice of St. Joseph County, Inc.
108 N. Main Street, #111
Suite #111
South Bend, IN 46601-1612
Telephone: (219)-237-0340 Fax: (219)-237-0349
R.N. home health aides, social services, bereavement counseling

nmc HOMECARE
1843 Commerce Drive
So. Bens, IN 46626
Telephone: (219)-289-8916
Fax: (219)-289-2686
Contact: Kathy Hammontree
National JCAHO-Accredited company providing a full range of Infusion and Respiratory therapies and specializing in the care

of HIV/AIDS patients. National Case Manager is also available at 800-445-1188

Visiting Nurse Association Home Care
P.O. Box 1615
South Bend, IN 46617-2878
Telephone: (219)-234-3181
Contact: Margaret Mynsberge - Director of Social Services
Health care; speech therapy

Medical Services

Memorial Hospital
615 North Michigan Street
South Bend, IN 46601-1087
Telephone: (219)-234-9041
Contact: Ella Goodman
Health Care

Michiana Community Hospital
2515 East Jefferson Blvd
South Bend, IN 46615-2619
Telephone: (219)-288-8311 Fax: (219)-282-3061
Contact: Steve Otto
Health Care

St. Joseph Medical Center
801 East LaSalle Street
P.O. Box 1935
South Bend, IN 46634
Telephone: (219)-237-7111
Contact: Dennis Heck
Health Care

St. Joseph Hospital - Mishawaka
215 West 4th Street
Mishawaka, IN 46544-1999
Telephone: (219)-259-2431
Contact: Marie Lureman
Pre & post test counseling

Starke County

County Health Depts

Starke County Health Department
Courthouse
Knox, IN 46534-1197
Telephone: (219)-772-9137
Contact: Florence Brentlinger - RN
HIV/AIDS education materials & referral service

Home Health Care

Starke Home Health Care
315 East Culver Road
Knox, IN 46534-2405
Telephone: (219)-772-6231 Fax: (219)-772-7656
Contact: Sandra Schroeder - Director
Skilled physical therapy, skilled nursing care

Steuben County

County Health Depts

Steuben County Health Department
317 S. Wayne St. #2A
Angola, IN 46703-1938
Telephone: (219)-665-2215
Contact: Jeri Easterday - Health Nurse
HIV Information

Tipton County

County Health Depts

Tipton County Health Department
First Floor-Courthouse
Tipton, IN 46072-9799
Telephone: (317)-657-8741 Fax: (310)-675-8741
Contact: Kathy Smith

Vanderburgh County

Home Health Care

Caremark Branch Network
4307 Vogel Road
Evansville, IN 47715
Telephone: (812)-474-1301 Fax: (812)-473-6028
Toll-Free: (800)-284-2425
Contact: ; Pamela Wilson - Nurse Manager
Clinical support and infusion therapy: Nutrition, Antimicrobials, Chemo.,Hematopoeti

Vigo County

Community Services

Indiana State University
Department of Counseling
Terra Haute, IN 47809
Telephone: (812)-237-3910 Fax: (812)-237-4348
Contact: Michael Schuff, Ph.D - Project Director
HIV testing & care coordination, counseling

Home Health Care

Homedco Infusion
Office C
1714 North 5th Street
Terre Haute, IN 47804
Telephone: (812)-232-5277 Fax: (800)-686-0267
Contact: Sam Shorter - Manager
Home infusion therapy, durable medical equipment & oxygen

Testing Sites

Union Hospital
1606 North 7th Street
TerreHaute, IN 47804-2780
Telephone: (812)-238-7540 Fax: (812)-238-7491
Contact: Myrna Dienhart
HIV testing, counseling & referrals

Wabash County

County Health Depts

Wabash County Health Department
Memorial Hall
Wabash, IN 46992
Telephone: (219)-563-0661
Contact: Jane Skeans
HIV/AIDS education materials

Wayne County

County Health Depts

Wayne County Health Department Nursing Division
Courthouse
Richmond, IN 47374
Telephone: (317)-973-9294
Contact: Jean Gifford
HIV Counseling/Testing/Info

Wells County

County Health Depts

Wells County Health Department
4th Floor Courthouse
Bluffton, IN 46714
Telephone: (219)-824-5006
Contact: R. Easley - RN
HIV/AIDS education materials

White County

County Health Depts

White County Health Department
County Building
P.O. Box 838
Monticello, IN 47960
Telephone: (219)-583-8254
Contact: Elsie Johnson, R.N.
HIV/AIDS education materials

IOWA

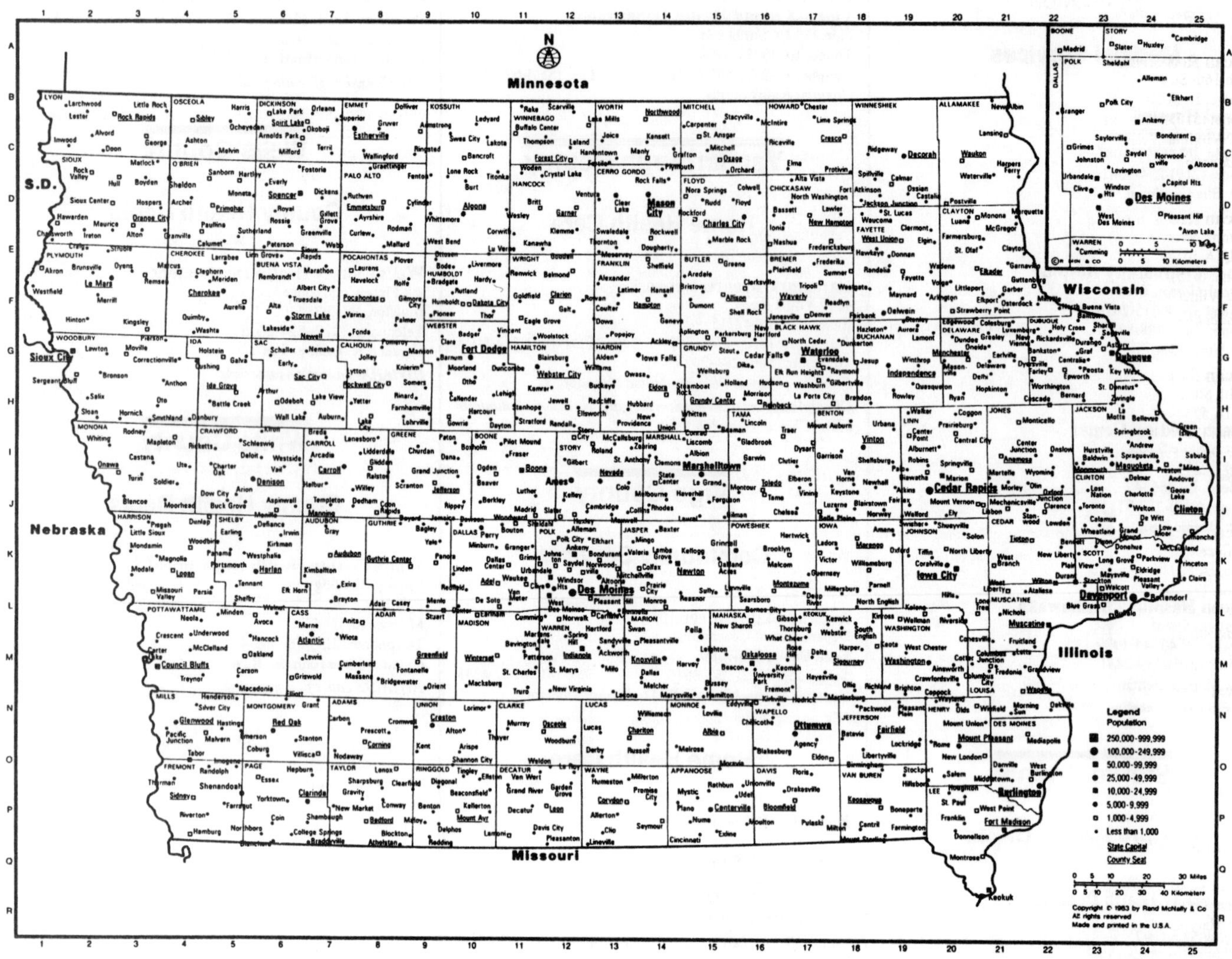

From City/County Planning Atlas Copyright 1989 by Reed McNally & Company, R.L. 90-S-28

Iowa

General Services

Education

American Red Cross
33 North 16th Street
Fort Dodge, IA 50501
Telephone: (515)-576-1911
Contact: Virginia Weiss
AIDS Education

American Red Cross
1520 Spring Street
Grinnell, IA 50112-1439
Telephone: (515)-236-5156
Contact: Wilma Vosburg
AIDS Education

American Red Cross
201 E. 4th Street
Vinton, IA 52349-1804
Telephone: (319)-472-4300   Fax: (319)-472-2302
Contact: David Happel
AIDS Education

American Red Cross, Hawkeye Chapter
2530 University Avenue
Waterloo, IA 50701
Telephone: (319)-234-6831   Fax: (319)-234-3668
Contact: Diane Solberg
AIDS Education

American Red Cross/AIDS Coalition
426 1/2 Fifth Street #B
Ames, IA 50010-6164
Telephone: (515)-232-6590
Contact: 515-232-5104
AIDS Education/Mental Health Services

American Red Cross/Dubuque Area Chapter
2400 Asbury Road
Dubuque, IA 52001-3071
Telephone: (319)-583-6451   Fax: (319)-583-0643
Contact: Mary Kay Schwind
AIDS Education

American Red Cross/East Page County
900 North 15th
Clarinda, IA 51632
Telephone: (712)-542-5268
Contact: Tammy Davis - Executive Secretary
AIDS Education

American Red Cross/Hawkeye Chapter
PO Box 1680
Waterloo, IA 50704
Telephone: (319)-234-6831   Fax: (319)-234-3668
Contact: Charles Baier
AIDS Education, (main office)

American Red Cross/North Lee County Chapter
709 9th Street
Fort Madison, IA 52627-4506
Telephone: (319)-372-1337
Contact: Laura Sutcliffe
AIDS Education

American Red Cross/South Lee County Chapter
410 Johnson Street
Keokuk, IA 52632
Telephone: (319)-524-3215
Contact: Raylene Guy
AIDS Education

Cass County Chapter
7 East 4th Street
Atlantic, IA 50022-1319
Telephone: (712)-243-4427
Contact: Joan Pauls
AIDS Education

Community Action
204 2nd Street East
Cresco, IA 52136
Telephone: (319)-547-4413
Emergency Services: Food, clothing, shelter

Madison County Extension Services
117 North 1st Street
Winterset, IA 50273-1501
Telephone: (515)-462-1001   Fax: (515)-462-1002
Education

Hotlines

Crisis Intervention
22 North Georgia
Mason City, IA 50401
Telephone: (515)-424-9133
24 Hour Crisis Line

State Health Departments

Iowa Department of Public Health, Division of Disease Prevention
Lucas Bldg., 1st Floor
Des Moines, IA 50319
Telephone: (515)-281-4938
Contact: Carolyn Jacobson - AIDS Program Mgr.

Statewide Services

Human Services
Iowa Building, 4th Floor
221 4th Avenue SE
Cedar Rapids, IA 52401
Telephone: (319)-398-3950   Fax: (319)-398-3513
Contact: 319-398-3525
Medicaid, food stamps

Iowa Department of Human Services
807 Court
PO Box 126
Harlan, IA 51537-1320
Telephone: (712)-755-3145
Medicaid, food stamps, AIDS waiver

Iowa Department of Human Services
417 East Kanesville Blvd.
Council Bluffs, IA 51503-4469
Telephone: (712)-328-5677
Financial Aid

SIEDA - Alcohol & Drug Services
PO Box 658
Ottumwa, IA 52501
Telephone: (515)-682-8741   Fax: (515)-682-2026
Substance Abuse Treatment serving Southern Iowa

St. Luke's Gordon Recovery Centers
2700 Pierce Street
Sioux City, IA 51104
Telephone: (712)-279-3960   Fax: (712)-279-3929
Statewide facility for substance abuse treatment

Adair County

Community Services

Neighborhood Service Center of Adair County
354 Public Square
Greenfield, IA 50849-1261
Telephone: (515)-743-2424
Emergency Services: Food, clothing, shelter

Home Health Care

Adair County Public Health
205A East Iowa Street
Greenfield, IA 50849-9454
Telephone: (515)-743-6173
Contact: Pam Deichmann
Nursing, hospice testing, referral

Adams County

Community Services

Adams County Ministerial Association
c/o Ken Rummer
Corning, IA 50841
Telephone: (515)-322-4152
Contact: Ken Rummer
Emergency Services: Food, clothing, shelter

Department of Human Services
Adams County Court House
Corning, IA 50841
Telephone: (515)-322-4031
Contact: Fred Shields
Financial Aid

Medical Services

Mercy Hospital
Rosary Drive
Corning, IA 50841
Telephone: (515)-322-3121   Fax: (515)-322-4872
Contact: Eva Breckenridge - In-Service Coordinator
Medical services

Allamakee County

Community Services

Department of Human Services
Courthouse
Waukon, IA 52172
Telephone: (319)-568-4583
Financial aid, food stamps, title 19, AIDS information

Relief Office
12th 1st Avenue NW
Waukon, IA 52172
Telephone: (319)-568-3591
Emergency services: food, clothing, shelter, drugs, medical, careutilities

Home Health Care

Allamakee Co. Public Health/Nursing and Homemaker Home Care
Health Aide Agency
Courthouse
Waukon, IA 52172
Telephone: (319)-568-2451
Contact: Arlene Ingles
Medical, nursing and home care services, testing

Medical Services

Veterans Memorial Hospital
22 1st Avenue Southeast
Waukon, IA 52172
Telephone: (319)-568-3411 Fax: (319)-568-6139
Medical Services

Appanoose County

Medical Services

St. Joseph's Mercy Hospital
RR #3
Centerville, IA 52544-9803
Telephone: (515)-437-4111 Fax: (515)-856-2273
Medical services, HIV testing, counseling, educational, speakers

Benton County

Community Services

Department of Human Services
114 E. 4th Street
Vinton, IA 52349-1757
Telephone: (319)-472-4759
Contact: Sandra Teach
Financial aide, food stamps, medical card

HACAP
202 East 4th Street
Vinton, IA 52349
Telephone: (319)-472-4761 Fax: (319)-472-4762
Contact: Jane Moffitt
Budget counseling, referral

Veterans Affairs
Courthouse
Vinton, IA 52349
Telephone: (319)-472-3150
Financial Aid

Home Health Care

Benton County Public Health Nursing
502 North 9th
Vinton, IA 52349-2254
Telephone: (319)-472-4705
Contact: Paula Hoppel
Nursing Services

Virginia Gay Hospital - Benton County Hospice
502 North 9th Avenue
Vinton, IA 52349-2299
Telephone: (319)-472-2348
Contact: Sandy Studebaker
Nursing Services

Black Hawk County

Community Services

Cedar AIDS Support System
2101 Kimball Avenue
Suite 401
Waterloo, IA 50702-5040
Telephone: (319)-292-1450
Contact: Stacy Frye
Buddy program, group, counseling

Department of Human Resources, Black Hawk County
Box 756
1407 Independence Road
Waterloo, IA 50704
Telephone: (319)-291-2436
Contact: Evan Klenk
Financial aid, food stamps, title 19

Family Service League
2530 University Avenue
Waterloo, IA 50701-3330
Telephone: (319)-235-6271 Fax: (319)-235-1380
Mental Health Services

Home Health Care

Covenant Medical Center
3421 W. 9th Street
Waterloo, IA 50702
Telephone: (319)-236-4085
Medical services, home care services

Homedco Infusion
P.O. Box 1351 (50704)
2530 Falls Avenue
Waterloo, IA 50701
Telephone: (319)-232-1525 Fax: (319)-236-0036
Nationwide experience in providing home infusion therapy to AIDS patients

Waterloo Visiting Nursing Association
2530 University Avenue
Waterloo, IA 50701-3330
Telephone: (319)-235-6201 Fax: (319)-232-7296
Nursing Services

Medical Services

Black Hawk Grundy Mental Health Center
3251 W. 9th Street
Waterloo, IA 50702
Telephone: (319)-234-2893 Fax: (319)-234-0354
Contact: Thomas Eachus - Mental Health Center
Mental health services

Peoples Community Health Clinic
403 Sycamore
Suite 2
Waterloo, IA 50703
Telephone: (319)-236-1332
Medical services, referrals & counseling

University of Northern Iowa Counseling
Student Services Center
Room 213
Cedar Falls, IA 50614
Telephone: (319)-273-2676
Mental health services, support & conseling

Boone County

Community Services

Boone Community Action, Inc.
721 Keeler St
Boone, IA 50036-2830
Telephone: (515)-432-5052
Contact: Gloria Hanson
Referrals to county services, emergency food pantry

Boone County Transportation
City Hall
Boone, IA 50036
Telephone: (515)-432-5038
Contact: Carol Lewiston - Director
Transportation Services

Salvation Army
503 Benton St
Boone, IA 50036-2932
Telephone: (515)-432-5770
Emergency Services: Food, clothing, shelter

Home Health Care

Boone Co Homemaker Health Aide Services & Meals on Wheels
Courthouse
1st Floor
Boone, IA 50036
Telephone: (515)-433-0534 Fax: (515)-432-8102
Medical Services, referrals from hospitals

Bremer County

County Health Depts

Bremer County Public Health
Courthouse
415 E. Bremer Avenue
Waverly, IA 50677
Telephone: (319)-352-5040
Home care for AIDS patients

Home Health Care

Bremer-Butler Hospice
406 W. Bremer Avenue
Waverly, IA 50677
Telephone: (319)-352-1274
Medical Services

Brmer Butler Hospice
406 W. Bremer Avenue
Suite C
Waverly, IA 50677-3432
Telephone: (319)-352-1274
Hospice care

Medical Services

Waverly Municipal Hospital
312 9th Street S.W.
Waverly, IA 50677-2619
Telephone: (319)-352-4120
Contact: Dixie Kramer - Infection Control Pract.
Medical Service

Buchanan County

Community Services

Department of Human Resources
1413 1st Street West
PO Box 408
Independence, IA 50644-2317
Telephone: (319)-334-6091
Financial Aid

Buena Vista County

Community Services

Department of Human Services
Courthouse Annex 311 5th Street
Storm Lake, IA 50588
Telephone: (712)-749-2536
Financial Aid

Upper Des Moines Opportunity Inc.
145 Old Creek Road
Storm Lake, IA 50588-9803
Telephone: (712)-732-1757
Emergency Services: Food, clothing, shelter

Butler County

Community Services

Department of Human Services
315 North Main Street
Allison, IA 50602-2030
Telephone: (319)-824-6941
Financial Aid

Department of Human Services
315 N. Main
PO Box 306
Allison, IA 50602
Telephone: (319)-267-2594
Contact: Debbie Huisinga
Financial aid, food stamps

Home Health Care

Butler County Public Health/Nursing Service
Courthouse
Allison, IA 50602
Telephone: (319)-267-2934
Medical and nursing services, home health care/referrals

Calhoun County

Community Services

Calhoun County Department of Health
515 Court Street
Rockwell City, IA 50579-1417
Telephone: (712)-297-8323 Fax: (712)-972-5309
Contact: Jane Condon
Financial Aid, Home Health Care

Calhoun County Sheriff Office
416 4th Street
Rockwell City, IA 50579
Telephone: (712)-297-7583
Emergency Services: Food, clothing, shelter

Commission of Veterans' Affairs
515 Court Street
Rockwell City, IA 50579-1417
Telephone: (712)-297-8632 Fax: (712)-297-5309
Financial Aid

Family Development Center
405 4th Street
Rockwell City, IA 50579-1413
Telephone: (712)-297-7721
Contact: Gail Wilson
Emergency Services: Food, clothing, shelter

County Health Depts

Calhoun County Department of Health
515 Court Street
Rockwell City, IA 50579-1417
Telephone: (712)-297-8323 Fax: (712)-297-5309
Home care, hospice, skilled nursing, education

Medical Services

Harvest Acres
2511 Sigourney Avenue
Rockwell City, IA 50579-9703
Telephone: (712)-297-8241 Fax: (712)-297-5394
Contact: Diane Patton - AID/HIV Educator
Substance abuse treatment & education

Carroll County

Community Services

Catholic Charities
409 1/2 W. 7th Street
Carroll, IA 51401-2320
Telephone: (712)-792-9597
Contact: Doreen Loeffelholz - Cheif Councelor
Mental Health

Community Opportunities, Inc.
603 W. 8th Street
PO Box 427
Carroll, IA 51401
Telephone: (712)-792-9266 Fax: (712)-792-5723
Emergency Services: Food, clothing, shelter

Department of Human Services
515 North Main Street
Carroll, IA 51401-2346
Telephone: (712)-792-4391 Fax: (712)-792-1310
Financial aid

Medical Services

Area XII Alcoholism & Drug Treatment Unit
322 W 3rd Street
Box 308
Carroll, IA 51401
Telephone: (712)-792-1344
Substance abuse and co-dependency treatment

Area XII Alcoholism and Drug Treatment Unit
518 North Clark
Carroll, IA 51401
Telephone: (712)-792-1344
Substance Abuse Treatment, HIV testing referrals

Manning Family Recovery Center
SA Abuse Treatment Unit
410 Main Street
Manning, IA 51455
Telephone: (712)-653-2072 Fax: (712)-653-2216
Contact: 712-653-2300 (crisis calls)
Statewide Substance Abuse Treatment

St. Anthony Regional Hospital
S. Clark Street
Carroll, IA 51401
Telephone: (712)-792-3581 Fax: (712)-792-2124
Contact: Katie Towers - Education Coordinator
Medical Services

Cass County

Community Services

Cass County General Assistance
Courthouse
Atlantic, IA 50022
Telephone: (712)-243-4424
Emergency Services: Food, clothing, shelter

Department of Human Services
Courthouse
Atlantic, IA 50022
Telephone: (712)-243-4401
Contact: Carol Gutchewsky
Financial aid, food stamps, AIDS waiver

Financial Aid for Lutherans/Lutheran Social Services
404 Poplar Street
Atlantic, IA 50022-1250
Telephone: (712)-243-2920
Contact: Deb Lamb
Counseling

Medical Services

Alcohol and Drug Assistance Agency
P.O. Box 34
320 Walnut
Atlantic, IA 50022-0034
Telephone: (712)-243-5091
Substance abuse treatment serving southwest Iowa

Cass County Memorial Hospital
1501 E. 10th Street
Atlantic, IA 50022-1936
Telephone: (712)-243-7560 Fax: (712)-243-7583
Contact: Kathryn Booth - Hospice Supervisor
Medical services, nursing, IV therapy, homemakers, transportation, nursing, 24 hour care

Southwest Iowa Mental Health Center
1408 E. 10th Street
Atlantic, IA 50022-1934
Telephone: (712)-243-2606 Fax: (712)-243-2688
Toll-Free: (800)-458-4403
Mental health services, individual counseling, family counseling, in-patient services, medications

Cedar County

Community Services

Cedar County Relief
Court House
Tipton, IA 52772
Telephone: (319)-886-2170
Financial Aid

Department of Human Services
101 Lynn Street
Tipton, IA 52772
Telephone: (319)-886-6036
Financial Aid

Train
519 Cedar Street
Tipton, IA 52772-1739
Telephone: (319)-886-3191
Emergency Services: Food, clothing, shelter

Home Health Care

Cedar County Hospice Care
Cedar County Court House
Tipton, IA 52772
Telephone: (319)-886-2226
Contact: Edie Himberling
Hospice care

Medical Services

Mid Eastern Iowa Community Mental Health Center
Cedar County Courthouse
Room B2
Tipton, IA 52772
Telephone: (319)-886-2405 Fax: (319)-338-7884
Contact: Laura Lovell - Office Coordinator
Mental health services, counseling for AIDS patients

Cerro Gordo County

Community Services

Cerro Gordo County Relief
220 N. Washington Avenue
Mason City, IA 50401-3254
Telephone: (515)-421-3083
Emergency Services: Food, Clothing, Shelter

Department of Human Services
22 North Georgia Avenue
Mason City, IA 50401-3435
Telephone: (515)-424-9977 Fax: (515)-424-1759
Contact: Oscar Fewins - Service Supervisor
Home healthcare, medical assistance, food stamps; emergency help forevicted

North Iowa Community Action Health Programs
P.O. Box 1627
Mason City, IA 50401-8627
Telephone: (515)-423-5044

Home Health Care

Cerro Gordo Community Health Nursing
Courthouse
220 N. Washington
Mason City, IA 50401
Telephone: (515)-421-3080
Contact: Susan Clarkson
Nursing, home care, HIV testing, counseling, referrals

Hospice of North Iowa
232 2nd Street, SE
Mason City, IA 50401-3906
Telephone: (515)-423-3508
Contact: Gloria Billings
Hospice care, North Iowa AIDS project, support groups

Medical Services

Cerro Gordo HHHA Service
Courthouse
220 N. Washington
Mason City, IA 50401
Telephone: (515)-421-3080 Fax: (515)-421-3158
Medical services, alternate HIV testing site, AIDS education

Mental Health Center of North Iowa
235 E Eisenhower Ave
PO Box 89A
Mason City, IA 50401-1562
Telephone: (515)-424-2075 Fax: (515)-424-9555
Contact: Ken Zimmeeman
Mental health services

Mental Health Center of North Iowa
235 E Eisenhower Ave
PO Box 89A
Mason City, IA 50401-1562
Telephone: (515)-424-2075 Fax: (515)-424-9555
Mental health services

Mental Health Center of North Iowa
235 S. Eisenhower Avenue
Mason City, IA 50401
Telephone: (515)-424-2075 Fax: (515)-424-9555
Mental health services

North Iowa Mercy Health
Center West Campus
Mason City, IA 50401-1562
Telephone: (515)-424-0440
Medical Services

North Iowa Mercy Health Center
84 Beaumont Drive
Mason City, IA 50401-2999
Telephone: (515)-424-7211 Fax: (515)-424-7827
Medical Services

Cherokee County

Community Services

Department of Human Services
239 West Maple
Cherokee, IA 51012-1852
Telephone: (712)-225-2588 Fax: (712)-225-4802
Financial and medical assistance

Salvation Army
111 North Fifth St
The Law Enforcement Center
Cherokee, IA 51012-1728
Telephone: (712)-225-6166
Emergency services: food, clothing, shelter with documentation of need.

Home Health Care

Cherokee County Public Health Nursing Service
Box B - Courthouse
Cherokee, IA 51012
Telephone: (712)-225-5580
Referrals, homecare & counseling

Medical Services

Plains Area Mental Health
724 North 1st
Cherokee, IA 51012-1207
Telephone: (712)-225-4111
Mental Health Services

Chickasaw County

Community Services

Chickasaw County Red Cross
101 North Locust Avenue
New Hampton, IA 50659
Telephone: (515)-394-5943
Emergency Services: Food, clothing, shelter

Department of Human Services
910 E. Main
New Hampton, IA 50659-1544
Telephone: (515)-394-4315
Food stamps, social services

Northeast Iowa Community Action Corporation
County Courthouse, 1st Fl
Box 205
New Hampton, IA 50659
Telephone: (515)-394-2007
Emergency Services: Food, clothing, shelter

Medical Services

St. Joseph's Community Hospital
308 North Maple Ave
New Hampton, IA 50659-1167
Telephone: (515)-394-4121 Fax: (515)-394-2328
Medical Services

Clarke County

Community Services

Clarke Community SCICAP Center
115 North Maine
Osceola, IA 50213-1214
Telephone: (515)-342-6516
Emergency Services: Food, clothing, shelter

Home Health Care

Clarke County Public Health
Courthouse
100 South Main
Osceola, IA 50213
Telephone: (515)-342-3724
Contact: Jean Gibbons - Director
Nursing Services

Medical Services

Crossroads Mental Health Center
820 N. Main Street
Osceola, IA 50213-1244
Telephone: (515)-342-4888
Mental Health Services

Clay County

Community Services

Clay County General Relief
300 W. Fourth Street
Spencer, IA 51301
Telephone: (712)-262-9438
Emergency Services: Food, clothing, shelter

Department of Human Services
215 W. Fourth Street
Box 3077
Spencer, IA 51301-3822
Telephone: (712)-262-3586
Financial aid, social services

Red Cross
407 1/2 Grand Avenue
Box 5277
Spencer, IA 51301
Telephone: (712)-262-1574
Emergency services: food, clothing, shelter, AIDS education

Home Health Care

Community Health Services
Spencer Municipal Hosp
114 E. 12th Street
Spencer, IA 51301
Telephone: (712)-264-6380
Medical services, hospice care

Medical Services

Northwest Iowa Mental Health
201 E. 11th Street
Spencer, IA 51301
Telephone: (712)-262-2922
Contact: Kim Wilson
Referrals and counseling

Spencer Municipal Hospital
114 E. 12th Street
Spencer, IA 51301-4300
Telephone: (712)-264-6198
Contact: Chris Van Kleer - Infection Control Nurse
Medical Services

Clayton County

Community Services

Department of Human Services
Clayton Co Office Bldg
429 High Street NE
Elkader, IA 52043
Telephone: (319)-245-1766
Financial aid

Home Health Care

Clayton County Public Health Nursing
County Office Building
PO Box 522
Elkader, IA 52043
Telephone: (319)-245-1145
Nursing Services

Medical Services

Central Community Hospital
Route 1 Box 269a
Elkader, IA 52043
Telephone: (319)-245-2250 Fax: (319)-245-2066
Medical Services

Clinton County

Community Services

New Directions, Inc.
217 6th Avenue South
Clinton, IA 52732-4305
Telephone: (319)-243-2124
Contact: Dan Bly
Substance Abuse Treatment, Counseling

Red Cross
1421 S. Bluff
Clinton, IA 52732-6551
Telephone: (319)-242-5223
Emergency Services: Food, clothing, shelter; AIDS education

Salvation Army
219 1st Avenue
Clinton, IA 52732-2015
Telephone: (319)-242-4502
Emergency Services: Food, clothing, shelter

Home Health Care

Amicare
562 Second Avenue South
Clinton, IA 52732
Telephone: (319)-243-7261
Contact: Karen Roode - Director
Homecare for AIDS patients

Medical Services

DeWitt Community Hospital
1118 11th Street
DeWitt, IA 52742-1296
Telephone: (319)-659-3241
Medical Services

Mental Health Center
320 Tucker Buildingh
Clinton, IA 52732
Telephone: (319)-243-5633 Fax: (319)-243-9567
Contact: Arthur Caerder - Executive Director
Mental Health Services

Crawford County

Community Services

Department of Human Services
107 S. Main Street
Denison, IA 51442-1958
Telephone: (712)-263-5668 Fax: (712)-263-4754
Emergency services: food, clothing, shelter, medical

Midwest Iowa Alcohol & Drug Abuse Center
1233 Broadway
Denison, IA 51442
Telephone: (712)-263-5065 Fax: (712)-263-6366
Contact: Joyce Harris
Substance Abuse Treatment, prevention & co dependency services

Home Health Care

Crawford County Public Health Nursing Service
Courthouse
PO Box 275
Denison, IA 51442
Telephone: (712)-263-9304
Nursing Services

Medical Services

West Iowa Community Mental Health Center
147 N. 7th Street
Denison, IA 51442-2457
Telephone: (712)-263-3172
Outpatient services

Dallas County

Community Services

Dallas County Coalition of Human Resources/Clothing Center
907 Main Street
Adel, IA 50003
Telephone: (515)-993-4531 Fax: (515)-993-5820
Contact: Marilyn Heikes - Director
Home care resources, resource directory, referrals to various socialservices

Department of Human Services
121 North 9th
PO Box 8
Adel, IA 50003-1443
Telephone: (515)-993-4264
Financial Aid

Veterans Affairs
801 Court Street
Adel, IA 50003-0056
Telephone: (515)-993-5809
Assistance with utilities, pensions; emergency food

Wear House
3rd & Otley
Perry, IA 50220
Telephone: (515)-465-2342
Emergency services: clothing & adult day care center

Home Health Care

Dallas County Public Health Nursing Service
618 10th Street
Perry, IA 50220
Telephone: (515)-993-3750
Contact: 515-465-2483
Nursing Services

Home Care Services, Inc.
907 Main Street
Adel, IA 50003
Telephone: (515)-993-3158
Transportation, meals on wheels, home care for AIDS patients

Medical Services

Dallas County Hospital
610 10th Street
Perry, IA 50220
Telephone: (515)-465-3547
Medical Services

Interim Health Care
600 1st Street
Perry, IA 50220-1803
Telephone: (515)-465-4057
Contact: Jackie Deets - Director of Health Care
Medical Services

West Central Mental Health
21111 W. Green
Adel, IA 50003
Telephone: (515)-993-4535
Toll-Free: (800)-321-7772
Contact: Jill Dannenbring
Mental Health Services

West Central Mental Health
2111 West Greene
Adel, IA 50003-1637
Telephone: (515)-993-4535
Mental Health Services

Davis County

Community Services

The Lord's Cupboard Distribution Center
107 North Davis
Bloomfield, IA 52537-1412
Telephone: (515)-664-2181
Emergency food services: Food, clothing, shelter

Home Health Care

Davis County PHN Service
105 South Pine
Bloomfield, IA 52537
Telephone: (515)-664-3629
Contact: Joanne Bride, BSN, RN - Nurse Administrator
Nursing Services

Medical Services

Davis County Hospital
507-09 N. Madison
Bloomfield, IA 52537
Telephone: (515)-664-2145
Medical Services

Decatur County

Home Health Care

Decatur County PHN Service
Courthouse
207 N. Main
Leon, IA 50144
Telephone: (515)-446-6518
Medical services, skilled nursing

Home care serviceervices
1401 Northwest Church Street
Leon, IA 50144
Telephone: (515)-446-4855
Medical Services

Medical Services

Decatur County Hospital
1405 NW Church St
Leon, IA 50144-1299
Telephone: (515)-446-4871
Contact: Pam Jackson - Director of Nursing
Medical Services

Decatur Medical Services
1404 NW Church
Leon, IA 50144-1297
Telephone: (515)-446-4855
Medical services, elderly home care

Delaware County

Community Services

Operation New View
222 South Franklin
Manchester, IA 52057
Telephone: (319)-927-4629
Referrals, utilities assistance

Home Health Care

Delaware County Community Health
709 W. Main
Manchester, IA 52057
Telephone: (319)-927-3232
Contact: Ext. 303
Medical services, home health care

Delaware County Public Health Nursing & Homemaker HHA
P.O. Box 359
Manchester, IA 52057-0359
Telephone: (319)-927-2584
Contact: Joyce Wahlford
Nursing Services

Des Moines County

Community Services

American Red Cross
Front & Jefferson
Burlington, IA 52601
Telephone: (319)-753-1970
Contact: Lynda Trustlow
Emergency services: food, clothing, shelter, HIV education

Salvation Army
217 South 3rd
Burlington, IA 52601-5520
Telephone: (319)-753-2038
Emergency Services: Food, clothing shelter

County Health Depts

Des Moines County Health Department
522 North Third Street
Burlington, IA 52601
Telephone: (319)-753-8215
Contact: Barbara Baker
Alternate Testing Sites

Medical Services

Desmoine City Health Center
522 N. 3rd Street
Burlington, IA 52601-5226
Telephone: (319)-753-8298
Nursing Services

Riverview Rehabilitation Center
602 N. 4th Street
Burlington, IA 52601-5026
Telephone: (319)-753-3633
Impatient/outpatient treatment

Southeastern Iowa Mental Health Center
407 N. 4th Street
Burlington, IA 52601-5229
Telephone: (319)-754-4618 Fax: (319)-754-4193
Mental Health Services

Woodlands Treatment Center
RR #1, Box 217
Burlington, IA 52601-9722
Telephone: (319)-753-0700
Substance Abuse Treatment

Dickinson County

Community Services

Upper Des Moines Opportunity
1609 18th Street
Spirit Lake, IA 51360
Telephone: (712)-336-1112
Contact: Laurie Ruth - Director
Emergency Services: Food, clothing, shelter

Home Health Care

Dickinson County Hospice
1713 Hill Avenue
Spirit Lake, IA 51360-1237
Telephone: (712)-336-4444
Contact: 712-336-2682

Hospice care

Dickinson Public Health Nursing Service
PO Box AB
Spirit Lake, IA 51360
Telephone: (712)-336-2682
Contact: Vivian C. Lynn - Administrator
Nursing Services

Medical Services

Dickinson County Memorial Hospital
2700 23rd Street
Hwy 71 South, Box AB
Spirit Lake, IA 51360
Telephone: (712)-336-1230
Medical services & surgical

Northwest Iowa Alcoholism & Drug Treatment Unit, Inc.
P.O. Box O
Spirit Lake, IA 51360
Telephone: (712)-336-4464 Fax: (712)-336-4306
Out-patient alcoholism & drug treatment counseling

Dubuque County

Community Services

Department of Human Services
Nesler Centre, Suite 140
Dubuque, IA 52004-0087
Telephone: (319)-557-8251 Fax: (319)-557-9177
Food stamps, title 19

Dubuque Regional AIDS Coalition
13th & Main
Dubuque, IA 52001
Telephone: (319)-589-4182
Contact: Kathleen Weber
AIDS coalition, education, volunteers

County Health Depts

Dubuque County Board of Health
13063 Seippel Road
Dubuque, IA 52002-9802
Telephone: (319)-557-7396
Medical Services

Home Health Care

Dubuque Visiting Nurses Association
P.O. Box 359
Dubuque, IA 52001-4825
Telephone: (319)-556-6200 Fax: (319)-556-4371
Contact: Julie McMahon
Alternate testing sites, medical services

Medical Services

Mercy Health Center
200 Mercy Drive
Dubuque, IA 52001-7360
Telephone: (319)-557-8331 Fax: (319)-589-9699
Toll-Free: (800)-637-2919
Contact: Kay Audever - Director of Health Education
Medical services, treatment center, support groups

Mercy Turning Point Treatment Center
Ste. 208, Prof.Arts Plaza
200 Mercy Drive
Dubuque, IA 52001
Telephone: (319)-589-8925 Fax: (319)-589-8162
Substance abuse treatment serving eastern Iowa

Substance Abuse Service Center
270 Nesler Center
Town Clock Plaza
Dubuque, IA 52001
Telephone: (319)-582-3784 Fax: (319)-582-4006
Contact: Diane Thomas - Executive Director
Substance Abuse Treatment

The Finley Hospital
350 North Grandview
Dubuque, IA 52001-6392
Telephone: (319)-582-1881 Fax: (319)-589-2621
Medical Services

Emmet County

Community Services

Emmet County Department of Human Services
220 South 1st Street
Estherville, IA 51334
Telephone: (712)-362-7237 Fax: (712)-362-7239
Financial aid, food stamps, title

Upper Des Moines Opportunity, Inc.
230 South 1st Street
Estherville, IA 51334
Telephone: (712)-362-2391
Emergency Services: Food, clothing, shelter

Home Health Care

Emmet County Public Health Nursing Service
609 1st Avenue North
1st Floor
Estherville, IA 51334
Telephone: (712)-362-2490
Nursing Services, HIV testing

Medical Services

Holy Family Hospital
826 North 8th Street
Estherville, IA 51334-1598
Telephone: (712)-362-2631 Fax: (712)-362-2636
Contact: Jeffrey Drop - President
Medical services

Fayette County

Community Services

Department of Human Services
129 A North Vine Street
West Union, IA 52175
Telephone: (800)-632-0014
Contact: 319-422-5634
Financial Aid

Northeast Iowa Community Action Corporation
P.O. Box 481
West Union, IA 52175-0481
Telephone: (319)-422-3354
Emergency Services: Food, clothing, shelter

Salvation Army of Fayette County
Arlington Branch
Oelwein State Bank
Arlington, IA 50606
Telephone: (319)-283-3361
Contact: Jens Nielson
Emergency Services: Food, clothing, shelter

Home Health Care

Fayette County Public Health Nursing Agency
114 North Bine Street
Box 516
West Union, IA 52175
Telephone: (319)-422-6061 Fax: (319)-422-6069
Homemaker/home health aide services, skilled nursing services

Homecare Helping Hand
P.O. Box 308
West Union, IA 52175
Telephone: (800)-632-0056
Rental & sale of durable medical equipment

Palmer Home Care
112 Jefferson
West Union, IA 52175
Telephone: (319)-422-3811 Fax: (319)-422-3664
Hospice, counseling

Medical Services

Mercy Hospital of Franciscan Sisters
201 8th Avenue SE
Oelwein, IA 50662
Telephone: (319)-283-2314 Fax: (319)-283-2318
Medical services, HIV testing

Northeast Iowa Mental Health Center
1297 South Frederick Ave.
Oelwein, IA 50662
Telephone: (319)-283-5774
Outpatient facility for Substance and Mental Health

Palmer Lutheran Health Center
112 Jefferson
West Union, IA 52175
Telephone: (319)-422-3811 Fax: (319)-422-3664
Medical Services

Floyd County

Community Services

Floyd County Department of Human Services
1206 S Main Street
P O Box 158
Charles City, IA 50616
Telephone: (515)-228-5713 Fax: (515)-228-6439
Financial aid, home care, social services, food stamps

Floyd County Relief Office
Courthouse 101 South Main
Charles City, IA 50616
Telephone: (515)-228-7111
Contact: Lois Litterer
Emergency Services: Food, clothing, shelter

Home Health Care

Community Nursing/Floyd County Memorial Hospital
711 Street
Charles City, IA 50616
Telephone: (515)-228-6830
Contact: Ext. 325
Nursing services, home health care

Floyd County Homemaker Home Health Aide Agency
1206 South Main
Charles City, IA 50616
Telephone: (515)-228-7432
Homecare for AIDS patients

Franklin County

Community Services

Hampton Community Food Pantry
PO Box 354
Hampton, IA 50441
Telephone: (515)-456-2192 Fax: (515)-456-4657
Contact: Kay Clay
Emergency services: food, annual clothing program (coats for kids)

Iowa Department of Human Services
P.O. Box 58
Hampton, IA 50441
Telephone: (515)-456-4763 Fax: (515)-456-4949
Financial aid, medical assistance

Home Health Care

Franklin County Public Health Nursing Service
Courthouse
Box 71
Hampton, IA 50441
Telephone: (515)-456-5629 Fax: (515)-456-2216
Nursing Services, homecare, home physical therapy

North Central Hospice
P.O. Box 27
Hampton, IA 50441
Telephone: (515)-456-2000 Fax: (515)-456-3449
Hospice care

Fremont County

Community Services

Department of Human Services
414 Clay Street
Sidney, IA 51652
Telephone: (712)-374-2512
Emergency services: food stamps, title 19

West Central Development Corp.
608 Clay Street
Sidney, IA 51652
Telephone: (712)-374-3367
Emergency services: food, clothing, shelter

Home Health Care

Public Health Nurse
820 Illinois
Box 357
Sidney, IA 51652
Telephone: (712)-374-2685
Contact: Becky Schaeffer
Nursing Services

Greene County

Community Services

Community Opportunities
Outreach Center
505 E. Lincolnway
Jefferson, IA 50129
Telephone: (515)-386-2719 Fax: (515)-386-2719
Emergency services

Department of Human Services
Courthouse
Jefferson, IA 50129
Telephone: (515)-386-2143
Social services

Medical Services

Greene County Medical Center
1000 W. Lincolnway St
Jefferson, IA 50129-1645
Telephone: (515)-386-2114
Medical Services

Grundy County

Home Health Care

Grundy County Public Health Nursing Service
704 H Avenue
Grundy Center, IA 50638-1410
Telephone: (319)-824-6312
Nursing Services

Guthrie County

Community Services

County Relief
Courthouse
200 North 5th Street
Guthrie Center, IA 50115
Telephone: (515)-747-2546
Contact: Connie Palmer
Emergency Services: Food, clothing, shelter

Family Development Center
103 North 3rd
Guthrie Center, IA 50115-1319
Telephone: (515)-747-3845 Fax: (515)-747-3845
Emergency Services: Food, clothing, shelter

Home Health Care

Guthrie County Public Health Nursing Services
102 South 4th Street
Guthrie Center, IA 50115-1640
Telephone: (515)-747-3972
Nursing Services, homecare speakers, health promotion visits

Medical Services

Guthrie County Hospital
710 North 12th Street
Guthrie Center, IA 50115
Telephone: (515)-747-2201
Medical Services

Hamilton County

Community Services

Department of Human Services
Courthouse
2300 Supion Street
Webster City, IA 50595-3191
Telephone: (515)-832-2231
Contact: Douglas Koons - Administration
Financial aid, food stamps, medical cards, counseling

Food Pantry/YOUR Inc.
915 High Street
P.O. Box 428
Webster City, IA 50595-2537
Telephone: (515)-832-6451 Fax: (515)-832-6451
Contact: Michael Bearden - Director
Provides referrals for emergency care: food, shelter & clothing

County Health Depts

Hamilton County Public Health Services
8201 Seneca Street
Webster City, IA 50595-2239
Telephone: (515)-832-9565 Fax: (515)-832-9554
Contact: Ms. Jackie Butter
Medical services

Hancock County

Community Services

Department of Human Services
Courthouse Annex
Garner, IA 50438
Telephone: (515)-923-3758
Contact: Connie Thompson
Financial aid, human services, AIDS waiver

Home Health Care

Hancock-Winnebago Homemaker Home Health Aide
Court House Annex
545 State Street
Garner, IA 50438
Telephone: (515)-923-2539
Home care, nursing services

Public Health Nursing Service/Hancock Co. Nursing Service
545 State Street
Garner, IA 50438
Telephone: (515)-923-3676
Nursing Services

Hardin County

Community Services

Alden Consignment, Unlimited
1201 Water
Alden, IA 50006
Telephone: (515)-859-7738
Contact: Julie Steward
Emergency Services: Clothing, household items, new & used furniture

Department of Human Services
County Office Building
1201 14th Avenue
Eldora, IA 50627
Telephone: (515)-858-3461 Fax: (515)-858-3465
Toll-Free: (800)-859-3048
Financial aid, food stamps, medical services

Harden COunty Food Shelf
1013 14th Street
Eldora, IA 50627-1604
Telephone: (515)-858-2577
Contact: Viloa Maymard
Food, paper & personal products

Red Cross of Hardin County
622 9th
Eldora, IA 50627
Telephone: (515)-858-5902
Emergency Services: Food, clothing, shelter

Home Health Care

Hardin County Community Nursing Service
County Office Building
Eldora, IA 50627
Telephone: (515)-858-3461
Contact: Jean Gehrke, R.N. - Nurse Administrator
Nursing, home care, infusion therapy

Medical Services

Ellsworth Municipal Hospital
110 Rocksylvania
Iowa Falls, IA 50126-2431
Telephone: (515)-648-4631
Medical Services

Harrison County

Community Services

Veterans Affairs
Courthouse
Logan, IA 51546
Telephone: (712)-644-3329
Contact: Royce Hildreth
Financial Aid

Home Health Care

Homemaker Service
Courthouse
Logan, IA 51546
Telephone: (712)-644-3437
Contact: Kathy Ried - Social Worker
Homemaker services, home care

Public Health Nursing Service
Courthouse
Logan, IA 51546
Telephone: (712)-644-2220 Fax: (712)-644-2643
Nursing Services

Medical Services

Family Health Office
Courthouse
Logan, IA 51546
Telephone: (712)-644-3436 Fax: (712)-644-2643
Medical services, referrals

Maternal and Child Health Services
Courthouse
Logan, IA 51546
Telephone: (712)-644-3436 Fax: (712)-644-2643
Contact: Sharon Barry - RNC Family Coordinator
Medical Services

Mental Health/Community Memorial Hospital
631 N. 8th
Missouri Valley, IA 51555-1102
Telephone: (712)-642-2784 Fax: (712)-642-2780
Contact: Rhonda Tomair - Director of Nursing
Mental health services & outpatient

Henry County

Community Services

Department of Human Services
202 North Jackson Street
Basement of HC Health Ctr
Mt. Pleasant, IA 52641
Telephone: (319)-986-5157
Financial aid, counseling, child care, in-home care, medical, AIDS & handicapped waivers

Fellowship Cup
205 North Jefferson St.
PO Box 713
Mt. Pleasant, IA 52641-2018
Telephone: (319)-385-3242
Food pantry, shelter for prisoner's families

Henry County Community Services
PO Box 652
Mt. Pleasant, IA 52641
Telephone: (319)-385-0790 Fax: (319)-385-0778
Contact: Shirley Chrisman - Director
Medical services, rent, utilities, medications

Howard County

Community Services

Department of Human Services
205 East 2nd street
Cresco, IA 52136
Telephone: (319)-547-2860
Financial aid, food stamps, Medicaid, family services

County Health Depts

Howard County Public Health
327 8 Avenue West
Cresco, IA 52136-1064
Telephone: (319)-547-2989
Contact: Cora Dunt - Nursing Administrator
Referrals, counseling

Medical Services

Howard County Hospital
235 8th Avenue West
Cresco, IA 52136
Telephone: (319)-547-2101 Fax: (319)-547-3448
Medical services, HIV testing, counseling, referrals, education,counseling, speakers

Humboldt County

Community Services

Department of Human Services
Courthouse, Gen Delivery
Dakota City, IA 50529-9999
Telephone: (515)-332-3383
Contact: Dough Koon
Emergency Services: Food, clothing, shelter

Wouk, Inc.
Humboldt County Court House
Dakota City, IA 50529-9999
Telephone: (515)-332-3631 Fax: (515)-332-1738
Emergency Services: Food & clothing

Home Health Care

Humboldt County Public Health Nursing
Courthouse
Dakota City, IA 50529-9999
Telephone: (515)-332-2492 Fax: (515)-332-1738
Nursing Services

Ida County

Community Services

Department of Human Services
Courthouse
Ida Grove, IA 51445
Telephone: (712)-364-2631
Contact: Lyle Fleshner
Financial Aid

Food Pantry/Mid-Sioux Opportunities
Courthouse
Ida Grove, IA 51445
Telephone: (712)-364-2175

Contact: Carolyn Bream
Emergency services: food, clothing, shelter

Ida County General Assistance
Courthouse
401 Moorehead
Ida Grove, IA 51445
Telephone: (712)-364-3498
Financial Aid

Iowa County

Community Services

Department of Human Services
P.O. Box 147
Marengo, IA 52301-0147
Telephone: (319)-642-5573
Contact: Sandra Teach - Area Director
Financial aide, food stamps, medical card

HACAP
P.O. Box 778
Williamsburg, IA 52361
Telephone: (319)-668-1812 Fax: (319)-668-1941
Contact: Barb Schaefer - Service Coordinator
Emergency services: fuel assistance, meals, clothing, shelter

Home Health Care

Public Health Nursing and Homemaker-Home Health Aide Service
Iowa County Health Dept.
RR#1, Box 15A
Williamsburg, IA 52361
Telephone: (319)-668-1021
Contact: Jodie Morrison
Homemaker - Home Health Aide Services

Medical Services

Iowa County Court House
c/o Marengo Memorial Hosp
P.O. Box 228
Marengo, IA 52301
Telephone: (319)-338-7884 Fax: (319)-338-7884
Mental health, counseling for AIDS patients

Marengo Memorial Hospital
P.O. Box 228
Marengo, IA 52301-0228
Telephone: (319)-642-5543 Fax: (319)-642-3748
Contact: Sue Faith - Director
Medical Services

Jackson County

Community Services

Jackson County Home and Community Health Service
Jackson County Public Hospital
700 West Grove
Maquoketa, IA 52060
Telephone: (319)-652-2474 Fax: (319)-652-5211
Contact: Basil Pannell - Infection Controll Coordinator
Substance abuse counseling, AIDS counseling, community education program

Operation New View
804 East Quarry
Maquoketa, IA 52060-2929
Telephone: (319)-652-5197
Emergency Services: Food, clothing, shelter, utilities

Home Health Care

Hospice of North Central Iowa
205 First Street, Northwest
Hampton, IA 40441
Telephone: (515)-456-2000
Hospice care, AIDS home care

Medical Services

Dubuque/Jackson Co Mental Health Center/Satellite Office
St. Johns Lutheran Church
204 N. Anna
Preston, IA 52069
Telephone: (319)-689-5306
Mental Health Services

Jackson County Hospital
700 West Grove
Maquoketa, IA 52060-2163
Telephone: (319)-652-2474
Medical Services

Jasper County

Community Services

Department of Human Services
Midtown Building
Newton, IA 50208
Telephone: (515)-792-1955
Contact: Judy Snook
Financial aid, food stamps, medical services

Salvation Army-Food Clothing-Shelter
219 North 2nd Avenue West
Newton, IA 50208
Telephone: (515)-792-6131
Emergency Services: Food, clothing, shelter

Medical Services

Central Iowa Foundation on Alcoholism & Drug Abuse
306 N 3rd Avenue East
Newton, IA 50208-3249
Telephone: (515)-792-2302
Substance abuse treatment; AIDS counseling

Skiff Medical Center
204 North Fourth Ave. E
PO Box 1006
Newton, IA 50208-3100
Telephone: (515)-792-5086
Medical Services

Jefferson County

Community Services

Jefferson County Department of Human Services
51 West Hempstead
PO Box 987
Fairfield, IA 52556-2832
Telephone: (515)-472-5011 Fax: (515)-472-3519
Toll-Free: (800)-642-6249
Food stamps, medical services

Jefferson County General Relief Programs
51 West Briggs
Fairfield, IA 52556
Telephone: (515)-472-3013
Contact: Blanch Hendricks - General Relief Director
Financial Aid

Home Health Care

Hospice of Jefferson County
PO Box 1783
Fairfield, IA 52556-1783
Telephone: (515)-472-8381
Contact: Nanette Conger
Hospice care

Jefferson County Public Health Nursing Service
2200 W. Jefferson Ave.
Fairfield, IA 52556-4231
Telephone: (515)-472-5929
Contact: Victoria J. McKeever - Nurse Administrator
Home care, IV therapy

Johnson County

Community Services

Department of Human Services
911 N. Governor Street
Iowa City, IA 52245-5921
Telephone: (319)-356-6050 Fax: (319)-337-2705
Financial aid, food stamps, disability

Iowa Center for AIDS Resources
320 E College Street
P.O. Box 2989
Iowa City, IA 52244
Telephone: (319)-338-2135
Support Groups

Mid-Eastern Council on Chemical Abuse
430 Southgate Avenue
Iowa City, IA 52240
Telephone: (319)-351-4357
Contact: Art Chut
Substance Abuse Treatment

Home Health Care

Iowa City Hospice, Inc.
613 E. Bloomington St
Iowa City, IA 52245
Telephone: (319)-351-5665
Hospice care

Visiting Nurse Association of Johnson County
R Plaza 485 Hwy 1 W.
Iowa City, IA 52246
Telephone: (319)-337-9686
Contact: Rosalie Rose
Nursing Services, social work, home health aide on call 24 hrs

Medical Services

ICARE (Iowa Center for AIDS Resources and Education)
P.O. Box 2989
Iowa City, IA 52244
Telephone: (319)-338-2135
Contact: Laura Hill
Medical Services

Iowa Student Health Service/University of Iowa
Steindler Building
Iowa City, IA 52242-0001
Telephone: (319)-335-8370 Fax: (319)-335-6659
Contact: Dr. Mary Khowassah
Medical services, HIV testing & counseling for students only

Mid-Eastern Council on Chemical Addiction
430 Southgate Avenue
Iowa City, IA 52240-4425
Telephone: (319)-351-4357 Fax: (319)-351-4907
Substance Abuse Treatment

Mid-Eastern Iowa Community Mental Health
505 E. College Street
Iowa City, IA 52240
Telephone: (319)-338-7884
Contact: Laura Lovell - Office Coordinator
Counseling for AIDS patients

Jones County

Community Services

Crisis Center
321 East 1st Street
Iowa City, IA 52230
Telephone: (319)-351-0140
Counseling/Suicide intervention/Prevention/AIDS information & referrals

Department of Human Services
500 West Main Street
Anamosa, IA 52205
Telephone: (319)-462-3557
Financial Services

Keokuk County

Community Services

Department of Human Services
RR #1, Box 308
Sigourney, IA 52591-9801
Telephone: (515)-622-2090 Fax: (515)-622-2286
Contact: Susan Rubis - Service Supervisor
Financial aid, in-home health care, state social worker, medicalassistance, food stamps, housing assistance

Home Health Care

Keokuk County Health Services
Courthouse
Sigourney, IA 52591
Telephone: (515)-622-3575 Fax: (515)-622-2286
Contact: Janice Moore - Administrator
Medical services, home health care

Medical Services

Keokuk County Health Center
1312 South Stewart Street
PO Box 286
Sigourney, IA 52591-9803
Telephone: (515)-622-2720 Fax: (515)-622-2720
Contact: Donna Brennenman
Medical services, long term care unit

Kewaunee County

Medical Services

St. Luke's Hospital
1026 A Avenue NE
5th Floor
Cedar Rapids, IA 54201-3026
Telephone: (319)-369-7740
Contact: Diane Rattner - Dir of Medical Social Services
Medical services, counseling for AIDS patients

Kossuth County

Community Services

Department of Human Services
Courthouse Annex
109 West State Street
Algona, IA 50511
Telephone: (515)-295-7771
Contact: Kathryn Lucas
Financial aid, general services

Home Health Care

Kossuth County Public Health Nursing Service
Courthouse Annex
109 W. State Street
Algona, IA 50511
Telephone: (515)-295-5602
Nursing Services

Medical Services

Kossuth County Hospital
Box 637
Hwy 169 South
Algona, IA 50511
Telephone: (515)-295-2451 Fax: (515)-295-7089
Medical Services

Lee County

Community Services

Lee County Department of Social Services
307 Bank Street
Box 937
Keokuk, IA 52632
Telephone: (319)-524-1052
Financial Aid

Social Services
933 Avenue H
PO Box 188
Fort Madison, IA 52627-4540
Telephone: (319)-372-3651
Financial aid, AIDS waiver

Linn County

Community Services

Area Substance Abuse Council
3601 16th Avenue SW
Cedar Rapids, IA 52404
Telephone: (319)-390-4611
Substance abuse treatment

Grant Area Red Cross
3601 42nd Street NE
Cedar Rapids, IA 52406-7111
Telephone: (319)-393-3500 Fax: (319)-393-1841
Contact: David Packard - AIDS/HIV Program Coordinator
Emergency services: food, clothing, shelter, support groups, buddysystem; financial aid through Ryan White; teen awareness program

HACAP Administrative Office
P.O. Box 789
Cedar Rapids, IA 52406-0789
Telephone: (319)-366-7631 Fax: (319)-366-0776
Toll-Free: (800)-332-5289
Emergency Services: Food, clothing, shelter

Rapids AIDS Project
3601 42nd Street NE
Cedar Rapids, IA 52402-7127
Telephone: (319)-393-9579
Contact: David Packard
AIDS coalition, financial services, social services, physician referrals,counseling

County Health Depts

Linn County Health Department
501 Thirteenth Street NW
Cedar Rapids, IA 52405-3700
Telephone: (319)-398-3551 Fax: (319)-364-7391
Contact: Vicki Smith
HIV testing and counseling

Home Health Care

Linn County Visiting Nurse Association
1201 3rd Avenue SE
Cedar Rapids, IA 52403-4009
Telephone: (319)-369-7990
Nursing Services

Medical Services

Area Substance Abuse Council
3601 16th Avenue SW
Cedar Rapids, IA 52404
Telephone: (319)-390-4611
Substance Abuse Treatment, Referrals and Counseling

Foundation II Crisis Center
1540 2nd Avenue SE
Cedar Rapids, IA 52403-2302
Telephone: (319)-362-2174
Contact: 800-332-4224 (24 hours)
Mental health services, counseling for crisis over phone only.

Mercy Family Practice Center
610 8th Street SE
Cedar Rapids, IA 52401-2196
Telephone: (319)-398-6170 Fax: (319)-398-6466
Contact: Ingrid McHugh - Nurse/Coordinator
Medical Services

Louisa County

Community Services

Human Services
317 Van Buren
Wapello, IA 52653-1222
Telephone: (319)-523-6351
Financial aid, AIDS waiver

Home Health Care

Louisa County Public Nursing Service
407 Washington St
Wapello, IA 52653-1431
Telephone: (319)-523-3981
Nursing services, home aides

Lucas County

Community Services

Department of Human Services
P.O. Box 735
Chariton, IA 50049-0735
Telephone: (515)-774-5071
Financial Aid

Home Health Care

Lucas County Public Health Nursing Service
123 S. Grand Street
PO Box 852
Chariton, IA 50049-1829
Telephone: (515)-774-4312 Fax: (515)-774-0444
Nursing Services

Lyon County

Community Services

Department of Human Services
803 South Green Street
Suite 2
Rock Rapids, IA 51246-1233
Telephone: (712)-472-3743
Financial aid, medical services

Medical Services

Merrill Pioneer Community Hospital
801 S. Greene
Rock Rapids, IA 51246-1988
Telephone: (712)-472-2591 Fax: (712)-472-2591
Medical Services

Madison County

Community Services

Department of Human Services
110 W. Green Street
Winterset, IA 50273
Telephone: (515)-462-2931
Contact: Ann Webers
Financial aid, AIDS hotline

Madison County Multipurpose Center
114 North 2nd Street
Winterset, IA 50273
Telephone: (515)-462-4704
Emergency Services: Food, clothing, shelter

Medical Services

Earlham Care--Winterset Office
602 E. Filmore St
Winterset, IA 50273-1355
Telephone: (515)-462-1143
Medical Services

Madison County Memorial Hospital
300 W Hutchings St
Winterset, IA 50273-2199
Telephone: (515)-462-2373 Fax: (515)-462-1948
Medical Services

Mahaska County

Community Services

Department of Human Services
P.O. Box 290
Oskaloosa, IA 52577-0290
Telephone: (515)-673-2396
Contact: Richard Johnson
Financial Aid

Marion County

Community Services

Community Action Center
305 S 3rd
Knoxville, IA 50138-2222
Telephone: (515)-842-6571
Emergency Services: Food, clothing, shelter

Department of Human Services
PO Box 191
Knoxville, IA 50138-0191
Telephone: (515)-842-5087
Contact: Margaret Carruthers
Financial aid, food stamps, medical services, cash grant, counseling

Knoxville Public Housing Agency
305 S. 3rd
Knoxville, IA 50138-2287
Telephone: (515)-828-7371
Rent Subsidy Assistance

Home Health Care

Hospice of Central Iowa
1202 W. Howard
Knoxville, IA 50138-3103
Telephone: (515)-828-7672
Contact: Maryjoe Romano
Hospice care

Marion County Public Health Nursing Service
Courthouse
1st Floor
Knoxville, IA 50138
Telephone: (515)-828-2238
Nursing services, homemaker services

Medical Services

Knoxville Area Community Hospital
1202 W. Howard Street
Knoxville, IA 50138-3103
Telephone: (515)-842-2151 Fax: (515)-842-3141
Medical services, HIV testing

Mater Medical Clinic
1202 W. Howard
Knoxville, IA 50138-3199
Telephone: (515)-828-7211 Fax: (515)-842-5686
Medical Services

South Central Mental Health
Pella Community Center
712 Union
Pella, IA 50219
Telephone: (515)-673-7406
Mental Health Services

Marshall County

Community Services

Churches United in Compassion and Concern

Marshalltown, IA 50158
Telephone: (515)-752-7537
Emergency Services: Food, clothing, shelter

Salvation Army
PO Box 482
Marshalltown, IA 50158
Telephone: (515)-753-5236
Emergency Services: Food, clothing, shelter

Social Security
202 West State Street
Marshalltown, IA 50158
Telephone: (515)-752-6376 Fax: (515)-752-7311
Social Security, disability

Substance Abuse Treatment Unit of Central Iowa
PO Box 1453
Marshalltown, IA 50158
Telephone: (515)-752-7217
Contact: 515-752-5421
Counseling

Home Health Care

Iowa River Hospice
P.O. Box 1086
Marshalltown, IA 50158
Telephone: (515)-753-7704 Fax: (515)-753-7379
Hospice care

Marshall County Nursing Service
Courthouse
3rd Floor
Marshalltown, IA 50158
Telephone: (515)-754-6353 Fax: (515)-754-6384
Nursing Services

Marshalltown Community Nursing Service
709 S. Center Street
PO Box 1202
Marshalltown, IA 50158-2833
Telephone: (515)-752-4611
Nursing Services

Mills County

Home Health Care

Mills County Public Health Nursing Services
107 E. Fourth Street
PO Box 518
Malvern, IA 51551
Telephone: (712)-624-8333
Contact: Barbara Kaiman
Nursing Services, Homemaker/Home Health Aide Services

Mitchell County

Community Services

Department of Human Services
115 North Main Street
PO Box 377
Osceola, IA 50461-1249
Telephone: (515)-342-6516
Financial aid, food stamps, child care

Medical Services

Mitchell County Care Facility
Route 3
Osage, IA 50461-9803
Telephone: (515)-732-3145
Residential care facility

Mitchell County Memorial Hospital
616 N. 8th Street
Osage, IA 50461-1498
Telephone: (515)-732-3781
Medical Services/Homemaker and Health Agency

Monona County

Community Services

Department of Human Services
Courthouse
610 Iowa
Onawa, IA 51040
Telephone: (712)-423-1921
Contact: Mark Mullin - Service Supervisor
Home health care, medical assistance, food stamps, fuel assistance

Home Health Care

Monona County Public Health Nursing Service
610 Iowa Avenue
Onawa, IA 51040-1699
Telephone: (712)-423-1773
Nursing Services

Medical Services

Burgess Memorial Hospital
1600 Diamond
Onawa, IA 51040-1548
Telephone: (712)-423-2311
Medical Services

Monroe County

Community Services

Helping Hand Center
710 Washington Avenue
Albia, IA 52531-2122
Telephone: (515)-932-5984
Emergency Services: Food, clothing, shelter

Home Health Care

Monroe County Public Health Nursing Service
Courthouse
Albia, IA 52531
Telephone: (515)-932-7191
Nursing services, home health aide

Medical Services

Monroe County Hospital
Route 3
Albia, IA 52531-9803
Telephone: (515)-932-2134
Medical Services

Montgomery County

Community Services

Department of Human Services
Courthouse
3rd Floor
Red Oak, IA 51566
Telephone: (712)-623-4838
Contact: Connie Timberman
Financial aid, food stamps, medical services

Home Health Care

Public Health Nursing Service
200 Coalbaugh
Red Oak, IA 51566
Telephone: (712)-623-4893
Nursing services, home health aides

Medical Services

Montgomery County Memorial Hospital
2301 Eastern Avenue
Red Oak, IA 51566-1799
Telephone: (712)-623-7000 Fax: (712)-623-7180
Contact: Terri Urban - Wellness Coordinator
Medical Services

Muscatine County

Community Services

Department of Human Services
120 East 3rd Street
4th Floor
Muscatine, IA 52761-4019
Telephone: (319)-263-9302
Financial aid, disability

Muscatine County Community Services
415 East 4th Mulberry
Muscatine, IA 52761
Telephone: (319)-263-7512
Contact: Nancy Nauman
Emergency Services: food, clothing, shelter; medical care, AIDS awareness,support group

Salvation Army
1000 Oregon
P.O. Box 208
Muscatine, IA 52761
Telephone: (319)-263-8272
Emergency Services: Food, clothing, shelter

Home Health Care

Community Home Care Inc.
614 Mulberry Avenue
Muscatine, IA 52761-3433
Telephone: (319)-264-5272
Home health care

Community Nursing Services
1609 Cedar Street
Muscatine, IA 52761-3426
Telephone: (319)-263-3325 Fax: (319)-263-6202
Nursing Services

Hospice of Muscatine
1518 Mulberry Avenue
Muscatine, IA 52761-3433
Telephone: (319)-264-9413 Fax: (319)-264-8614
Hospice care

Medical Services

Community Medical Services
1616 Cedar Street
Muscatine, IA 52761-3461
Telephone: (319)-263-0122
Child/maternal health

Muscatine General Hospital
1518 Mulberry Avenue
Muscatine, IA 52761-3499
Telephone: (319)-264-9100 Fax: (319)-264-8641
Contact: Vickie Charlton - Infectious Disease
Medical Services

O'Brien County

Community Services

Department of Human Services
PO Box 400
Primghar, IA 51245-0400
Telephone: (712)-757-5135
Contact: Paula Heckenlively
Financial aid, food stamps, AIDS waiver

Home Health Care

Northwest Iowa Home Health Care
255 North Welch Avenue
Primghar, IA 51245
Telephone: (712)-757-3905
Nursing Services

Medical Services

Baum-Harmon Memorial Hospital
255 N. Welch Avenue
Primghar, IA 51245
Telephone: (712)-757-3905
Medical Services

Osceola County

Community Services

Department of Human Services
230 9th Street
Sibley, IA 51249-1801
Telephone: (712)-754-3622 Fax: (712)-754-2301
Contact: Paula Heckenlively - Service Supervisor
In-home healthcare program, administered by state social worker, medicalassistance, food stamps; emergency help for evicted

Medical Services

Osceola Community Health Services
110 Cedar Lane
Sibley, IA 51249-1055
Telephone: (712)-754-4611
Medical Services

Page County

Community Services

Department of Human Services
121 S. 15th Suite C
Clarinda, IA 51632-2245
Telephone: (712)-542-5111
Financial aid, general services

Department of Human Services
P.O. Box 569
Shenondoah, IA 51601
Telephone: (712)-246-4167
Financial Aid

Home Health Care

Page County Public Health Nursing
109 N. Sycamore
Shenandoah, IA 51601-1229
Telephone: (712)-246-2223
Nursing services, home health care

Medical Services

Clarinda Municipal Hospital
17th & Wells
Clarinda, IA 51632
Telephone: (712)-542-2176 Fax: (712)-542-3380
Medical Services, Testing, Counseling

Palo Alto County

Community Services

Department of Human Services
2105 Main Street
Emmetsburg, IA 50536
Telephone: (712)-852-3523 Fax: (712)-852-3524
Financial Aid

Harmony House
2308 Main Street
Emmetsburg, IA 50536-1553
Telephone: (712)-852-4612
Emergency Services: Food, clothing, shelter

Home Health Care

Palo Alto Public Health Nursing
3201 1st Street
Emmetsburg, IA 50536-2599
Telephone: (712)-852-3522
Nursing care

Plymouth County

Community Services

Mid Sioux Opportunity, Inc.
418 Marion Street
Box 390
Remsen, IA 51050
Telephone: (712)-786-2001 Fax: (712)-786-3250
Toll-Free: (800)-859-2001
Emergency Services: Food, clothing, shelter

Medical Services

Plains Area Mental Health
P.O. Box 70
Semars, IA 51031
Telephone: (712)-364-3500 Fax: (712)-546-4624
Mental Health Services, Referrals and Counseling

Pocahontas County

Community Services

Department of Human Services
23 3rd Avenue NE
Box F
Pocahontas, IA 50574-1614
Telephone: (712)-355-3565
Contact: Ren Walrod
Financial Aid

Home Health Care

Pocahontas County Public Nursing Service
Courthouse
Pocahontas, IA 50574
Telephone: (712)-335-4142
Nursing Services

Polk County

Community Services

American Red Cross - Central Iowa
2116 Grand Ave
Des Moines, IA 50312
Telephone: (515)-244-6700
Contact: Lynn Laws; 800-445-2437 -
Financial services, social services, physician referrals, buddy & volunteerprograms

Buddy Program-American Red Cross
2116 Grand Avenue
Des Moines, IA 50312-5368
Telephone: (515)-244-6700
Mental health services, emotional support

NCA/Central Assessment Center
1446 Martin Luther King Parkway
Des Moines, IA 50314
Telephone: (515)-244-2297
Substance Abuse Treatment, Referral Services and Counseling

Polk County Department of Social Services
111 Court Avenue
Room 230
Des Moines, IA 50309
Telephone: (515)-286-3434
Emergency Services: Food, clothing, shelter

Veterans Administration
210 Walnut Street
Des Moines, IA 50309-2198
Telephone: (515)-284-0219
Toll-Free: (800)-827-1000
Contact: Norman Bauer
Financial Aid

Home Health Care

Caremark Homecare Branch Network
2332 Rocklyn Drive
Urbandale, IA 50322-4935
Telephone: (515)-270-0123 Fax: (515)-270-9767
in-home IV therapy

Homedco Infusion
11224 Aurora Avenue
Des Moines, IA 50322-7905
Telephone: (515)-270-2400 Fax: (515)-270-0014
Nationwide experience in providing home infusion therapy to AIDS patients

Hospice of Central Iowa
3619 1/2 Douglas Avenue
Des Moines, IA 50310-5345
Telephone: (515)-274-3400 Fax: (515)-271-1302
Hospice care, Cavanaugh house

nmc HOMECARE
108 Fifth Avenue SW
Altoona, IA 50009
Telephone: (515)-967-7633
Fax: (515)-967-5459
Contact: Gail Mc Nurlen
National JCAHO-Accredited company providing a full range of Infusion and Respiratory therapies and specializing in the care of HIV/AIDS patients. National Case Manager is also available at 800-445-1188

Universal Home Health Care, Inc.
1500 30th Street
Suite 2004
West Des Moines, IA 50265
Telephone: (515)-223-3000 Fax: (515)-223-3074
Toll-Free: (800)-593-0104
Contact: Linda Behrens
Nursing Services, home health aid.

Medical Services

Broadlawns Medical Center
1801 Hickman Road
Des Moines, IA 50314-1597
Telephone: (515)-282-2200
Contact: 515-282-5752
Medical Services

Iowa Lutheran Hospital/University at Penn
700 East University Avenue
Des Moines, IA 50316
Telephone: (515)-263-5612
Contact: Mary Rex Roat
Treatment of infectious diseases

Westside Community Hospital
48th & Franklin
Des Moines, IA 50310
Telephone: (515)-271-6000
Medical Services

Pottawattamie County

Community Services

Human Services
417 E. Kanesville
Council Bluffs, IA 51503
Telephone: (712)-328-5689 Fax: (712)-322-7607
Financial Aid

Salvation Army
28 North 7th Street
Council Bluffs, IA 51501-0759
Telephone: (712)-328-2088
Emergency Services: Food, clothing,

County Health Depts

Council Bluffs City Health Department
209 Pearl Street
Council Bluffs, IA 51503
Telephone: (712)-328-3194
Contact: Linda McQuinn
Alternate testing sites-HIV testing

Home Health Care

Visiting Nurses of Pottawattamie County
119 South Main Street
Suite 350
Council Bluffs, IA 51503
Telephone: (712)-328-2636
Contact: Mary Murphy
Nursing services, counseling, screening, AIDS waiver

Medical Services

Mercy Mental Health Center
427 Kanesville Boulevard
Council Bluffs, IA 51501-4481
Telephone: (712)-328-2609
Mental Health Services

Poweshiek County

Community Services

Human Services Department
819 Commercial Street
Grinnell, IA 50112-2144
Telephone: (515)-236-3149
Financial aid, food stamps, AIDS waiver

Mid-Iowa Community Action Outreach Office
834 Broad Street
Grinnell, IA 50112-2100
Telephone: (515)-236-3923
Emergency Services: Food, clothing, shelter

Poweshiek County Relief Department
302 E. Main
Box 177 COurthouse
Montezuma, IA 50171
Telephone: (515)-623-3061
Financial Aid

Home Health Care

Grinnell Regional Medical Center
210 4th Avenue
Grinnell General Hospital
Grinnell, IA 50112-1833
Telephone: (515)-236-7511
Medical Services

Ringgold County

Community Services

Congregate Meals
Main Street
Tingley, IA 50863
Telephone: (515)-772-4499
Emergency Services: Food, clothing, shelter

Department of Human Services
Ringgold Co. Courthouse
Mount Ayr, IA 50854
Telephone: (515)-464-2247
Contact: Kris Baudyuch
Financial aid, food stamps, medical AIDS waiver

Neighborhood Center
202 North Taylor
Mount Ayr, IA 50845
Telephone: (515)-464-2401
Emergency services: food, clothing, shelter

Sac County

Community Services

Family Development Center
1708 West Main
Sac City, IA 50583-2429
Telephone: (712)-662-3236
Emergency Services: Food, clothing, shelter

General Relief - Human Services
Courthouse
Sac City, IA 50583
Telephone: (712)-662-4552
Contact: Peggy Dettmann
Financial Aid

Sac County Department of Human Services
Courthouse Annex
100 S. State Street
Sac City, IA 50583
Telephone: (712)-662-4782
Financial aid, medical services

Home Health Care

Sac County Public Health Nursing Service
Courthouse Annex
100 S. State Street
Sac City, IA 50583
Telephone: (712)-662-4785
Nursing services, home health aides

Scott County

Community Services

Quad Cities AIDS Coalition
605 N. Main Street
Room 6A
Davenport, IA 52803-5243
Telephone: (319)-324-8638
Support group, referrals, education

County Health Depts

Scott County Health Department
Bicentennial Bdg, Floor 5
428 Western Avenue
Davenport, IA 52801
Telephone: (319)-326-8618
Contact: Roma Taylor
HIV alternate test sites, partner notification

Home Health Care

Caremark Homecare Branch Network
1008 West 35th Street
Davenport, IA 52806-5827
Telephone: (319)-386-3220 Fax: (319)-386-4715
Contact: Kevin Cahill - Pharmacy/Ops. Manager
In-home IV infusion therapy

Visiting Nurse Association
PO Box 4346
Davenport, IA 52808-1318
Telephone: (319)-324-5274 Fax: (319)-323-9551
Contact: Tom Moen
Out-of-hospital care

Medical Services

Center for Alcohol & Drug Services, Inc.
1523 S. Fairmount
Davenport, IA 52802
Telephone: (319)-322-2667
Substance abuse treatment, prevention, emergency services

Medical Pavillon
1351 W. Central Park Ave
Davenport, IA 52806-1889
Telephone: (319)-383-2646
Referrals for treatment & counseling

St. Luke's Hospital
1227 E. Rusholme
Davenport, IA 52803-2498
Telephone: (319)-326-6512
Infectious control department

Sioux County

Community Services

Church Food Pantry
407 Albany Avenue SE
Orange City, IA 51041-1627
Telephone: (712)-737-4430
Emergency services: food

Iowa Department of Human Services
215 Central Avenue SE
PO Box 270
Orange City, IA 51041-1739
Telephone: (712)-737-2943 Fax: (712)-737-3564
Financial aid, food stamps

Mid-Sioux Opportunities
323 N. Main
Sioux Center, IA 51250
Telephone: (712)-722-3611
Contact: Hawarden: 712-552-1724
Emergency Services: Food, clothing, shelter, fuel assistance

Home Health Care

Publical Homecare Aide Service
211 Central Avenue South East
Orange City, IA 51041
Telephone: (712)-737-2971 Fax: (712)-737-3564
Medical services, home care, nursing

Sioux County Public Health Nursing Service
Courthouse
211 Central Avenue, SE
Orange City, IA 51041
Telephone: (712)-737-2971
Nursing Services

Medical Services

Bethesda Midwest
209 1 Street NE
Orange City, IA 51041-1443
Telephone: (712)-737-2635
Mental Health Services

Hegg Memorial Health Center
1202 21st Avenue
Rock Valley, IA 51247
Telephone: (712)-476-5305 Fax: (712)-476-5305
Medical Services

Orange City Municipal Hospital and Hospice of Sioux County
400 Central Avenue
Orange City, IA 51041
Telephone: (712)-737-4984 Fax: (712)-737-5252
Medical Services

Sioux Center Community Hospital and Community Health Enrich.
605 South Main Avenue
Sioux Center, IA 51250
Telephone: (712)-722-1271 Fax: (712)-722-0787
Toll-Free: (800)-722-1922
Medical Services

Story County

Community Services

Ames Health & Welfare Services
1120 Marston Avenue
Ames, IA 50010-5863
Telephone: (515)-232-0472
Emergency Services: Food, clothing, shelter

Bethesda Clothing Room
1517 Northwestern
Ames, IA 50010-5271
Telephone: (515)-232-6256
Emergency Services: Food, clothing, shelter

Legal Aid
937 6th Street
Nevada, IA 50201-2046
Telephone: (515)-382-2471
Legal Aid

Social Security Administration
6th & Kellog
Box 1608/ Post Office Bdg
Ames, IA 50010
Telephone: (515)-233-2484 Fax: (515)-233-2487
Social Security, disability

Home Health Care

Mary Greeley Medical Center
117 11th Street
Ames, IA 50010
Telephone: (515)-239-2011
Medical Services

Homeward Hospice
117 11th Street
Ames, IA 50010-5707
Telephone: (515)-239-2314 Fax: (515)-239-6891
Toll-Free: (800)-529-4610
Hospice care

Medical Services

Center for Adiction Recovery
511 Duff Avenue
Suite B
Ames, IA 50010-6391
Telephone: (515)-232-3206 Fax: (515)-232-3780
Toll-Free: (800)-286-3205
Contact: David Sahr - Director
Substance Abuse Treatment

Central Iowa Mental Health Center
1212 McCormick Avenue
Ames, IA 50010-6809
Telephone: (515)-232-5811
Mental Health Services

Tama County

Community Services

Mid-Iowa Community Action
219 W. 4th Street
Tama, IA 52339
Telephone: (515)-484-4713
Emergency Services: food, shelter

Home Health Care

Tama County Health Service
129 W. High St
Toledo, IA 52342-1319
Telephone: (515)-484-4788
Contact: Norma Jackson, RN - Public Health Nurse Admin
Medical services by skilled nurses, home visits

Taylor County

Community Services

Department of Human Services
309 Main St
Bedford, IA 50833-1319
Telephone: (712)-523-2129
Contact: Darla FIne
Financial Aid

Union County

Community Services

Department of Human Services
Courthouse
Lower Level
Creston, IA 50801
Telephone: (515)-782-8502
Financial Aid

MATURA Action Corporation with Centers in Lenox & Bedford
203 W. Adams
Creston, IA 50801-3106
Telephone: (515)-782-8431 Fax: (515)-782-6287
Emergency Services: Clothing, food, and shelter

Meals on Wheels
Greater Community Hosp
1700 W. Townline

Creston, IA 50801
Telephone: (515)-782-7091
Emergency services: food

Southern IA Regional Housing
219 N. Pine St
Creston, IA 50801-2413
Telephone: (515)-782-8585 Fax: (515)-782-8900
Emergency Services: Food, clothing, shelter

Home Health Care

Green Valley Hospice
1700 West Town Lane
Creston, IA 50801
Telephone: (515)-782-7091 Fax: (515)-782-2192
Contact: Kay Kinsella - Administrator
Hospice care

Medical Services

Greater Community Hospital and Green Valley Hospice
1700 W. Townline
Creston, IA 50801-1051
Telephone: (515)-782-7091
Contact: Marly Scherlin
Medical services, home care, hospice care, outpatient

Van Buren County

Community Services

Department of Human Services
Courthouse
Box 458
Keosauqua, IA 52565
Telephone: (319)-293-3791
Financial Aid

Home Health Care

Van Buren County Public Nursing Service
PO Box 122C
RR#2 Hwy 1 North
Keosauqua, IA 52565
Telephone: (319)-293-3431 Fax: (319)-293-6250
Contact: Cyndi Munson
Nursing Services

Wapello County

Community Services

Department of Human Services
116 East 3rd
Box 457
Ottumwa, IA 52501-2903
Telephone: (515)-682-8793 Fax: (515)-682-7828
Contact: Marge Fayre - Service Supervisor
In home healthcare program administered by state social worker, medicalassistance, food stamps; emergency help for evicted

SIEDA - Alcohol & Drug Services
PO Box 658
Ottumwa, IA 52501-0658
Telephone: (515)-682-8741
Contact: Roy D. Forgy
Drug & alcohol services/home care, family services, housing stabilization family development

Social Security Administration
51 West Hempstead
PO Box 987
Ottumwa, IA 52501
Telephone: (515)-472-5011
Financial Aid

Home Health Care

Hospice of Wapello County
312 East Altavista
Ottumwa, IA 52501
Telephone: (515)-682-0684
Medical Services, Hospice Care

Ottumwa Public Health Nursing Service
108 East Main Street
Ottumwa, IA 52501
Telephone: (515)-683-0671 Fax: (515)-682-5434
Contact: Cindy Ritz - Nurse Administrator
Home health care

Wapello County Public Health Nursing
108 East Main Street
PO Box 158
Ottumwa, IA 52501-2904
Telephone: (515)-685-4671
Contact: Cindy Rite
Nursing Services

Warren County

Community Services

Department of Human Services
901 East Iowa
Indianola, IA 50125-1413
Telephone: (515)-961-5353 Fax: (515)-961-4420
Contact: Karen DeVore - Service Supervisor
Home health care, medical assistance, food stamps; emergency help forevicted

Helping Hand
P.O. Box 45
Indianola, IA 50125
Telephone: (515)-961-3864
Community services

Home Health Care

Homemaker Health Aide Service
103 West 1st Avenue
Indianola, IA 50125-2420
Telephone: (515)-961-1064 Fax: (515)-961-1013
Home Care

Warren County Health Services
103 West 1st Street
Indianola, IA 50125-2420
Telephone: (515)-961-1074 Fax: (515)-961-1013
Contact: Linda Shaver
Nursing services, home care aides

Medical Services

Mental Health Services
103 West First Ave
Indianola, IA 50125-2420
Telephone: (515)-243-5181 Fax: (515)-961-1074
Contact: Larry Sanzter
Mental health services & counseling

Washington County

Medical Services

Washington County Hospital
400 E. Park Street
Washington, IA 52353
Telephone: (319)-653-5481
Contact: Jean Baumert - Infectious Control Nurse
Medical Services

Wayne County

Community Services

Department of Human Services
Courthouse
PO Box 465
Corydon, IA 50060
Telephone: (515)-872-1820
Contact: Jim Steffensmier - Service Supervisor
Home healthcare, state social worker, medical assistance, food stamps;emergency help for evicted

Home Health Care

Wayne County PHNS
417 Southeast Street
PO Box 102
Corydon, IA 50060
Telephone: (515)-872-1167 Fax: (515)-872-2260
Contact: Denise Conway
Nursing services, home health aides

Medical Services

Loan Closet
American Legion Bldg.
100 East Jefferson
Corydon, IA 50060
Telephone: (515)-872-1282
Loans medical equipment

Wayne County Hospital/HHHA
417 SE Street
Corydon, IA 50060
Telephone: (515)-872-2260 Fax: (515)-872-1329
Contact: Steve Hand
Medical Services

Webster County

Community Services

Commission of Veterans Affairs
County Courthouse
330 1st Avenue North
Fort Dodge, IA 50501
Telephone: (515)-576-1561
Emergency Services: Food, clothing, shelter

Department of Human Services
24 N. 9th Street
Box 837
Fort Dodge, IA 50501
Telephone: (515)-955-6353
Contact: Nancy Alcron
Financial aid, AIDS waiver

North Central Iowa Mental Health Center
720 South Kenyon Road
Fort Dodge, IA 50501
Telephone: (515)-955-7171
Counseling, referrals & education programs.

Salvation Army
126 N. 7th Street
Box 100
Fort Dodge, IA 50501
Telephone: (515)-576-1281
Emergency Services: Food, clothing, shelter

Home Health Care

Webster County Public Health Nursing Service
330 First Avenue N
Fort Dodge, IA 50501
Telephone: (515)-573-4107
Contact: Kitty Webster
Nursing Services

Medical Services

North Central Alcoholism/Research Foundation
726 South 17th Street
Fort Dodge, IA 50501
Telephone: (515)-576-7261
Substance abuse treatment serving north central Iowa

North Central Iowa Mental Health Center
720 South Kenyon Road
Fort Dodge, IA 50501
Telephone: (515)-955-7171
Mental Health Services

Winnebago County

Community Services

Department of Human Services
216 South Clark Street
Forest City, IA 50436-1810
Telephone: (515)-582-3271
Contact: Kathy Saber
Financial aid, medical services

Home Health Care

Public Health Nursing
216 S. Clark
Forest City, IA 50436
Telephone: (515)-582-4763
Nursing services, home care aides

Medical Services

Forest City Regional Medical Center
Route 1
PO Box 289
Forest City, IA 50436
Telephone: (515)-582-2904 Fax: (515)-582-5417
Medical Services

Winneshiek County

Home Health Care

Winneshiek County Public Health Nursing Service
201 W. Main St
Decorah, IA 52101-1775
Telephone: (319)-382-4662
Contact: Marlene Fenstermann
Nursing services, AIDS education

Medical Services

CompreCare
104 West Water Street
Decorah, IA 52101-1806
Telephone: (319)-382-8495
Medical Services

NE Iowa Mental Health Center
P.O. Box 349
Decorah, IA 52101-0349
Telephone: (319)-382-3649
Mental health service, substance abuse treatment

Winneshiek County Memorial Hospital and Healthland Health
901 Montgomery
Decorah, IA 52101-2399
Telephone: (319)-382-2911
Contact: Sally Bachman
Medical Services

Woodbury County

Community Services

A.I.D. (Assistance, Information, Direction) Center
206 6th Street
Sioux City, IA 51101-1208
Telephone: (712)-252-1861
Emergency Services: Food, clothing, shelter

Bargain Center
1001 7th Street
Sioux City, IA 51103-1913
Telephone: (712)-255-0575
Emergency Services: Clothing

Meals on Wheels
2720 Stone Park Blvd
Sioux City, IA 51104-3734
Telephone: (712)-279-3217
Emergency Services: Food

Salvation Army
P.O. Box 783
Sioux City, IA 51102-0783
Telephone: (712)-255-8836
Emergency Services: Food, clothing, shelter

Soup Kitchen
703 W. 5th Street
Sioux City, IA 51103-3719
Telephone: (712)-258-0027
Emergency Services: Food

Home Health Care

Alternative Home Care
220 S. Fairmount Street
Sioux City, IA 51107-1224
Telephone: (712)-274-7676
Nursing and other home health care

Amicare Home Health Services
500 11th Street
Sioux City, IA 51105-1427
Telephone: (712)-233-1137 Fax: (712)-233-1123
Toll-Free: (800)-383-4545
Nursing Services/Hospice

nmc HOMECARE
1925 Geneva St
Sioux City, IA 51103
Telephone: (712)-252-1678
Fax:(712)-252-1241
Contact: Pam Angerhofer
National JCAHO-Accredited company providing a full range of Infusion and Respiratory therapies and specializing in the care of HIV/AIDS patients. National Case Manager is also available at 800-445-1188

Siouxland Easter Seals Society
504 4th Street
Sioux City, IA 51101-1602
Telephone: (712)-258-5523
Contact: Mary Ann Coltey, RN, BAS
Nursing services, home health, physical therapy

Medical Services

Marian Health Center
801 5th Street
Sioux City, IA 51101-1399
Telephone: (712)-279-2296 Fax: (712)-279-2034
Contact: Ed Vanbramer - MD
Medical services

St. Luke's Regional Medical Center
2720 Stone Park Blvd
Sioux City, IA 51104-3734
Telephone: (712)-279-3500 Fax: (712)-279-7983
Medical services, mental health

Worth County

Community Services

Northwood Ministrial Association
First Lutheran Church
309 9th Street North
Northwood, IA 50459
Telephone: (515)-324-2984
Contact: Mark Gravdal
Emergency services: Food

Home Health Care

Worth County Public Health Nursing Service
849 Central Avenue
Northwood, IA 50459-1519
Telephone: (515)-324-1741 Fax: (515)-324-2195
Contact: Nancy Faber
Nursing services, AIDS education

Wright County

Community Services

Meals on Wheels
Belmond Community Hosp
403 1st Street Southeast
Belmond, IA 50421
Telephone: (515)-444-3223
Contact: Iola Tulp
Emergency services: food

Wright County Department of Human Services
115 First Street SE
Clarion, IA 50525-1401
Telephone: (515)-532-6645 Fax: (515)-532-2761
Contact: Douglas Koons
Financial Aid

Home Health Care

Wright County Public Health Nurses/Homemakr Home Health Aide
115 1st Street SE
Clarion, IA 50525-1401
Telephone: (515)-532-3461 Fax: (515)-532-3762
Contact: Alice Rector
Nursing Services and Homemaker Home Health Aide Services

KANSAS

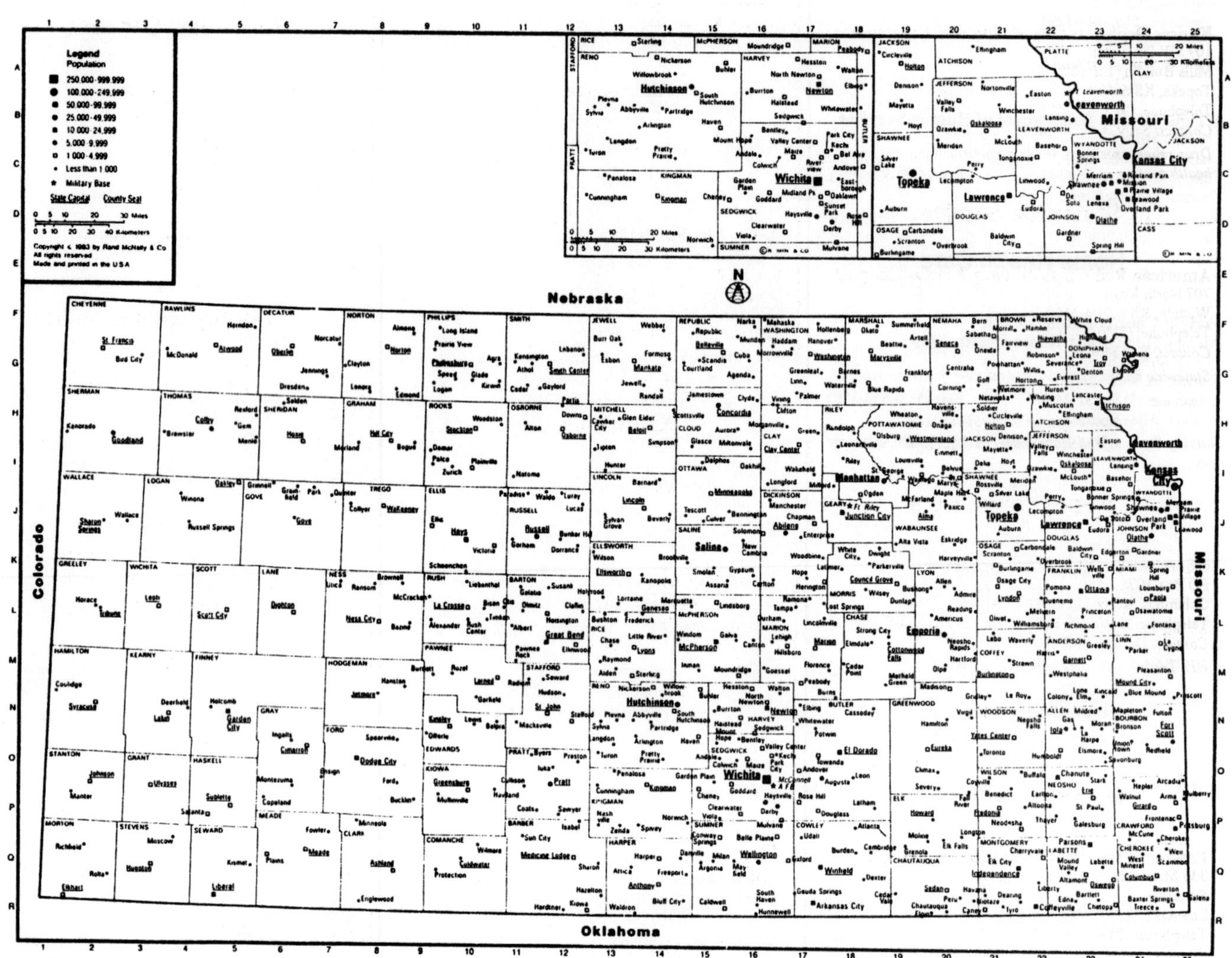

From City/County Planning Atlas Copyright 1989 by Reed McNally & Company, R.L. 90-S-28

Kansas

General Services

State Health Departments

Kansas Department of Health and Environment
109 SW 9th Street
Mills Building Ste 605
Topeka, KS 66620
Telephone: (913)-296-5587
Contact: Sally Finney Brazier - Director
Drug reimbursement, case management, home & community health care

Statewide Services

American Red Cross/Midway Kansas Chapter
707 North Main
Wichita, KS 67203-3669
Telephone: (316)-265-6601
Contact: Bev Morlan
Statewide Red Cross referral and educational services.

Cherokee County

Home Health Care

Cherokee County Health Department
PO Box 107
Columbus, KS 66725-0107
Telephone: (316)-429-3087 Fax: (316)-429-3623
Contact: Dolores Mulnix
HIV Testing and Counseling

Douglas County

County Health Depts

Lawrence/Douglas County Health Department
336 Missouri
Suite 201
Lawrence, KS 66044-1395
Telephone: (913)-843-0721
Contact: Ann Ailor
HIV testing & counseling

Home Health Care

Hospice Care in Douglas County
336 Missouri-Lower Level
Lawrence, KS 66044
Telephone: (913)-749-5006
Contact: Kay Metzger - Director
Home health care, hospice care in hospitals & nursing homes

Medical Services

Bert Nash Mental Health Center
336 Missouri
Suite 202
Lawrence, KS 66044-1390
Telephone: (913)-843-9192 Fax: (913)-843-5858
Contact: Sandra Shaw
Counseling

Ellis County

Testing Sites

Hays Planned Parenthood
122 East 12th Street
Hays, KS 67601-3608
Telephone: (913)-682-2434
Contact: Marian Shapiro - Director
Counseling, HIV Testing, Education, Public Speaking.

Ford County

Testing Sites

Dodge City Family Planning Clinic
811 North 2nd
Box 1152
Dodge City, KS 67801-5230
Telephone: (316)-225-1933
Contact: Twila M. Helfrich
HIV Testing and Counseling

Geary County

Medical Services

USA Meddac
Attn. H.S.X.X. - D.C.C.S.
Fort Riley, KS 66442
Telephone: (913)-239-7107 Fax: (913)-239-7632
Contact: Capt. Carper
Clinical Services, Education

Johnson County

County Health Depts

Johnson County Health Department
301-B South Clainbome
Olathe, KS 66062
Telephone: (913)-791-5660
Contact: Carol Stehly
HIV testing & counseling

Johnson County Health Department
301B Clairbome Rd
Olathe, KS 66062-1724
Telephone: (913)-791-1580
Contact: Beverly Wharton
Home health care, trasnportation, IV therapy, Ryan White Title II funding

Johnson County Health Department
6000 Lamar
Room 140
Mission, KS 66202-3299
Telephone: (913)-791-5660 Fax: (913)-791-5670
Contact: Phyllis Ball
Health Care and Education

Home Health Care

nmc HOMECARE
9301 W 53rd St
Merriam, KS 66203
Telephone: (913)-384-2100
Fax:(913)-384-5903
Contact: Gary Hamilton
National JCAHO-Accredited company providing a full range of Infusion and Respiratory therapies and specializing in the care of HIV/AIDS patients. National Case Manager is also available at 800-445-1188

Medical Services

Johnson County Mental Health
6000 Lamar Ave
Shawnee Mission, KS 66202-3299
Telephone: (913)-831-2550 Fax: (913)-791-5652
Contact: David Weibe
Counseling, support group

Kiowa County

County Health Depts

Kiowa County Health Department
211 East Florida
Greensburg, KS 67054-2294
Telephone: (316)-723-2136
Contact: Mitzi Hesser, RN
Health Care and Education, HIV referrals

Leavenworth County

County Health Depts

Leavenworth County Health Department
620 Olive St
Leavenworth, KS 66048-2653
Telephone: (913)-684-0730 Fax: (913)-684-0491
Contact: Linda Lobb
Health Care and Education

Medical Services

Northeast Kansas Mental Health & Guidance Center
818 N. Seventh Street
Leavenworth, KS 66048-1496
Telephone: (913)-682-5118 Fax: (913)-682-4664
Contact: Mark Boling, M.D.
Mental Health

Mc Pherson County

County Health Depts

McPherson County Health Department
1001 North Main
McPherson, KS 67460-4227
Telephone: (316)-241-1753
Contact: Carolyn Weddle
Health care and education, HIV counseling & testing

Phillips County

County Health Depts

Phillips County Health Department
Courthouse Annex
784 6th Street
Phillipsburg, KS 67661
Telephone: (913)-543-2179
Contact: Linda Shelton
AIDS prevention, adolescents & community; testing

Reno County

Community Services

Department of Social & Rehabilitation Services
PO Box 2978
Hutchinson, KS 67504-2978
Telephone: (316)-663-5731 Fax: (316)-663-7868
Contact: Judy Winters
Support Group/Rehabilitation

The Medical Center
1100 North Main
Hutchinson, KS 67501-4496
Telephone: (316)-663-2151
Contact: Anthony C. Beauchamp
Counseling for those referred from HIV Testing Sites

County Health Depts

Reno County Health Department
209 W. 2nd
Hutchinson, KS 67501-5232
Telephone: (316)-665-2900
Contact: Dana Hutchinson
Health care & AIDS education, support groups

Riley County

County Health Depts

Riley County/Manhattan Health Department
2030 Tecumseh Road
Manhattan, KS 66502-3541
Telephone: (913)-776-4779
Contact: Joan Smith
HIV Support Groups.

Saline County

County Health Depts

Salina-Saline County Health Dept.
300 West Ash
Salina, KS 67401-2335
Telephone: (913)-827-9376
Contact: Del Mierblein
Health care, HIV testing & education

Home Health Care

Hospice of Salina Inc.
333 S. Santa Fe
PO Box 2238
Salina, KS 67402
Telephone: (913)-825-1717 Fax: (913)-825-4949
Contact: Kim Fair
Home and intermediate health care, terminal care

St. John's Regional Health Center
139 N. Penn
Salina, KS 67401-3057
Telephone: (913)-827-5591 Fax: (913)-823-4358
Contact: Barbara Knight
Home and intermediate health care

Sedgwick County

Community Services

Family and Friends of Persons with AIDS
St Johns Episcopal Church
409 N Topeka
Wichita, KS 67202
Telephone: (316)-684-4890
Contact: Jody Thompson
Support group for family & friends

County Health Depts

Wichita/Sedgwick County Health Department
1900 East 9th
Wichita, KS 67214-3115
Telephone: (316)-268-8401
Contact: Patsy Abshier, Patricia McDonald -
AIDS education, HIV testing

Home Health Care

Hospice of Wichita/Connect Care
P.O. Box 3267
Wichita, KS 67201-3267
Telephone: (316)-265-9441
Home and Intermediate Health Care; Other Support

Testing Sites

University of Kansas School of Medicine CBCT
1010 North Kansas
Wichita, KS 67214
Telephone: (316)-261-2622
Contact: Dr. Donna Sweet
Research, testing, counseling

Seward County

County Health Depts

Seward County Health Department
102 West 2nd Street
Liberal, KS 67901-3445
Telephone: (316)-624-3804 Fax: (316)-624-3808
Contact: Hope Alvarez
Health Care and Education

Shawnee County

Community Services

Apostolic Church of Jesus Christ
2420 Bellview Street
Topeka, KS 66605-1750
Telephone: (913)-266-7102
Contact: Aletha Cushinberry - Pastor
Counseling; spiritual worship

Shawnee County Medical Society
1027 Southwest Gage
Topeka, KS 66604
Telephone: (913)-234-5668
Referral service

The Menninger Foundation
5800 SW 6th
Topeka, KS 66606-9699
Telephone: (913)-273-7500 Fax: (913)-273-8625
Mental Health

County Health Depts

Topeka/Shawnee County Health Department
1615 W. 8th
Topeka, KS 66606
Telephone: (913)-233-8961
Contact: Dr. Mary Tawadros
Health Care & Education

Medical Services

VA Medical Center/Colmery-O'Neil
2200 Gage Boulevard
Topeka, KS 66622-0001
Telephone: (913)-272-3111 Fax: (913)-271-4309
Contact: Ramona Brice
Medical Services for any Military Personnel

Sherman County

County Health Depts

Sherman County Health Department
919 Main Street
Goodland, KS 67735-2940
Telephone: (913)-899-5627
Contact: Sara Veselik
Health Care and AIDS Education

Wyandotte County

County Health Depts

Kansas City-Wyandotte County Health Department
619 Ann Avenue
Kansas City, KS 66101-3038
Telephone: (913)-321-4803
Contact: Edward Beasely - MPA Assistant Administrator
Health care, education, epidimeology, STD, pediatrics, lab, dental

Home Health Care

Caremark Homecare Branch Network
Cambridge Business Park
112 Greystone
Kansas City, KS 66103
Telephone: (913)-321-0714
Contact: Diana Winslow - Nurse Manager

Medical Services

Department of Preventive Medicine/KU Medical Center
4125 Rainbow Boulevard
Kansas City, KS 66103-3110
Telephone: (913)-588-2772 Fax: (913)-588-2780
Contact: Tom D.Y. Chin
AIDS epidemiology, prevention & control.

Family Health Services
1401 Southwest Boulevard
Kansas City, KS 66103-1828
Telephone: (913)-262-0550 Fax: (913)-262-0000
Contact: Sharon D. Lee - Director; Lydia A. Moore -
Health Care and Education

KENTUCKY

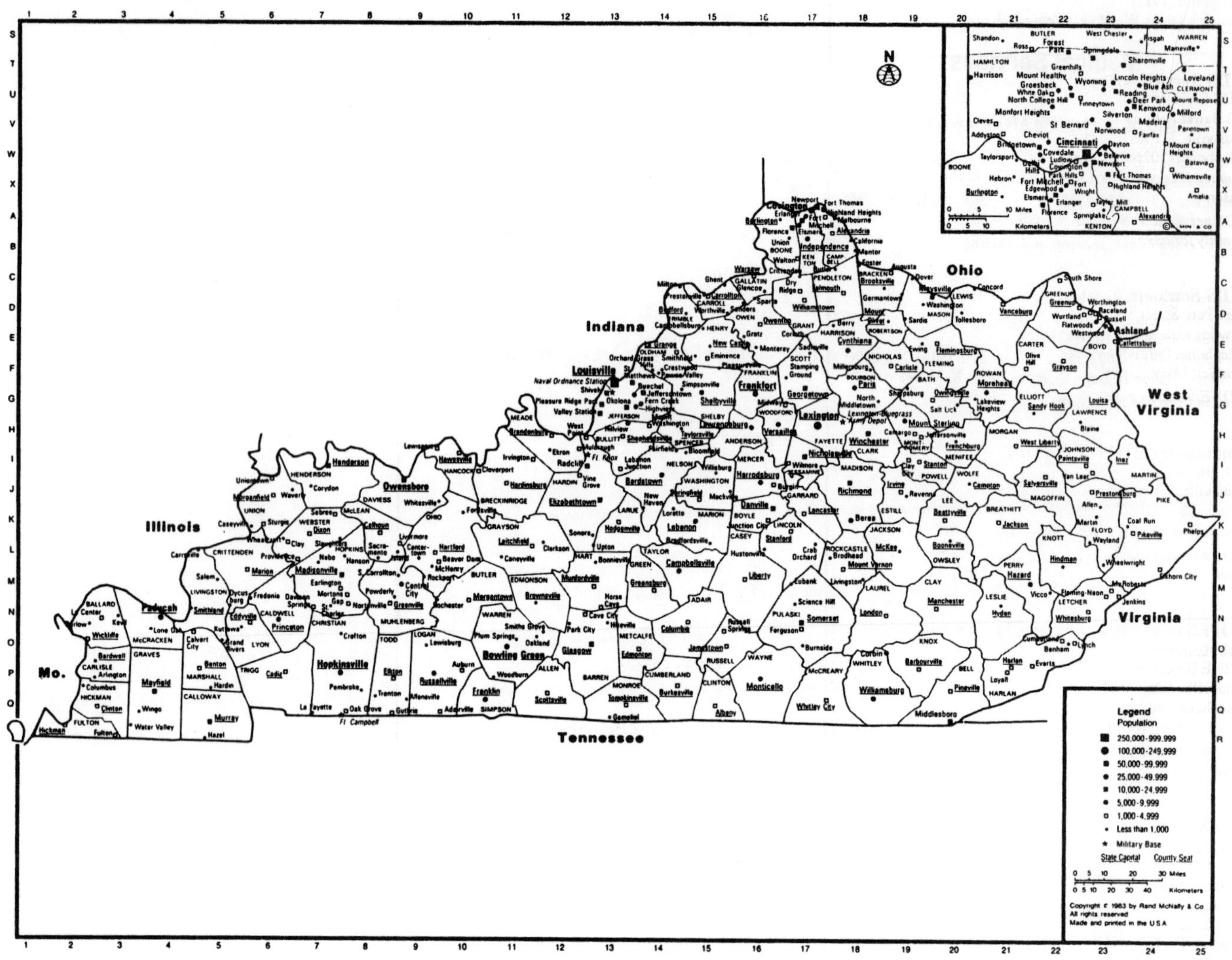

From City/County Planning Atlas Copyright 1989 by Reed McNally & Company, R.L. 90-S-28

Kentucky

General Services

Education

AIDS Services Center
AIDS Services Center
810 Barret Avenue
Louisville, KY 40204
Telephone: (502)-625-5490 Fax: (502)-574-5497
Contact: Christopher Davis - Executive Assistant; Howard Mason
AIDS prevention education, library, newsletter, education & monthly forums.

AIDS Southern Kentucky
1539 Park Street
Bowling Green, KY 41011
Telephone: (502)-745-6151
Contact: Mary Hazard
AIDS Education and Prevention.

Community Health Trust, Inc.
P.O. Box 4277
Louisville, KY 40204
Telephone: (502)-454-0306
Contact: Stephen A. Schneller
AIDS education, prevention, grants, services, financial assistance

COPES (Council on Prevention and Education: Substances)
1228 E Breckinridge
Louisville, KY 40204
Telephone: (502)-538-6820
Contact: Kim Roberts
Information on AIDS and other drug and alchohol related issues.

ERASE Project/Educ. Research for Aids and Sex Education
Kentucky State University
Hathaway Hall #215
Frankfort, KY 40601
Telephone: (502)-227-5988
Contact: Dr. Betty Griffen - Chair Person
Teacher training for certification

Jefferson County Health Department
AIDS/HIV Prevention Prgm
400 East Gray Street
Louisville, KY 40202
Telephone: (502)-625-6520
Contact: Collin C. Schwoyer
AIDS/HIV education

Kentuckiana Hemophilia Foundation
982 Eastern Parkway
Louisville, KY 40217-1566
Telephone: (502)-634-8161
Contact: Cyndthia Hall
Education and information for those with hemophilia.

Kentuckiana People with AIDS Coalition
810 Barret Avenue
Louisville, KY 40204
Telephone: (502)-625-5490 Fax: (502)-574-5497
Contact: Jamie Rittenhouse - Executive Director
HIV education and support

Northern KY AIDS Consortia
610 Medical Village Drive
823 Scott Street
Edgewood, KY 41017
Telephone: (606)-291-0770
Contact: Lynn Coomer
Advocacy, HIV prevention education, case management

Presbyterian AIDS Network, PHEWA
100 Witherspoon
Louisville, KY 40202
Telephone: (201)-846-1510
Contact: Mark Wendorf
AIDS issues and education

Hotlines

Kentucky HIV/AIDS Information
Kentucky HIV/AIDS Education Program
275 E. Main Street
Frankfort, KY 40621
Telephone: (606)-564-2500

State Health Departments

Kentucky Department for Health Services, Division of Epidemiology
275 E. Main Street
Frankfort, KY 40621KY
Telephone: (502)-574-5490
Contact: Reginald Finger - Director, Div. of Epidemiology

Kentucky Department of Health Services, AIDS/HIV Prevention Program
Frankfort, KY 40601
Telephone: (502)-564-6539
Contact: Jeff Vessels - Supervisor, AIDS
Prevention education, information

Statewide Services

Department for Social Services Office
P.O. Box 415
New Castle, KY 40050-0415
Telephone: (502)-845-2922
Contact: Keith Gunnels
Referrals

Adair County

County Health Depts

Adair County Center
904 Westlake Drive
Columbia, KY 42728-1147
Telephone: (502)-384-2286 Fax: (502)-384-4800
Social services, child protective services, medicaid, referrals, foodstamps, HIV testing

Home Health Care

Family Home Health
Grand Lane
Columbia, KY 42728-1527
Telephone: (502)-384-6411
Contact: Julie Davis
Family home health care

Westlake Home Health
P.O. Box 468
Columbia, KY 42728
Telephone: (502)-384-4753
Contact: Renne Mccloud

Allen County

County Health Depts

Allen County Health Department
207 East Locust
P.O. Box 128
Scottsville, KY 42164-0128
Telephone: (502)-237-4423 Fax: (502)-237-4777
Contact: Vesper Jones - Administrator
Home health aides, AIDS coordinator, physical therapy

Home Health Care

Allen-Monroe County Health Department
Home Health Agency
East Locust, P.O. Box 128
Scottsville, KY 42164
Telephone: (502)-237-4423 Fax: (502)-237-4777
Contact: Joyce Mansfield, RN
Health services, referrals

Anderson County

County Health Depts

Anderson County Health Department
208 South Main Street
Lawrenceburg, KY 40342-1110
Telephone: (502)-839-4551
Contact: Garland VanZant - Administrator; Lewis Wash, M.D. - Chairman
Counseling & testing.

Ballard County

County Health Depts

Ballard County Center
U.S. Highway 60
P.O. Box 357
LaCenter, KY 42056
Telephone: (502)-665-5432
Contact: Jim Cantrell
HIV counseling & testing.

Barren County

County Health Depts

Barren County Health Center
P.O. Box 1464
218 South Liberty Street
Glasgow, KY 42142-1464
Telephone: (502)-651-8321
Contact: Faye Smith
HIV testing & counseling.

Bell County

County Health Depts

Bell County Center - Branch Office
N 20th Street, City Hall
P.O. Box 160
Middlesboro, KY 40965
Telephone: (606)-248-2862
Contact: Susan Gulley
Counseling, testing

Bourbon County

County Health Depts

Bourbon County Health Department
341 East Main Street
Paris, KY 40361-2198
Telephone: (606)-987-1915 Fax: (606)-987-3230
Contact: Central Bluegrass: 987-7493; Lisa Levy, M.D. Chairperson
Testing & counseling

Boyle County

County Health Depts

Boyle County Health Department
448 South Third Street
P.O. Box 398
Danville, KY 40423-0398
Telephone: (606)-236-2053 Fax: (606)-236-2863
Contact: Harold Yankey - Administrator; Honorable Mary Pendygraft - Chairperson
Counseling & testing

Home Health Care

Heritage Hospice, Inc.
P.O. Box 1213
337 W. Broadway
Dansville, KY 40422-1213
Telephone: (606)-236-2425 Fax: (606)-236-6152
Contact: Andy Baker
In-home care

Bracken County

Community Services

Bracken County Center
Frankford Street
P.O. Box 117
Brooksville, KY 41004
Telephone: (606)-735-2157
Contact: Tim Stump - Director of Public Health
Social services, testing, counseling

Breathitt County

County Health Depts

Breathitt County Health Department
1133 Main Street
P.O. Box 730
Jackson, KY 41339-1141
Telephone: (606)-666-5274
Contact: Angie Reynolds, R.N - Acting Amin. Assistant; John C. Rice, D.M.D. - Chairman
Social Services

Breckinridge County

Community Services

Communicare Clinic
Route 1, Box 82
Mattlingly Prof. Building
Hardinsburg, KY 40143-9715
Telephone: (502)-756-5816
Mental Health Servicesand counseling HIV

Dept. for Social Services Office
P.O. Box 426
U.S. Highway 60
Hardinsburg, KY 40143-0426
Telephone: (505)-756-2196
Contact: Robert Boone
Social services

Home Health Care

Breckenridge County Home Health
Lincoln Trail Dist Health
Old US 60
Hardinsburg, KY 40143
Telephone: (502)-756-5461

Testing Sites

Breckinridge County Center
Courthouse, Public Square
P.O. Box 456
Hardinsburg, KY 40143
Telephone: (502)-756-5121
Contact: Monica Jarboe, R.N.
HIV testing (anonymous & confidential), counseling, referrals, education

Bullitt County

County Health Depts

Bullitt County Health Department
181 Lees Valley Road
P.O. Box 278
Shepherdsville, KY 40165-5902
Telephone: (502)-543-2415
Contact: Edmund J. Fitzgibbons - Administrator; James R. Cundiff, M.D. - Chairman
Social services, HIV testing (confidential), referrals, counseling

Butler County

Community Services

Dept. for Social Services Office
111 North Tyler
P.O. Box 279
Morgantown, KY 42261-8434
Telephone: (505)-526-3833
Referrals, counseling, foster care

County Health Depts

Butler County Health Center
104 North Warren Street
P.O. Box 99
Morgantown, KY 42261-7924
Telephone: (502)-526-3221
Contact: Sandra Martin, RN
HIV testing (anonymous & confidential), counseling, referrals

Caldwell County

Home Health Care

Western Kentucky IV Services Inc. - O.P.T.I.O.N. Care
108 East Washington St
Princeton, KY 42445-2250
Telephone: (800)-877-0345
Contact: Steve P'Pool - President
Home IV and Nutritional Services

Testing Sites

Caldwell County Center
310 Hawthorne Street
P.O. Box 327
Princeton, KY 42445-1622
Telephone: (502)-365-6571
Contact: Raymond Giannini; Beckie Buchaan -
Education, HIV testing (confidential & anonymous), counseling, referrals

Calloway County

County Health Depts

Calloway County Center
701 Olive Street
P.O. Box 1115
Murray, KY 42071-1944
Telephone: (502)-753-3381 Fax: (502)-759-1711
Contact: B.J. Weathers, R.N. - Supervisor
Anonymous HIV testing, counseling, referrals, literature

Campbell County

County Health Depts

Campbell County Center
12 East Fifth Street
Newport, KY 41071-1618
Telephone: (606)-431-1704
Contact: Alice Nelter, R.N.
Anonymous HIV testing counseling, referrals, education, STD counseling.

Carlisle County

Testing Sites

Carlisle County Center
East Court Street
P.O. Box 96
Bardwell, KY 42023
Telephone: (502)-628-5431
Contact: Anne Reed, R.N.
HIV testing (anonymous & confidential) counseling, referrals

Carroll County

County Health Depts

Carroll County Center
401 11th Street
P.O. Box 98
Carrollton, KY 41008-1451
Telephone: (502)-732-6641
Contact: Kathy Harvey, R.N.
Anonymous HIV testing, counseling, referrals, education, STD education.

Carter County

County Health Depts

Carter County Center
U.S. 60 East
P.O. Box 919
Grayosn, KY 41143
Telephone: (606)-474-5100
Contact: Loretta Murphy, R.N.
Social services; anonymous HIV testing, counseling, education, referrals.

West Carter Center
Hitchins Avenue
P.O. Box 728
Olive Hill, KY 41164
Telephone: (606)-286-6000
Contact: Ellen Blevin - Coordinator
Social Services; HIV testing, counseling, education, referrals.

Casey County

County Health Depts

Casey County Center
Route 2, Sharp Drive
P.O. Box 778
Liberty, KY 42539-0778
Telephone: (606)-787-6911 Fax: (606)-787-2507
Contact: Susan Hoskins, R.N.
Social services; anonymous HIV testing, counseling, education, referrals,literature.

Home Health Care

Lake Cumberland Home Health
Route 1, Box 5-A
Liberty, KY 42539-9821
Telephone: (606)-787-9224
Skilled nursing, physical therapy, speech therapy, occupationaltherapy, personal care and home making

Christian County

County Health Depts

Christian County Health Department
1700 Canton Street
P.O. Box 647
Hopkinsville, KY 42240-1923
Telephone: (502)-887-4160
Contact: Anita Simmons - Acting Admin. Assistant; William C. Dew, D.M.D. - Chairman
Social services, testing & counseling, prenatal care

Clark County

Community Services

Bluegrass East Comeprehensive Mental Health Care Center
26 North Highland
Winchester, KY 40391-2024
Telephone: (606)-744-2562
Contact: Ron Kibbey
AIDS counseling; mental health clinic

Dept. for Social Services Office
11 South Highland Street
Winchester, KY 40391-0335
Telephone: (606)-745-4771
Contact: Sherman Weider
Referrals

County Health Depts

Clark County Health Department
400 Professional Avenue
Winchester, KY 40391-1184
Telephone: (606)-744-4482
Contact: Len Midden - Adminsitrator; Mark Barrett, M.D. - Chairman
Social services, testing & counseling for AIDS; general prenatal care family planning, immunizations

Home Health Care

Clark County Health Department
Home Health Agency
400 Professional Avenue
Winchester, KY 40391-1184
Telephone: (606)-744-1488
HIV testing/counseling, home health; physical, occupational & speechtherapy; social services

Hospice East, Inc.
1107 West Lexington Ave.
Winchester, KY 40391-1165
Telephone: (606)-745-3500
Contact: Carol Richardson - Director
Home care services for terminally ill patients in Clark & Powell counties.

Clay County

County Health Depts

Clay County Center
100 South Court Street
Manchester, KY 40962-1284
Telephone: (606)-598-2425 Fax: (606)-598-1546
Contact: Kathy Fields
Social Services; anonymous HIV testing, counseling, referrals, education,literature.

Clinton County

County Health Depts

Clinton County Health Center
201 Twin Lake Medical Arts
P.O. Box 383
Albany, KY 42602
Telephone: (606)-387-5711
Contact: Kathy Bernanrd, RN - County AIDS Coordinator
HIV testing, counseling

Cumberland County

Community Services

Dept. for Social Services Office
Smith Street
P.O. Box 372
Burkesville, KY 42717
Telephone: (606)-864-3834
Contact: Frances Abston

County Health Depts

Cumberland County Center
Celina Street
P.O. Box 412
Burkesville, KY 42717-9415
Telephone: (502)-864-2206 Fax: (502)-864-1232
Contact: Jean Bishop
Referrals, HIV testing, counseling, education, literature.

Cumberland County Health Department
Branch Office
P.O. Box 412
Burcksville, KY 42717
Telephone: (502)-864-2206
Contact: Sandra Hoots
Referrals, HIV testing, counseling, education, literature

Estill County

County Health Depts

Estill County Health Department
River Drive, Highway #52
P.O. Box 115
Irvine, KY 40336
Telephone: (606)-723-5181
Social services, testing & counseling, prenatal care, TB testing

Fayette County

Community Services

AIDS Volunteers of Lexington
214 W Maxwell St
PO Box 431
Lexington, KY 40585-0431
Contact: Pam Goldman
Support group, buddy system, hotline & speakers

Dept. for Social Services Office
120 West High Street
Lexington, KY 40508-1207
Telephone: (606)-252-3587
Contact: Ben McClellan
Social services

County Health Depts

Lexington-Fayette County Health Department
650 Newtown Pike
Lexington, KY 40508-1113
Telephone: (606)-252-2371
Contact: Margaret Levin - Counselor
Social/support services, counseling, testing, referrals

Home Health Care

Bluegrass Home Health Lexington/Fayette County Health Dept
650 Newton Pike
Lexington, KY 40508-1113
Telephone: (606)-252-2371
Contact: Maria Raab

Hospice of the Bluegrass
2312 Alexandria Dr.
Lexington, KY 40504-3277
Telephone: (606)-276-5344
Contact: Gretchen M. Brown
For terminally ill patients (less than 6 months), home care.

O.P.T.I.O.N Care
501 Darby Creek Road
Suite 5
Lexington, KY 40509
Telephone: (606)-263-1103 Fax: (606)-263-1214
Contact: Janet Wilson
Home IV and Nutritional Services

Fleming County

County Health Depts

Fleming County Health Department
Court Square
Flemingsburg, KY 41041-1399
Telephone: (606)-845-6511
Contact: Donald Colgan - Administrator
Social services; education, seminars, testing

Floyd County

Community Services

Appalacian Research and Defense Fund
28 North Front Street
Prestonburg, KY 41653
Telephone: (606)-886-3876 Fax: (606)-886-3704
Contact: John Rosenberg
Legal aid referrals

County Health Depts

Floyd County Health Department
21 Front Street
P.O. Box 188
Prestonburg, KY 41653
Telephone: (606)-886-2788
Social services, HIV testing & counseling

Franklin County

Community Services

Dept. for Social Services Office
102 Metro Street
Frankfort, KY 40601-1985
Telephone: (502)-564-3540 Fax: (502)-564-6425
Contact: Sally Bowzer
Investigative cases, foster care, HIV/AIDS policy, 24 hour service,referral

County Health Depts

Franklin County Health Department
100 Glenns Creek Road
Frankfort, KY 40601-2363
Telephone: (502)-564-7647
Contact: Freddie Goins - Administrator; O.M. Patrick, M.D. - Chairman
Social Services

Home Health Care

Franklin County Health Department
Home Health Agency
124 West Todd
Frankfort, KY 40601
Telephone: (502)-223-1744
Contact: 502-223-2017 nights & wkends,
Home health aides, all therapies, medical & social services, medicalsupplies.

Fulton County

Community Services

Fulton County Center
West Fulton Office
402 Troy
Hickman, KY 42050
Telephone: (502)-236-2825
Contact: Kay Shaw
Social Services

Garrard County

Community Services

Garrard County Center
104 South Campbell Street
Lancaster, KY 40444-1208
Telephone: (606)-792-2462 Fax: (606)-792-3147
Social Services

Grant County

Community Services

Dept. for Social Services Office
202 North Main Street
Williamsport, KY 41097-1110
Telephone: (606)-824-4471
Contact: Judy Curry

County Health Depts

Grant County Center
234 Barnes Road
Williamstown, KY 41097
Telephone: (606)-824-5074
Contact: Linda Boulin
Social services; health services, HIV information, referral, testing

Graves County

County Health Depts

Graves County Center
North 7th & Lockridge
P.O. Box 414
Mayfield, KY 42066
Telephone: (502)-247-3553
Contact: Peggy Hayes
Social services, health services

Grayson County

County Health Depts

Grayson County Center
124 East White Oak Street
P.O. Box 176
Leitchfield, KY 42754-1447
Telephone: (502)-259-3141
Contact: Philys Anderson
Health services, HIV/AIDS testing

Green County

Community Services

Green County Center
103 South First Street
Greensburg, KY 42743-1501
Telephone: (502)-932-4341
Contact: June Burton - District Director
Social services, pre & post testing for HIV, health service

Home Health Care

Lake Cumberland Home Health
702 Columbia Hwy.
Suite A
Greensburg, KY 42743-1027
Telephone: (502)-932-7427
Contact: Sharon Watson, RN
Skilled nursing, home speech therapy, medical & physical therapy

Greenup County

County Health Depts

Greenup County Health Department
U.S. 23; P.O. Box 377
Greenup, KY 41144
Telephone: (606)-473-9838
Contact: Curtis Hieneman - Acting Admin. Assistant; J.G. Boggs, M.D. - Chairman
Social services; health services

Hancock County

Community Services

Hancock County Center
Harrison Street
P.O. Box 275
Hawesville, KY 42348
Telephone: (502)-927-8803
Contact: Denise Long - Nursing Supervisor
Social services, health service, testing & counseling for HIV/AIDS

Hardin County

Community Services

Hardin County Center
Woodland Drive-Layman Ln
P.O. Box 250
Elizabethtown, KY 42701
Telephone: (502)-765-6196
Contact: Barbara Kealford
Social Services

Home Health Care

Hospice of Central Kentucky
105 Ricg Road
Elizabethtown, KY 42702
Telephone: (502)-737-6300
In-home nursing, hospice care

Hospice of Central Kentucky
P.O. Box 2149
Elizabethtown, KY 42702-0368
Telephone: (502)-737-6300
Contact: Stephen R. Connor, PhD
Home health care, bereavement support

Harlan County

County Health Depts

Harlan County Center
403 Clover Street
P.O. Box 309
Harlan, KY 40831-0309
Telephone: (606)-573-4820 Fax: (606)-573-6128
Social Services

Harrison County

Community Services

Social Security Administration Office
604 West Main Street
Human Resources
Fort Mitchell, KY 47117
Telephone: (606)-567-7281
Contact: Ruby Roberts
Financial assistance

Hart County

County Health Depts

Hart County Center
505 Fairground Road
P.O. Box 65
Munfordville, KY 42765
Telephone: (502)-524-2511
Social Services

Henderson County

County Health Depts

Henderson County Center
438 Fifth Street
P.O. Box 13
Henderson, KY 42420-3052
Telephone: (502)-826-3951
Contact: Billye Ruth Staples - RN
HIV testing; pre & post test counseling, follow-up referrals, youthawareness & AIDS/HIV education program

Henry County

Community Services

Seven Counties Mental Health Servives, Inc.
P.O. Box 193
Emminence, KY 40019-0193
Telephone: (502)-845-2928 Fax: (502)-589-8614
Contact: Carol Carrits - Director
Education, preventive care HIV/AIDS, referral

Home Health Care

North Central District Health Department
Home Health Agency
P.O. Box 358
New Castle, KY 40050
Telephone: (502)-845-2761
Contact: Mary Ann Bright

Hickman County

County Health Depts

Hickman County Center
370 South Washington St.
Clinton, KY 42031-1324
Telephone: (502)-653-6110
Contact: Janie Holder, RN
HIV testing, pre & post test counseling, follow-up referrals, youthawareness & AIDS/HIV education program

Hopkins County

County Health Depts

Hopkins County Health Department
412 North Kentucky Ave.
P.O. Box 1266
Madisonville, KY 42431-1711
Telephone: (502)-821-5242
Contact: Jack Morris - Adminsitrator; Honorable Hanson Slaton - Chairman
HIV testing; pre & post test counseling; follow up referrals, youthawareness & AIDS/HIV education program

Jackson County

County Health Depts

Jackson County Center
Highway 421
P.O. Box 250
McKee, KY 40447
Telephone: (606)-287-8421
Contact: Diana Lakes - RN
HIV testing; pre & post test counseling; follow-up referrals, youthawareness & AIDS/HIV education program

Jefferson County

Community Services

ACLU AIDS Task Force
425 West Muhammed Ali Blvd.
Louisville, KY 40202
Telephone: (502)-581-1181
Legal information and advocacy, educational services & referrals

Glade House - Community Health Trust
AIDS Services Center
810 Barret Avenue
Louisville, KY 40204
Telephone: (502)-634-1789
Contact: Steve Schneller
Transitional facility for persons with AIDS.

Human Resources Cabinet,Division of Disability Determination
7th and West Jefferson
Louisville, KY 40202
Telephone: (502)-588-4404
Contact: Emileen Tindle
Medical determination of disabilities after Social Security application.

Kentucky Lawyer Referral Service
707 West Main Street
Louisville, KY 40202
Telephone: (800)-372-2999
A Service of the Louisville Bar Association.

Kentucky Lawyer Referral Service
707 West Main Street
Louisville, KY 40202
Telephone: (800)-372-2999
A Service of the Louisville Bar Association.

Kentucky Lawyer Referral Service
707 West Main Street
Louisville, KY 40202
Telephone: (800)-372-2999
A Service of the Louisville Bar Association.

Kentucky Minority AIDS Council
c/o Lincoln Foundation
233 West Broadway
Louisville, KY 40202
Telephone: (502)-585-4733 Fax: (502)-585-9648
Contact: Sam Robinson

Formed to prevent the spread of AIDS in the black community.

Legal Aid Society
Urban County Govemment Center
810 Barret Avenue-Suite 652
Louisville, KY 40204-2354
Telephone: (502)-574-8199 Fax: (502)-574-5497
Contact: Jeffrey Been
Legal Counsel services for civil cases for persons living with HIV and AIDS

Mothers and Others
AIDS Services Center
810 Barret Avenue Room 266-B
Louisville, KY 40204
Telephone: (502)-944-6120
Support group for mother and others who have a loved one with AIDS

Fred Schloemer Counseling Services
204 Executive Park
Sherbum Lane
Louisville, KY 40207
Telephone: (502)-895-3386
Counseling for individuals, couples and families for AIDS related issues.

United Way Information and Referral
Metro United Way
334 East Broadway
Louisville, KY 40202
Telephone: (502)-583-2821 Fax: (502)-583-0330
Contact: Rob Reifsnyder - President
Information and referrals.

County Health Depts

Jefferson County Health Depart., STD Clinic
850 Barret Avenue, #301
Louisville, KY 40204
Telephone: (502)-625-6699
Information, STD services

Louisville-Jefferson County Health Department
P.O. Box 1704
Louisville, KY 40201-1704
Telephone: (502)-574-6530 Fax: (502)-574-5734
Contact: David R. Cundiff, M.D., M.P.H - Director, Mason Rudd - Chairman
Social Services, HIV/STD Testing and Counseling.

Home Health Care

Caretenders
9200 Shelbyville Road
Louisville, KY 40222-8505
Telephone: (502)-896-2281
Contact: Bernice Wygal
Skilled nursing,In-home IV therapy,home health aides,Accepts Medicaid,Medicare.

Olsten Kimberly Quality Care
100 Mallard Creek Road
Suite 300
Louisville, KY 40207-4802
Telephone: (502)-893-8888
Contact: Debbie Kennedy
Skilled nursing, in-home therapy, home health aides

Olsten Kimberly Quality Care
710 Executive Park
Louisville, KY 40207-4675
Telephone: (502)-895-4213
Contact: Dana Fallot
Skilled nursing, in-home IV therapy, home health aides

Visiting Nurses Association
101 W. Chestnut
Louisville, KY 40202-3807
Telephone: (502)-584-2456 Fax: (502)-584-8059
Toll-Free: (800)-346-4577
Contact: Elizabeth Runyon
Skilled nursing, home health aides, IV therapy

Medical Services

KY Hemophilia Program / Brown Cancer Center
529 South Jackson Street
Louisville, KY 40202
Telephone: (502)-582-8479
Contact: Mary Maraso
Testing & counseling, referrals

KY Hemophilia Program / KY Program for Handicapped Children
982 Eastern Parkway
Louisville, KY 40217-1566
Telephone: (502)-588-4459 Fax: (502)-595-3175
Contact: Donna Vaughn , MSW
HIV information

Testing Sites

Planned Parenthood of Louisville, Inc.
1025 S Second Street
Louisville, KY 40203-0855
Telephone: (502)-584-2471 Fax: (502)-584-2476
Contact: Rosalind Heinz
HIV screening, AIDS/risk prevention education, counseling

Jessamine County

County Health Depts

Jessamine County Health Department
215 East Maple Street
Nicholasville, KY 40356-1527
Telephone: (606)-885-4149
Contact: Joanne Morgan
HIV/AIDS Health Services

Johnson County

County Health Depts

Johnson County Health Department
Second and Wood Streets
P.O. Box 111
Paintsville, KY 41240
Telephone: (606)-789-2590 Fax: (606)-789-8888
Contact: Patricia Pelphrey - Administrative Specialist
HIV testing/counseling

Home Health Care

Hospice of Big Sandy, Inc.
236 College Street
Red-Brown-William Bldg.
Paintsville, KY 41240
Telephone: (606)-789-3841 Fax: (606)-789-1527
Toll-Free: (800)-998-9144
Contact: Claire Arsanault
In home care

Hospice of Big Sandy, Inc.
PO Box 1747
Paintsville, KY 41240
Telephone: (606)-789-1527 Fax: (800)-998-9144
Contact: Calire Aresenault - Executive Director
Home care for the terminally ill, nursing care, bereavement counseling,social services

Johnson/Magoffin County Home Health Agency
Home Health Agency
P.O. Box 111, 2nd & Wood Street
Paintsville, KY 41240
Telephone: (606)-789-2596 Fax: (606)-789-3244
Contact: Anna Bowen, RN - Coordinator
Nursing, AIDS assistant, home making chores, speech therapy

Kenton County

County Health Depts

North Kentucky District Health Department
Health Education Division
610 Medical Village Drive
Edgewood, KY 41017
Telephone: (606)-341-4264 Fax: (606)-341-2631
Contact: Cathy-Kuntel Mains
AIDS prevention education, case management

Home Health Care

St. Elizabeth Medical Center Hospice
2002 Madison Avenue
Covington, KY 41014-1585
Telephone: (606)-292-4256 Fax: (606)-292-4120
Contact: Becky Fritz
Home health aides, physical therapy

Testing Sites

Kenton County Center
912 Scott Street
Covington, KY 41011-3142
Telephone: (606)-581-3886
Contact: Karen Gamer,LPN
Social services; anonymous, free HIV testing; counseling,referrals, education

Kenton County Health Center
912 Scott Street
Covington, KY 41011-2447
Telephone: (606)-291-0770
Contact: Eric Washington
Anonymous testing, counseling, referrals, education

Knott County

Testing Sites

Knott County Center
West Main Street
Highway 60
Hindman, KY 41822
Telephone: (606)-785-3144
Contact: Ella Sexton, R.N.
HIV testing (anonymous & confidential), counseling, referrral, education

Knox County

County Health Depts

Knox County Health Department
Liberty Street
P.O. Box 1689
Barbourville, KY 40906-0897
Telephone: (606)-546-3486
Contact: Judy Kelly, R.N.
HIV testing (anonymous & confidential), counseling, referral, education

Larue County

County Health Depts

Larue County Center
215 East Main St
Hodgenville, KY 42748-1305
Telephone: (502)-358-3844 Fax: (502)-358-4239
Contact: Joyce Walsh, R.N.
Social services; anonymous HIV testing, referrals, education

Home Health Care

Larue County Home Health
215 East Main Street
Hodgenville, KY 42748-1305
Telephone: (502)-358-3155 Fax: (502)-358-4539
Contact: Susie Shelley - Home Health Director
Skilled mursing, home health aides, physical therapy, speech therapy

Laurel County

County Health Depts

Cumberland Valley District Health Department
Branch Office
Regional State Office Bld
London, KY 40741
Telephone: (606)-598-5564 Fax: (606)-598-6615
Contact: Martha Blair
AIDS education, STD counseling, HIV testing & counseling.

Laurel County Health Department
310 West Third
London, KY 40741-1899
Telephone: (606)-864-5187
Contact: Ruth Gaines - Administrator
Social Services

Lawrence County

Testing Sites

Lawrence County Center
1080 Meadowbrook Lane
P.O. Box 596
Louisa, KY 41230
Telephone: (606)-638-4389
Contact: Phyllis Ward, R.N.
HIV testing (anonymous & confidential), counseling, referrals

Lee County

Community Services

Lee County Center
Center Street
P.O. Box 587
Beattyville, KY 41311
Telephone: (606)-464-2492
Social Services

Letcher County

County Health Depts

Leslie County Center
Comer Broadway & Webb
P.O. Box 300
Whitesburg, KY 41858
Telephone: (606)-672-2393
Contact: Jean Hoskins - RN
HIV testing; pre & post test counseling, follow-up referrals, youthawareness & AIDS/HIV education program

Lewis County

County Health Depts

Lewis County Health Department
905 Fairland Drive
P.O. Box 219
Vanceburg, KY 41179
Telephone: (606)-796-2632
Contact: Linda Stafford - Acting Admin. Assistant; Eugena Forman, R.N. - Chairperson
Social Services

Lincoln County

Community Services

Dept. for Social Services Office
PO Box 358 Stanford
Stanford, KY 40484
Telephone: (606)-365-3551
Contact: Kathy Hill
Referrals & counseling

County Health Depts

Lincoln County Health Department
44 Healthway
Stanford, KY 40484
Telephone: (606)-365-3106
Contact: Charles E. Crase, M.D. - Chairman
Testing & counseling

Livingston County

County Health Depts

Livingston County Center
124 State Street
P.O. Box 128
Smithland, KY 42081
Telephone: (502)-928-2193 Fax: (502)-928-2098
Contact: Linda Belt - Coordinator
Anonymous HIV testing, counseling, referrals, education.

Livingston County Center
124 State Street
P.O. Box 128
Smithland, KY 42081
Telephone: (502)-928-2193 Fax: (502)-928-2098
Contact: Linda Belt
Screening, anonymous HIV testing, referrals, counseling.

Logan County

County Health Depts

Logan County Center
151 South Franklin Street
Russellville, KY 42276-1934
Telephone: (502)-726-8341
Contact: Georgia Davis, R.N.
Social services; anonymous HIV testing, counseling, referrals, education.

Lyon County

County Health Depts

Lyon County Center
Fairview Ave. & Hillwood
P.O. Box 96
Eddyville, KY 42038
Telephone: (502)-388-9763 Fax: (502)-388-5941
Contact: Beverly Jones, ARNP
Social services; anonymous HIV testing, counseling, referrals, literature

Madison County

Community Services

Social Security Administration Office
620 University Shopping Center
Richmond, KY 40475
Telephone: (606)-624-5714
Contact: Gerry Hunt - Branch Manager

County Health Depts

Madison County Health Department
Boggs Lane
P.O. Box 906
Richmond, KY 40476
Telephone: (606)-623-7312
Contact: Dolly Lynch, R.N.
HIV testing (anonymous & confidential), counseling, referral, education

Home Health Care

Hospice of the Kentucky River
210 St. George Street
Richmond, KY 40475
Telephone: (606)-624-8820 Fax: (606)-624-9230
Care for terminal ill

Madison County Health Department
Mepco Home Health Agency
214 Boggs Lane, PO Box 906
Richmond, KY 40475
Telephone: (606)-623-3441 Fax: (606)-623-5910
Contact: Mary Lou Whitt - Coordinator
Skilled nursing, physical therapy, speech therapy, occupational therapy,& home health care aides

Magoffin County

County Health Depts

Magoffin County Health Department
723 Parkway Drive
P.O. Box 610
Salyersville, KY 41465-9740
Telephone: (606)-349-6212
Contact: Kathy Hembree - Administrator
HIV testing, counseling, group education, referrals, literature.

Marion County

Community Services

Marion County Center
516 North Spalding
Lebanon, KY 40033-1023
Telephone: (502)-692-3393
Social Services

Home Health Care

Marion County Health Center, Marion/Washington County Home Health
516 North Spalding Avenue
Lebanon, KY 40033-1023
Telephone: (502)-692-9705 Fax: (502)-358-4239
Contact: Susie Shelley - Home Health Director
Skilled nursing, home health aides, physical & speech therapy, Medicaidwaiver

Marshall County

County Health Depts

Marshall County Health Department
307 East 12th Street
Benton, KY 42025-1525
Telephone: (502)-527-1496 Fax: (502)-527-5321
Contact: Susie Tynes - Acting Administrator
Social services, HIV testing & counseling center

Martin County

County Health Depts

Martin County Health Department
Main Street
P.O. Box 354
Inez, KY 41224
Telephone: (606)-298-7752
Contact: Jane Bond - Administrator
Social Services

Home Health Care

Martin County Home Health
P.O. Box 1289
Inez, KY 41224-1289
Telephone: (606)-298-7748 Fax: (606)-298-3922
Toll-Free: (800)-377-6244
Contact: Mary Kolotar - Unit Coordinator
Home health agency: skilled nurses, RN, certified nurses aides

Mason County

County Health Depts

Mason County Center
120 West Third Street
P.O. Box 266
Maysville, KY 41056-1013
Telephone: (606)-564-9447
Social Services

McCracken County

Community Services

Paducah-McCracken County Center
916 Kentucky Avenue
P.O. Box 2357
Paducah, KY 42002-1955
Telephone: (502)-444-9631
Contact: Jim Cantrell
Social services, case management services, assistance for income-eligiblepersons

McCreary County

County Health Depts

McCreary County Center
P.O. Box 208
Whitley City, KY 42653-0208
Telephone: (606)-376-2412 Fax: (606)-376-3815
Social Services

McLean County

Testing Sites

McLean County Center
310 West Seventh Street
Calhoun, KY 42327-2046
Telephone: (502)-273-3062
HIV testing

Meade County

Testing Sites

Meade County Center
520 Fairway Drive
Brandenburg, KY 40108-0306
Telephone: (502)-422-3988
Testing and counseling

Menifee County

Testing Sites

Menifee County Center
Main Street
P.O. Box 106
Frenchburg, KY 40322
Telephone: (606)-768-2151
HIV testing & counseling

Mercer County

Testing Sites

Mercer County Center
411 North Greenville St.
Harrodsburg, KY 40330-1202
Telephone: (606)-734-4522
Contact: West Bluegrass: 748-5242
Testing

Monroe County

County Health Depts

Monroe County Health Department
P.O. Box 247
Tompkinsville, KY 42167-0247
Telephone: (502)-487-6782
Contact: Charlotte Turner - Acting Admin. Assistant
Testing & counseling

Montgomery County

Testing Sites

Montgomery County Center
117 Civic Center
Mt. Sterling, KY 40353-1400
Telephone: (606)-498-3808
Testing & counseling

Morgan County

County Health Depts

Morgan County Health Center
493-A Riverside Dr.
West Liberty, KY 41472
Telephone: (606)-743-3744
Contact: Donna Payne
Health care-HIV testing

Muhlenberg County

County Health Depts

Muhlenberg County Health Department
Legion Drive
P.O. Box 148
Central City, KY 42330
Telephone: (502)-754-3200

Contact: Jeanette Williams - Administrative Specialist
Testing and pre-test counseling

Nelson County

County Health Depts

Nelson County Health Department
325 South Third Street
Bardstown, KY 40004-1046
Telephone: (502)-348-3222
Contact: Shirley Martin, R.N. - Acting Admin. Assistant
Testing, pre- & post-test counseling

Home Health Care

Hospice of Nelson County
P.O. Box 471
118 E. Broadway
Bardstown, KY 40004-0471
Telephone: (502)-348-3660   Fax: (502)-349-1292
Contact: Sharon Bade
Nursing, social services, testing, AIDS volunteers, family bereavementcounseling

Nazareth Home Health
P.O. Box 47
Nazareth, KY 40048
Telephone: (502)-348-1585   Fax: (502)-348-1527
Contact: Mary Ellen Ritchie
Statewide call 1-800-633-9844.

Nicholas County

Testing Sites

Nicholas County Center
2330 Concrete Road
Carlisle, KY 40311
Telephone: (606)-289-2188
Testing and counseling

Oldham County

Community Services

Seven Counties Mental Health Services
1919 Highway 53
P.O. Box 233
LaGrange, KY 40031
Telephone: (502)-589-8600   Fax: (502)-589-8614
Contact: Carol Carrits - Director
Referrals, education, preventive care

County Health Depts

Oldham County Health Department
Highway 146
P.O. Box 53
LaGrange, KY 40031
Telephone: (502)-222-3516   Fax: (502)-222-0816
Contact: Paul Cuffe - Acting Admin. Assistant; Mr. Jere Kiesel - Chairman
Referrals, counseling, testing

Owen County

Home Health Care

Three Rivers District Health Dept.
North Main Park, Rt 5
327 North Main Park, Route 5
Owenton, KY 40359
Telephone: (502)-484-3412   Fax: (502)-484-0834
Contact: Debra Chapman
Skilled nursing, physical therapy

Three Rivers District Health Dept. Home Health Agency
327 North Main Street
Suite 5
Owenton, KY 40359
Telephone: (502)-484-3412
Contact: Debbie Chapman
AIDS/HIV Health Care Services

Testing Sites

Owen County Center
Route 4, Box 12
Highway 22E
Owenton, KY 40359-9402
Telephone: (502)-484-5736   Fax: (502)-484-3413
Contact: Mary Francis Hardin
Testing, counseling, referrals, community education

Owsley County

Testing Sites

Owsley County Center
Highway 28
P.O. Box 220
Booneille, KY 41314
Telephone: (606)-593-5181   Fax: (606)-593-6082
Contact: Deana Mc Intosh
Screening, counseling and referrals

Perry County

Testing Sites

Perry County Center
239 Lovern Street
P.O. Box 599
Hazard, KY 41701-1793
Telephone: (606)-436-2196
Contact: Kentucky River: 439-2361
Testing, pre-test and post-test counseling

Pike County

Home Health Care

Home Health Care Services, Inc.
546 South Mayo Trail
Pikeville, KY 41501-1546
Telephone: (606)-432-2111   Fax: (606)-437-1000
Contact: Robin McPeer
Home health: hospice

Powell County

County Health Depts

Powell County Health Department
376 North Main Street
P.O. Box 460
Stanton, KY 40380-2171
Telephone: (606)-663-4360
Contact: Linda Fagan, M.D. - Health Officer
Testing & counseling

Pulaski County

County Health Depts

Pulaski County Center
500 Bourne Avenue
Somerset, KY 42501-1916
Telephone: (606)-679-4416
HIV testing & counseling

Home Health Care

Hospice of Lake Cumberland
108 College Street
P.O. Box 651
Somerset, KY 42502-0651
Telephone: (606)-679-4389
Contact: Tom Adams
Nursing services, 24 hour on call, home maker & personal care, socialservices, chaplain

Lake Cumberland Home Health
310 Langdon Street
Somerset, KY 42501
Telephone: (606)-679-7439
Contact: Susan Wilson
1-800-432-9838 for outlying area codes: health care

Robertson County

County Health Depts

Robertson County Health Department
Main Street
P.O. Box 72
Mt. Olivet, KY 41064
Telephone: (606)-724-5222
Contact: Gladys Sweeney G. Wayne Buckler - Chairman
Referral services

Rockcastle County

Testing Sites

Rockcastle County Center
Richmond Street
PO Box 840
Mt. Vernon, KY 40456-0840
Telephone: (606)-256-2242
Testing, counseling

Rowan County

Community Services

Dept. for Social Services Office
P.O. Box 203, Rte 27
Harrison Square
Cynthiana, KY 40351-0203
Telephone: (606)-885-9541
Contact: Bonita Watson
Child and adult protection

Russell County

Home Health Care

Home Health - Lake Cumberland
P.O. Box 573
Russell Springs, KY 42642-0573
Telephone: (502)-866-3230
Contact: Isabell Flanagan
AIDS/HIV Home Health Care Services

Home Health-Lifeline, Lake Cumberland Medical Arts Boulevard
Dowell Road
Russell Springs, KY 42642
Telephone: (502)-866-4100 Fax: (502)-866-4104
Toll-Free: (800)-765-4103
Contact: Christina Jessee,RN
Skill nursing, physical therapy, speech, in home nursing

Testing Sites

Russell County Center
New Annex of Courthouse
P.O. Box 378
Jamestown, KY 42629-0378
Telephone: (502)-343-2181
Testing & counseling

Shelby County

Community Services

Seven Counties Mental Health Services
P.O. Box 136
24 Village Plaza
Shelbyville, KY 40065-0136
Telephone: (502)-633-5683
Contact: Carrol Carrits - Director
Education, referrals, preventive care HIV/AIDS

County Health Depts

Shelby County Center
419 Washington Street
P.O. Box 254
Shelbyville, KY 40065-1127
Telephone: (502)-633-1231
Contact: Donna Harpeo
HIV testing & counseling, pre-natal care, family planning, STD &immunizations

Home Health Care

Olsten Kimberly Quality Care
Village Plaza Center
Shelbyville, KY 40065
Telephone: (502)-633-0678
Contact: Judy Fallis
Home care for AIDS patients

Simpson County

Testing Sites

Simpson County Center
P.O. Box 365
Franklin, KY 42135-0365
Telephone: (502)-586-8261
Contact: Cindy Phillips - Nurse
HIV testing, counseling, STD programs

Spencer County

Community Services

Dept. for Social Services Office
P.O. Box 352
Taylorsville, KY 40071-0352
Telephone: (502)-477-8807
Contact: Barbara Domingo

Seven Counties Mental Health Services
Spencer County Center
Reasor Avenue
Taylorsville, KY 40071
Telephone: (502)-477-2577
Contact: Carrol Carrits - Director
Education, referrals, preventive care

Testing Sites

Spencer County Center
Main Street
P.O. Box 175
Taylorsville, KY 40071
Telephone: (502)-477-8146
Contact: Kay Watts - Nurse
HIV testing, counseling

Taylor County

Testing Sites

Taylor County Center
407 East First Street
P.O. Box 68
Campbellsville, KY 42718-1836
Telephone: (502)-465-4191
Contact: Susan Sowards - Nurse Supervisor
HIV testing and counseling

Todd County

County Health Depts

Todd County Health Department
205 McReynolds
P.O. Box 305
Elkton, KY 42220
Telephone: (502)-265-2362
Contact: Libby Harris - Administrator, Cecil Mallory - Chairman
HIV testing and counseling

Trigg County

County Health Depts

Trigg County Center
196 Main Street
P.O. Box 191
Cadiz, KY 42211-9117
Telephone: (502)-522-8121
Social services, AIDS testing, counseling

Trimble County

Community Services

Dept. for Social Services Office Human Services
275 East Main Street
6th Floor
Bedford, KY 40006-0246
Telephone: (502)-255-7274
Social services

County Health Depts

Trimble County Center
Millers Lane
P.O. Box 250
Bedford, KY 40006
Telephone: (502)-255-7701
Contact: Nancy Hason - Nurse
Free testing and counseling

Union County

County Health Depts

Union County Center
218 West McElroy
P.O. Box 88
Morganfield, KY 42437
Telephone: (502)-389-1230
Contact: Dennis Brinkly
Testing, counseling

Warren County

Community Services

Barren River District Health Department - Central Office
1133 Adams Street
P.O. Box 1157

Bowling Green, KY 42102-1157
Telephone: (502)-781-8039
Contact: Melinda Overstreet - HIV Care Coordinator; Honorable Donald Houchin - Chairman
Case managers, assistance with home care insurance, mental healthcounseling

Cumberland Trace Legal Services
1032 College Street
Box 1776
Ellingreen, KY 42102-1776
Telephone: (502)-782-1924
For low-income

Testing Sites

Barren River District Health Department
P.O. Box 1157
Bowling Green, KY 42102-1157
Telephone: (502)-781-2490 Fax: (502)-796-8946
Contact: Melinda J. Overstreet - HIV Care Coordinator
Medical clinic; STD/HIV testing & counseling

Wayne County

Home Health Care

Lifeline Home Health
1 South Creek Drive
Suite 118
Monticello, KY 42633
Telephone: (606)-348-6000 Fax: (606)-348-7270
Toll-Free: (800)-999-2321
Contact: Kim Gooch

Medical Services

Lake Cumberland Clinical Services
P.O. Box 786
Highway 1275
Monticello, KY 42633-0786
Telephone: (606)-348-9318
Mental Health Services

Webster County

Community Services

Webster County Center
College and Clayton Ave.
P.O. Box 109
Dixon, KY 42409
Telephone: (502)-639-9315
Contact: Carolyn Bemette
Social Services

Whitley County

County Health Depts

Whitley County Health Department
North Second Street
P.O. Box 147
Williamsburg, KY 40769
Telephone: (606)-549-3380
Contact: Ray Kennedy - Administrator

Whitley County Health Department
Corbin Branch
P.O. Box 1221
Corbin, KY 40702
Telephone: (606)-528-5613
Social Services

Woodford County

County Health Depts

Woodford County Health Department
229 North Main Street
Versailles, KY 40383
Telephone: (606)-873-4541
Contact: Deborah Acker
Social Services; testing & counseling

LOUISIANA

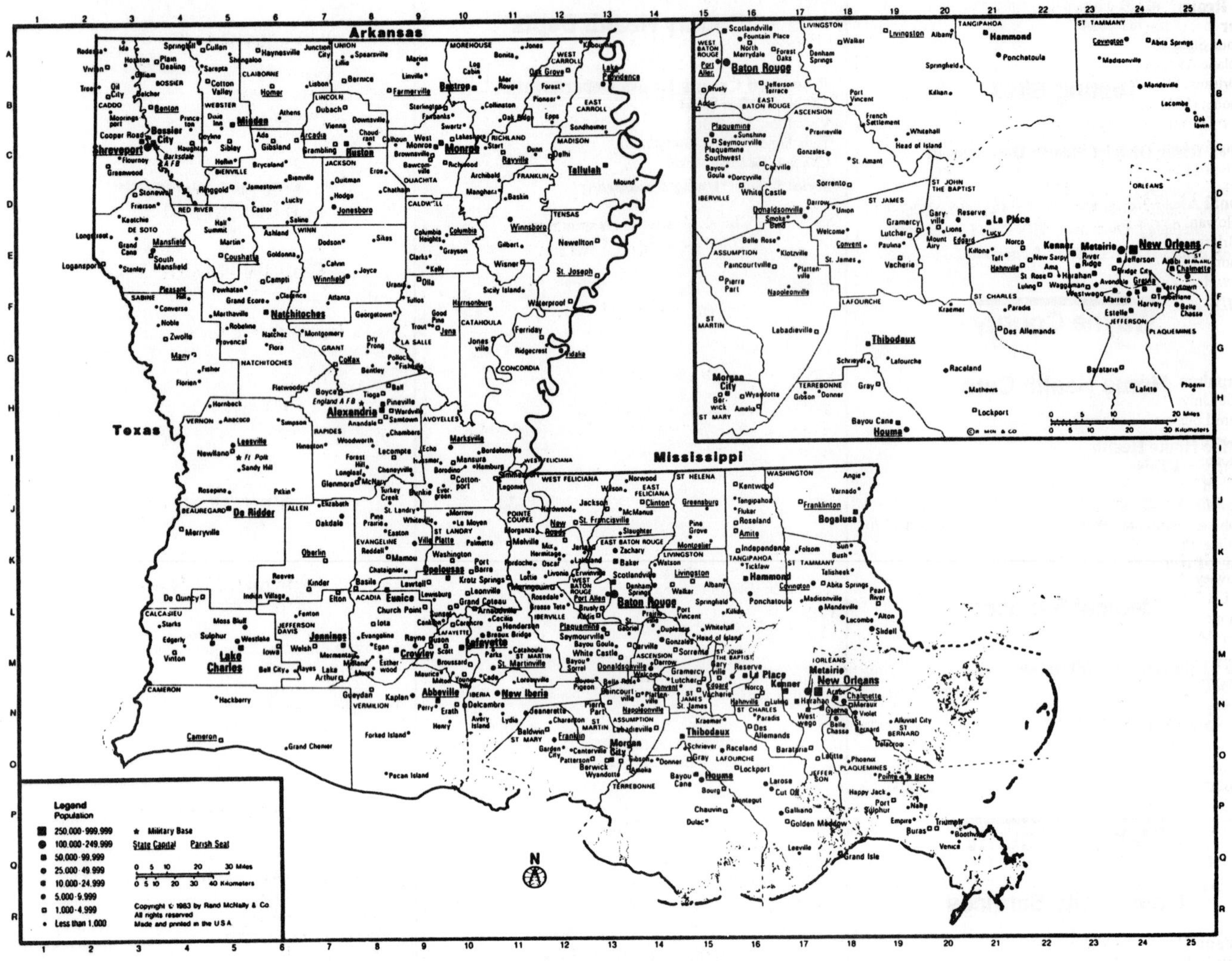

From City/County Planning Atlas Copyright 1989 by Reed McNally & Company, R.L. 90-S-28

Louisiana

General Services

Education

Delta Region AIDS Education and Training Center
Louisiana State Univ.
542 Tulane Avenue
New Orleans, LA 70112
Telephone: (504)-568-3855 Fax: (504)-568-7893
Contact: Dr. William R. Brandon, M.D.
Training for health care professionals

Regional AIDS Interfaith Network
1000 Howard Avenue
New Orleans, LA 70113
Telephone: (504)-523-3755 Fax: (504)-523-0007
Contact: Ron Vnger
HIV/AIDS education for churches, volunteers serve on care teams

Tangipahoa AIDS
Box 568 University Station
Southern Louisiana University
Hammond, LA 70402
Telephone: (504)-549-2194 Fax: (504)-549-3477
Contact: Dr. David Blackwell - Director
Public & Prof. education

Whole Health Outreach, Inc.
100 Rowley Blvd.
Arabi, LA 70032
Telephone: (318)-271-9110
Contact: Mary Calabresi - Project Director
Speakers bureau, AIDS prevention education & training, supportgroup, referrals

State Health Departments

Louisiana Department of Health and Hospitals
325 Loyola Avenue-Rm 618
New Orleans, LA 70160
Telephone: (504)-568-5005
Contact: Dr. Louise McFarland
Counseling, education, referrals, HIV testing, treatment

Louisiana Dept. of Health HIV/AIDS Services
325 Loyola Avenue
Room 618
New Orleans, LA 70112
Telephone: (504)-568-7415
Contact: Van Jenkins - Director

Acadia Parish

County Health Depts

Acadia Parish Health Unit
530 West Mill Street
Crowley, LA 70526-5509
Telephone: (318)-788-7507
AIDS testing

Allen Parish

County Health Depts

Allen Parish Health Unit
601 5th St. Courthouse
P.O. Drawer 160
Oberlin, LA 70655-0160
Telephone: (318)-639-4390
Contact: Diane Flowers
HIV testing, counseling, STD education

Allen Parish Health Unit
107 South 12th St.
Oakdale, LA 71463-2932
Telephone: (318)-335-1147
AIDS testing & counseling

Ascension Parish

County Health Depts

Ascension Parish Health Unit
901 Catalpa Street
Donaldsonville, LA 70346-2437
Telephone: (504)-474-2004 Fax: (504)-474-2060
Contact: Joyce Jones
HIV testing & counseling, referrals

Ascension Parish Health Unit
1024 SE Ascension Complex
Gonzales, LA 70737-4263
Telephone: (504)-644-4582
AIDS testing

Assumption Parish

County Health Depts

Assumption Parish Health Unit
1258 Highway 1008
Napoleonville, LA 70390
Telephone: (504)-369-6031
Contact: Cordy Talbot
STD testing

Avoyelles Parish

County Health Depts

Avoyelles Parish Health Unit
109 Government St.
Marksville, LA 71351-2933
Telephone: (318)-346-2586
Contact: Nancy Johnson
Child health services

Beauregard Parish

County Health Depts

Beauregard Parish Health Unit
116 Evangeline St.
P.O. Box 327
De Ridder, LA 70634-0327
Telephone: (318)-463-4486
Contact: Brenda Vallery
AIDS testing

Bienville Parish

County Health Depts

Bienville Parish Health Unit
P.O. Box 276
Arcadia, LA 71001-0276
Telephone: (318)-263-2125
Contact: Jo Phoenix
AIDS testing

Bossier Parish

County Health Depts

Bossier Parish Health Unit
700 Benton Road
P.O. Box 5608
Bossier City, LA 71111-5608
Telephone: (318)-741-7314
Contact: Betty Prince
AIDS testing

Caddo Parish

Community Services

Young Women's Christian Association
AIDS Minority Outreach
700 Pierre Street
Shreveport, LA 71103
Telephone: (318)-226-8717
Contact: Nellie Davis - Coordinator
HIV testing & counseling; student outreach, education

County Health Depts

Caddo Parish Health Unit
102 East Industrial Loop
Vivian, LA 71082-2920
Telephone: (318)-375-2808
Contact: Emma Ganz
HIV testing & counseling

Caddo Parish Health Unit
1035 Creswell
P.O. Box 3008
Shreveport, LA 71101
Telephone: (318)-676-5222 Fax: (317)-676-5221
Contact: Williams Glins
HIV testing & counseling

Home Health Care

Caremark Branch Network
2210 Line Avenue
Suite 207
Shreveport, LA 71104
Telephone: (318)-686-9616 Fax: (318)-226-4716
Toll-Free: (800)-727-3303
Contact: Robert Baucum - Operations Manager; Wylie Shores - Pharmacy/Ops Manager

Clinical support and infusion therapy: nutrition, antimicrobials, chemo.,hematopoeti

Medical Services

Louisiana State University Medical Center
Viral Disease Clinic
1534 Elizabeth, Ste. 420
Shreveport, LA 71101
Telephone: (318)-227-5060
Contact: Janet Landon, RN - Supervisor
Referrals to home health, social services

Testing Sites

Shreveport Regional TB Clinic
1035 Creswell Street
Shreveport, LA 71101
Telephone: (318)-227-5225
Contact: Bill Stutson
HIV testing

Calcasieu Parish

County Health Depts

Calcasieu Parish Health Unit
721 E. Prien Lake Rd
P.O. Box 3169
Lake Charles, LA 70601-8694
Telephone: (318)-478-6020
HIV testing; pre & post-test counseling, early intervention clinic for HIV+

Caldwell Parish

County Health Depts

Caldwell Parish Health Unit
HC 74, Box 28
Columbia, LA 71418-9803
Telephone: (318)-649-2393
Contact: Connie McCants
HIV testing, referrals, counseling, community health services

Cameron Parish

County Health Depts

Cameron Parish Health Unit
Courthouse Square
P.O. Box 930
Cameron, LA 70631
Telephone: (318)-775-5368
Contact: Susan Dupont
HIV testing, counseling, referrals, community health care

Catahoula Parish

County Health Depts

Catahoula Parish Health Unit
309 Short Street
P.O. Box 240
Harrisonburg, LA 71340-0240
Telephone: (318)-744-5261 Fax: (318)-744-5344
Contact: Dorothy Evans
Immunization, STD, family planning

Claiborne Parish

County Health Depts

Claiborne Parish Health Unit
624 West Main St.
Homer, LA 71040-3418
Telephone: (318)-927-6127 Fax: (318)-927-6362
Contact: Doris Harvey
HIV testing & counseling

Concordia Parish

County Health Depts

Concordia Parish Health Unit
905 Mississippi Avenue
P.O. Box 826
Ferriday, LA 71334-0826
Telephone: (318)-757-8632
Contact: Carolyn Lushute
HIV testing, STD & TB control, education

Concordia Parish Health Unit
P.O. Box 826
Ferriday, LA 71334-0826
Telephone: (318)-336-5519
Contact: Emma Nelson, RN
Counseling

De Soto Parish

County Health Depts

Desoto Parish Health Unit
P.O. Box 312
Mansfield, LA 71052-0312
Telephone: (318)-872-0472
Contact: Marie Hicks
Family planning, child health clinic, STD, referrals

East Baton Rouge Parish

County Health Depts

E. Baton Rouge Parish Health Unit
353 N. 12th Street
PO Box 3017
Baton Rouge, LA 70802-4612
Telephone: (504)-342-1707
Contact: Marguerite Walker
Referrals, child health, TB clinic

Medical Services

Hemophilia Program
446 N. 12th Street
Baton Rouge, LA 70802-4613
Telephone: (504)-342-6451 Fax: (504)-342-4707
Contact: JoAnn Patin
Factor & medical supplies needed

Testing Sites

Baton Rouge Regional TB Clinic
353 N. 12th St.
Baton Rouge, LA 70802-4612
Telephone: (504)-342-1798
Contact: Meretta Wilson
HIV testing

East Carroll Parish

County Health Depts

E. Carroll Parish Health Unit
407 Second Street
Lake Providence, LA 71254-2699
Telephone: (318)-559-2012
Contact: Luanna Starks, R.N. - AIDS Coordinator
HIV testing; pre & post-test counseling; early intervention clinic for HIV+

East Feliciana Parish

County Health Depts

East Feliciana Parish Health Unit
Marston Street
PO Box 227
Clinton, LA 70722
Telephone: (504)-683-8551
Contact: Charlotte Minor - Office Manager
HIV testing; pre & post-test counseling; early intervention clinic for HIV+

Evangeline Parish

County Health Depts

Evangeline Parish Health Unit
309 Second Street
Mamou, LA 70554-3603
Telephone: (318)-468-5903
Contact: Peggy Thomas, R.N. - Public Health Nurse
HIV testing, individual pre & post-test counseling

Evangeline Parish Health Unit
415 W. Cotton St.
P.O. Box 369
Ville Platte, LA 70586-4441
Telephone: (318)-363-1135
Contact: Lima Fuselier, R.N. - Nursing Supervisor
HIV testing; pre & post-test counseling, early intervention clinic forHIV+,referrals

Franklin Parish

County Health Depts

Franklin Parish Health Unit
704 Jackson St.
P.O. Box 547
Winnsboro, LA 71295-2115
Telephone: (318)-435-2143
Contact: Mary Cannon, R.N. - Nursing Supervisor
HIV testing; pre & post-test counseling; early intervention clinic for HIV+

Grant Parish

County Health Depts

Grant Parish Health Unit
513 8th Street
PO Box 232
Colfax, LA 71417-1523
Telephone: (318)-627-3133
Contact: Betty Vercher
Public Health

Iberia Parish

County Health Depts

Iberia Parish Health Unit
121 W. Pershing St.
Courthouse Annex
New Iberia, LA 70560
Telephone: (318)-373-0021
Contact: Elizabeth Landry
Testing & counseling

Iberville Parish

County Health Depts

Iberville Parish Health Unit
58-300 Meriam Street
Plaquemine, LA 70764-0444
Telephone: (318)-687-9021
Contact: Mary Anthony
STD clinic, adult health services, HIV testing

Jackson Parish

County Health Depts

Jackson Parish Health Unit
319 Sixth St.
PO Box 87
Jonesboro, LA 71251-3405
Telephone: (318)-259-6601
Contact: Gayle Sullivan
HIV testing and counseling

Jefferson Parish

County Health Depts

Jefferson Parish Health Unit
111 N. Causeway Blvd.
PO Box 652
Metairie, LA 70001-5450
Telephone: (504)-838-5100
Contact: Jerrell Mathison, M.D.
HIV testing & counseling

Jefferson Parish Health Unit - Harvey
1901 8th Street
Harvey, LA 70058
Telephone: (504)-361-6526
Contact: Mary Green
Child health clinic, STD clinic

Home Health Care

Curaflex Infusion Services
524 Elmwood Park Blvd
#110
New Orleans, LA 70123-3339
Telephone: (504)-733-7300 Fax: (504)-734-7854
Contact: Reed Stephen
Home IV therapy: TPN, Enteral, IV Antibiotics, Aerosolized/IV Pentamidine

Jefferson Davis Parish

County Health Depts

Jefferson Davis Parish Health Unit
314 Church Street
P.O. Box 317
Jennings, LA 70546-0317
Telephone: (318)-824-2193
Contact: Lena Fruge
Statistics, nursing services, testing & counseling

La Salle Parish

County Health Depts

Lasalle Parish Health Unit
305 N. 1st Street
P.O. Box 17
Jena, LA 71342
Telephone: (318)-992-4842
Contact: Marie Wooten
HIV testing, home care, clinic

Lafayette Parish

Community Services

Lafayette CARES
605 W. St. Mary
P.O. Box 91446
Lafayette, LA 70509
Telephone: (318)-233-2437 Fax: (318)-235-4178
Toll-Free: (800)-354-2437
Contact: Gene Dolese
Telephone counseling, support groups, HIV testing & counseling, financialassistance & case management

Home Health Care

Caremark Branch Network
118 Toledo Drive
Lafayette, LA 70506
Telephone: (318)-237-2593 Fax: (318)-233-4536
Contact: Charmaine DuPre - District Manager
Clinical support & infusion therapy: nutrition, antimicrobials, chemo.,hematopoeti

Medical Services

Lafayette Regional TB Clinic
2100 Jefferson Street
Lafayette, LA 70501
Telephone: (318)-262-5616 Fax: (318)-262-5399
Contact: Karen Fuselier
Family planning, STD

Testing Sites

Lafayette Parish Health Unit
2100 Jefferson Street
Building B
Lafayette, LA 70501-8522
Telephone: (318)-262-5616 Fax: (318)-262-5399
Contact: Lois Breaux
HIV testing & counseling; child care, TB clinic

Lafourche Parish

County Health Depts

Lafourche Parish Health Unit
2535 Veterans Blvd.
Thibodaux, LA 70301
Telephone: (504)-447-0921
Contact: Betty Hebert - RN
HIV testing & counseling, STD, home care

Lafourche Parish Health Unit
133 West 112th Street
Cucoff, LA 70345
Telephone: (504)-632-5567
Contact: Sheila Gros
HIV counseling, home care

Medical Services

Teche Regional TB Clinic
206 E. Third Street
Thibodaux, LA 70302-3312
Telephone: (504)-447-0916 Fax: (504)-447-0920
Contact: Marcia Waguespack

Lincoln Parish

County Health Depts

Lincoln Parish Health Unit
405 E. Georgia Ave.
P.O. Box 869
Ruston, LA 71273-0869
Telephone: (318)-251-4120
Contact: JoAnn Grafton
Testing & counseling

Livingston Parish

County Health Depts

Livingston Parish Health Unit
8393 Flordia Blvd.
P.O. Box 1487
Denham Springs, LA 70727-7806
Telephone: (504)-665-2489
Contact: Pat Hennessey, RN
HIV testing & counseling

Livingston Parish Health Unit
20140 Iowa Street
P.O. Box 365
Livingston, LA 70754
Telephone: (504)-686-7017
Contact: Flora Bush
Public health, home care, child care, HIV testing & counseling

Madison Parish

County Health Depts

Madison Parish Health Unit
606 Depot St.
Tallulahph, LA 71282-3833
Telephone: (318)-574-3311
Contact: Altrechiea Hutto
Home care, HIV testing & counseling, child care, public education

Morehouse Parish

County Health Depts

Morehouse Parish Health Unit
1006 North Washington St
Bastrop, LA 71220-3010
Telephone: (318)-283-0806
Contact: Melanie Dew
STD testing, immunizations, TB control, HIV testing

Natchitoches Parish

County Health Depts

Natchitoches Parish Health Unit
625 Bienville St Ext.
P.O. Box 489
Natchitoches, LA 71457-0489
Telephone: (318)-357-3132
Contact: Bea Smith, RN
STD/HIV counseling & testing

Orleans Parish

Community Services

Project Lazarus
P.O. Box 3906
New Orleans, LA 70177
Telephone: (504)-949-3609 Fax: (504)-944-7944
Contact: Hugh McCabe - Director
Residence for people with AIDS

United Services for AIDS
938 Lafayette Street
Suite 419
New Orleans, LA 70113
Telephone: (504)-523-3755
Funding for housing

Medical Services

Charity Hospital
1532 Tulane Avenue-C100
New Orleans, LA 70112
Telephone: (504)-568-5304 Fax: (504)-568-6393
Contact: Ted Wisniewski, M.D. - Administrator
Medical care, counseling for AIDS patients

Childrens Hospital of New Orleans
Pediatric AIDS Program
200 Henry Clay Avenue
New Orleans, LA 70117
Telephone: (504)-524-4611 Fax: (504)-523-2084
Contact: Michael Kaiser, M.D. - Program Director, M. Beth Scalco, BCSW - Program Coordinator
Case Mgt, Advocacy, Health Ed., Pediatric AIDS Program

Louisiana Department of Health & Hospitals
HIV Program Office
1542 Tulane Avenue
New Orleans, LA 70112
Telephone: (504)-568-7041
Contact: Ted Wisniewski - M.D.

Orleans Parish Family Planning Clinic
1800 N. Broad
New Orleans, LA 70160-2340
Telephone: (504)-942-8255
Contact: Emelda Williams
Testing & counceling for HIV

Testing Sites

NO/AIDS Task Force
1407 Decatur Street
New Orleans, LA 70116
Telephone: (504)-522-2458
Contact: Torie Kranze
Testing, counseling

Planned Parenthood of Louisiana
4018 Magazine St.
New Orleans, LA 70115-2749
Telephone: (504)-897-9212 Fax: (504)-897-9234
Contact: Terri Bartlett - Director
HIV testing & counseling, risk reduction education

Ouachita Parish

County Health Depts

Ouachita Parish Health Unit
2913 Desiard St.
P.O. Box 4460
Monroe, LA 71201-7207
Telephone: (318)-362-3400
Contact: Dr. Shelly Jones - Medical Director
HIV testing; pre & post-test counseling; early intervention clinic forthose diagnosed HIV-positive

Ouachita Parish Health Unit
413 Natchitoches St.
West Monroe, LA 71291-3196
Telephone: (318)-362-3428
Contact: Cheryl Rountree
HIV testing-pre & post counseling

Home Health Care

nmc HOMECARE
1355 Louisville Ave
Monroe, LA 71201
Telephone: (318)-323-8972
Fax:(318)-387-9015
Contact: Billy Amos
National JCAHO-Accredited company providing a full range of Infusion and Respiratory therapies and specializing in the care of HIV/AIDS patients. National Case Manager is also available at 800-445-1188

Testing Sites

Monroe Regional TB Clinic
2913 DeSiard Street
Monroe, LA 71203-7207
Telephone: (318)-362-3445
Contact: Sharon Liner
Referrals, early intervention course

Northeast Regional Office
2913 Betin Street
Monroe, LA 71201-7257
Telephone: (318)-362-5252
Contact: Billie J. Strickland
Testing & counseling, nursing services, clinic

Plaquemines Parish

County Health Depts

Plaquemines Parish Health Dept.
3706 Main Street
Belle Chasse, LA 70037-3099
Telephone: (504)-394-3510
Referrals

Pointe Coupee Parish

County Health Depts

Pointe Coupee Parish Health Unit
282 B Hospital Road
New Roads, LA 70760
Telephone: (504)-638-7320
Contact: Laveene Aguillard
HIV testing, counseling, AIDS education

Rapides Parish

County Health Depts

Rapides Parish Health Unit
P.O. Box 5918
Alexandria, LA 71307-5918
Telephone: (318)-487-5282
Contact: Pauline Bennett - Public Health Nurse
HIV testing; pre & post-test counseling; early intervention clinic for HIV+

Medical Services

Region 6 - Regional VD Clinic
1335 Jackson Street
Alexandria, LA 71306-6930
Telephone: (318)-487-5270 Fax: (318)-487-5338
Contact: Gary Gresham
Pre & post test counseling

Red River Parish

County Health Depts

Red River Parish Health Unit
2015 Red Oak Road
P.O. Box 628
Coushatta, LA 71019-9505
Telephone: (318)-932-4087
Contact: Dianne Milner
HIV testing

Richland Parish

County Health Depts

Richland Parish Health Unit
205 S. Eugene St.
P.O. Box 666
Rayville, LA 71269-2627
Telephone: (318)-728-4441
Contact: O'Darria Clem
HIV testing

Sabine Parish

County Health Depts

Sabine Parish Health Unit
245 Highland Drive
PO Box 398
Many, LA 71449-0398
Telephone: (318)-256-4105 Fax: (318)-256-4144
Contact: Brenda Leo, RN
General health - HIV testing & counseling

Saint Bernard Parish

County Health Depts

St. Bernard Parish Health Unit
2712 Palmisano Blvd.
Chalmette, LA 70043-3624
Telephone: (504)-278-7410
Contact: Charlene Clemens
STD testing

Saint Charles Parish

County Health Depts

St. Charles Parish Health Unit
201 Post Drive
Luling, LA 70070-9507
Telephone: (504)-785-2314
Contact: Leola Zeringue
HIV testing, counseling

Home Health Care

Caremark Branch Network
Westside One - Suite 100
115 James Drive West
St. Rose, LA 70087
Telephone: (504)-466-5932 Fax: (504)-468-8310
Toll-Free: (800)-628-2477
Contact: Gerald Lanclos - Branch Manager, Jamie Poche - Operations Manager, Jennifer Hartenstein - Pharmacy/Ops Manager
Clinical support and infusion therapy: nutrition, antimicrobials, chemo.,hematopoeti

Critical Care America
190 James Drive East
Eastside One, Ste 100
St Rose, LA 70087
Telephone: (504)-468-8200 Fax: (504)-469-1182
Toll-Free: (800)-444-3944
Contact: Terry Fayer
Coordinate & integrate all clinical & psychosocial services for HIV+

HNS, Inc.
125 James Drive West
Suite 140
St. Rose, LA 70087
Telephone: (504)-464-6100 Fax: (504)-464-6164
Toll-Free: (800)-872-4467
Contact: Frank Hebert
Home Infusion Therapy, In-home Nursing and Attendant Care, P.T. Services, Pentamidine

Saint Helena Parish

County Health Depts

St. Helena Parish Health Unit
N. Second Street
P.O. Box 428
Greensburg, LA 70441
Telephone: (504)-222-6178
Contact: Betty Lee
Rural health clinic

Saint James Parish

County Health Depts

St. James Parish Health Unit
2430 Louisiana Ave
PO Box 387
Lutcher, LA 70071-0387
Telephone: (504)-869-4441
Contact: Jay Bienvenu
Testing

St. James Parish Health Unit
Highway 20
29170 Health Unit Sq.
Vacherie, LA 70090
Telephone: (504)-265-2181
STD clinics

Saint John The Baptist Parish

County Health Depts

St. John Parish Health Unit
Courthouse, E. 3rd St.
P.O. Box 83
Edgard, LA 70049
Telephone: (504)-497-8726

St. John Parish Health Unit
473 Central Avenue
P.O. Drawer P
Reserve, LA 70084
Telephone: (504)-536-2128
Contact: Francis McDonald
HIV testing, counseling clinic

Saint Landry Parish

County Health Depts

St. Landry Parish Health Unit
Sunset Strip - Hwy 93
PO Box 57
Sunset, LA 70584
Telephone: (318)-662-5260
Testing & referral

St. Landry Parish Health Unit
131 City Avenue
PO Box 1167
Eunice, LA 70535-1167
Telephone: (318)-457-2767
HIV testing, counseling, referrals, clinic

St. Landry Parish Health Unit
Havard St.
PO Box 404
Melville, LA 71353
Telephone: (318)-623-4941

Medical Services

St. Landry Parish Health Unit
308 West Bloch St.
PO Box 552
Opelousas, LA 70571-0552
Telephone: (318)-948-0220
Contact: Irene Stagg
Referrals for testing and medical aid, prevention clinic

Saint Martin Parish

County Health Depts

St. Martin Parish Health Unit
415 St. Martins Street
St. Martinsville, LA 70582
Telephone: (318)-332-2857
Testing, referrals & counseling

Testing Sites

St. Martin Parish Health Unit
415 St. Martin Street
St. Martinville, LA 70582
Telephone: (318)-394-3097
Contact: Faye Sonnier
HIV testing and counseling

St. Martin Parish Health Unit
205 North Main Street
Breaux Bridge, LA 70517-5095
Telephone: (318)-332-2857
Contact: Katherine Guidry - Nurse
HIV testing and counseling

Saint Mary Parish

County Health Depts

St. Mary Parish Health Unit
800 First St.
Franklin, LA 70538-4910
Telephone: (318)-828-0410
Contact: Joanna LeBlanc
General health - HIV testing

Testing Sites

St. Mary Parish Health Unit
301 Third Street
Morgan City, LA 70380-3524
Telephone: (504)-380-2441
Contact: Joanna LeBlanc - Supervisor of Nursing
HIV testing, counseling, child health care, TB testing

Saint Tammany Parish

County Health Depts

St. Tammany Parish Health Unit - Covington
200 Covington Center
Suite 2
Covington, LA 70433
Telephone: (504)-893-6208
Contact: Gwendolyn Boothe - RN
HIV early intervention, testing & counseling

Testing Sites

St. Tammany Parish Health Unit
333 Bouscaren St.
PO Box 850
Slidell, LA 70459-3419
Telephone: (504)-646-6445
Contact: Doris Olsen - RN
Testing & counseling

Tangipahoa Parish

Testing Sites

Tangipahoa Parish Health Unit
1600 N. Morrison Blvd.
Hammond, LA 70401-1530
Telephone: (504)-543-4030
Contact: Nolan Richardson
Testing & counseling

Tensas Parish

Testing Sites

Tensas Parish Health Unit
133 Plank Road
P.O. Box 77
St. Joseph, LA 71366
Telephone: (318)-766-3513 Fax: (318)-766-9090
Contact: Pauline Patton
Testing, counseling, referrals

Terrebonne Parish

Testing Sites

Terrebonne Parish Health Unit
600 Polk St.
Houma, LA 70361-4154
Telephone: (504)-857-3601 Fax: (504)-857-3607
Contact: Linda Porche RN
Testing and counseling

Union Parish

Testing Sites

Union Parish Health Unit
1002 Marion Hwy
P.O. Box 516
Farmerville, LA 71241-9212
Telephone: (318)-368-3156 Fax: (318)-368-3831
Contact: Faith Brantley
Testing, counseling, referrals

Vermilion Parish

County Health Depts

Vermilion Parish Health Unit
419 North Cushing Ave
Kaplan, LA 70548-4123
Telephone: (318)-643-7467
Contact: Mona Fruge
Referrals

Vermilion Parish Health Unit
406 Seventh St.
Gueydan, LA 70542-4106
Telephone: (318)-536-6072
Referral & counseling

Vernon Parish

County Health Depts

Vernon Parish Health Unit
406 W. Fertitta Blvd
P.O. Box 1471
Leesville, LA 71496-1471
Telephone: (318)-238-6410 Fax: (318)-238-6447
Contact: Bob Westmoreland
Referrals, counseling, educational programs

Washington Parish

County Health Depts

Washington Parish Health Unit
1104 Bene Street
P.O. Box 524
Franklinton, LA 70438-1135
Telephone: (504)-839-5646
Contact: Audrey Thomas
Testing & counseling

Webster Parish

County Health Depts

Webster Parish Health Unit
111 Murrell Ave
P.O. Box 814
Minden, LA 71058-0814
Telephone: (318)-371-3030
Contact: Debra Vogel
HIV testing

Webster Parish Health Unit
218 First St. NE
Springhill, LA 71075-3218
Telephone: (318)-539-4314
Testing & counseling

West Baton Rouge Parish

Testing Sites

West Baton Rouge Parish Health Unit
685 Louisiana
P.O. Box 227
Port Allen, LA 70767-2144
Telephone: (504)-342-7525 Fax: (504)-383-3552
Contact: Bernadine DeJean
Testing & referral

West Carroll Parish

County Health Depts

W. Carroll Parish Health Unit
Koerner & Beale Streets
P.O. Box 306
Oak Grove, LA 71263
Telephone: (318)-428-9361
Contact: Dora Sowell
Testing, counseling, referral

West Feliciana Parish

County Health Depts

W. Feliciana Parish Health Unit
5154 Burnette Road
PO Box 1928
St.Francisville, LA 70775
Telephone: (504)-635-3644
Contact: Deanna Shipp
Testing

Winn Parish

County Health Depts

Winn Parish Health Unit
301 W. Main St.
P.O. Box 111
Winnfield, LA 71483
Telephone: (318)-628-2148
Contact: Inez Anyan
Testing & counseling

MAINE

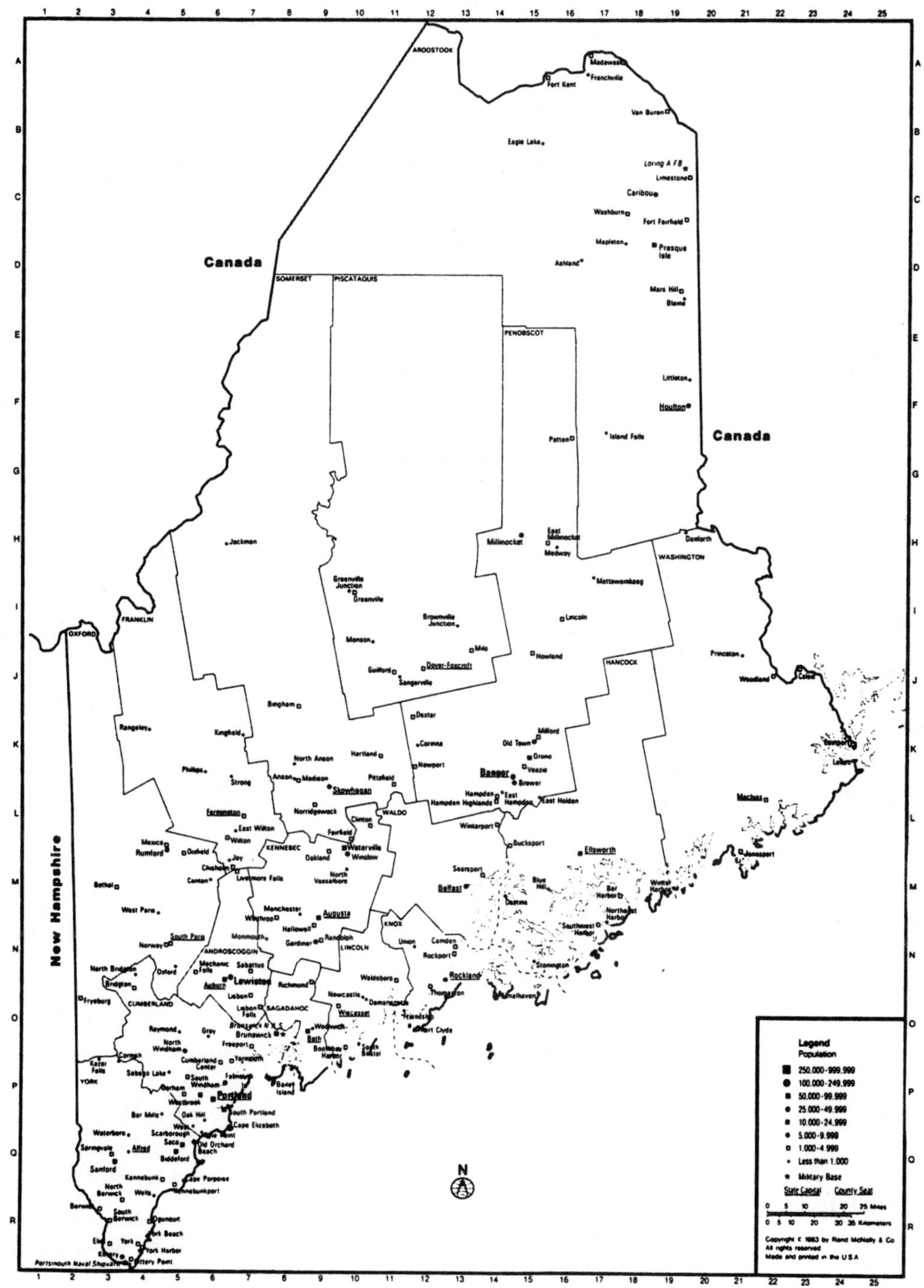

From City/County Planning Atlas Copyright 1989 by Reed McNally & Company, R.L. 90-S-28

Maine

General Services

Education

American Red Cross
524 Forest Avenue
Portland, ME 04101-1591
Telephone: (207)-874-1192
Information about antibody testing, blood transfusions, education.

Department of Education
State House Station 23
Augusta, ME 04333-0001
Telephone: (207)-287-5926
Contact: Joni Foster
Information/HIV/AIDS curricula, materials, policies for public schools.

Waldo- Knox AIDS Coalition
PO Box 956
Belfast, ME 04915-0956
Telephone: (207)-338-1427
Contact: Nan Stone
Education, Advocacy, Referrals, Support

Statewide Services

Maine Department of Human Services
State House Station 11
Augusta, ME 04333
Telephone: (207)-287-5060
Contact: Tom Bancroft - AIDS Coordinator
Advocacy, acute care, home health, income assistance, mental health, other

Androscoggin County

Home Health Care

nmc HOMECARE
60 Pine Street
Lewiston, ME 04240
Telephone: (207)-784-0057
Fax: (207)-786-4171
Contact: Susan Amundsen
National JCAHO-Accredited company providing a full range of Infusion and Respiratory therapies and specializing in the care of HIV/AIDS patients. National Case Manager is also available at 800-445-1188

Testing Sites

STD Clinic
One Auburn Center
PO Box 70
Auburn, ME 04212-0070
Telephone: (207)-795-4019 Fax: (207)-795-4021
Anonymous AIDS/HIV antibody testing and counseling sites

Aroostook County

Community Services

Northern Maine Medical Center
143 East Main Street
Fort Kent, ME 04743-1497
Telephone: (207)-834-3155 Fax: (207)-834-3155
Contact: Joanne Fortin
AIDS information clearinghouse, education, speakers & support services.

Testing Sites

Health First
PO Box 1116
Presque Isle, ME 04769
Telephone: (207)-764-3721
Contact: Jackie Allen
Anonymous AIDS/HIV Antibody Counseling & Testing Sites

Cumberland County

Community Services

The AIDS Project
22 Monument Square
5th Floor
Portland, ME 04101-4031
Telephone: (207)-774-6877 Fax: (207)-879-0761
Contact: Deborah Shields
Anonymous HIV Testing & Counseling, community education, case management,statewide hotline.

Home Health Care

AIDS Lodging House
233 Oxford Street
P.O. Box 3820
Portland, ME 04104
Telephone: (207)-874-1000
Contact: Rick Bouchard - Director
Housing for people with AIDS/HIV

Caremark
136 US Route 1, Suite 4
Scarborough, ME 04074
Telephone: (207)-885-5600
Contact: Deborah Miller - General Manager, Kim Krauss - Branch/Operations Mgr.
Clinical Support and Infusion Therapy: nutrition,antimicrobials, chemo., hematopoeti

HNS, Inc.
160 C. Larrabee Road
Westbrook, ME 04092
Telephone: (207)-856-2266
Contact: John Leonard
Home infusion therapy, attendants, nurses, pentamidine, pharmacy, counseling

Medical Services

Public Health Division/AIDS Case Management Program
389 Congress St, Rm 307
Portland, ME 04101
Telephone: (207)-874-8300
Contact: Jodi Fickett
AIDS Case Management Services/Portland Residents Only

Testing Sites

Portland STD Clinic
Portland City Hall
3rd Floor
Portland, ME 04101-2991
Telephone: (207)-874-8452 Fax: (207)-874-8649
Contact: Nate Nickerson
Anonymous AIDS/HIV Antibody Counseling & Testing Sites

Hancock County

Testing Sites

Downeast Family Planning
P.O. Box 1087
Ellsworth, ME 04605
Telephone: (207)-667-5304 Fax: (207)-667-6117
Toll-Free: (800)-492-5550
Contact: Vyvyenne Ritchie
Anonymous AIDS/HIV Antibody Counseling & Testing Sites

Kennebec County

Community Services

Bureau of Child & Family Services
State House Station #11
Augusta, ME 04333-0001
Telephone: (207)-287-5060 Fax: (207)-626-5555
Contact: Tom Bancroft - AIDS Coordinator
AIDS Case Management Services

County Health Depts

Kennebec Valley Regional Health Agency
P.O. Box 1568
Waterville, ME 04903-1568
Telephone: (207)-873-1127 Fax: (207)-873-2059
Contact: Mike Giles
Case management, advocacy, referrals, HIV testing

Knox County

Testing Sites

MidCoast Family Planning
22 White Street
PO Box 866
Rockland, ME 04841
Telephone: (207)-594-2551
Contact: Tory Levteman
Anonymous AIDS/HIV Antibody Counseling & Testing Sites

Penobscot County

Community Services

Eastern Maine AIDS Network
263 State Street
Bangor, ME 04401
Telephone: (207)-990-3626
Contact: Sally Lou Patterson
AIDS case management services, support groups, referrals, education

Testing Sites

Bangor STD Clinic
103 Texas Ave
Bangor, ME 04401
Telephone: (207)-947-0700 Fax: (207)-945-4384
Contact: Patty Miles
Anonymous AIDS/HIV counseling & testing sites, HIV health maintenanceclinic

York County

Testing Sites

York County STD Clinic
11 Hills Beach Road
Biddeford, ME 04005
Telephone: (207)-282-1516 Fax: (207)-282-6133
Contact: Patricia Rothoff
Anonymous AIDS/HIV Antibody Counseling & Testing Sites

MARYLAND

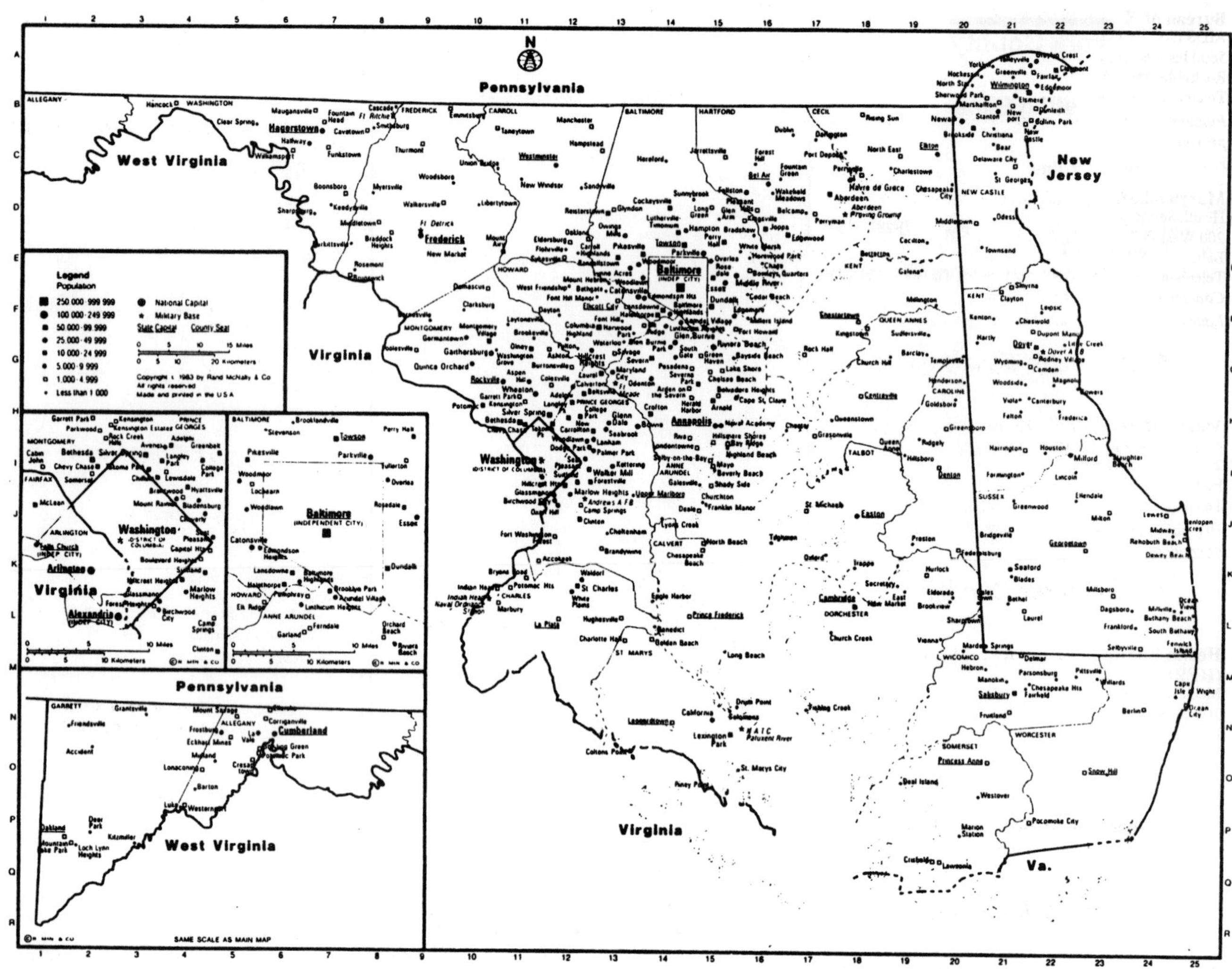

From City/County Planning Atlas Copyright 1989 by Reed McNally & Company, R.L. 90-S-28

Maryland

General Services

Education

Bureau of Health Professions
AIDS ETC Program
5600 Fishers Lane, Rm 4C03
Rockville, MD 20857
Telephone: (301)-443-6364
Funding agency for centers, AIDS education for healthcare providers

Maryland State Department of Education
Health Services
200 West Baltimore Street
Baltimore, MD 21201
Telephone: (410)-333-2819 Fax: (410)-333-2423
Contact: Debbie Somerville
Education materials related to AIDS prevention.

State Health Departments

Maryland Dept. of Health & Mental Hygiene, AIDS Administration
201 West Preston Street
Baltimore, MD 21201
Telephone: (410)-225-6707 Fax: (410)-333-5954
HIV policy, drug assistance, counseling, testing, education, referralhotline

Statewide Services

Health Education & Resource Organization (HERO)
Medical Arts Building
101 W. Read Street #825
Baltimore, MD 21201
Telephone: (410)-685-1180
AIDS information care

Anne Arundel County

Community Services

American Red Cross, Mid-Atlantic Region
7272 Park Circle Drive
Ste. 150
Hanover, MD 21076
Telephone: (410)-712-7600
Contact: Ray W. Brown - Chairman

Medical Services

Anne Arundel Health Department
3 Truman Parkway
Annapolis, MD 21401
Telephone: (410)-222-7108
Case management, HIV information, testing on Wednesdays

Baltimore County

Community Services

Department of Human Resources, Project Home
311 W. Saratoga Street
Room 566
Baltimore, MD 21201-3500
Telephone: (410)-333-0148 Fax: (410)-333-0392
Contact: April Seitz - AIDS Specialist
Case management, and supportive housing for PWA's

County Health Depts

Baltimore County Health Department
1538 Country Ridge Lane
Essex, MD 21221
Telephone: (410)-887-0246
Contact: Betty Miner
Anonymous HIV testing (3rd Thurs 2-4pm); confidential HIV testing(every Thurs. 5-6:30pm)

Baltimore County Health Department
1 Investment Pl.
11th Floor
Towson, MD 21204
Telephone: (410)-887-3740
Contact: Eileen Foster
Confidential testing, counseling, clinic

Home Health Care

Caremark
1039 North Calvert Street
Baltimore, MD 21202
Telephone: (410)-752-4489 Fax: (410)-720-6085
Toll-Free: (800)-523-1435
Contact: Brian Ford - RN CPN
Clinical support and infusion therapies: nutrition, antimicrobials, chemo.,hematopoeti

Medical Services

Chase-Brexton Clinic
101 W Read St
Baltimore, MD 21201-4915
Telephone: (410)-837-2050 Fax: (410)-837-2071
Full range of medical services

Johns Hopkins Hospital
600 North Wolfe St
Wilmer 300
Baltimore, MD 21205
Telephone: (410)-955-2966 Fax: (410)-955-2924
Contact: Dr. Douglas Jabs
Treat CMV retinitis, referrals

University of Maryland at Baltimore, Infectious Diseases
10 South Pine St
Baltimore, MD 21201
Telephone: (301)-328-7560
Contact: Sylvia Scherr
HIV care unit, parent/child clinic, education

University of Maryland School of Medicine
29 South Green Street
Baltimore, MD 21201
Telephone: (410)-328-5711 Fax: (410)-328-4430
Contact: Dr. David Wheeler
Medical care, testing

University of Maryland School of Medicine (Pediatrics)
31 South Green Street
Room 220
Baltimore, MD 21201
Telephone: (410)-706-8220
Clinical service, testing, social services

University of Maryland, Pediatric Immunology
31 South Green Street
Room 206
Baltimore, MD 21201
Telephone: (410)-706-8220
Medical services, education

Testing Sites

Chase - Brexton Clinic, Inc.
101 West Reed Street
Suite 211
Baltimore, MD 21201
Telephone: (410)-837-2050 Fax: (410)-837-2071
Contact: David Shippee - Executive Director; Jack Neville, Jr. - Director of Counseling
HIV testing, AIDS services

Calvert County

County Health Depts

Calvert County Health Department
Route 4
Prnce Frederick, MD 20678
Telephone: (410)-535-5400
Contact: Carol Prince
Anonymous office counseling & testing services

Caroline County

County Health Depts

Caroline County Health Department
301 Randolph Street
Denton, MD 21629
Telephone: (410)-479-2860 Fax: (410)-479-4871
Contact: Michelle Camper
Total case managment

Carroll County

County Health Depts

Carroll County Health Department
540 Washington Rd
Westminster, MD 21157
Telephone: (410)-876-4967 Fax: (410)-876-4998
Contact: Mrs. Middleton
Counseling, testing, support groups, case managements

Cecil County

County Health Depts

Cecil County Health Department
401 Bow Street
Elkton, MD 21921
Telephone: (410)-996-5550 Fax: (410)-996-5179
Contact: Paulette Husfelt
Anonymous counseling & testing, AIDS case management

Charles County

County Health Depts

Charles County Health Department
Garrett Street
PO Box 640
LaPlata, MD 20646
Telephone: (301)-934-9577 Fax: (301)-934-1658
Contact: Faye Grillo
HIV/AIDS testing & counseling; case management, education, home & communitybased services, HIV newsletter, partner notification, outreach

Dorchester County

County Health Depts

Dorchester County Health Department
751 Woods Road
Cambridge, MD 21613
Telephone: (410)-228-3223 Fax: (410)-228-9319
Contact: Lisa Lee
AIDS testing & counseling; clinics for sexually transmitted diseases

Frederick County

County Health Depts

Frederick County Health Department
350 Montevue Lane
Frederick, MD 21702
Telephone: (301)-694-1752 Fax: (301)-698-9161
Contact: Trisha Grove
Counseling & testing, clinic, case management

Medical Services

Frederick Memorial Hospital
West 7th Street
Frederick, MD 21701
Telephone: (301)-698-3300 Fax: (301)-698-3292
Contact: Jenny Boyer

Garrett County

County Health Depts

Garrett County Health Department/Interagency Council on AIDS
253 N. 4th Street
Oakland, MD 21550
Telephone: (301)-334-1523 Fax: (301)-334-1014
Contact: Carol Clark
Home health agency, shelter & financial services

Harford County

County Health Depts

Harford County Health Department
119 S. Hayes Street
PO Box 797
Bel Air, MD 21014
Telephone: (410)-838-1500
Contact: Louise Treheme L.C.S.W.
Confidential counseling/testing, case management, clinic

Harford County Health Department
34 N. Philadelphia Blvd.
Aberdeen, MD 21001
Telephone: (410)-273-5626 Fax: (410)-879-6823
Contact: Cheri Fansler
Confidential counseling & testing, case management services, supportgroups, partner notification, satellite clinic associated with the JohnsHopkins

Howard County

Community Services

Family Life Center
10451 Twin Rivers Road
Columbia, MD 21044-2387
Telephone: (410)-997-3557 Fax: (410)-964-1791
Contact: Paula LaSalle
Counseling for Patients Only

Howard County Health Department, Addictions Services Center
3545 Ellicott Mills Drive
Ellicott City, MD 21043-4548
Telephone: (301)-465-0127
Contact: Frank McGloin
Individual, Family and Group Counseling; Support Groups

County Health Depts

Howard County Health Department
9525 Durness Lane
Laurel, MD 20723
Telephone: (301)-880-5888
Contact: Betty Pike
HIV testing & counseling

Howard County Health Department
10650 Hickory Ridge Road
Columbia, MD 21044
Telephone: (410)-313-2333 Fax: (410)-313-6103
Contact: Mary Mazzuca
Testing, counseling, information, partner notification, disabilityservices, case management

Home Health Care

AIDS Alliance of Howard County & Hospice
5537 Twin Knolls Road
Suite 433
Columbia, MD 21045
Telephone: (410)-730-5072 Fax: (410)-730-5284
Contact: Nancy Weber
Hospice, volunteer support, referrals

Caremark Connection Network
7168 Columbia Gateway Dr.
Suite C
Columbia, MD 21046
Telephone: (410)-720-6060 Fax: (410)-720-6085
Contact: Diane Chmel - Branch Manager
Clinical support and infusion therapies: Nutrition, Antimicrobials, Chemo.,Hematopoeti

HNS, Inc.
9730 Patuxent Woods Drive
Columbia, MD 21046
Telephone: (410)-381-0770 Fax: (410)-381-6240
Toll-Free: (800)-446-4467
Contact: Stephanie Amey
Home Infusion Therapy

Hospice Services of Howard County
5537 Twin Knolls Road
Suite 433
Columbia, MD 21045
Telephone: (410)-730-5072 Fax: (410)-730-5284
Contact: Lynn Hottle
Support in Home, Hospital, or Nursing Home; Information, Referrals

New England Critical Care
7150 Columbia Gateway Dr.
Columbia, MD 21046-2101
Telephone: (410)-720-6500 Fax: (410)-720-6220
Toll-Free: (800)-826-6445
Contact: Jeanne Lynn
Superior, quality traditional and innovative infusion therapies in home

nmc HOMECARE
6935-A Oakland Mills Rd
Columbia, MD 21045
Telephone: (410)-381-5802
Fax: (410)-381-9161
Contact: Alex Monger
National JCAHO-Accredited company providing a full range of Infusion and Respiratory therapies and specializing in the care of HIV/AIDS patients. National Case Manager is also available at 800-445-1188

Visiting Nurse Association
4785 Dorsey Hall Drive
Suite 112
Ellicott City, MD 21042-7728
Telephone: (301)-465-1955
Contact: Mary Brubaker
Complete Home Health Care, Hospice Services

Testing Sites

Columbia Health Center
10630 Little Patuxent Pk.
Columbia, MD 21044
Telephone: (410)-313-7500 Fax: (410)-313-6108
Contact: Mary Lou Mazzuca

HIV counseling & testing

Kent County

County Health Depts

Kent County Health Department
125 South Lynchnurg Street
Chestertown, MD 21620
Telephone: (410)-778-1350
Contact: Mary Moore
HIV testing & counseling

Medical Services

Kent and Queen Anne's Hospital
Infectious Disease Dept
Chestertown, MD 21620
Telephone: (410)-778-3300 Fax: (410)-778-7657
Contact: Donna Saunders
HIV testing and counseling, all infectious disease

Montgomery County

Community Services

Second Genesis
7910 Woodmont Avenue
Suite 500
Bethesda, MD 20814
Telephone: (301)-656-1545 Fax: (301)-656-9313
Contact: Bernice Thomas - Health Educator
AIDS/HIV personnel counseling

County Health Depts

Montgomery County Health Department
2000 Dennis Avenue
Silver Spring, MD 20902-4192
Telephone: (301)-271-7681
Contact: Tina Clark - Health Educator
Clinical services, case mgt, ed/outreach, social services & home care

Montgomery County Health Department; Office on AIDS
2000 Dennis Avenue
Silver Springs, MD 20902
Telephone: (301)-217-7681 Fax: (301)-217-1754
Contact: Carol Jordan
Diagnosis evaluation, case management, social services, support groups,buddies

Home Health Care

Holy Cross Hospice Home Care
9805 Dameron Drive
Silver Springs, MD 20902-5797
Telephone: (301)-565-1171
Contact: Jill Audett
Limited inpatient hospice, in-home hospice care, skilled nursing, counseling.

Holy Cross Hospital of Silver Spring
1500 Forest Glen Road
Silver Spring, MD 20910
Telephone: (301)-905-0100 Fax: (301)-905-1011

Prince George's County

County Health Depts

Prince Georges County Health Department
Communicable Disease
3003 Hospital Drive
Cheverly, MD 20785
Telephone: (301)-386-0210
Testing site (anonymous).

Home Health Care

Homedco Infusion
12400 Kiln Court
Beltsville, MD 20705
Telephone: (800)-252-0740
Contact: Elaine Jakubowski
Infusion therapy for in-home HIV/AIDS patients.

nmc HOMECARE
513 Commerce Drive
Upper Marlboro, MD 20772
Telephone: (301)-390-8400
Fax: (301)-390-7110
Contact: Mariellen Lowry
National JCAHO-Accredited company providing a full range of Infusion and Respiratory therapies and specializing in the care of HIV/AIDS patients. National Case Manager is also available at 800-445-1188

Queen Anne's County

County Health Depts

Queen Anne County Health Department
206 N. Commerce Street
Centreville, MD 21617
Telephone: (410)-758-0720 Fax: (410)-758-2838
Contact: Marianne Thompson
Public health services

Saint Mary's County

County Health Depts

St. Mary's County Health Department
Peabody Street
P.O. Box 316
Leonardtown, MD 20650-0316
Telephone: (301)-475-4316 Fax: (301)-475-4350
Contact: Diana McKinney - R.N., B.S.
Public health services.

Somerset County

County Health Depts

Somerset Health Department
4327 Crisfield Highway
Westover, MD 21871
Telephone: (410)-651-0822 Fax: (410)-651-2985
Contact: Marsha East
Public health services.

Medical Services

Edward W McCready Memorial Hospital
Hall Highway
Crisfield, MD 21817
Telephone: (410)-968-1200 Fax: (410)-968-3005
Contact: Debby Cullen
Treatment & referrals

Talbot County

County Health Depts

Talbot County Health Department
100 S. Hanson Street
Easton, MD 21601
Telephone: (410)-822-2292 Fax: (410)-822-2583
Contact: Carol Hansen
Public health services.

Washington County

County Health Depts

Washington County Health Department
1302 Pennsylvania Avenue
Hagerstown, MD 21742
Telephone: (301)-791-3232
Contact: Sandra Walters
HIV testing, AIDS education

Wicomico County

County Health Depts

Wicomico County Health Department
300 W. Carroll Street
Salisbury, MD 21801
Telephone: (410)-543-6943 Fax: (410)-543-6975
Contact: Karen Satterlee
Public health services.

Worcester County

County Health Depts

Worcester County Health
PO Box 249 Street
6040 Public Landing Road
Snow Hill, MD 21863
Telephone: (410)-632-1110 Fax: (410)-632-0906
Contact: Jane Apson - MD
Anonymous HIV testing-education, partner notification, case management

Worcester County Health Department
400-A Walnut Street
Pocomoke, MD 21851
Telephone: (410)-957-2005
Contact: Bertha Shockley
HIV testing, case management

MASSACHUSETTS

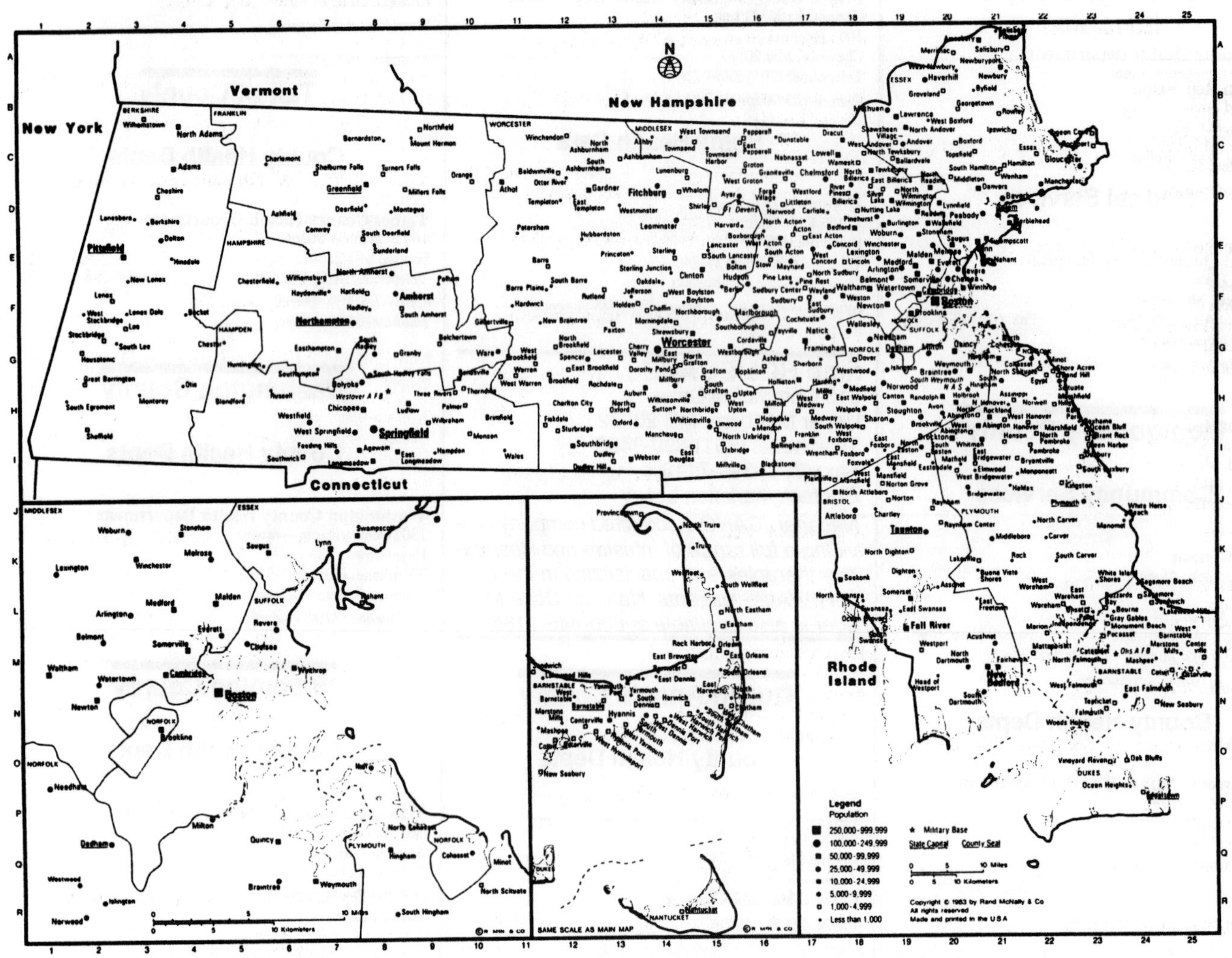

From City/County Planning Atlas Copyright 1989 by Reed McNally & Company, R.L. 90-S-28

Massachusetts

General Services

Education

American Red Cross
61 Medford Street
Somerville, MA 02143
Telephone: (617)-623-0053 Fax: (617)-623-0355
Contact: Hedi Hemlein
Statewide educational services, homeless students

American Red Cross - Berkshire County Chapter
P.O. Box 644
Pittsfield, MA 01202-0644
Telephone: (413)-442-1506 Fax: (413)-448-6051
Contact: Kathleen Phillips
Educational services

American Red Cross - Pioneer Valley Chapter
235 Chestnut Street
Springfield, MA 01103
Telephone: (413)-737-4306 Fax: (413)-785-0929
Contact: Jean Hobbie - Director
Educational services

Bridge Over Troubled Waters
47 West Street
Boston, MA 02111-1223
Telephone: (617)-423-9575
Contact: Barbara Whelan
Educational services & HIV testing

Central Massachusetts Area Health Education Center
50 Lake Avenue
Worcester, MA 01604
Telephone: (508)-756-6676
Contact: Gail Lewis - Health Director
Publishes Resource Directory for Central Massachusetts

Community Health Program
112 Packard Avenue
Tufts University
Medford, MA 02155
Telephone: (617)-381-3233 Fax: (617)-628-5800
Contact: Seymour Bellin - Director
Courses for Community health programs

Fenway Community Health Center Mental Health Department
7 Haviland Street
Boston, MA 02115-1817
Telephone: (617)-267-7573
Contact: Rob Johnson - Coord. HIV Educ. & Support Grp
AIDS education and group services

General Videotex Corporation/Delphi Information Network
1030 Massachusetts Ave.
Cambridge, MA 02138
Telephone: (800)-544-4005
Databases, Electronic Media

Greater Gardner AIDS Task Force
161A Chestnut Street
Gardner, MA 01440-2703
Telephone: (508)-632-1350 Fax: (508)-632-1350
Contact: Janet Lauricalla - Facilitator
Education, information and referrals, pre-test screening for HIV

Harvard University, School of Public Health
8 Story Street
Cambridge, MA 02138
Telephone: (617)-432-1090
Contact: Rick Marlink - Director
AIDS educational program, AIDS in the workplace

Health Awareness Services of Central Massachusetts
71 Elm Street
Worcester, MA 01609-2310
Telephone: (508)-756-7123 Fax: (508)-756-8922
Contact: Heather Robinson - AIDS Health Educator, Jerry Cheney - Adolescent Health Care
Educational and outreach services; Targets youth and youth servingprofessionals

Health Care of Southeastern Massachusetts
728 Brockton Ave.
Abington, MA 02351-2114
Telephone: (617)-857-1025 Fax: (617)-857-1754
Contact: Beverly Wright
AIDS education

Health Care of Southeastern Massachusetts
728 Brockton Avenue
PO Box 2127
Abington, MA 02351
Telephone: (617)-857-1025 Fax: (617)-857-1754
Contact: Sheldon Bar
SE Mass Educational Services

Health Quarters, Inc.
19 Broadway Street
Beverly, MA 01915-4417
Telephone: (508)-927-9824 Fax: (508)-922-5904
Northeast Mass educational services

Healthworks, A Family Life Resource Center, Inc.
77 E. Merrimack Street
Lowell, MA 01852-2747
Telephone: (508)-459-6871
Contact: Donna Morse
Educational services, counseling prevention for individuals, offices alsoin Lawrence and Haverhill

International Deaf-Tek, Inc.
PO Box 2431
Framingham, MA 01701-0424
Telephone: (508)-620-1777
Contact: Brenda Monene - President
Electronic mail service, schools, service providers agency, organizations,university programs

JSI Research & Training
210 Lincoln Street
Boston, MA 02111
Telephone: (617)-482-9485 Fax: (617)-482-0617
Contact: Lori Kiel - HIV AIDS Program Manager
Statewide HIV educational services and training for health care workers

Massachusetts Hospital Association
5 New England Exec Park
Burlington, MA 01803
Telephone: (617)-272-8000 Fax: (617)-270-5238
Contact: Lois Kinzer - Director
Statewide educational services

Massachusetts Nurses Association
340 Turnpike Street
Canton, MA 02021
Telephone: (617)-821-4625 Fax: (617)-821-4445
Statewide educational services

Massachusetts Prevention Center
24 Crecent Street
Suite 301
Waltham, MA 02154
Telephone: (617)-893-0111 Fax: (617)-647-2675
Contact: Marsha Lazar - Director
Training, consultation & technical assistance

New England AIDS Education and Training Center
320 Washington Street
Brookline, MA 01234
Telephone: (617)-566-2283 Fax: (617)-566-2994
Contact: Kelly Fattman
Education for health care providers

New England AIDS Etc: University of Massachusetts
55 Lake Avenue North
Worcester, MA 01655-0001
Telephone: (617)-566-2283 Fax: (617)-566-2994
Contact: Program Director - Michael E. Huppert
Educational Services

Northern Educational Service/ETHOS III AIDS Program
756 State Street
Springfield, MA 01109-4116
Telephone: (413)-737-8523 Fax: (413)-737-5446
Contact: Jay Griffin - Director
Community prevention programs, outreach, counseling, testing, speakers,case management, support groups

Orrian Enterprises
91 Main Boulevard
Shrewsbury, MA 01545-3151
Telephone: (508)-842-3464 Fax: (508)-842-3464
Contact: Gail Army - President
AIDS education

The Psychological Center's Prevention Network
488 Essex Street
Lawrence, MA 01840-1245
Telephone: (508)-688-2323
Contact: Lebron Zoriada
NE Mass community services

Tri-Prevention First/North Central Alcoholism Commission
100 Grove Street
Worcester, MA 01605-2608
Telephone: (508)-752-8083 Fax: (508)-798-9857
Contact: Kirsten Nicholas
Central Mass educational services; prevention training & referrals

Hotlines

International Institute of Greater Lawrence, Inc.
LIFE/AIDS Project
45 Canal Street
Lawrence, MA 01840
Telephone: (508)-687-0981
Contact: Rafael Abislaiman
Community services & hotline

Massachusetts AIDS Hotline

In-State only (800)-235-2331

State Health Departments

Massachusetts Department of Public Health
150 Tremont Street
11th Floor
Boston, MA 02111
Telephone: (617)-727-0368 Fax: (617)-272-6943
Publication's on AIDS, HIV testing and referrals

Massachusetts Department of Public Health
150 Tremont Street
Boston, MA 02111-1126
Telephone: (617)-727-0368
Contact: John Auerbach - AIDS Program Director
Alternative Testing and Seropositive support

Massachusetts State Dept. of Health
150 Tremont Street
11th Floor
Boston, MA 02111
Telephone: (617)-727-0368 Fax: (617)-727-6496
Contact: Maryette Guerra - AIDS Coord.

Statewide Services

AIDS Action Committee
131 Clarendon Street
Boston, MA 02116
Telephone: (617)-437-6200 Fax: (617)-437-6445
Toll-Free: (800)-235-2331
Contact: Larry Kessler
Statewide educational services/support group & hotline, Legal services

Massachusetts Department of Public Welfare
627 Main Street
Worcester, MA 01608
Telephone: (508)-792-7200
Financial Services

Massachusetts Department of Public Welfare
600 Washington Street
Boston, MA 02111-1704
Telephone: (617)-348-5500 Fax: (617)-348-8590
Contact: Rick Vogel - Director of AIDS Services
State Resources Agency

Barnstable County

Community Services

Cape Cod AIDS Council
592 Main St. Connection
Hyannis, MA 02601
Telephone: (508)-778-5111 Fax: (508)-778-5127
Contact: George Hodgon
Referrals, counseling, home assistance, transportation

Provincetown AIDS Support Group
96-98 Bradford Street
PO Box 1522
Provincetown, MA 02657
Telephone: (508)-487-9445 Fax: (508)-487-0565
Contact: Alice M Foley
Counseling, transportation, entitlement adovacy

Medical Services

Cape Cod Hospital
27 Park Street
Hyannis, MA 02601
Telephone: (508)-771-1800
SE Mass medical services, counseling, referrals, psychiatric care

Berkshire County

Community Services

Berkshire Council on Alcoholism and Addictions
Doyle Detoxification
793 North Street
Pittsfield, MA 01201
Telephone: (413)-499-0337
Contact: Doreen Rainer
Medical assessment, treatment for withdrawal, counseling and referral

Counseling Center in the Berkshires
232 First Street
Pittsfield, MA 01201-4749
Telephone: (413)-499-4090
Contact: Dr. John Messerschmitt
Counseling and Support Groups

Home Health Care

Homedco Infusion
1450 East Street
Pittsfield, MA 01201-5319
Telephone: (413)-443-4788 Fax: (413)-443-0437
Nationwide experience in providing home infusion therapy to AIDS patients

Hospice of Northern Berkshire, Inc.
PO Box 171
North Adams, MA 01247-0171
Telephone: (413)-664-6526
Contact: Anna Singleton
Hospice supportive services to terminally ill patients and their families

Hospice of South Berkshire
PO Box 428
Great Barrington, MA 01230-0428
Telephone: (413)-528-4786 Fax: (413)-528-3279
Hospice supportive services to terminally ill patients and their families

Medical Services

Berkshire Mental Health
333 East Street
Pittsfield, MA 01201-5392
Telephone: (413)-499-0412 Fax: (413)-448-2198
Contact: Ray Breen; Angie Buchaver -
Counseling and Support Groups/Sliding fee

Bristol County

Community Services

New Bedford Area Center for Human Services
337 Union Street
New Bedford, MA 02741
Telephone: (508)-990-8280 Fax: (508)-991-5153
Contact: Adrienne McGowan
Educational services, counseling

Project Care/AIDS Advocacy Center
PO Box A-2097
337 Union Street
New Bedford, MA 02741
Telephone: (508)-990-8280 Fax: (508)-991-5153
Contact: Adrian McGowan
Testing, counseling & education

Home Health Care

Community Nurses Association of Fairhaven
40 Centre Street
Fairhaven, MA 02719-2932
Telephone: (508)-992-6278 Fax: (508)-992-6591
Contact: Evelyn Ellis
SE Mass Home Health Care Services

Hospice of Community Health Agency
141 Park Street
Attleboro, MA 02703-3020
Telephone: (508)-222-0118 Fax: (508)-226-8936
Hospice suppor for terminally ill patients and their families

Hospice of St. Luke's Hospital
101 Page Street
New Bedford, MA 02740-3464
Telephone: (508)-997-1515 Fax: (508)-997-1515
Contact: Edith Vaughn
Hospice supportive services to terminally ill patients and their families

Testing Sites

New Bedford Health Department
100 Brock Avenue
New Bedford, MA 02744-1317
Telephone: (508)-991-6174 Fax: (508)-991-6291
Medical services, TB testing

Stanley Street Treatment & Resource Center/Project AWARE
386 Stanley Street
Fall River, MA 02720-6009
Telephone: (508)-679-5222 Fax: (508)-674-3699
Toll-Free: (800)-937-3610
Contact: Pauline T. Smith
Southeast Massachusetts community services, HIV testing and counseling;case management, support groups, outreach programs, education, multilingual

Essex County

Community Services

Cape Ann AIDS Task Force
22 Popular Street
Gloucester, MA 01930-4832
Telephone: (508)-281-9771 Fax: (508)-281-9779
Contact: Sheryl Knutsen
Northeast Mass community services

Center for Addictive Behaviors
27 Congress Street
Salem, MA 01970-5594
Telephone: (508)-745-8890
Prevention center, counseling, education, referrals, training

Community Action, Inc.
25 Locust Street
Haverhill, MA 01832-5689
Telephone: (508)-373-1971
Fuel assistance, housing, family day care

Marblehead Community Counseling Center
Growth & Learning Center
66 Clifton Avenue
Marblehead, MA 01945
Telephone: (617)-631-8273
Drug-free Counseling Services (Outpatient)

Project Cope, Inc.
117 North Common Street
Lynn, MA 01905-4299
Telephone: (617)-581-9270
Drug-free counseling, inpatient long term care, halfway house

Home Health Care

Hospice Program of the VNA of Greater Lynn
16 City Hall Square
Lynn, MA 01901
Telephone: (617)-598-2454
Hospice supportive services to terminally ill patients and their families

Visiting Nurses Association of Lynn
16 City Hall Square
Lynn, MA 01901
Telephone: (617)-598-2454 Fax: (617)-598-2454
Contact: Mary DeVeau
NE Mass Home Health Care Services

Medical Services

Center for Addictive Behaviors - Detox Unit
P.O. Box 500
Hathorne, MA 01937-0305
Telephone: (508)-777-2121 Fax: (508)-774-4814
Medical assessment, treatment for withdrawal, counseling and referral

Franklin County

Home Health Care

Hospice in Franklin County
164 High Street
Greenfield, MA 01301-2691
Telephone: (413)-772-0211 Fax: (413)-774-4438
Contact: Joanne Schlunk
Hospice supportive services to terminally ill patients and their families

Hampden County

Community Services

Child and Family Services
367 Pine Street
Springfield, MA 01105-1998
Telephone: (413)-737-1426 Fax: (413)-739-9988
Contact: Douglas Allan
Counseling and support groups for HIV families & children

Kate's Kitchen
264 Elm Street
Holyoke, MA 01040
Telephone: (413)-532-0233 Fax: (413)-536-9109
Contact: Bob Goushea
Serves one hot meal daily, 7 days a week to anyone in need

The Grey House
22 Sheldon Street
Springfield, MA 01107-1915
Telephone: (413)-734-6696
Contact: Mary Jeanne Tash - Executive Director
Emergency food & clothing, youth after school programs, elder care

Urban Ministry/Council of Churches
32 Ridgewood Place
Springfield, MA 01105
Telephone: (413)-733-2149 Fax: (413)-733-9817
Contact: Rev. Ann Geer
Advocacy, counseling, support groups

Westfield Counseling Center of Providence Hospital
41 Church Street
Westfield, MA 01085-2805
Telephone: (413)-568-3368
Contact: Karen Walsh-Pio
Drug-free counseling services (outpatient)

Westfield Counseling Center of Providence Hospital
41 Church Street
Westfield, MA 01085-2805
Telephone: (413)-568-3368
Contact: Karen Walsh-Pio
Substance abuse counseling, AIDS education

Home Health Care

Curaflex/Clinical Homecare
111 Park Avenue
West Sprngfield, MA 01089-1900
Telephone: (413)-733-4193 Fax: (413)-736-4450
Toll-Free: (800)-533-8059
Contact: Dr. Harrison Willcutts - Vice President
Home Infusion Therapy

Holyoke Visiting Nurses
330 Whitney Avenue
Suite 500
Holyoke, MA 01041-2028
Telephone: (413)-534-5691 Fax: (413)-538-7168
Contact: Debra Patulak
Hospice life care services to terminally ill patients and their families

Homedco
120 Carando Drive
Springfield, MA 01104
Telephone: (413)-736-4529 Fax: (413)-732-4029
Toll-Free: (800)-332-0722
Contact: Eleanor McCarthy
Respiratory, HME, infusion therapy, pharmacy services, AIDS education

Medical Services

Alcohol and Substance Abuse Program
210 Elm Street
Holyoke, MA 01040-4302
Telephone: (413)-538-9400
Contact: Vincent Tobin
Medical assessment, treatment for withdrawal, counseling and referral

Alcoholism Services of Greater Springfield
1400 State Street
Springfield, MA 01109-2550
Telephone: (413)-736-0334
Contact: Ann Shea
Medical assessment, treatment for withdrawal, counseling and referral

Center for Partial Hospitization
20 Hospital Drive
Holyoke, MA 01040
Telephone: (413)-534-2626 Fax: (413)-536-8224
Contact: Carmel Steger
Group counseling, short term intensive therapy, substance abuse &psychiatric

Gandara Mental Health Center, Inc.
1985 Main Street
Springfield, MA 01107
Telephone: (413)-736-8328 Fax: (413)-746-4270
Contact: Hector Slores
Counseling, case management, meal programs

Providence Hospital Substance Abuse Treatment Program
First Step
1233 Main Street
Holyoke, MA 01040-4317
Telephone: (413)-536-7383 Fax: (413)-539-2406
Toll-Free: (800)-292-9275
Contact: Ron Basil
Detoxification from opiates, medical evaluation, counseling & referral

Providence Hospital's Health & Hospital Services
210 Elm Street
Holyoke, MA 01040-4317
Telephone: (413)-538-9400
Western Massachusetts medical services

Hampshire County

Community Services

AIDS Care/Hampshire County
P.O. Box 1087
Northampton, MA 01061
Telephone: (413)-586-5394 Fax: (413)-584-9615
Contact: Reed Ide
Support volunteers, referrals, case management for people with HIV or AIDS

Family Planning Council of Western Mass., Inc.
16 Center Street
Northampton, MA 01060-3905
Telephone: (413)-586-2016 Fax: (413)-586-0212
Toll-Free: (800)-750-2016
Contact: Luz Pena - Till Director
Outreach education, HIV counseling & testing, support services

Valley Human Services, Inc.
96 South Street
Ware, MA 01082-1698
Telephone: (413)-967-6241 Fax: (413)-967-9807
Contact: Evelyn Glichman - Director
Drug-free Counseling Services (Outpatient)

Western Massachusetts Food Bank
P.O. Box 160
Hatfield, MA 01038-0160
Telephone: (413)-247-9738
Contact: Mary Lou Joyner - Office Manager
Clearinghouse for redistributing surplus foods to other non-profit groups.

Hillsborough County

Home Health Care

Caremark
9 Cedarwood Drive
Unit #3
Bedford, MA 03110
Telephone: (603)-644-3255
Toll-Free: (800)-544-1052
Contact: Anne DuPont - Sales Mgr.- HIV; John Stofko - Branch Mgr.
Clinical Support and Infusion Therapies: Nutrition, Antimicrobials, Chemo.,Hematopoeti

Middlesex County

Community Services

Arlington Youth Consultation Center
12 Prescott Street
Arlington, MA 02174-3016
Telephone: (617)-646-5880 Fax: (617)-641-5478
Contact: Patsy Kraemer - Director
Drug-free Counseling Services (Outpatient)

CASPAR Intervention Center
245 Beacon Street
Somerville, MA 02143-3635
Telephone: (617)-628-6300 Fax: (617)-628-6810
Contact: Kathy Wilkins - Director
Medical assessment, treatment for withdrawal, counseling and referral

Concilio Addictions Program
105 Windsor Street
Cambridge, MA 02139-3606
Telephone: (617)-661-8001 Fax: (617)-661-8008
Contact: Richard Osorio - Supervisor
AIDS counseling & outreach program

Haitian-American Culture Center
432 Columbia Street
Cambridge, MA 02141-3606
Telephone: (617)-621-0014 Fax: (617)-621-0575
Contact: Jean R Richard - Executive Director

Hispanic AIDS Resource Center
555 Merrimack Street
Lowell, MA 01854-4014
Telephone: (508)-970-2697
NE Mass educational services & hotline

North Charles Institute for the Addictions
260 Beacon Street
Somerville, MA 02143-3594
Telephone: (617)-661-5700 Fax: (617)-868-4840
Contact: Patrick Griswold - AIDS Coordinator
Counseling for AIDS patients, methodane maintenance, AIDS education &yearly AIDS updates

Planned Parenthood League
99 Bishop Richard Allen Drive
Cambridge, MA 02139-3496
Telephone: (617)-492-0518 Fax: (617)-661-9212
Toll-Free: (800)-682-9218
Contact: Susan Newsome - Associate Director

Region West Family Counseling Service
74 Walnut Park
Newton, MA 02158-1492
Telephone: (617)-965-6200 Fax: (617)-965-6203
Contact: Maurice Soulis - Social Worker
Drug-free Counseling & Family Services, Outpatient Mental Health

Tri-City Community Mental Health and Retardation Center
140 A. Ferry Street
Malden, MA 02148
Telephone: (617)-397-2000 Fax: (617)-397-0439
Contact: Anne P. Umana - Executive Director
Counseling and Support Groups/Sliding fee

Home Health Care

HNS, Inc.
Woodland Park II
8 Park Drive, Suite 9
Westford, MA 01886
Telephone: (508)-692-6305 Fax: (508)-692-6834
Contact: John Leonard - Manager
Home infusion therapy, in-home nursing and attendant care, physical therapyservices, pentamidine, referrals, case management

Home Hospice Care of Whidden Memorial Hospital
103 Garland Street
Everett, MA 02149-5095
Telephone: (617)-381-7111 Fax: (617)-381-7195
Contact: Jeanne Leydon - Manager
Home & hospice comprehensive care for patients and their families.

Homedco Infusion
260-D Fordham Road
Wilmington, MA 01887
Telephone: (508)-657-8443 Fax: (508)-657-8582
Contact: Distribution Supervisor
Respiratory, HME, Infusion Therapy

Hospice Care
21 Maple Street
Arlington, MA 02174-4903
Telephone: (617)-648-3172 Fax: (617)-279-4677
Contact: Sheila Scott - Director
Hospice supportive services to terminally ill patients and their families

Hospice of Cambridge
186 Alewife Brook Parkway
Suite 206
Cambridge, MA 02138-1126
Telephone: (617)-547-2620 Fax: (617)-876-2526
Contact: Arlene Lowney - Director
Hospice supportive services to terminally ill patients and their families

Hospice Program, Emerson Hospital
Old Road to Nine Acre
Concord, MA 01742
Telephone: (508)-369-1400 Fax: (508)-287-3651
Contact: Paul Montgomery - Coordinator
Hospice supportive services to terminally ill patients and their families

Nashoba Nursing Service/Nashoba Associated Boards of Health
Central Avenue
Ayer, MA 01432
Telephone: (508)-772-3337 Fax: (508)-772-7248
Toll-Free: (800)-698-3307
Contact: Mary S. Licquirish - Q.A. Manager
Homemaker, home care, companions

NETWORK Curaflex Health Services
293 Boston Post Road West
Marlborough, MA 01752
Telephone: (800)-334-3988
Contact: Nancy Seretta - General Manager
Home Infusion Therapy

Visiting Nurse Association of Cambridge
186 Alewife Brook Pkwy
Suite 206
Cambridge, MA 02138
Telephone: (617)-547-2620 Fax: (617)-547-2329
Contact: Nancy Kinlin;
Home health care

Visiting Nurse Association of Greater Lowell, Inc.
336 Central Street
PO Box 1965
Lowell, MA 01853-2115
Telephone: (508)-459-9343 Fax: (508)-459-0981
Contact: Anne Paquette - Coordinator
Hospice supportive services to terminally ill patients and their families

Medical Services

Bay Colony Health Services
800 West Cummings Park
Suite 1200
Woburn, MA 01801-6504
Telephone: (617)-935-3025 Fax: (617)-935-7805
Contact: Tim Conor - Director
Specializing in treatment of chemical dependency

Somerville Hospital - Division of Community Health
125 Lowell Street
Somerville, MA 02145-1414
Telephone: (617)-623-8686 Fax: (617)-628-4213

Contact: Charles Kaplan - Manager
Greater Boston area medical services

South Middlesex Addiction Services
3 Merchant Road
PO Box 606
Framingham, MA 01701-7401
Telephone: (617)-237-1811 Fax: (508)-620-2493
Contact: Betsy Fontes - Director
Medical assessment, treatment for withdrawal, counseling and referral

Nantucket County

Medical Services

Nantucket AIDS Network
Nantucket Cottage Hospital
Nantucket, MA 02554
Telephone: (508)-228-3955 Fax: (508)-325-5597
Contact: Cheryl Bartlett - HIV Coordinator
Hospice/HIV services, support groups, home care, inpatient

Norfolk County

Community Services

Back Bay Counseling Service
1368 Beacon Street
#109 Coolidge Corner
Brookline, MA 02146
Telephone: (617)-739-7860
Counseling

Bay State Community Services
15 Cottage Ave.
Quincy, MA 02169-5215
Telephone: (617)-471-8400 Fax: (617)-376-8910
Contact: Bill Spinks
Community services & support groups

Needham Youth Department
Town Hall
1471 Highland Avenue
Needham, MA 02192
Telephone: (617)-455-7500
Contact: Thomas Engelman
Drug-free Counseling Services (Outpatient)

New England Hemophilia Association
180 Rustcraft Road
Dedham, MA 02026-4547
Telephone: (617)-326-7645 Fax: (617)-329-5122
Contact: Education & Services Coor
Information liaison for hemophiliacs with AIDS, direct services

Northern Berkshire MHA
85 Main Street
Suite 500
North Adams, MA 02147-3406
Telephone: (413)-664-4541 Fax: (413)-662-3311
Contact: Kelly Morandi; Majorie Cohan
Drug-free Counseling Services (Outpatient)

Home Health Care

Good Samaritan Hospice of the Archdiocese of Boston
310 Allston Street
Brighton, MA 02146
Telephone: (617)-566-6242 Fax: (617)-566-3055
Hospice services to terminally ill patients and their caregivers

Hospice of the South Shore, Inc.
100 Bay State Drive
Braintree, MA 02184-5534
Telephone: (617)-843-0947 Fax: (617)-843-6465
Contact: Karen Riley - Director
Bereuement services, support group for AIDS patients, home health aides,social group worker, chaplain

Neponset Valley Hospice
3 Edgewater Street
Norwood, MA 02062
Telephone: (617)-769-8282 Fax: (617)-762-0718
Toll-Free: (800)-425-8282
Contact: Joanne Smith
Hospice supportive services to terminally ill patients and their families

VNA/Hospice Community Services/Faulkner Hospice Services
1100 High Street
Dedham, MA 02026-5798
Telephone: (617)-566-1507 Fax: (617)-455-6869
Contact: MaryLou McLean
Hospice supportive services to terminally ill patients and their families

Medical Services

Mass Regional Prevention Center
15 Cottage Ave.
Quincy, MA 02169-5216
Telephone: (617)-471-8400 Fax: (617)-376-8910
Contact: Melanie Snook
Greater Boston area medical services

Quincy Detox Center
120 Whitwell Street
Quincy, MA 02169-1815
Telephone: (617)-472-1484
Medical assessment, treatment for withdrawal, counseling and referral

Plymouth County

Community Services

Hingham Health Department
7 East Street
Hingham, MA 02043
Telephone: (617)-741-1466 Fax: (617)-740-0239
Medical services

Middleboro/Lakeville MHC
94 South Main Street
Middleboro, MA 02346
Telephone: (508)-947-6100
Drug-free Counseling Services (Outpatient)

Pathways Prevention Center
109 Rhode Island Road
Route 79
Lakeville, MA 02347
Telephone: (508)-946-3444 Fax: (508)-946-1187
Contact: Arthur Bowles
SE Mass community services, Training, Education

Home Health Care

Brockton Visiting Nurse Association
1280 Belmont Street
Brockton, MA 02401-4402
Telephone: (508)-587-2121 Fax: (508)-584-8780
Contact: Mary Lou McNiff
Hospice supportive services to terminally ill patients and their families

Medical Services

Alcoholism Intervention Center at Brockton
686 North Main Street
Brockton, MA 02401-2444
Telephone: (508)-584-9210
Contact: Jack Mazzotti
Medical assessment, treatment for withdrawal, counseling and referral

Suffolk County

Community Services

Action for Boston Community Development
178 Tremont Street
Boston, MA 02111-1017
Telephone: (617)-357-6810
Contact: Henry Vera Garcia
Greater Boston area community services

Alliance for Young Families
30 Winter Street
11th Floor
Boston, MA 02108
Telephone: (617)-482-9122 Fax: (617)-482-9129
Contact: Joan Tighe
Greater Boston area community services

Boston AIDS Consortium/Harvard School of Public Health
718 Huntington Avenue
Boston, MA 02115-6023
Telephone: (617)-432-0885 Fax: (617)-432-2494
Contact: Timothy Palmer
Referrals

Brookside Community Health Center
3297 Washington Street
Jamaica Plain, MA 02130-2655
Telephone: (617)-522-4700
Community health services & support group

Coalition for Legal Rights of the Disabled
11 Beacon Street
Suite 925
Boston, MA 02108
Telephone: (617)-723-8455 Fax: (617)-723-9125
Toll-Free: (800)-872-9992
Contact: Dan Aheam
Legal Services & Advocacy, consists of over two dozen advocacy groups

Cognitive Behavior Therapist
29 Commonwealth Avenue
Suite 809
Boston, MA 02116
Telephone: (617)-262-6269
Contact: Robert Haas - L.I.C.S.W.
AIDS/HIV counseling

Crittenton Hastings House
10 Perthshire Road
Boston, MA 02135-1798
Telephone: (617)-782-7600 Fax: (617)-254-7966
Contact: Karren Van-Unen - Health Director
Residential programs for pregnant and parenting teenagers,counseling, nutrition, child care

First AIDS Project
5 Washington Street
Roxbury, MA 02121
Telephone: (617)-427-1008 Fax: (617)-445-2291
Greater Boston area community services, HIV counseling & support

Gay and Lesbian Advpcates amd Defenders
P. O. Box 218
Boston, MA 02112
Telephone: (617)-426-1350 Fax: (617)-426-3594
Legal Services & Advocacy

Greater Boston Food Bank
99 Atkinson Street
Boston, MA 02118-1039
Telephone: (617)-427-5831 Fax: (617)-427-0146
Contact: Westy Egmont
Clearinghouse for redistributing surplus foods to other non-profit groups.

Haitian Multi-Service Center/Haitian AIDS Project
12 Bicknell Street
Dorchester, MA 02121-4102
Telephone: (617)-436-2848 Fax: (617)-287-0284
Greater Boston area community services & support groups-for AIDS/HIV

Kenmore Healing Arts Center
25 Huntington Avenue
Suite 609
Boston, MA 02116-2605
Telephone: (617)-267-6525
Individual, couple and group therapy, referrals, AIDS counseling

Life Lines AIDS Prevention Project for the Homeless
c/o Shattuck Shelter
170 Morton Street
Jamaica Plain, MA 02130
Telephone: (617)-522-8110 Fax: (617)-524-4709
Community services

Martha Eliot Health Center
33 Bickford Street
Jamaica Plain, MA 02130-1499
Telephone: (617)-522-5300 Fax: (617)-983-9478
Community services & support group

Massachusetts Department of Social Services
24 Farnsworth Street
Boston, MA 02210
Telephone: (617)-727-0900 Fax: (617)-261-7437
Contact: Sue Tobin, RN
Services for infants with AIDS

Multicultural AIDS Coalition
801 Tremont St.
Boston, MA 02118
Telephone: (617)-442-1622 Fax: (617)-442-6622
Contact: Barbara Gomes-Beach
Technical assistance, outreach, advocacy for AIDS-related agencies.

Noodle Island Multi Service
14 Porter Street
East Boston, MA 02128-1654
Telephone: (617)-569-7310 Fax: (617)-569-7890
Drug-free Counseling Services (Outpatient)

Reaching Out to Chelsea Adolescents
144 Washington Avenue
Chelsea, MA 02150-3903
Telephone: (617)-889-5210
Greater Boston area

Veterans Administration
JFK Fed Bldg, Gov't Ctr
Dept of Vet Affairs
Boston, MA 02203
Telephone: (617)-227-4600
Contact: Albert Evans
Call for VA benefits information & regional phone numbers.

Home Health Care

Visiting Nurse Association of Boston
75 Arlington Street
Boston, MA 02116-3941
Telephone: (617)-577-7900
Contact: Beverly Wancho
Greater Boston area home health care services & support groups

Medical Services

Addiction Treatment Center of New England
77 F Warren Street
Brignton, MA 02135
Telephone: (617)-254-1271 Fax: (617)-787-4279
Contact: Harvey Kautman
Detoxification from opiates, medical evaluation, counseling & referral

Bay Cove Substance Abuse Center/Clinic
66 Canal Street
Boston, MA 02114
Telephone: (617)-474-0460 Fax: (617)-474-0461
Contact: Elizabeth Bredin
Detoxification from opiates, medical evaluation, counseling & referral

Beth Israel Social Services/Counseling Clinic
330 Brookline Avenue
Boston, MA 02115
Telephone: (617)-735-4634
Contact: Susan Burnstein - Director
AIDS/HIV primary care, AIDS clinical trials, homecare, women's health,mental health counseling, emergency

Boston City Hospital, Division of Psychiatry
ACC 4
818 Harrison Avenue
Boston, MA 02118
Telephone: (617)-534-4228 Fax: (617)-534-4517
Contact: Abraham Fingold - Program Director
Comprehensive Counseling for patients recieving primary health care atBoston City Hospital

Boston Detox
Lemul Shattuck Building
170 Morton Street 12th Floor
Jamaica Plaine, MA 02130
Telephone: (617)-983-3710 Fax: (617)-983-9380
Contact: Fred Walker
Medical assessment, treatment for withdrawal, counseling and referral

Carney Hospital
2100 Dorchester Avenue
Boston, MA 02124-5666
Telephone: (617)-296-4000 Fax: (617)-296-7759
Contact: Ann Killion
Medical services, primary care

Children's Hospital
AIDS Program
300 Longwood Avenue
Boston, MA 02115
Telephone: (617)-735-6832 Fax: (617)-730-0660
Contact: Kenneth McIntosh, M.D. - Clinical Trials Coord.
AIDS Treatment, Evaluation Services; Drug, Pharmaceutical Research

Codman Square Health Center
6 Norfolk Street
Dorchester, MA 02124-3550
Telephone: (617)-825-9660 Fax: (617)-825-0328
Contact: Rudy Padilla
Greater Boston area

Dimock Community Health Center
55 Dimock Street
Roxbury, MA 02119-1029
Telephone: (617)-442-8800 Fax: (617)-445-0091
HIV services programs, substance abuse, out patient program, halfway houses

Geiger Gibson Community Health Center
250 Mt. Vernon Street
Dorchester, MA 02125-3220
Telephone: (617)-288-1140 Fax: (617)-288-3910
Contact: Peggy McSharry
Medical, dental, mental health; free anonymous HIV testing

Lemuel Shattuck Hospital
170 Morton Street
Jamaica Plain, MA 02130-3782
Telephone: (617)-522-8110
Inpatient/Outpatient specialty care, statewide education services andsupport group

Massachusetts General Hospital
WACC Building
15 Parkman
Boston, MA 02114-2622
Telephone: (617)-726-6772 Fax: (617)-726-7541
Contact: Dr. Jonathon Worth
Psychiatric care for people with AIDS

North End Community Health Center
332 Hanover Street
Boston, MA 02113-1997
Telephone: (617)-742-9570
Pediatric and adult medicine, mental health and home care

Project TRUST - Boston City Hospital
818 Harrison Avenue
Boston, MA 02118-2999
Telephone: (617)-534-4495 Fax: (617)-445-0988
Contact: Rhoda Creamer
HIV testing and counseling, primary care clinic, treatment for uninsured

South End Community Health Center
400 Shawmut Avenue
Boston, MA 02118-2097
Telephone: (617)-425-2000 Fax: (617)-425-4080
Contact: Nadine Beck
Medical services & support group

Southern Jamaica Plain Health Center
687 Centre Street
Jamaica Plain, MA 02130-2556
Telephone: (617)-278-0710 Fax: (617)-524-5170
Contact: Steven Cadwell
Greater Boston area medical services

The Ethopian Family Center, Inc.
140 Clarendon Street
Suite 601
Boston, MA 02116-5137
Telephone: (617)-424-9305 Fax: (617)-351-7615
Medical services & support group

Uphams Corner Neighborhood Health Center
500 Columbia Road
Dorchester, MA 02125-2322
Telephone: (617)-287-8000 Fax: (617)-282-8625
Medical services

Worcester County

Community Services

AIDS Pastoral Care Network (APCN)
25 Crescent Street
Worcester, MA 01605-2406
Telephone: (508)-757-8385 Fax: (508)-842-8821
Contact: Brother William Callahan - Chairman

AIDS Project Worcester
305 Shrewsbury Street
Worcester, MA 01604-4012
Telephone: (508)-755-3773
Contact: Jim Volkes - HIV Director
HIV Antibody Testing, Community & Support Services, Food and Transportation

AIDS Support Group
191 Pakachoag Street
Auburn, MA 01501-2567
Telephone: (508)-755-8718 Fax: (508)-795-1603
Contact: Gina T. Colorio - Reverand
Support Group

Catholic Charities
15 Ripley Street
Worcester, MA 01610-2598
Telephone: (508)-798-0191 Fax: (508)-797-5659
Contact: Bilingual Social Worker
Mental Health Services, Substance Abuse Services

Chirho-Lambda Counseling Service
P.O. Box 17187
Main Street Station
Worcester, MA 01601-7187
Telephone: (508)-795-1118
Contact: Rev George McDermott
Pastoral care, support groups, education, gay & lesbian counseling,transgender counseling

Morning Star Metropolitan Community Church
231 Main St.
Cherry Valley, MA 01611-3143
Telephone: (508)-791-2294 Fax: (508)-892-4320
Contact: Scott Spaulding
Pastoral Care, Support Groups, Mental Health Care, Education, AIDS/HIV Ministry

The Mustard Seed/Catholic Worker House
93 Piedmont Street
Worcester, MA 01609
Telephone: (508)-754-7098
Soup Kitchen, Free Nursing Clinic, Homeless Outreach, Advocacy Program

The Salvation Army
630 Main Street
Worcester, MA 01608-2021
Telephone: (508)-756-7191
Contact: Major Robert A. Dries - Clergy
Community & Support Services, Pastoral Care, Financial Services; referrals& counseling

University of Mass Medical Center/Ambulatory Psychiatry AIDS
55 Lake Avenue North
Worcester, MA 01655
Telephone: (508)-856-2537 Fax: (508)-856-5981
Contact: Patrick Fairchild, MD
Mental Health Services, Support Group, Services for HIV testing,counseling, referrals, case management

Worcester Area Community Services
P.O. Box 226 Greendale Station
Worcester, MA 01606
Telephone: (508)-756-4354 Fax: (508)-752-1379
Contact: Jim Murphy - Program Director
Health Care Providers, HIV Antibody Testing, Nutritional Services

Worcester Children's Friend Society
21 Cedar Street
Worcester, MA 01609-2524
Telephone: (508)-753-5425 Fax: (508)-757-7659
Contact: Dr. Sheila Rosenblatt - Program Director
Community & Support Services, Mental Health Services, Education

Worcester Pastoral Counseling Center
4 Caroline Street
Worcester, MA 01604-3810
Telephone: (508)-757-0376
Contact: David Dolron - Executive Director
Referrals, counseling & education with mental health services, pastoralcare

Home Health Care

Critical Care America
50 Washington Street
Westborough, MA 01581
Telephone: (508)-836-3610 Fax: (508)-870-5935
Toll-Free: (800)-344-5500
Contact: Don Steen - President
Coordinate & integrate all clinical & psychosocial services for HIV+

Interim Health Care
1233 Main Street
Worcester, MA 01603-1817
Telephone: (508)-792-5900 Fax: (508)-754-5167
Contact: Administrator
Health Care Services, Home Health Care, Medicare/Medicaid, Physical Therapy

Nurses House Call
324 Grove Street
Worcester, MA 01605
Telephone: (508)-753-4780 Fax: (508)-752-1597
Contact: Lynn McCann - Administrator
Health Care Providers, Home Health Care, Pediatric Services

Pernet Family Health Service
237 Millbury Street
Worcester, MA 01610-2177
Telephone: (508)-755-1228
Contact: Director
Health Care, Home Health Care, Hospice Care, Pediatric Services

Visiting Nurse Association of Auburn, Inc.
41 South Street
Auburn, MA 01501-2851
Telephone: (508)-832-5749 Fax: (508)-832-3046
Contact: Deanna Goggins - Director
Health Services, Home Health Care, Hospice, Pediatric Services, Education

Wachusett Home Health Agency
43 Harvard Street
Wister, MA 01609-2586
Telephone: (508)-754-0052 Fax: (508)-752-3781
Contact: Karen Diamnond - Director
Home Health Care: certified, non-profit, skilled home health professionals

Medical Services

Amethyst Point
232 Chandler Street
Worcester, MA 01609-2928
Telephone: (508)-753-3975
Contact: Arlene Dorischild
Holistic Health Services

Great Brook Valley Health Center, Inc.
19 Tacoma Street
Worcester, MA 01605-3544
Telephone: (508)-852-1805
Health, pediatric, nutritional services, HIV testing, case management

Medical Center of Central Massachusetts Memorial
119 Belmont Street
Worcester, MA 01605-2982
Telephone: (508)-793-6611 Fax: (508)-793-6412
Contact: Dr. Mark Keroack - Chariman, HIV Advisory Gr
Health care providers, HIV antibody testing, home health care, infectiousdisease specialists

PRO HEALTH, Division of Montachusett Opportunity Council
689 Main Street
Fitchburg, MA 01420-4398
Telephone: (508)-345-4366 Fax: (508)-348-1425
Contact: Joyce Ryan - Director
Health care, nutrition, pediatric services, mental health services,education, HIV testing

Spectrum Addicition Services Inc.
155 Oak Street
Westborough, MA 01581-3317
Telephone: (508)-366-5202 Fax: (508)-898-1570
Contact: Dr. Seymour Solomon
Health Services, HIV Antibody Testing, Nutritional Services, Mental Health

U Mass Medical School/Research Dept of Ob/Gyn & Pediatrics
55 Lake Avenue North
Worcester, MA 01655-0001
Telephone: (508)-856-3107 Fax: (508)-856-5016
HIV Antibody Testing, Pediatric Services, Support Groups (women), Education

University of MA Medical Center
Infectious Disease Division
55 Lake Avenue North
Worcester, MA 01655-0001
Telephone: (508)-856-2659 Fax: (508)-856-5981
Contact: Joan Avotto
Health care provider, counseling, diagnostic & therapeutic services forHIV testing, counseling for HIV

University of Massachusetts Medical Center/Pediatric Immunology
55 Lake Avenue North
Worcester, MA 01655-0001
Telephone: (508)-856-3947 Fax: (508)-856-5500
Contact: Director
Pediatric Services

Testing Sites

City of Worcester, Dept of Public Health, Hep B/AIDS Div
25 Meade St.
Worcester, MA 01610-2715
Telephone: (508)-799-8568 Fax: (508)-799-8544
Contact: Susan Sereti
Hotline/HIV Antibody Testing, Education, Referrals

MICHIGAN

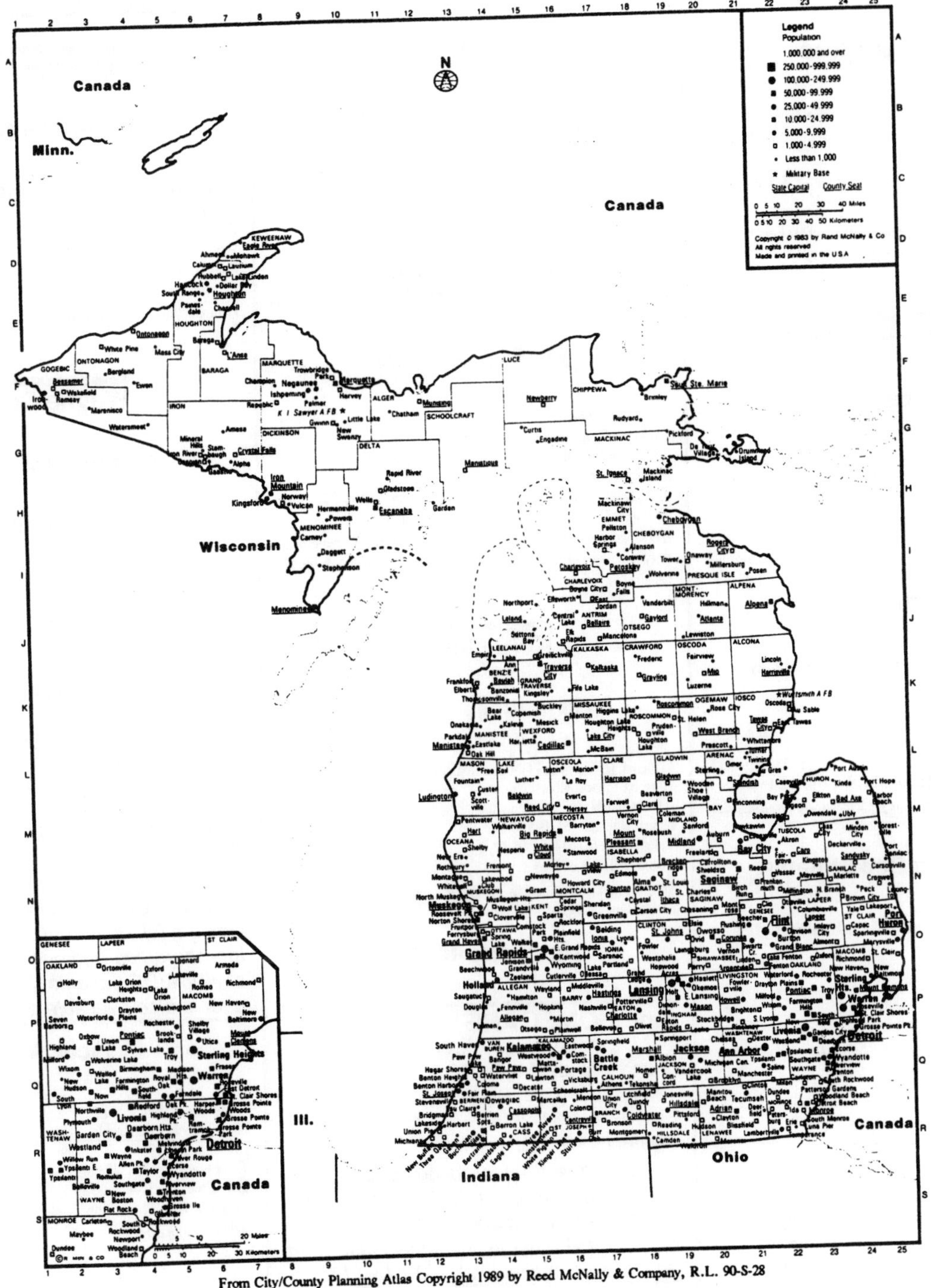

From City/County Planning Atlas Copyright 1989 by Reed McNally & Company, R.L. 90-S-28

Michigan

County

Medical Services

Sault Ste. Marie Tribe of Chippewa Indians Health Services
Health Services
Kincheloe, MI
Telephone: (906)-495-5615
Contact: Russ Vizina
HIV testing (anonymous & confidential) counseling, referral, HIVprevention, case management, primary care health provider, (tribal members)

General Services

Education

Michigan Department of Education School Program Services
P.O. Box 30008
Lansing, MI 48909
Telephone: (517)-373-2589
AIDS Education program

Hotlines

Lesbian-Gay Male Program Office and Gay Hotline
University of Michigan
3116-3118 Michigan Union
Ann Arbor, MI 48109-1349
Telephone: (313)-763-4186 Fax: (313)-747-4133
Contact: Jim Toy - Coordinator M.S.W.; Billie Edwards -
Counseling, Education, Advocacy, Community Organization Services, Referral

State Health Departments

Michigan Department of Public Health, Office of AIDS Prevention
Bureau of Infectious Disease
Lansing, MI 48909
Telephone: (517)-335-8371
Contact: Randall S. Pope - Chief
Prevention, Counseling, Testing, Education, Workshops, Technical Assistance

Michigan Department of Public Health-Pediatric AIDS Program
3423 North Logan Street
P.O. Box 30195
Lansing, MI 48909
Telephone: (517)-335-8900 Fax: (517)-335-9222
Contact: George Anderson - Office of Child Health
Prevention training, drug abuse, AIDS education

Chippewa County

Medical Services

Michigan Inter-tribal Council
Field Health Office
Watertower Drive
Kincheloe, MI 49788
Telephone: (906)-495-2289 Fax: (906)-492-7322
Contact: Charlotte Hewitt
Educational, outreach & referrals

Genesee County

Community Services

Urban League of Flint
5005 Lawndale Drive
Flint, MI 48503-1890
Telephone: (313)-789-7611 Fax: (313)-787-4518
Contact: Tracy Peterson
Counseling, hospital visitation & support services, education, literature

Isabella County

Medical Services

Nimkee Memorial Clinic
Saginaw Chippewa Indian Tribe
2591 South Leahton
Mt. Pleasant, MI 48858
Telephone: (517)-772-3767 Fax: (517)-772-3700
Contact: Diana Marshall - AIDS Coordinator
HIV testing (anonymous), counseling, referrals, case management, healthcare, education, outreach services & mental health.

Kent County

Community Services

Grand Rapids AIDS Resource Center
1414 Robinson Road S.E.
P.O. Box 6603
Grand Rapids, MI 49506
Telephone: (616)-459-9177 Fax: (616)-459-3432
Contact: Jan Koopman
Support services, buddy program, counseling, food bank, education, andlegal referrals

Home Health Care

nmc HOMECARE
607 Cascade West Prkwy SE
Grand Rapids, MI 49546
Telephone: (616)-954-2600
Fax: (616)-954-2609
Contact: Matt Berry
National JCAHO-Accredited company providing a full range of Infusion and Respiratory therapies and specializing in the care of HIV/AIDS patients. National Case Manager is also available at 800-445-1188

Oakland County

Home Health Care

nmc HOMECARE
1575 Woodward Ave # 114
Bloomfield Hills, MI 48302
Telephone: (313)-332-1111
National JCAHO-Accredited company providing a full range of Infusion and Respiratory therapies and specializing in the care of HIV/AIDS patients. National Case Manager is also available at 800-445-1188

Washtenaw County

Community Services

Hemophilia Foundation of Michigan
411 Huron View Boulevard
Suite 101
Ann Arbor, MI 48103-2997
Telephone: (313)-761-2535 Fax: (313)-761-3267
Contact: Susan Bigari - Patient Services Coordinator
Counseling, Hospital Visitation, Support Services & Education

Wayne County

Community Services

Michigan Protective and Advocacy Services
292 00 Vassar Blvd.venue
Suite 501
Livonia, MI 48152
Telephone: (313)-473-2990 Fax: (313)-473-4104
Contact: Jay Kaplan - Attorney Advocate
Legal rights for HIV patients

Home Health Care

nmc HOMECARE
9282 General Dr, Suite 120
Plymouth, MI 48170
Telephone: (313)-459-3780
Fax: (313)-459-2028
Contact: Ruth Ann Pendergrast
National JCAHO-Accredited company providing a full range of Infusion and Respiratory therapies and specializing in the care of HIV/AIDS patients. National Case Manager is also available at 800-445-1188

Medical Services

New Health Center
28550 Five Mile Road
Livonia, MI 48154
Telephone: (313)-522-5801 Fax: (313)-427-8270
Toll-Free: (313)-427-2550
Contact: Bev Thompson
AIDS treatment unit

MINNESOTA

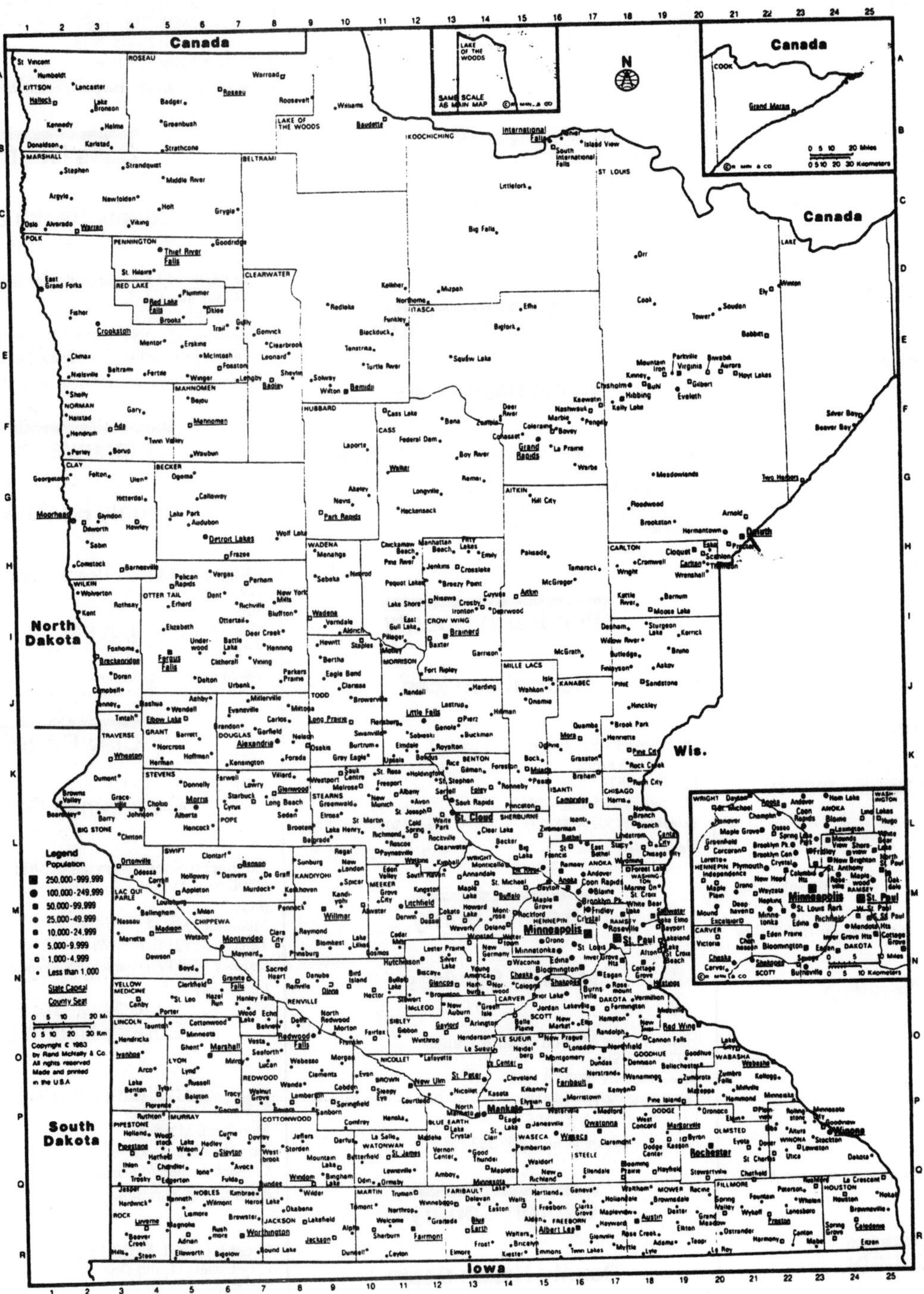

From City/County Planning Atlas Copyright 1989 by Reed McNally & Company, R.L. 90-S-28

Minnesota

General Services

Education

American Red Cross
11 Dell Place
eapolis, MN 55403-3296
Telephone: (612)-871-7676
Contact: Joe Larson
AIDS education

Community Action Council
15025 Glazier Avenue
Apple Valley, MN 55124-6300
Telephone: (612)-431-2112
Contact: Rita Mueller
AIDS education

Hotlines

AIDS Interfaith Council of Minnesota
Minnesota AIDS Project
2025 Nicollet Ave So #200
Minneapolis, MN 55404
Telephone: (612)-870-7773 Fax: (612)-870-8650
Contact: Loraine Teel - Executive Director
Tollfree hotline: 1-800-248-AIDS; case management

County Social Services
P.O. Box 718
Faribault, MN 55021-0718
Telephone: (507)-334-0031
24-hour Hotline: 1-800-422-1286

State Health Departments

Minnesota Department of Health, AIDS/STD Prevention Services
717 SE Delaware Street
P.O. Box 9441
Minneapolis, MN 55440-9441
Telephone: (612)-623-5698 Fax: (612)-623-5743
Contact: Jill DeBoer
Information & disease prevention services for HIV/STD infected and relatedpersons

Statewide Services

Minnesota AIDS Project
2025 Nicollet Avenue
Suite #200
Minneapolis, MN 55404-2555
Telephone: (612)-870-7773
Contact: Roy Schmidt
Referrals, case management, legal services, housing & education

Aitkin County

County Health Depts

Aitkin County Public Health Nursing Service
204 First Street, North West
Aitkin, MN 56431
Telephone: (218)-927-4357 Fax: (218)-927-7210
Contact: Lynne Kellerman
Education, in-home care

Becker County

Home Health Care

Multi County Nursing Services
P.O. Box 701
Detroit Lakes, MN 56501-0701
Telephone: (218)-847-9224
Contact: Nancy Bauer
Home care

Multi-County Nursing Service
1000 8th Street SE
P.O. Box 701
Detroit Lakes, MN 56501-2839
Telephone: (218)-847-9224
Contact: Tammi Stalberger
Public health home care.

Big Stone County

Home Health Care

Big Stone County Countryside Public Health
217 NW Third Street
Ortonville, MN 56278-1416
Telephone: (612)-839-6135
Contact: Barb Schnaser, RN
Home care services, education

Blue Earth County

Medical Services

Immanuel - St. Joseph's Hospital
1025 Marsh Street
P.O. Box 8673
Mankato, MN 56002-4795
Telephone: (507)-625-4031 Fax: (507)-325-2926
Medical services

Brown County

Medical Services

Sioux Trails Mental Health Center
1407 South State
New Ulm, MN 56073-3715
Telephone: (507)-354-3181 Fax: (507)-354-3181
Toll-Free: (800)-247-2809
24-hour emergency call 1-800-247-2809

Carlton County

County Health Depts

Carlton County Health Services
30 North 10th Street
Cloquet, MN 55720-1605
Telephone: (218)-879-4511
Contact: Karen Wunderlich, P.H.N. - Health Services Director
Home care for children, elderly, AIDS patients

Carver County

County Health Depts

Carver County Community Health Service
540 E. 1 Street
Waconia, MN 55387-1601
Telephone: (612)-448-3435 Fax: (612)-442-4493
Contact: Mary Lou Jirik
Public health, pre- and post- counseling, homecare

Cass County

County Health Depts

Cass County Community Health Center
P.O. Box 40
Walker, MN 56484
Telephone: (218)-547-3300 Fax: (218)-547-2855
Contact: Jeanine Frenzel - Health Director
Home care, hospice, referrals, resources for AIDS.

Chippewa County

County Health Depts

Chippewa County Health Department
719 North Seventh Street
Suite 308
Montevideo, MN 56265-1398
Telephone: (612)-269-2174
Educational programs, videos, pamphlets.

Clay County

Community Services

Lutheran Social Service of Minnesota
627 Center Avenue
Suite 3
Moorhead, MN 56560-1918
Telephone: (218)-236-1494 Fax: (218)-236-0836
Contact: Gail Peterson - AIDS Counselor
Counseling

County Health Depts

Clay County Health Department
715 11th Street North
Moorhead, MN 56560
Telephone: (218)-299-5222
Contact: Joanne Jorgenson
AIDS testing and counseling.

West Central AIDS Project
Clay County Health Dept.
715 North 11th Street
Moorhead, MN 56560
Telephone: (218)-299-5220
Contact: Iva Thielges
HIV testing, counseling, preventive education, referrals

Home Health Care

Clay-Wilkin CHS
715 Eleven Street North
Moorhead, MN 56560-2025
Telephone: (218)-299-5224
Contact: Iva Thielges
Home health care

Clearwater County

Home Health Care

Clearwater County Health Department-Nursing Service
175 4th Street Northwest Route 3
Box 46A
Bagley, MN 56621-0479
Telephone: (218)-694-6581
Contact: Cindy Schuppert
Visiting nurses

Cook County

Home Health Care

Cook County Public Health Nursing Service
411 West 2nd Street
Grand Marais, MN 55604
Telephone: (218)-387-2282
Contact: Rosemary A. Lamson - PHN Director
AIDS education, HIV testing, home health care & public health nursing

Crow Wing County

Community Services

The Counseling Center
523 North 3rd Street
Brainerd, MN 56401
Telephone: (218)-828-7606 Fax: (218)-828-3103
Toll-Free: (800)-828-7379
Contact: Yvonne Jacobs - Clinical Supervisor
Serves HIV+ clients

Home Health Care

Crow Wing County Health Services
322 Laurel Street
Brainerd, MN 56401
Telephone: (218)-828-3973
Contact: Linda S. Hamilton
Referrals, home health care, public education

Dakota County

County Health Depts

Dakota County Public Health Department
14955 Galaxie Avenue
Apple Valley, MN 55124-8579
Telephone: (612)-891-7500 Fax: (612)-891-7473
Contact: Barbara J. Schroeder
Child health care, immunizations

Home Health Care

Caremark
1355 Mendota Heights Road
Suite 240
Mendota Heights, MN 55120
Telephone: (612)-452-5600 Fax: (612)-452-9531
Toll-Free: (800)-624-8142
Contact: Laurie Johnson
CLINICAL SUPPORT AND INFUSION THERAPY: Nutrition, Antimicrobials, Chemo., Hematopoeti

Douglas County

Home Health Care

Douglas County PHNS
3401 South Broadway
Alexandria, MN 56308
Telephone: (612)-763-5438
Contact: Doreen Hanson, RN
Home-health care & hospice care.

Faribault County

County Health Depts

Faribault County, F&M Human Service Center
County Office Building
P.O. Box 217
Blue Earth, MN 56013
Telephone: (507)-526-3265
Contact: Constance Leland
Mental & public health, income maintenance, child protection, & familyservices.

Fillmore County

Home Health Care

Fillmore County Public Health Nursing
Courthouse
P.O. Box 84
Preston, MN 55965
Telephone: (507)-765-3898
Contact: Sharon Serfling
Home-health agency, educational & family health programs.

Goodhue County

County Health Depts

Goodhue County Health Department
419 Bush Street
Red Wing, MN 55066-2500
Telephone: (612)-388-0433
Contact: Vicki Iocco
Nursing service, family health & AIDS education.

Grant County

County Health Depts

Grant County Health Department
10 1st Northwest
P.O. Box 120
Elbow Lake, MN 56531-4698
Telephone: (218)-685-4461
Contact: Lorys L. Westburg
Screening, home care

Hennepin County

Community Services

AIDS Ministry Program- Archdiocese of St. Paul & Minneapolis
Riverside Medical Center
Riverside at 25th Ave. S.
Minneapolis, MN 55454
Telephone: (612)-337-4345
24 hour answering

Aliveness Project
730 East 38th Street
Minneapolis, MN 55407-2572
Telephone: (612)-822-7946 Fax: (612)-822-9668
Contact: Kevin Sitter - President of the Board
HIV/AIDS outreach program; foodshelf, home delivery, therapy, seminars

Bridge for Runaway Youth
2200 Emerson Avenue South
Minneapolis, MN 55405-2628
Telephone: (612)-377-8800 Fax: (612)-377-6426
Contact: Thomas Sawyer - Executive Director
Shelter, referrals, family planning, self-help groups regarding HIV/AIDS

First Universalist Church of Minneapolis
3400 Dupont Avenue South
Minneapolis, MN 55408
Telephone: (612)-825-1701 Fax: (612)-825-8879
Contact: Reverend Terry Sweetser
Community outreach

Friends for Lesbian and Gay Concerns
2756 Aldrich Avenue South
Minneapolis, MN 55405
Telephone: (612)-333-2548
Contact: David Anderson
Religious organization (Quaker)

Harbor Lights Salvation Army
1010 Currie Avenue
Minneapolis, MN 55403
Telephone: (612)-338-0113 Fax: (612)-338-4717
Contact: Major David Dalberg
Homeless shelter, chemical dependency treatment, housing, HIV testingonFridays only

Lutheran Social Service
2414 Park Avenue
Minneapolis, MN 55404-2599
Telephone: (612)-774-9507
Contact: Betchen Oberdorser
Mental health counseling, youth and teen program

Minneapolis Youth Diversion Program
1905 3rd Avenue South
Minneapolis, MN 55404-2720
Telephone: (612)-871-3613 Fax: (612)-871-3628
HIV testing, counseling of families or partners, preventive health care,education

Minnesota AIDS Project (MAP)
2025 Nicollet Avenue S.
Minneapolis, MN 55404
Telephone: (612)-870-7773 Fax: (612)-870-8650
Appropriate and caring services

County Health Depts

Hennepin County Community Health Department
525 Portland Avenue South
Level 3
Minneapolis, MN 55415-1569
Telephone: (612)-348-2741
Contact: Vicki Thelen
Counseling, testing, case management, HIV education, outreach programs

Hennepin County Community Health Department
Red Door Clinic
525 Portland Avenue
Minneapolis, MN 55415
Telephone: (612)-348-6363 Fax: (612)-348-3830
AIDS Testing and counseling.

Home Health Care

Becklund Home Health Care
8421 Wayzata Boulevard
Suite 100
Golden Valley, MN 55426-1344
Telephone: (612)-544-0315
Home health services

Critical Care America
811 West 106th Street
Bloomington, MN 55420
Telephone: (612)-884-9551 Fax: (612)-884-1722
Toll-Free: (800)-422-1281
Contact: Christina Wittchow
Coordinate & integrate all clinical & psychosocial services for HIVhome infusion

HNS, Inc.
14700 28th Ave. North
Suite 90
Plymouth, MN 55447
Telephone: (612)-557-9296 Fax: (612)-557-0650
Contact: Joe Bauer
Home infusion therapy, in-home nursing and attendant care, physical therapy

Hospital Home Care
2450 - 26th Avenue South
Minneapolis, MN 55406-1245
Telephone: (612)-721-2491
Contact: Marylou Irving
Home health care

Interim Health Care
5131 Edina Industrial Blvd.
Suite 290
Edina, MN 55439
Telephone: (612)-832-9434 Fax: (612)-832-9560
Contact: Cheryl Stadler
Home health aides, homemaker service

Methodist Hospital Home Care Service/Hospice
6500 Excelsior Boulevard
St. Louis Park, MN 55426-4700
Telephone: (612)-932-6087
Home care & hospice program

Metro Visiting Nurse Association
2021 E. Henepin Avenue
Suite 230
Minneapolis, MN 55413
Telephone: (612)-673-2700 Fax: (612)-673-2931

North Memorial Medical Center Hospice
3300 Oakdale Avenue North
Robbinsdale, MN 55422
Telephone: (612)-520-5770
Contact: Connie Holden

Park Nicollet Medical Center
2525 Chicago Avenue South
Minnepaolis, MN 55404
Telephone: (612)-871-1024 Fax: (612)-871-9220
Contact: Kiran Belani,M.D.
Treatment for pediatric infectious diseases

Medical Services

Healing Point
5251 Chicago Avenue
Richfield, MN 55417
Telephone: (612)-822-5636
Contact: Edith Davis
Acupuncture treatment

Hemophilia Center at The University of Minnesota
Box 713 - UMHC
Minneapolis, MN 55455
Telephone: (612)-626-6455 Fax: (612)-625-4955
Toll-Free: (800)-688-5252
Contact: Nigel Keyopsicker
Range of services including AIDS treatment for people with hemophilia

Nancy Page Program
245 South Clifton Avenue
Minneapolis, MN 55403-3467
Telephone: (612)-870-3787
Contact: Richard Stasik
Rule 36 program

Pilot City Health Center
1349 Penn Avenue North
Minneapolis, MN 55411-3094
Telephone: (612)-348-6000 Fax: (612)-348-2131
Contact: Howard Johnson
Dental and medical care

The Doctors
1436 W. Lake Street
Minneapolis, MN 55408-2645
Telephone: (612)-824-1772 Fax: (612)-824-8191
Medical service, HIV clinic

University of Minnesota Hospital and Clinics
Harvard and E. River Rd.
P.O. Box 707
Minneapolis, MN 55455
Telephone: (612)-626-6222 Fax: (612)-626-3028
Medical services, HIV clinic

Testing Sites

Neighborhood Involvement Program
2431 South Hennepin Ave.
Minneapolis, MN 55405-2605
Telephone: (612)-374-3125 Fax: (612)-374-3323
Contact: Daniel Haugen - President/Exec. Director
Red Door Clinic conducts confidential HIV testing, counseling

Red Door Health Clinic Gen.
525 Portland Avenue South
Minneapolis, MN 55415
Telephone: (612)-347-2437
Provides confidential HIV/STD testing and counseling.

Isanti County

County Health Depts

Isanti County Health
1557 South Highway 293
Cambridge, MN 55008
Telephone: (612)-689-4071
Contact: Rita Jensenanz - Administrative Assistant
Home health care, disease prevention, counseling, AIDS workshop

Itasca County

Community Services

Itasca County Human Services
Courthouse
123 NE 4th Street
Grand Rapids, MN 55744
Telephone: (218)-327-2851
Contact: Lora Mathison
Prevention & education for civic groups, support group, referrals

Kanabec County

Home Health Care

Kanabec County Public Health Nursing Service
18 North Vine Street
Mora, MN 55051-1351
Telephone: (612)-679-2282 Fax: (612)-679-9994
Contact: Wendy Thompson
Referrals, counseling.

Kandiyohi County

Community Services

Lutheran Social Services
Regional Offices
333 Litchfield Avenue South West
Willmar, MN 56201
Telephone: (612)-235-5411 Fax: (612)-235-2601
Contact: Rick Loesth
Referral services

County Health Depts

Kandiyohi County Community Health
905 Litchfield Avenue W.
Willmar, MN 56201
Telephone: (612)-235-4785
Contact: Michelle D. Then
AIDS information and education, home care

Home Health Care

Rice Memorial Hospital
301 Becker Avenue SW
Willmar, MN 56201-3395
Telephone: (612)-235-4543 Fax: (612)-231-4852
Medical care

Medical Services

Willmar Regional Treatment Center
North Highway 71
Willmar, MN 56201
Telephone: (612)-231-5100 Fax: (612)-231-5329
Contact: Gregory Spartz
Serves HIV+ clients

Le Sueur County

Home Health Care

Le Sueur County Public Health Nursing Service
88 South Park
Le Center, MN 56057
Telephone: (612)-357-2251
Contact: Kathy Ruhland - PHN
Home health services

Lyon County

Community Services

Southwest Minnesota AIDS Project
109 South 5th Street
Marshall, MN 56258-1934
Telephone: (507)-537-9264
Information, referrals, buddy system

County Health Depts

Lincoln, Lyon Merry, Pipestone Counties Community Health Services
1210 East College Drive
Suite 800
Marshall, MN 56258-2010
Telephone: (507)-537-6713
Contact: Ellie Martin-Trautman - Director
Resource referral educational services

Mahnomen County

County Health Depts

Mahnomen County Health Department
P.O. Box 226
Mahnomen, MN 56557
Telephone: (218)-935-2527
Contact: Betty Aanerud
Information & counseling

Marshall County

Home Health Care

Marshall County Public Health Nursing Service
109 South Minnesota St.
Warren, MN 56762-1461
Telephone: (218)-745-5154
Contact: Diana Kostrzewski
Home care agency services

Mc Leod County

Home Health Care

McLeod County Public Health Nursing Service
804 Eleventh Street
Glencoe, MN 55336
Telephone: (612)-864-3185 Fax: (612)-864-3410
Contact: Jean Johnson, ON
Education, home care

Meeker County

County Health Depts

Meeker County Public Health Nursing Service
101 South Gorman
Litchfield, MN 55355-3398
Telephone: (612)-693-2882 Fax: (612)-693-9185
Contact: Ann Jensen
Presentations, education, referrals, in home nursing services.

Morrison County

Home Health Care

Morrison County Public Health Nursing Service
200 East Broadway Street
Little Falls, MN 56345-3594
Telephone: (612)-632-6665 Fax: (612)-632-0294
Contact: Maryjude Hoeffel; Bonnie Paulson
Homecare, hospice

Mower County

Community Services

Mower County Human Services
1005 North Main Street
Austin, MN 55912
Telephone: (507)-437-9483
Contact: Bruce Henricks - Director
Home care, AIDS/HIV resource person, community awareness, education, taskforce

Murray County

County Health Depts

Murray County Health Department
2711 Broadway Avenue
Slayton, MN 56172-1313
Telephone: (507)-836-6148 Fax: (507)-836-8999
Contact: Lenore Wendorf
Education, referrals

Nicollet County

Home Health Care

Nicollet County Nursing Service
501 S. Minnesota Avenue
St. Peter, MN 56082
Telephone: (507)-931-6800 Fax: (507)-931-9220
Home health service

Nobles County

County Health Depts

Nobles County Health Department
P.O. Box 757
315 Tenth Street
Worthington, MN 56187-0757
Telephone: (507)-372-8263 Fax: (507)-372-8223
Contact: Georgia M. Entenza
Home care

Medical Services

South Western Mental Health Agency
1024 Seventh Avenue
Worthington, MN 56187
Telephone: (507)-376-4141
Contact: Dr. Kathleen Christensen
Outpatient primary chemical dependency program for residents of 4 counties,counseling, referrals

Norman County

Home Health Care

Norman County
16 East 3rd Avene North
Room 107
Ada, MN 56510
Telephone: (218)-784-7499
Contact: Karen Mitteness
Home care services

Olmsted County

County Health Depts

Olmsted County Health Department
1650 Fourth Street SE
Rochester, MN 55904-4700
Telephone: (507)-285-8360
Contact: Mary Wellik
HIV counseling & testing

Home Health Care

Comfort Home Health Care
2311 Highway 52N
West Frontage Road
Rochester, MN 55901-1633
Telephone: (507)-281-2332
Home health care

Medical Services

Family Service Rochester
903 West Center Street
Rochester, MN 55902-6278
Telephone: (507)-287-2040 Fax: (507)-287-2063
Contact: Larry Lindstrom - Social Worker III
Family & couple counseling

Otter Tail County

Community Services

Fergus Falls Ministerium
Box 713
Fergus Falls, MN 56538
Telephone: (218)-739-8580
Contact: Kurtis Alvin Rotto
Task force

County Health Depts

Otter Tail County Health Department
Courthouse
Fergus Falls, MN 56537
Telephone: (218)-739-2271
Contact: Phyllis G. Knutson
HIV testing & counseling home care, public education

Home Health Care

Home Health Care Department
Perham Memorial
665-3rd Street SW
Perham, MN 56573
Telephone: (218)-346-4500 Fax: (218)-346-4540
Contact: Gen Keranen - R.N.
Home health care

Pennington County

County Health Depts

Red Lake County Health Department
Courthouse
P.O. Box 616
Thief River Falls, MN 56701
Telephone: (218)-681-5950
Contact: Carol Borchert
Educational services, prevention

Medical Services

Inter-County PHN
Courthouse, Box 616
Thief River Falls, MN 56701
Telephone: (218)-681-5950
Contact: Susan Olson
Public health nursing education

Pine County

Home Health Care

Pine County PHN Service
210 6th Street
Pine City, MN 55063-1423
Telephone: (612)-629-6781
Contact: Kaye Kotek
Home health care

Pipestone County

County Health Depts

Pipestone County Health Department
416 S. Hiawatha Avenue
Pipestone, MN 56164-1566
Telephone: (507)-537-6713
Contact: Ellie Trautman
Home health, educational services

Polk County

Home Health Care

Polk County PHN Service
1500 University Avenue
Box 403
Crookston, MN 56716-1159
Telephone: (218)-281-3385
Contact: Ellen J. O'Connor
Home care

Ramsey County

Community Services

Critical Care Services, Incorporated
336 Chester Street
St. Paul, MN 55107-1203
Telephone: (612)-228-6800 Fax: (612)-228-6832
Contact: Theresa Stecher
Transportation Services

First Call For Help - St. Paul
166 East 4th Street
Suite 310
St. Paul, MN 55101-1448
Telephone: (612)-291-4666
Information, referrals, education

Hemophilia Foundation, National
1821 University Avenue
Suite S145
St. Paul, MN 55104
Telephone: (612)-641-1324 Fax: (612)-641-1336
Contact: Elizabeth Klein
Emergency financial assistance, support, presentations, education,referrals

Ramsey County Human Services
160 East Kellogg Blvd.
Suite 330
St. Paul, MN 55101
Telephone: (612)-227-3292

County Health Depts

Ramsey County Public Health Department
50 Kellogg Blvd. West
#930
St. Paul, MN 55102-1657
Telephone: (612)-298-5971
Contact: Rob Fulton
Educational programs

Home Health Care

Health Span Home Care and Hospice
3030 Centere Point Drive
Roseville, MN 55113
Telephone: (612)-545-2003
Contact: Teddy Petersen (628-4281)
Home care & hospice

In Home Health
2250 County Road C W
Roseville, MN 55113-2504
Telephone: (612)-633-6522 Fax: (612)-633-5733
Home care

Staff Builders Service, Inc.
2610 University Avenue
Suite 510
St. Paul, MN 55114
Telephone: (612)-642-1130 Fax: (612)-642-1633
Home health care

Medical Services

Children's Hospital of St. Paul
345 North Smith Avenue
St. Paul, MN 55102-2392
Telephone: (612)-220-6760
Contact: Dr. Richard Anderson
Testing & counseling for pediatric HIV

Hamm Memorial Psychiatric Clinic
555 Park Street
St. Paul, MN 55103-2110
Telephone: (612)-224-0614
Mental health counseling, AIDS counseling

Model Cities Health Center
430 North Dale
St. Paul, MN 55103-2225
Telephone: (612)-222-6029 Fax: (612)-228-9878
Contact: Linda Atlas
Medical care

Vet Center
2480 University Avenue
St. Paul, MN 55114-1796
Telephone: (612)-644-4022 Fax: (612)-725-2234
Contact: Ernest Boswell
Case management, advocacy, crisis intervention, grief counseling, support group

Wellspring Naturopathic Clinic
1365 Englewood Avenue
St. Paul, MN 55104-1952
Telephone: (612)-644-4436
Natural & homopathic treatments

Testing Sites

North End Health Center
135 Manitoba (at Rice)
St. Paul, MN 55117-5400
Telephone: (612)-489-8021 Fax: (612)-489-9402

Contact: Nancy Briggs
Testing & general medical services

St. Paul Division of Public Health
555 Cedar Street
Room 111 Clinic
St. Paul, MN 55101
Telephone: (612)-292-7752 Fax: (612)-222-2770
Testing and counseling.

St. Paul-Ramsey Medical Center
640 Jackson Street
St. Paul, MN 55101
Telephone: (612)-221-1280 Fax: (612)-221-8616
Contact: Dr. Keith Henry
HIV/AIDS clinical and testing services, home care team

West Side Community Health Center
153 Concord Street
St. Paul, MN 55107-2295
Telephone: (612)-222-1816 Fax: (612)-222-1305
Contact: Faith O'Neill
HIV testing & counseling; STD testing

Redwood County

Home Health Care

Redwood County Public Health Nursing Service
141 North Highway 101
P.O. Box 189
Redwood Falls, MN 56283-1403
Telephone: (507)-637-2969
Contact: Genie Simow, PHN
Visiting RN's, bereavement referrals, counseling, public health resources,educational services

Renville County

Home Health Care

Renville County Public Health Nursing Service
500 Depue Avenue East
Olivia, MN 56277-1334
Telephone: (612)-523-2570
Contact: Nancy A. Sperl
Home care

Roseau County

Home Health Care

Roseau County Public Health Nursing Service
7155 Delmure Drive
Roseau, MN 56751
Telephone: (218)-463-3211
Contact: MaryAnna Pelowki
Homecare agency, resource & referral

Saint Louis County

County Health Depts

St. Louis County Health Department
222 East Superior
Duluth, MN 55802
Telephone: (218)-725-5200 Fax: (218)-725-5297
Contact: Larry Sundberg
Case management, HIV/AIDS education

Medical Services

Duluth Community Health Center
Two East Fifth Street
Duluth, MN 55805
Telephone: (218)-722-1497 Fax: (218)-722-7239
Testing, individual therapy, group support, children's support, education

St. Luke's Hospital Outpatient Mental Health Clinic
915 East First Street
Duluth, MN 55805-2193
Telephone: (218)-726-5506 Fax: (218)-726-5181
Contact: Donna Churchill
Serves HIV+ clients, mental health

Stearns County

County Health Depts

Benton County Health Department
1139 Franklin Avenue
Box 661
St. Cloud, MN 56302-1211
Telephone: (612)-253-8440
Contact: Pat Rudie
Home care services, education

Medical Services

St. Cloud Hospital
1406 6th Avenue North
St. Cloud, MN 56301-1901
Telephone: (612)-251-2700 Fax: (612)-656-7058
Contact: Steven M. Vincent, PhD - Licensed Psychologist
Counseling

Testing Sites

Central Minnesota AIDS Project
810 West St. Germain
Suite 305
St. Cloud, MN 56301
Telephone: (612)-259-1909
HIV testing

Steele County

County Health Depts

Steele County Public Health Nursing
590 Dunnell Drive
Box 890
Owatonna, MN 55060-4751
Telephone: (507)-451-4400
Contact: Dee-Ann Petty John - Health & Education Director
Public health services, home care, research counselors, education, andresource center

Stevens County

Home Health Care

Stevens-Traverse Public Health
210 Atlantic Avenue
400 East First Street
Morris, MN 56267
Telephone: (612)-589-1313
Contact: Sandra Tubbs
Home care-immunization, hospice

Stevens-Traverse Public Health Nursing Service
210 Atlantic Avenue
Morris, MN 56267-1321
Telephone: (612)-589-2294
Contact: Margie Nelson - Public Health Nurse

Swift County

Home Health Care

Swift County, Countryside Public Health
620 Atlantic Avenue
P.O. Box 265
Benson, MN 56215-1851
Telephone: (612)-843-4546
Contact: Julie Jensen - Dir of Public Nursing
General home care

Todd County

Home Health Care

Todd County Public Health Nursing Service
Courthouse Annex
119 S. Third Street
Long Prairie, MN 56347
Telephone: (612)-732-4440 Fax: (612)-732-6233
Contact: Bonnie Conner
Home care

Testing Sites

Greater Staples Hospital Care Center
401 East Prarie Avenue
Staples, MN 56479
Telephone: (218)-984-1515
Hospital care, HIV testing

Wabasha County

County Health Depts

Wabasha County Health Department
107 East Third Street
Wabasha, MN 55981-1453
Telephone: (612)-565-3334
Contact: Laurie Hodgson, PHN
Home care, child care

Wadena County

County Health Depts

Wadena County Health Department
Courthouse
415 South Jefferson
Wadena, MN 56482
Telephone: (218)-631-1344
Contact: Janet M. Mattson, P.H.N.
Home care, AIDS education, child health care

Waseca County

Home Health Care

Public Health Nursing
300 N. State Street
Suite 3
Waseca, MN 56093
Telephone: (507)-835-0685
Contact: Shirley Lundquist - R.N., P.H.N
Nursing care for HIV and AIDS patients, education

Watonwan County

County Health Depts

Watonwan County, FMW Human Service Center
720 First Avenue
P.O. Box 31
St. James, MN 56081-1779
Telephone: (507)-375-3294
Contact: Laura Kramer
Community health, social services

Medical Services

Madelia Clinic
4 East Main Street
Madelia, MN 56062-1841
Telephone: (507)-642-3255
Family practice

Wilkin County

Home Health Care

Wilkin County Public Health Nursing Service
Courthouse
P.O. Box 127
Breckenridge, MN 56520
Telephone: (218)-643-4722
Contact: Glee W. Dodson
Home health care, home aides care

Winona County

Home Health Care

Winona County CHS
Courthouse
171 West Third Street
Winona, MN 55987
Telephone: (507)-457-6400
Contact: Lynn Theurer - Coordinator
Home health care

Yellow Medicine County

Home Health Care

Countryside Public Health Service
868 Prentice Street
Granite Falls, MN 56241
Telephone: (612)-564-3010
Contact: Laurie Dieken
Home health care & home maker services

MISSISSIPPI

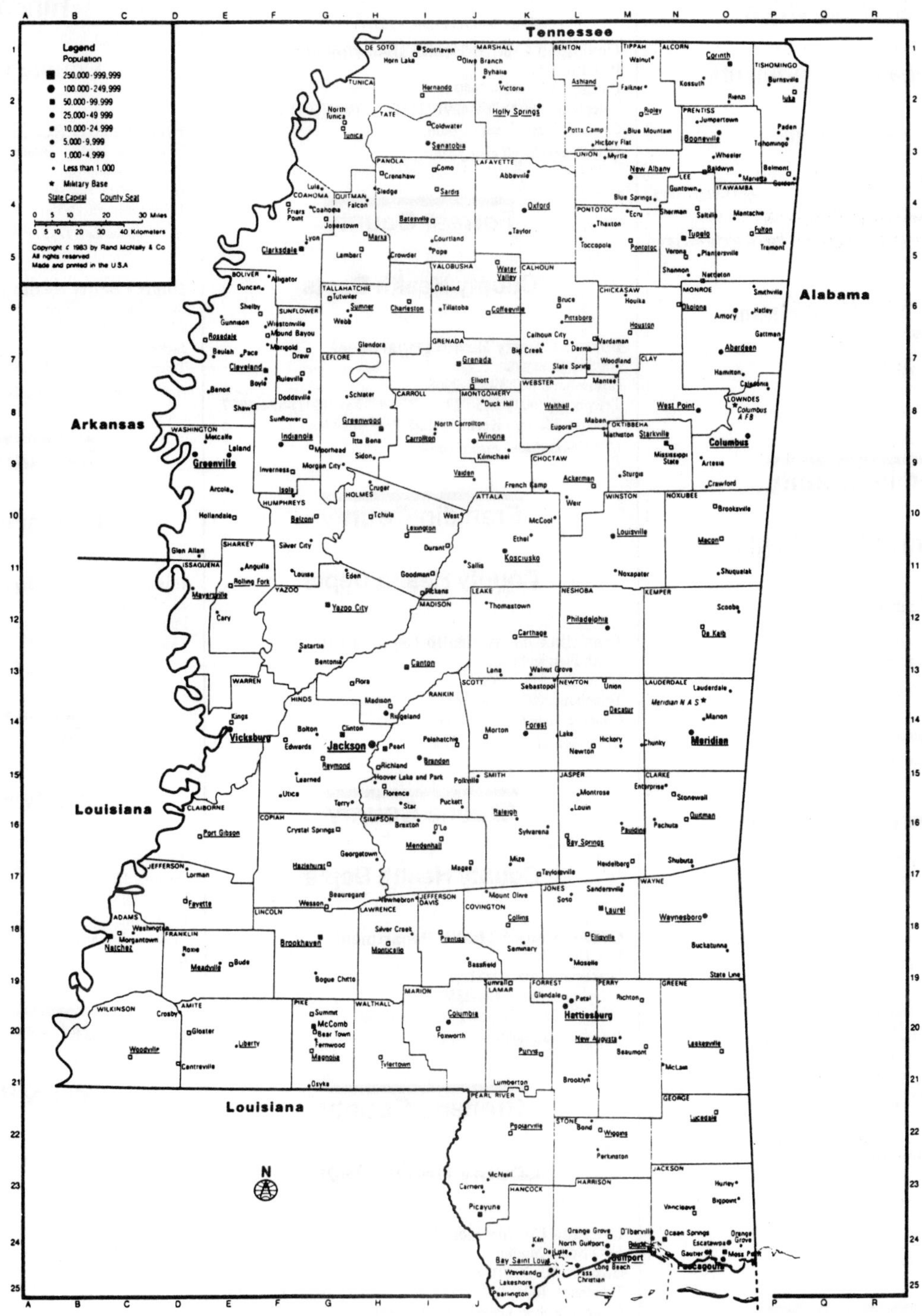

From City/County Planning Atlas Copyright 1989 by Reed McNally & Company, R.L. 90-S-28

Mississippi

General Services

State Health Departments

Mississippi Department of Health
2423 North State Street
Jackson, MS 39215
Telephone: (601)-960-7725 Fax: (601)-960-7909
Contact: Letitia Shaw - Ryan White Care Coordinator
Drug program, counseling, community based services, prevention

Mississippi State Department of Health
HIV/AIDS Prevention Program
P.O. Box 1700
Jackson, MS 39215-1700
Telephone: (601)-960-7723
Contact: Mary Jane Coleman - R.N., Director

Amite County

County Health Depts

Amite County Health Department
P.O. Box 209
Liberty, MS 39645-0209
Telephone: (601)-657-8351
HIV Counseling/Testing Site

Benton County

County Health Depts

Benton County Health Department
Jct. 370 & 5 West
Ashland, MS 38603
Telephone: (601)-224-6442
HIV Counseling/Testing Site

Bolivar County

County Health Depts

Bolivar County Health Department
Box 550
Cleveland, MS 38732
Telephone: (601)-843-2706
Contact: Harold Otis - DIS
HIV Counseling/Testing Site

Clarke County

County Health Depts

Clarke County Health Department
426 Highway 512
Quitman, MS 39355
Telephone: (601)-776-2149
HIV Counseling/Testing Site

Covington County

County Health Depts

Covington County Health Department
P.O. Box 940
Collins, MS 39428-0940
Telephone: (601)-765-4291 Fax: (601)-765-2888
Contact: Jessie Dees - Coord.
HIV Counseling/Testing Site

Forrest County

County Health Depts

Forrest County Health Department
5008 Highway 42
Hattiesburg, MS 39401-2908
Telephone: (601)-583-0291 Fax: (601)-584-4057
Contact: Marilyn Keene - AIDS Program Mgr.
HIV Counseling/Testing Site

Franklin County

County Health Depts

Franklin County Health Department
South First and Oak
Meadville, MS 39653
Telephone: (601)-384-5871
Contact: June Cotton - Coord. Nurse
HIV Counseling/Testing Site

Greene County

County Health Depts

Greene County Health Department
P.O. Box 130
Leakesville, MS 39451-0130
Telephone: (601)-394-2389 Fax: (601)-394-5294
Contact: Sandy Hayberg - Coord. Nurse
HIV Counseling/Testing Site

Grenada County

County Health Depts

Grenada County Health Department
1241 South Mound
Grenada, MS 38901-4597
Telephone: (601)-226-3711 Fax: (601)-227-1168
Contact: Robert Davies - STD Coord.
HIV Counseling/Testing Site

Harrison County

County Health Depts

Harrison County Health Department
Broad Avenue & 15th
Gulfport, MS 39501
Telephone: (601)-863-1036 Fax: (601)-864-6084
Contact: Dot Hilton - Coord. Nurse
HIV Counseling/Testing Site

Hinds County

County Health Depts

Hinds County Health Department
Nakoma S. Health Center
1999 Hwy 80
Jackson, MS 39204
Telephone: (601)-354-6007
HIV Counseling/Testing Site

Hinds County Health Department
South Jackson Clinic
1500 Terry Road, Bldg E
Jackson, MS 39204
Telephone: (601)-355-6377
HIV Counseling/Testing Site

Itawamba County

County Health Depts

Itawamba County Health Department
110 Crane Street
Fulton, MS 38843-1713
Telephone: (601)-862-3710
HIV Counseling/Testing Site

Jackson County

County Health Depts

Jackson County Health Department
Hospital Road
Pascagoula, MS 39567
Telephone: (601)-762-1117 Fax: (601)-762-5934
Contact: Edwina White - Infection Control Nurse
HIV Counseling/Testing Site

Jefferson County

County Health Depts

Jefferson County Health Department
Poindexter Street
PO Box 446
Fayette, MS 39069
Telephone: (601)-786-3061
Contact: Linda Sanders - Coord. Nurse
HIV Counseling/Testing Site

Jefferson Davis County

County Health Depts

Jeff Davis County Health Department
Box 517
Prentiss, MS 39474
Telephone: (601)-792-5135 Fax: (601)-792-8916
HIV Counseling/Testing Site

Jones County

County Health Depts

Jones County Health Department
P.O. Box 2487
Laurel, MS 39442-2487
Telephone: (601)-426-3258 Fax: (601)-425-9384
Contact: Linda Sanders - Coord. Nurse
HIV Counseling/Testing Site

Kemper County

County Health Depts

Kemper County Health Department
Highway 16 West
Po Box 96
DeKalb, MS 39328
Telephone: (601)-743-5865 Fax: (601)-743-9964
HIV Counseling/Testing Site

Lafayette County

County Health Depts

Lafayette County Health Department
P.O. Box 1395
Oxford, MS 38655
Telephone: (601)-234-5231
HIV Counseling/Testing Site

Lamar County

County Health Depts

Lamar County Health Department
207 Main Street
Purvis, MS 39475
Telephone: (601)-794-8504 Fax: (601)-794-8796
Contact: Pamela Miller - Coord. Nurse
HIV.Counseling/Testing Site

Lawrence County

County Health Depts

Lawrence County Health Department
Courthouse Circle
PO box 246
Monticello, MS 39654
Telephone: (601)-587-2561
Contact: Cindy Wilson - Coord. Nurse
HIV Counseling/Testing Site

Leake County

County Health Depts

Leake County Health Department
P.O. Box 573
Carthage, MS 39051-0573
Telephone: (601)-267-3072 Fax: (601)-267-6277
Contact: Marie Carraway - Coord. Nurse
HIV Counseling/Testing Site

Lee County

Medical Services

North Mississippi Medical Center
830 South Gloster
Tupelo, MS 38801-4996
Telephone: (601)-841-3158 Fax: (601)-841-3552
Contact: Carole Moore

Leflore County

County Health Depts

Leflore County Health Department
2600 Browning Road
Greenwood, MS 38930
Telephone: (601)-453-0284
Contact: Sharen Gerrity - Coord. Nurse
HIV Counseling/Testing Site

Lincoln County

County Health Depts

Lincoln County Health Department
1212 N. Park Lane NE.
Brookhaven, MS 39601
Telephone: (601)-833-3314 Fax: (601)-833-5150
Contact: Joyce Woods - Coord. Nurse
HIV Counseling/Testing Site

Lowndes County

County Health Depts

Lowndes County Health Department
1112 Military Road
Columbus, MS 39701-4196
Telephone: (601)-328-6091 Fax: (601)-328-7355
Contact: Amy Wallace - Coord. Nurse
HIV Counseling/Testing Site

Madison County

County Health Depts

Madison County Health Department
317 North Union Street
Canton, MS 39046
Telephone: (601)-859-3316
Contact: Judy Ward - Coord. Nurse
HIV Counseling/Testing Site

Noxubee County

County Health Depts

Oktibbeha County Health Department
Yates Street
Starkville, MS 39739
Telephone: (601)-323-4565 Fax: (601)-323-2667
Contact: Mamita Henderson - Coord. Nurse
HIV Counseling/Testing Site

Panola County

County Health Depts

Panola County Health Department
Highway 51 South
Batesville, MS 38606
Telephone: (601)-563-4616 Fax: (601)-563-6304
Contact: Pam White - Coord. Nurse
HIV Counseling/Testing Site

Perry County

County Health Depts

Perry County Health Department
Courthouse Annex
New Augusta, MS 39462
Telephone: (601)-964-3288 Fax: (601)-964-3289
Contact: Ann Garner - Coord. Nurse
HIV Counseling/Testing Site

Pike County

County Health Depts

Pike County Health Department
P.O. Box 645
McComb, MS 39648
Telephone: (601)-684-1030 Fax: (601)-684-5990
Contact: Annie Brent - Coord. Nurse
HIV Counseling/Testing Site

Pontotoc County

County Health Depts

Pontotoc County Health Department
341 Ridge Road
PO Box 248
Pontotoc, MS 38863
Telephone: (601)-489-1241
Contact: Jan Rowan - Coord. Nurse
HIV Counseling/Testing Site

Rankin County

Home Health Care

nmc HOMECARE
10 River Bend Place
Jackson, MS 39208
Telephone: (601)-936-4828
Fax: (601)-936-2059
Contact: Billy Everett
National JCAHO-Accredited company providing a full range of Infusion and Respiratory therapies and specializing in the care of HIV/AIDS patients. National Case Manager is also available at 800-445-1188

Tallahatchie County

County Health Depts

Tallahatchie County Health Department
209 S. Pleasant St.
Charleston, MS 38921
Telephone: (601)-647-3404 Fax: (601)-647-2689
HIV Counseling/Testing Site

Tippah County

County Health Depts

Tippah County Health Department
116 Hospital St.
Ripley, MS 38663
Telephone: (601)-837-3084
Contact: MArtha Grisham - Coord. Nurse
HIV Counseling/Testing Site

Tishomingo County

County Health Depts

Tishomingo County Health Department
1505 Bettydale Street
Iuka, MS 38852-1112
Telephone: (601)-423-6100
Contact: Edna Tapt - Coord. Nurse
HIV Counseling/Testing Site

Walthall County

County Health Depts

Walthall County Health Department
433 Beulah Avenue
Tylertown, MS 39667-2703
Telephone: (601)-876-4924
Contact: Becky Hillburn - Coord. Nurse
HIV Counseling/Testing Site

Warren County

County Health Depts

Warren County Health Department
807 Monroe Street
Vicksburg, MS 39180-2529
Telephone: (601)-636-4356
Contact: Salena Greenee - Coord. Nurse
HIV Counseling/Testing Site

Washington County

County Health Depts

Washington County Health Department
1633 Hospital St.
Greenville, MS 38701
Telephone: (601)-332-8177 Fax: (601)-378-8853
Contact: Betty Watkins - Coord. Nurse
HIV Counseling/Testing Site

MISSOURI

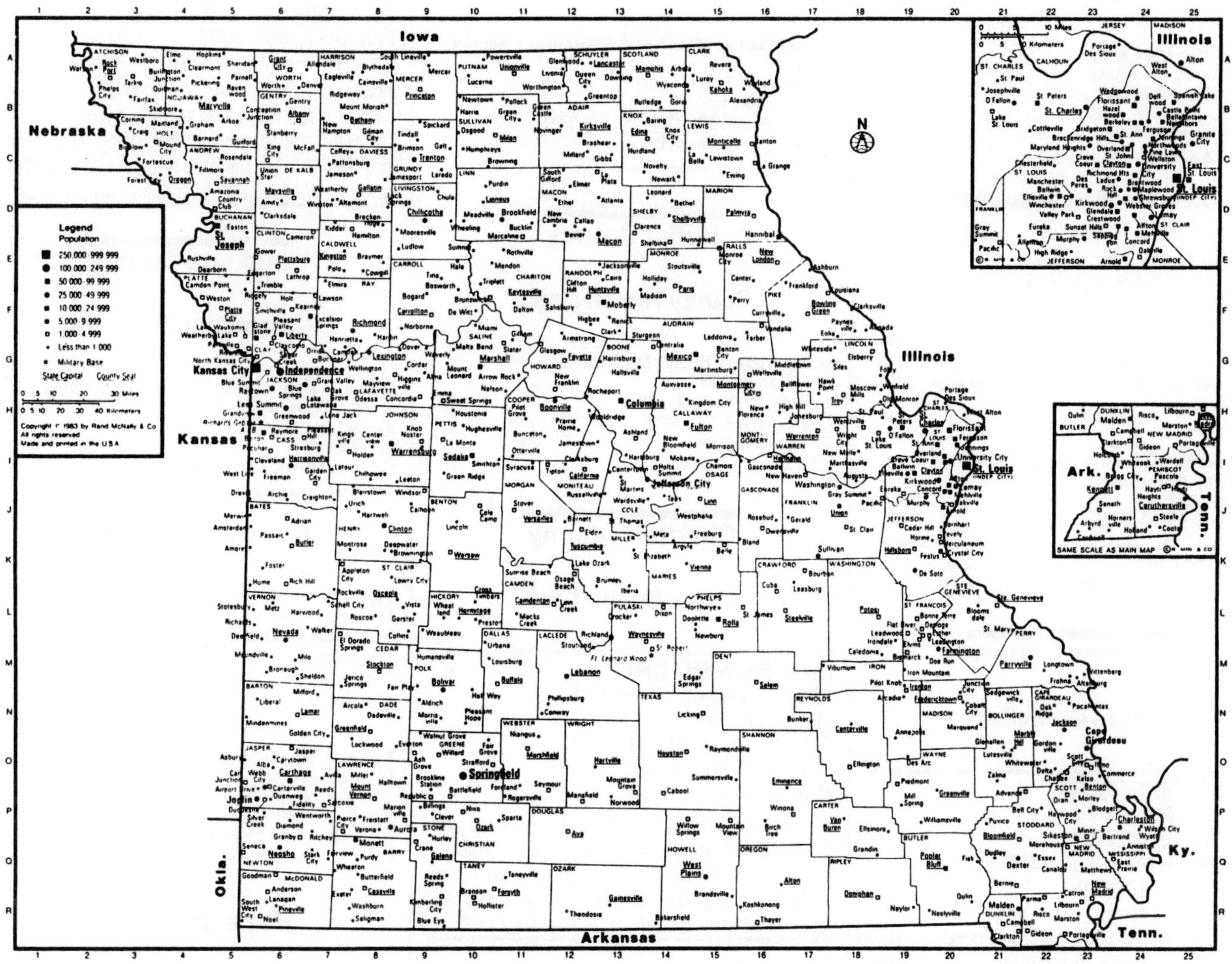

From City/County Planning Atlas Copyright 1989 by Reed McNally & Company, R.L. 90-S-28

Missouri

General Services

Education

KCVA Medical Center
4801 Linwood Boulevard
Kansas City, MO 64128
Telephone: (816)-861-4700
Contact: Glenn R. Hodges Ext. 3205
Medical & Educational Services

State Health Departments

Missouri Department of Health
Bureau of Special Health Care Needs
1730 East Elm Street
Jefferson City, MO 65101
Telephone: (314)-751-6002 Fax: (314)-751-6447
Contact: Les Hancock
Dental care, medical care, case management, transportation & some housing

Missouri Department of Health Bureau of STD/HIV Prevention
P.O. Box 570
Jefferson City, MO 65102
Telephone: (314)-751-6438 Fax: (314)-751-6447
Contact: Bill Huber
Thirteen counseling and HIV testing sites

Andrew County

Home Health Care

nmc HOMECARE
910 Woodbine
St. Joseph, MO 64506
Telephone: (816)-233-6477
Fax: (816)-233-9229
Contact: Gary Hamilton
National JCAHO-Accredited company providing a full range of Infusion and Respiratory therapies and specializing in the care of HIV/AIDS patients. National Case Manager is also available at 800-445-1188

Boone County

County Health Depts

Columbia-Boone County Health Department
600 E. Broadway
Columbia, MO 65205
Telephone: (314)-874-7355
Contact: Ms. Beau Whitlock
HIV Testing/Counseling Site

Home Health Care

O.P.T.I.O.N. Care
3210 East Pointe Drive
Columbia, MO 65201
Telephone: (314)-875-1230 Fax: (314)-874-8012
Contact: Gregory Steinhoff - Administrator
Home IV and Nutritional Services

Buchanan County

Testing Sites

Department of Health and Community Service - Clinic
904 South 10th Street
St. Joseph, MO 64503
Telephone: (816)-271-4725 Fax: (816)-271-4682
Contact: Penney Moore, RN
HIV testing/counseling site, care coordination

Butler County

County Health Depts

Butler County Health Department
1618 N. Main Street
Poplar Bluff, MO 63901-3499
Telephone: (314)-785-8478
Contact: Edith Helsel
HIV Testing/Counseling Site

Chariton County

Home Health Care

nmc HOMECARE
614 W. Jackson, Suite 100
Mexico, MO 65286
Telephone: (314)-581-1721
Fax: (314)-581-5868
Contact: Rheba Ryan
National JCAHO-Accredited company providing a full range of Infusion and Respiratory therapies and specializing in the care of HIV/AIDS patients. National Case Manager is also available at 800-445-1188

Cole County

County Health Depts

Cole County Health Department
210 Adams Street
Jefferson City, MO 65101
Telephone: (314)-636-2181
Contact: Ivah Braun - RN
HIV Testing/Counseling Site

Greene County

County Health Depts

Springfield-Greene County Health Department
227 E Chestnut Expressway
Springfield, MO 65802
Telephone: (417)-864-1686 Fax: (417)-864-1099
Contact: Robin Alton
HIV Testing/Counseling Site

Home Health Care

nmc HOMECARE
2102 West Vista
Springfield, MO 65807
Telephone: (417)-881-6994
Fax: (417)-881-2021
Contact: Patricia Skjerve
National JCAHO-Accredited company providing a full range of Infusion and Respiratory therapies and specializing in the care of HIV/AIDS patients. National Case Manager is also available at 800-445-1188

Jackson County

Community Services

Grace & Holy Trinity Episcopal Cathedral
415 W. 13th Street
Kansas City, MO 64105-1427
Telephone: (816)-474-8260
Contact: J. Earl Kavanaugh; Charmaine Fowler
AIDS task force, counseling, care

County Health Depts

Jackson County Health Department
313 South Liberty St
Independence, MO 64050-3899
Telephone: (816)-881-4424
Contact: Joan Kolichett - Dept. Director
Free HIV testing and counseling site

Kansas City Missouri Health Department
HIV/AIDS Program
1423 East Linwood Blvd., 2nd Floor
Kansas City, MO 64109
Telephone: (816)-923-2600
Contact: Ernest Williams - Counseling & Testing Coord.
HIV testing

Home Health Care

Curaflex Infusion Services
7076 Universal Avenue
Kansan City, MO 64120
Telephone: (816)-483-9400 Fax: (816)-483-3669
Toll-Free: (800)-695-2872
Contact: John Frick - General Manager
Home IV therapy: TPN, Enteral, IV Antibiotics, Aerosolized/IV Pentamidine

Good Samaritan Project
3030 Walnut Street
Kansas City, MO 64108
Telephone: (816)-561-8784
Contact: Ina Pope
Home health care and support group; answering machine after 10:00pm

O.P.T.I.O.N. Care of Kansas City
6123 E. Connecticut Ave.
Kansas City, MO 64120-1346
Telephone: (816)-241-1001
Contact: Greg Mitchell
Home IV and Nutritional Services

Medical Services

Samuel V. Rogers Community Health Center
825 Euclid Street
Kansas City, MO 64124
Telephone: (816)-474-4920 Fax: (816)-474-6475
Contact: Tom Reynolds
Medical support, treatment, counseling, testing, education

Swope Parkway Clinic
4900 Swope Clinic
Kansas City, MO 64130
Telephone: (816)-923-5800 Fax: (816)-923-9210
Contact: Francis Nunley
Medical support, counseling, testing, education, case management

Truman Medical Center/Gold Medicine Infectious Disease Ctr.
2301 Holmes
Kansas City, MO 64108-2677
Telephone: (816)-556-3554 Fax: (816)-283-4554
Contact: Rose Faman
Medical services, counseling, treatment, testing

Testing Sites

Kansas City Free Health Clinic
2 East 39th Street
Kansas City, MO 64111
Telephone: (816)-231-8895
Contact: Karen Mitchell - HIV Program Director
Anonymous testing, medical/dental care, case management, psychotherapy, support

Jasper County

Community Services

St. John's Region Medical Ctr/4-State Community AIDS Project
2727 McClellan Blvd.
Joplin, MO 64804
Telephone: (417)-781-2727 Fax: (417)-625-2958
Contact: Anthony Wilson - Market Promotion Coordinator
Support group for AIDS patients; hospice

County Health Depts

Joplin City Health Department
513 Kentucky Avenue
Joplin, MO 64801
Telephone: (417)-623-6122
Contact: Laura Hurn, R.N.
HIV Testing/Counseling Site

Home Health Care

nmc HOMECARE
1602 East 20th Street
Joplin, MO 64804
Telephone: (417)-782-1939
Fax: (417)-782-9337
Contact: Patricia Skjerve
National JCAHO-Accredited company providing a full range of Infusion and Respiratory therapies and specializing in the care of HIV/AIDS patients. National Case Manager is also available at 800-445-1188

Macon County

County Health Depts

Macon County Health Department
1131 Jackson
Macon, MO 63552-2020
Telephone: (816)-385-4711
Contact: Grace Osman - RN
HIV Testing/Counseling Site

Saint Francois County

County Health Depts

St. Francois County Health Department
1025 W. Main Street
Park Hills, MO 63601-2079
Telephone: (314)-431-1947
Contact: Jane Hartrup - RN
HIV Testing/Counseling Site

Saint Louis County

Home Health Care

Caremark Connection Network
3795 Rider Trail South
Earth City, MO 63045
Telephone: (314)-344-9949 Fax: (314)-344-0006
Contact: Dan Shine - Operations Director; Penny Pritchard - Branch Manager
Clinical support & infusion therapy: nutrition, antimicrobials, chemo.,hematopoeti

Curaflex Infusion Services
4010 Wedgeway Court
St Louis, MO 63045
Telephone: (800)-765-5757 Fax: (314)-291-3386
Contact: Dan Kraemer - General Manager
Home IV therapy: TPN, Enteral, IV Antibiotics, Aerosolized/IV Pentamidine,referrals

Homedco Infusion
934 South HIghway Drive
St Louis, MO 63026
Telephone: (314)-349-2227 Fax: (314)-349-4876
Home infusion therapy for AIDS patients

nmc HOMECARE
1901 Beltway Drive
St. Louis, MO 63114
Telephone: (314)-426-7171
Fax: (314)-428-3658
Contact: Steve Kymens
National JCAHO-Accredited company providing a full range of Infusion and Respiratory therapies and specializing in the care of HIV/AIDS patients. National Case Manager is also available at 800-445-1188

Testing Sites

Metro St. Louis AIDS Program, St. Louis County Health Dept.
6065 Helen Avenue
St. Louis, MO 63134-2013
Telephone: (314)-522-6410
Contact: Debra Lueckerath
HIV Testing/Counseling Site

Saint Louis City (city) County

Home Health Care

Caremark Connection Network
4362 Forrest Park Ave
St. Louis, MO 63108
Telephone: (314)-533-8454
Contact: Alida Merrill - Operations Manager
Clinical support & infusion therapy: nutrition, antimicrobials, chemo.,counseling, education, support group

Medical Services

Washington University School of Medicine
4511 Forest Park Avenue
Suite 304
St. Louis, MO 63108
Telephone: (314)-454-0058 Fax: (314)-361-5231
Contact: Diana Bose
Treatment of infectious diseases & drug research

Saline County

County Health Depts

Saline County Public Health Office
P.O. Box 218
Marshall, MO 65340
Telephone: (816)-886-3434
Contact: Billie Vardiman, BSN
HIV testing, high-risk only

Texas County

Home Health Care

nmc HOMECARE
201 South Grand
Houston, MO 65483
Telephone: (417)-967-3818
Fax: (417)-967-3765
Contact: Patricia Skjerve
National JCAHO-Accredited company providing a full range of Infusion and Respiratory therapies and specializing in the care of HIV/AIDS patients. National Case Manager is also available at 800-445-1188

MONTANA

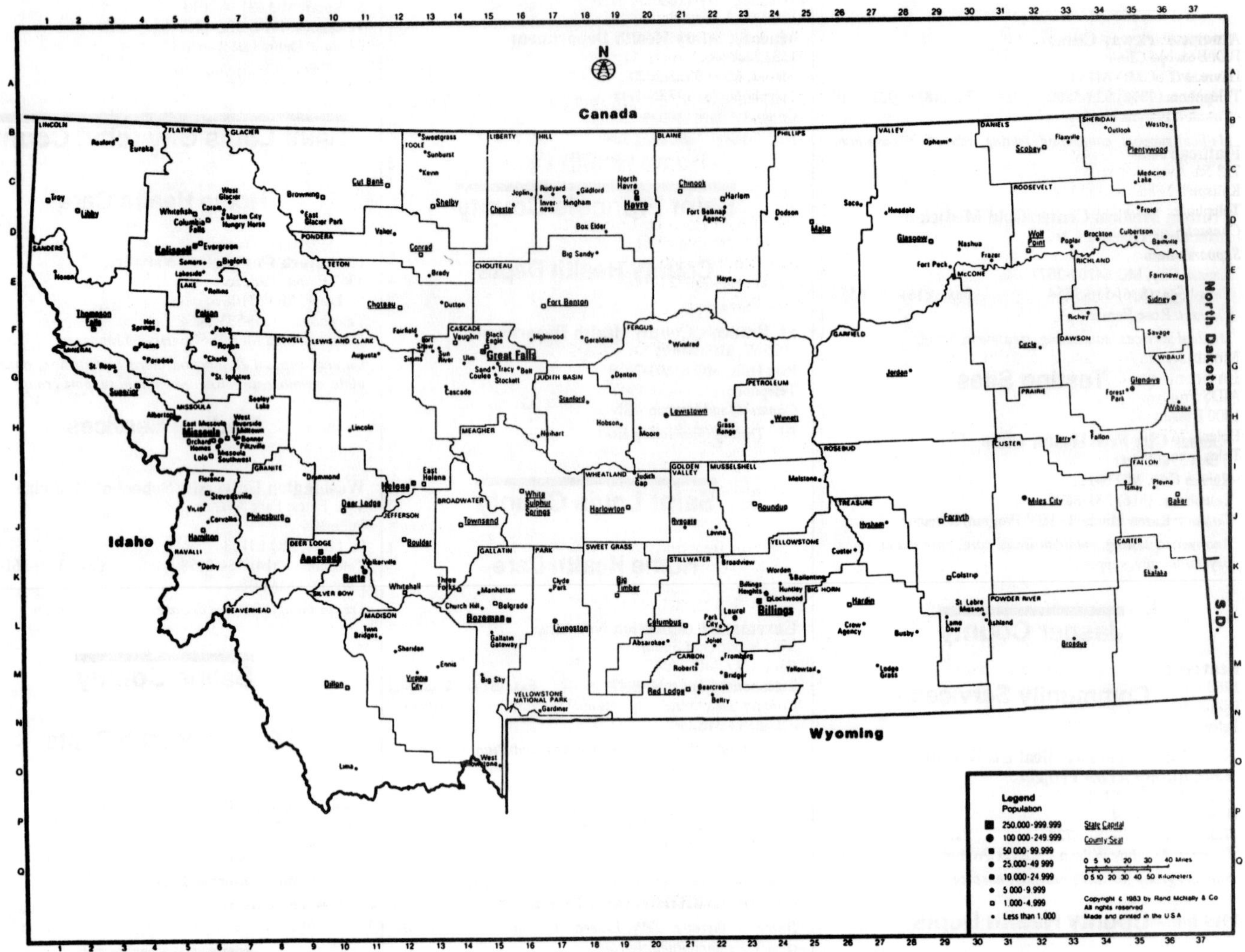

From City/County Planning Atlas Copyright 1989 by Reed McNally & Company, R.L. 90-S-28

Montana

General Services

Education

American Red Cross - Havre
P.O. Box 1449
Havre, MT 50501-1449
Telephone: (406)-265-6356

Flathead AIDS Council
723 5th Avenue East
Kalispell, MT 59901-5347
Telephone: (406)-756-5684
Contact: Cheryl Lowe
Support network, HIV education

State Health Departments

Montana Department of Health and Environmental Services
AIDS Program
1400 Broadway
Helena, MT 59620
Telephone: (406)-444-2454 Fax: (406)-444-2606
Contact: Bruce Desonia - AIDS/STD Program Mgr.

Beaverhead County

County Health Depts

Beaverhead County Health Department
1260 South Atlantic
Dillon, MT 59725-2713
Telephone: (406)-683-4771

Blaine County

Medical Services

PHS Indian Hospital

Harlem, MT 59526
Telephone: (406)-353-2651
Contact: John Tilley, MD - AIDS Coordinator

Cascade County

Community Services

Community Helpline
113 6th Street North
Great Falls, MT 59401
Telephone: (406)-453-6511
Info and referral

Samaritans of Montana
1114 5th Ave S
P.O. Box 1903
Great Falls, MT 59405-2230
Telephone: (406)-454-0402
Contact: Fletcher Wideman
HIV/AIDS counseling, education

Social Security Administration (SSA)
119 First Avenue North
Great Falls, MT 59401-3732
Telephone: (406)-761-0661
Assistance with SSDI, info and referral related to disability

County Health Depts

Cascade City-County Health Department
1130 17th Avenue South
Great Falls, MT 59405-4598
Telephone: (406)-761-1190
Contact: Carol Keaster
HIV Counseling & Testing, Health Education & Risk Reduction Site

Home Health Care

Gift of Life Hospice-Columbus
125 Northwest Bypass H
Great Falls, MT 59405-4389
Telephone: (406)-727-3333
Home-based care

Medical Services

Columbus Hospital
500 15th Avenue South
Great Falls, MT 59403
Telephone: (406)-727-3333
Acute care medical facility

Montana Deaconess Medical Center - Hospital
1101 26th Street South
Great Falls, MT 59405-5161
Telephone: (406)-791-5571
Acute care medical facility

Northwest Medical Offices
401 15th Ave South
Great Falls, MT 59405-4396
Telephone: (406)-727-1770
Comprehensive private-pay medical, clinical services

Dawson County

Community Services

Dawson County Welfare Dept.
218 West Bell St
Glendive, MT 59330-1644
Telephone: (406)-365-3364
General assistance

County Health Depts

Dawson County Health Department, AIDS Task Force
207 West Bell St
Glendive, MT 59330-1694
Telephone: (406)-365-5213
Contact: Camille Spitzer, Jeanne Seifert
HIV counseling, testing, referrals, partner notification, education andrisk reduction

Medical Services

Dawson County Family Planning
Glendive Medical Clinic
107 Dilworth, #5
Glendive, MT 59330
Telephone: (406)-365-2935
Health care clinic, STD risk reduction and infection prevention (pm only)

Fergus County

County Health Depts

Musselshell County Health Department
404 4th Avenue South
Lewistown, MT 59457
Telephone: (406)-538-7466

Medical Services

Fergus County Nurses Office
712 West Main
Courthouse
Lewistown, MT 59457-2562
Telephone: (406)-538-5624

Testing Sites

Central Montana Family Planning
618 W. Main Street
Suite 203
Lewistown, MT 59457
Telephone: (406)-538-8811
Contact: Sue Irvin
Counseling and Testing Site for HIV

Flathead County

Community Services

First Call For Help - Help Network
P.O. Box 2969
Kalispell, MT 59903-2969
Telephone: (406)-752-6565
Information and referral, networking

County Health Depts

Flathead City-County Health Department
723 5th Avenue East
Kalispell, MT 59901
Telephone: (406)-756-5684
Contact: Wendy Doely
HIV Counseling & Testing, Health Education & Risk Reduction Site

Home Health Care

Flathead County Home Health Care
First and Main Bldg
Kalispell, MT 59901
Telephone: (406)-752-6453
Information and referral, networking

Flathead Hospice
1280 Burns Way
Kalispell, MT 59901-3110
Telephone: (406)-752-8667

Medical Services

Flathead Valley Chemical Dependency Clinic
P.O. Box 7115
Kalispell, MT 59904-0115
Telephone: (406)-756-6453 Fax: (406)-756-8546
Contact: Mike Cummings

Information & Referral, Networking

North Valley Hospital & Extended Care Center
6575 Highway 93 South
Whitefish, MT 59937
Telephone: (406)-862-2501
Information & Referral - Networking

Pathways, Inc.
200 Heritage Way
Kalispell, MT 59901-3180
Telephone: (406)-756-3950 Fax: (406)-756-3957
Toll-Free: (800)-843-2890
Contact: Rick Johnson
Information & Referral, Networking

Gallatin County

Community Services

Southern Montana AIDS Coalition
108 Sourdough Ridge
Bozeman, MT 59715
Telephone: (406)-994-5231
Contact: David Gay - Chair
HIV education, advocacy and support

Home Health Care

Gallatin Hospice
915 Highland Blvd.
Bozeman, MT 59715-4618
Telephone: (406)-587-5683
Home-based care for terminally ill, counseling/support

Medical Services

Montana State University - Student Health Service
MSU Campus
Bozeman, MT 59717
Telephone: (406)-994-2311 Fax: (406)-994-2504
Contact: James Mitchell
Walk-in clinical health services

Testing Sites

Bridger Clinic
300 N. Willson Avenue
Suite 2001
Bozeman, MT 59715-3551
Telephone: (406)-587-0681
Contact: Shelly Videon
HIV Counseling & Testing, Health Education & Risk Reduction Site

Glacier County

County Health Depts

Glacier County Health Department
1210 East Main
Cut Bank, MT 59427
Telephone: (406)-873-2924

Medical Services

PHS Indian Hospital
Po Box 760
Browning, MT 59417
Telephone: (406)-338-6100
Contact: Judy Maeda, RN - AIDS Coordinator
Counseling and Medical Services

Hill County

Community Services

Rocky Boy (Bureau of Indian Affairs) Social Services
P.O. Box 664
Rocky Boy Route
Box Elder, MT 59521
Telephone: (406)-395-4282
Economic and general assistance

County Health Depts

Hill County Health Department
300 Fourth Avenue
Havre, MT 59501
Telephone: (406)-265-5481
Contact: Kathy Mader, RN
HIV counseling & testing site, task force, HIV education

Medical Services

Golden Triangle Mental Health
P.O. Box 1658
Havre, MT 59501-1658
Telephone: (406)-265-9639
Mental health services

Northern Montana College - Student Health Service
Cowan Hall, Room 213
Havre, MT 59501
Telephone: (406)-265-3783
Contact: Sue Swann - Director of Student Affairs
Clinical/infirmary services for students, AIDS information

Jefferson County

County Health Depts

Jefferson County Health Department
P.O. Box 41
Whitehall, MT 59759-0423
Telephone: (406)-287-3249

Lewis And Clark County

County Health Depts

Lewis & Clark City-County Health Department AIDS Program
1930 9th Ave
Helena, MT 59601
Telephone: (406)-443-2584 Fax: (406)-443-0459
Contact: Paula Block
Community education, risk reduction, HIV testing

Medical Services

St Peter Community Hospital
2475 Broadway
Helena, MT 59601-4999
Telephone: (406)-442-2480
Acute care facility

Mc Cone County

County Health Depts

McCone County Health Department
P.O. Box 199
Circle, MT 59215-0199
Telephone: (406)-485-3425

Mineral County

County Health Depts

Mineral County Health Department
P.O. Box 488
Superior, MT 59872-0488
Telephone: (406)-822-3321

Missoula County

Medical Services

Providence Center - St. Patrick Hospital Dependency Programs
Providence Center
902 N Orange Street
Missoula, MT 59802
Telephone: (406)-543-7271
Counseling, inpatient treatment

St Patrick Hospital
500 West Broadway
Missoula, MT 59802-4008
Telephone: (406)-543-7271
Information & referral, networking

University of Montana - Student Health Service
634 Eddy Ave
Missoula, MT 59812-0001
Telephone: (406)-243-2122
Counseling and mental health, treatment of STDs, medical/dental services

Vet Center
500 N Higgins Avenue
Missoula, MT 59802-4535
Telephone: (406)-721-4918
Walk-in & by appt counseling center, info & referral

Park County

County Health Depts

Park County Health Department
414 East Callender St
Livingston, MT 59047-2799
Telephone: (406)-222-6120

Phillips County

County Health Depts

Phillips County Health Department
Phillips County Library
P.O. Box 309
Malta, MT 59538
Telephone: (406)-654-2521

Pondera County

County Health Depts

Pondera County Health Department
809 Sunset Boulevard
Conrad, MT 59425-1717
Telephone: (406)-278-3247

Powder River County

County Health Depts

Powder River County Health Department
P.O. Box 325
Broadus, MT 59317-0325
Telephone: (406)-436-2297

Roosevelt County

Medical Services

PHS Indian Health Center
PO Box 67
Poplar, MT 59255
Telephone: (406)-768-3491 Fax: (406)-768-3603
Contact: Donna Mae Snodgrass
Medical services

Rosebud County

County Health Depts

Rosebud County Health Department
251 N 17th Avenue
P.O. Box 388
Forsyth, MT 59327
Telephone: (406)-356-2156

Sanders County

County Health Depts

Sanders County Health Department
P.O. Box 519, Courthouse
Thompson Falls, MT 59873-0519
Telephone: (406)-827-4395

Sheridan County

County Health Depts

Sheridan County Health Department
100 West Laurel
Plentywood, MT 59254
Telephone: (406)-765-2310

Silver Bow County

Medical Services

Ridgeview Treatment Center
2500 Continental Drive
Butte, MT 59701-6565
Telephone: (406)-496-5400 Fax: (406)-782-7829
Contact: Marilyn Holm
Inpatient alcohol & drug treatment

St James Community Hospital
400 South Clark
Butte, MT 59701-2395
Telephone: (406)-782-8361
Acute care hospital, HIV counseling

Testing Sites

Family Services/HIV Testing and Counseling
25 West Front Street
Butte, MT 59701
Telephone: (406)-723-6507 Fax: (406)-723-7245
Contact: Gan Cossel, RN
HIV Counseling & Testing, Health Education, Risk Reduction Site

Stillwater County

Medical Services

Stillwater County Community Hospital
44 West 4th Ave North
P.O. Box 959
Columbus, MT 59019
Telephone: (406)-322-5316

Sweet Grass County

County Health Depts

Sweet Grass Community Health
Sweet Grass Community Hospital
P.O. Box 1228
Big Timber, MT 59011
Telephone: (406)-932-5917

Teton County

County Health Depts

Teton County Health Department
914 4th Street NW
P.O. Box 335
Choteau, MT 59422
Telephone: (406)-466-2562

Toole County

County Health Depts

Toole County Health Department
Courthouse
Shelby, MT 59474
Telephone: (406)-434-5372

Treasure County

County Health Depts

Treasure County Health Department
P.O. Box 201
Hysham, MT 59038-0272
Telephone: (406)-342-5886

Valley County

County Health Depts

Valley County Health Department
Courthouse Annex
Glasgow, MT 59230
Telephone: (406)-288-8221

Wibaux County

County Health Depts

Wibaux County Health Department
Courthouse
P.O. Box 117
Wibaux, MT 59353
Telephone: (406)-795-2434

Yellowstone County

County Health Depts

Yellowstone City-County Health Department
Courthouse, Room 308
P.O. Box 35033
Billings, MT 59107
Telephone: (406)-256-2757

Medical Services

Deering Community Health Center
123 South 27th Street
Billings, MT 59101-4206
Telephone: (406)-256-6821 Fax: (406)-256-6829
Contact: Ron Seibel
HIV Counseling & Testing, Health Education, Risk Reduction Site

Mental Health Center
1245 N 29th Street
Billings, MT 59101-0183
Telephone: (406)-252-5658
Outpatient mental health

NEBRASKA

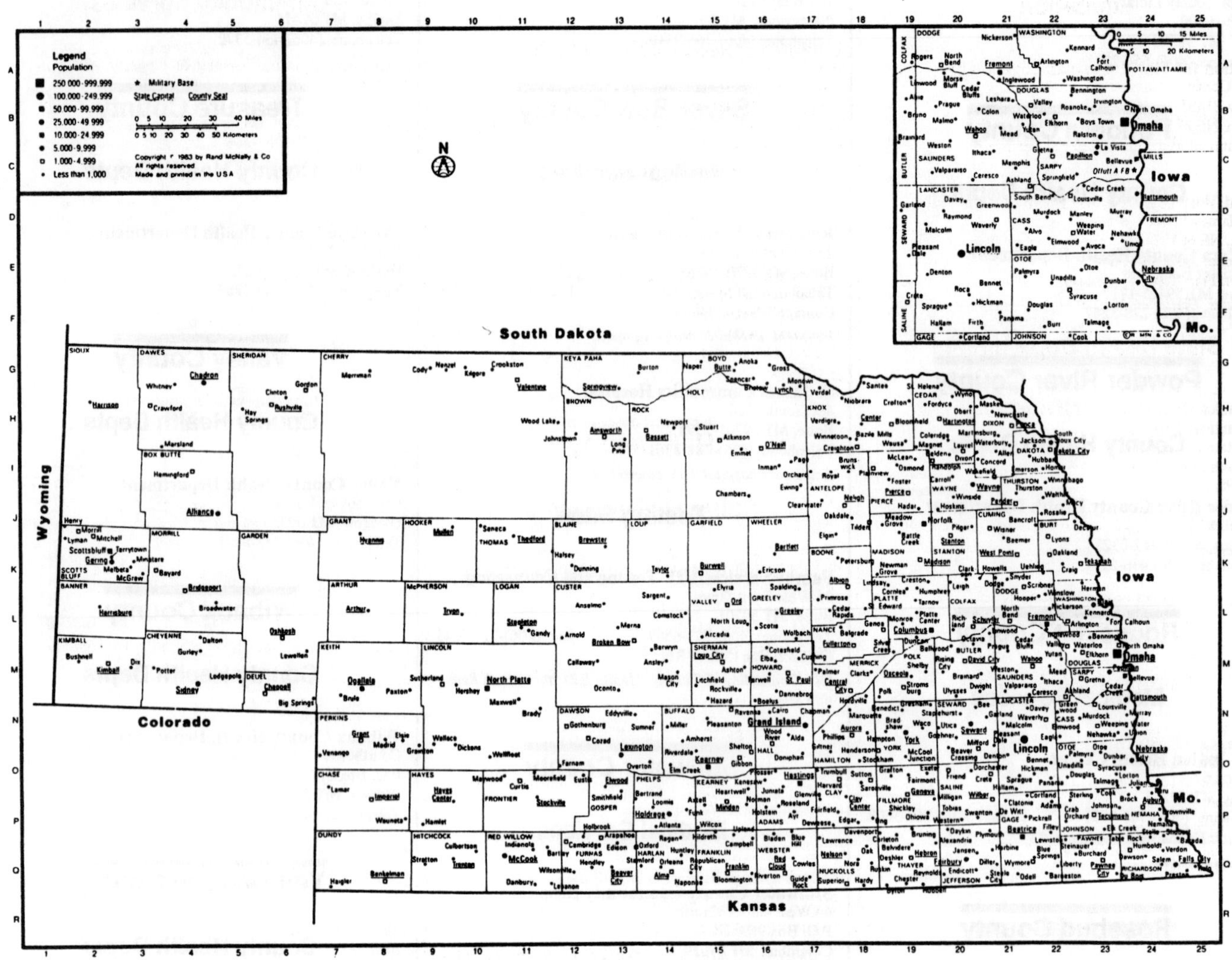

From City/County Planning Atlas Copyright 1989 by Reed McNally & Company, R.L. 90-S-28

Nebraska

General Services

Education

Coalition for Gay & Lesbian Civil Rights
Health Concerns Committee
PO Box 81455
Lincoln, NE 68509
TEducational Materials & Referral Services

United Way of Midlands/ First Call for Help
1805 Harney Street
Omaha, NE 68102
Telephone: (402)-444-6666
Contact: Fran Condon - Director
Databases, Electronic Media

State Health Departments

Nebraska Department of Health, AIDS Prevention Program
Craft State Office Bldg.
200 South Silber Street
North Platte, NE 69101
Telephone: (308)-535-8134
Contact: Virginia Wilkinson - AIDS Program Director
Confidential AIDS testing site, counseling.

Douglas County

Community Services

Nebraska AIDS Project
3624 Leavenworth St
Omaha, NE 68105
Telephone: (402)-342-6367 Fax: (402)-342-9073
Contact: Gary George
HIV testing, counseling,(free/anonymous), referrals, education, casemanagement, hotline (800-782-2437-9-11 M-F, 6-11 Sat/Sun)

Home Health Care

Critical Care America
3315 N 107th Street
Omaha, NE 68134
Telephone: (402)-493-6322 Fax: (402)-496-7025
Toll-Free: (800)-274-2144
Contact: Debbie Swanson - Dir. Nursing
Coordinate & integrate all clinical & psychosocial services for HIV+

Homedco Infusion
P.O.Box 27569
Omaha, NE 68127-0569
Telephone: (402)-553-8009
Contact: Mike Adams
Home infusion therapy for AIDS patients

nmc HOMECARE
8603 G. Street
Omaha, NE 68127
Telephone: (402)-339-7572
Fax: (402)-339-1904
Contact: Tara Stratman
National JCAHO-Accredited company providing a full range of Infusion and Respiratory therapies and specializing in the care of HIV/AIDS patients. National Case Manager is also available at 800-445-1188

Medical Services

University of Nebraska Medical Center
HIV Clinic
600 South 42nd Street
Omaha, NE 68198-5400
Telephone: (402)-559-4420 Fax: (402)-559-5581
Contact: Dr. Susan Swindells
AIDS Medical treatment & Research Center

Testing Sites

Nebraska AIDS Etc, Univ of NE Med Ctr
600 South 42nd Street
Omaha, NE 68198-5400
Telephone: (402)-559-6681 Fax: (402)-559-5581
Contact: Deb Brown
HIV clinic

Hall County

County Health Depts

Grand Island/Hall County Health Department
105 East 1st Street
Grand Island, NE 68801-6022
Telephone: (308)-381-5175
Contact: Mary Hem
Free AIDS testing and counseling (confidential), support groups

Home Health Care

nmc HOMECARE
143 Roberts Street
Grand Island, NE 68802
Telephone: (308)-381-7030
Fax: (308)-381-4786
Contact: Tara Stratman
National JCAHO-Accredited company providing a full range of Infusion and Respiratory therapies and specializing in the care of HIV/AIDS patients. National Case Manager is also available at 800-445-1188

Holt County

Home Health Care

nmc HOMECARE
P.O. Box 873 320 East Douglas St.
O'Neill, NE 68763
Telephone: (402)-336-1619
Contact: Pam Angerhofer
National JCAHO-Accredited company providing a full range of Infusion and Respiratory therapies and specializing in the care of HIV/AIDS patients. National Case Manager is also available at 800-445-1188

Lancaster County

Community Services

Jean Durgin-Ilene/Parents & Friends of Lesbians & Gays
PO Box 4374
Lincoln, NE 68504-0374
Telephone: (402)-435-4688
AIDS Support Group

Lincoln Urban Ministries
215 Centennial Mall South
Room 408
Lincoln, NE 68508-1813
Telephone: (402)-474-3017
Contact: Rev. Dr. Norman Leach
Pastoral care & AIDS Healing Services

Nebraska Department of Social Services
1050 North Centennial Mall South
Suite 350
Lincoln, NE 68505
Telephone: (402)-471-7000
Contact: Tam Goodmen Carndy
Financial resources; education & referral services, assistance withMedicaid

County Health Depts

Lincoln-Lancaster County Health Department
2200 St. Mary's Avenue
Lincoln, NE 68502-3749
Telephone: (402)-471-8065
Contact: Tim Timons
Free AIDS testing and counseling (confidential)

Home Health Care

Homedco Infusion
1631 Cushman Drive
Lincoln, NE 68506
Telephone: (402)-434-2950 Fax: (402)-434-2963
Toll-Free: (800)-347-5946
Contact: Tom Danek
Home infusion therapy for AIDS patients

Lincoln County

Home Health Care

nmc HOMECARE
509 E 7th, Suite 5
No. Platte, NE 69101
Telephone: (308)-532-2366
Contact: Tara Stratman
National JCAHO-Accredited company providing a full range of Infusion and Respiratory therapies and specializing in the care

of HIV/AIDS patients. National Case Manager is also available at 800-445-1188

Nemaha County

County Health Depts

Nemaha County Health Department
1824 North Street
Auburn, NE 68305-2341
Telephone: (402)-274-4549
Contact: Kay Oestmann - R.N.
Free AIDS testing and counseling confidential

Scotts Bluff County

Testing Sites

Scotts Bluff County Health Department
County Administration Bdg
Gering, NE 69341
Telephone: (308)-635-3866
Contact: Bill Wineman
Free AIDS testing and counseling (confidential)

NEVADA

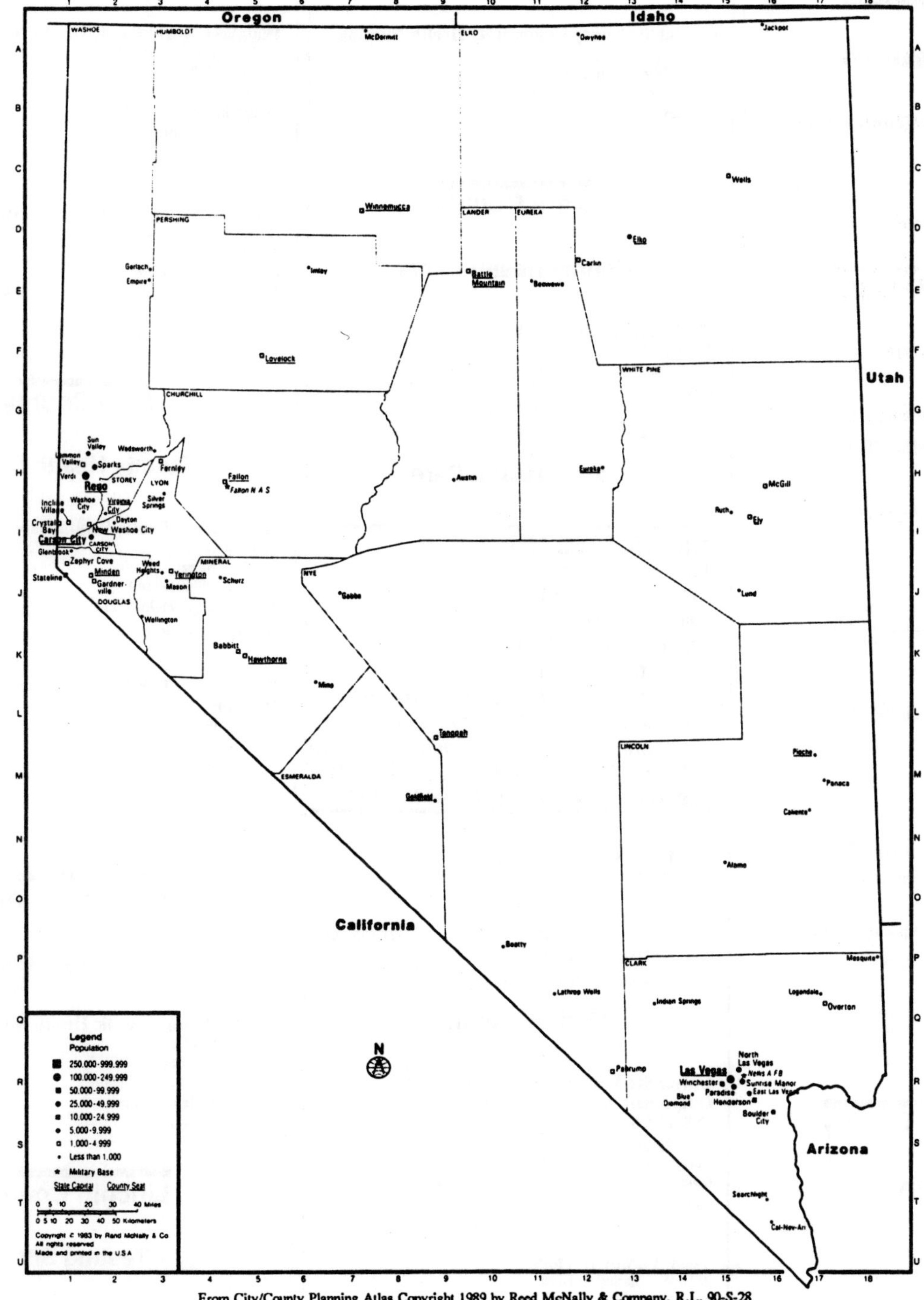

From City/County Planning Atlas Copyright 1989 by Reed McNally & Company, R.L. 90-S-28

Nevada

General Services

Education

American Red Cross, Clark County Chapter
1819 E. Charleston Blvd.
Las Vegas, NV 89104-1936
Telephone: (702)-384-1225
Contact: Bill Hanagarne
Education, Pamphlets, Resource Center

University of Nevada Las Vegas
Graduate Nursing Program
4505 S. Maryland Parkway
Las Vegas, NV 89154
Telephone: (702)-739-3415
Contact: Vicky Carwein - Association Professor
Education, Pamphlets, Resource Center

State Health Departments

Nevada State Health Department
Division of STD/AIDS
505 East King Street
Carson City, NV 89710
Telephone: (702)-687-4804
Contact: Dr. John Yacenda - Program Manager, HIV/AIDS; Bill Hill - Surveillance Coord.; Pam Walton - Ryan White Care Coord.
Drug assistance, home health care

Statewide Services

AID for AIDS in Nevada
1111 Desert Lane
Las Vegas, NV 89102-2305
Telephone: (702)-369-2326
Contact: Gregory Durrett, MBA - Executive Director
Free HIV testing, pre/post counseling, education, referrals

State of Nevada, Bureau of Alcohol and Drug Abuse
505 East King Street
Carson City, NV 89710-0001
Telephone: (702)-885-4790
Contact: Tim Moen - Program Analyst
Information

Carson City County

Medical Services

Pediatric Dental Services
314 W. 5th Street
Carson City, NV 89701-4604
Telephone: (702)-882-1111 Fax: (702)-882-1120
Contact: Raymond B. Graber, DDS

Testing Sites

Carson City Public Health Nursing
1711 N. Roop Street
Carson City, NV 89701-3113
Telephone: (702)-887-2195
Contact: Maggie Holloway
Testing, Counseling

Churchill County

Testing Sites

Churchill County Community Health Nursing
85 N. Taylor
Fallon, NV 89406-2750
Telephone: (702)-423-4434
Contact: Janet Swan
Testing, Counseling

Clark County

County Health Depts

Clark County Health District
P.O. Box 4426
Las Vegas, NV 89127-0426
Telephone: (702)-383-1202 Fax: (702)-383-1446
Contact: Rick Reich - AIDS Services Coord.
Video Tapes, Publications, Pamphlets, Resource Center

Home Health Care

nmc HOMECARE
3321 Sunrise Ave
Las Vegas, NV 89101
Telephone: (702)-438-2273
Fax: (702)-438-1875
Contact: Karen Thornton
National JCAHO-Accredited company providing a full range of Infusion and Respiratory therapies and specializing in the care of HIV/AIDS patients. National Case Manager is also available at 800-445-1188

O.P.T.I.O.N Care of Nevada
3900 W Charleston Blvd
Suite Z
Las Vegas, NV 89102-1628
Telephone: (702)-258-0011 Fax: (702)-258-3668
Contact: Marfie Niemyer - AIDS Coordinator
Home IV and Nutritional Services

Medical Services

University Medical Center, AIDS Unit Outpatient & Inpatient Services
1800 W. Charleston Blvd.
Las Vegas, NV 89102
Telephone: (702)-383-2000 Fax: (702)-383-3641
Contact: Ed Davis, Ph.D. - Support Group Co-Facilitator
Support Groups, Medical Services

Vegas Family Doctors
2810 W. Charleston Blvd
Suite F-54
Las Vegas, NV 89102-1921
Telephone: (702)-870-0808 Fax: (702)-870-3275
Contact: Kathryn Crooks, MD
Complete, comprehensive medical care, testing and referrals

Douglas County

Testing Sites

Douglas County Public Health Nursing
1433 Hwy 395 Gardnerville
P.O. Box 218
Minden, NV 89423
Telephone: (702)-782-9038
Contact: Irene Best
Testing, Counseling

Douglas County Public Health Nursing
(175 Hwy. 50, Stateline)
P.O. Box 11849
Zephyr Cove, NV 89448
Telephone: (702)-588-6921 Fax: (702)-588-9214
Contact: Pat Thomas
Testing, counseling, referral

Elko County

County Health Depts

Elko County Public Health Department
Medical Clinic
762 14th Street
Elko, NV 89801-3349
Telephone: (702)-738-7211
Testing, Counseling

Elko County Public Health Nursing-Wells Division
148 Fourth Street
P.O. Box 353
Wells, NV 89835
Telephone: (702)-752-3216
Contact: Colleen Folwell
Testing, Counseling

Lander County

Testing Sites

Lander County Public Health Nursing
6th Humboldt 98-11
Battle Mountain, NV 89820
Telephone: (702)-635-2386
Contact: Helen Thompson
Testing, Counseling

Lincoln County

Testing Sites

Lincoln County Public Health Nursing
(Hospital Complex Hwy 93)
360 Lincoln Street
Caliente, NV 89008
Telephone: (702)-726-3123
Contact: Mary Jean
Testing, Counseling

Lyon County

County Health Depts

Lyon County Public Health Nursing
555 East Main Street
P.O. Box 988
Fernley, NV 89408
Telephone: (702)-351-1301
Contact: Dr. John Yacenda
Testing, Counseling

Mineral County

County Health Depts

Mineral County Public Health Nursing
(331 First Street)
P.O. Box 1477
Hawthorne, NV 89415
Telephone: (702)-945-3657
Contact: Connie Torres
Testing, Counseling

Nye County

Testing Sites

Nye and Esmeraldo County Public Health Nursing
565 Erie Main
P.O. Box 409
Tonopah, NV 89049
Telephone: (702)-482-6659
Contact: Catherine Shelton
Testing, Counseling

Nye County Public Health Nursing
Co. Comp. Bldg Hwy 160
P.O. Box 160
Pahrump, NV 89041
Telephone: (702)-727-5750
Contact: Marilyn Gallivan
Testing, Counseling

Pershing County

Testing Sites

Pershing County Public Health Nursing
535 Western Avenue
PO Box 1166
Lovelock, NV 89419
Telephone: (702)-273-2041
Contact: Vener Anoran
Testing, Counseling

Washoe County

Community Services

Nevada AIDS Foundation/Bridges in Consciousness
P.O. Box 478
Reno, NV 89504-0478
Telephone: (702)-329-2437 Fax: (702)-329-9144
Information, Residence Program, Counseling, Referrals

County Health Depts

Washoe County District Health Depart., HIV Early Intervention
1001 East 9th Street
Reno, NV 89520-0027
Telephone: (702)-328-2404
Contact: Dr. Nancy Rody - AIDS Coordinator
Information, Testing, HIV+ Early Intervention Clinic

Home Health Care

Caremark Connection Network
1380 Greg Street
Suite 217
Sparks, NV 89431
Telephone: (702)-355-3300
Contact: Dan Stames - Branch Manager
Clinical Support and Infusion Therapies: Nutrition, Antimicrobials, Chemo.,Hematopoeti

St. Mary's Home Care Services and Hospice Program
235 West 6th Street
Reno, NV 89520-0108
Telephone: (702)-789-3046 Fax: (702)-789-3909
Contact: Donna Shilinsky - Director
Home Health Care, Hospice

Medical Services

Spanish Springs Medical Group
1015 Spanish Springs Rd.
Sparks, NV 89431-9403
Telephone: (702)-359-3466 Fax: (702)-359-3548
Contact: Katherine Bennett, M.D.
Medical Examinations

St. Mary's Regional Medical Center
235 W. 6th Street
Reno, NV 89520-0108
Telephone: (702)-323-2041 Fax: (702)-789-3679
Medical Services

Veterans Administration Medical Center
1000 Locust
Reno, NV 89520-0111
Telephone: (702)-786-7200 Fax: (702)-328-1464
Contact: Terry Rycker
Medical Services

Washoe Professional Center
75 Pringle Way
Suite 608
Reno, NV 89502-1490
Telephone: (702)-348-7781 Fax: (702)-329-2567
Contact: David L. Diedrichsen, M.D.
Medical Examinations, Counseling

White Pine County

Testing Sites

White Pine County Public Health Nursing
995 Campton Street
Ely, NV 89301-1987
Telephone: (702)-289-2107 Fax: (702)-289-8842
Testing, Counseling

NEW HAMPSHIRE

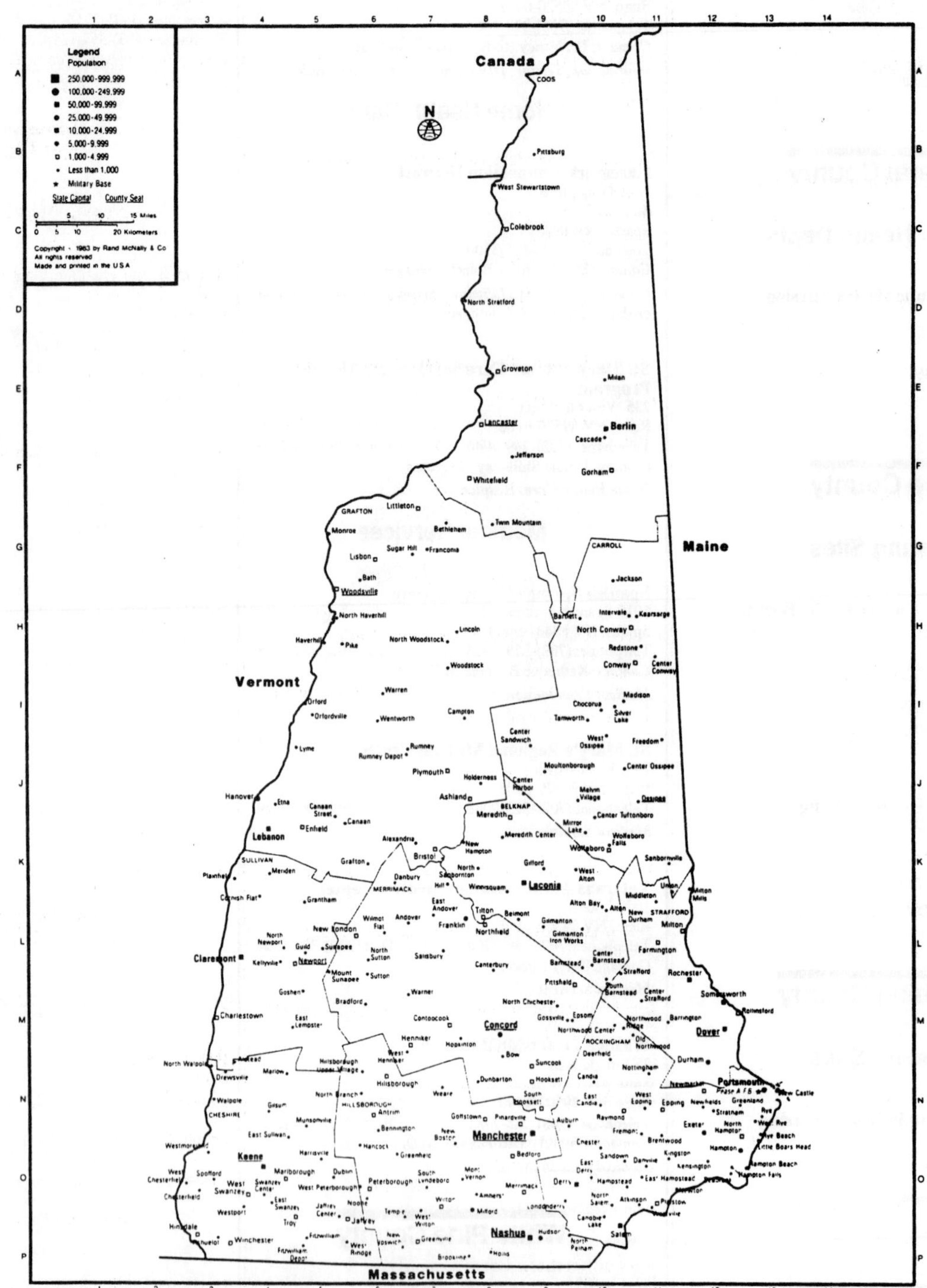

From City/County Planning Atlas Copyright 1989 by Reed McNally & Company, R.L. 90-S-28

New Hampshire

General Services

Hotlines

New Hampshire AIDS Hotline

,In-state only (800)-752-2437
8:30am to 4:30pm

New Hampshire AIDS Information Line

In-state only (800)-639-1122
9 am to 10 pm daily

New Hampshire Spanish Hotline

In state only (800)-344-7432

New Hampshire Teens AIDS Hotline

In state only (800) 344-7432
Wed., Thurs. 6 pm to 9 pm

State Health Departments

New Hampshire Division of Public Health, AIDS/HIV Division
6 Hazen Drive
Concord, NH 03301
Telephone: (603)-271-4502

Statewide Services

Bureau of Disease Control/ HIV/AIDS Program
6 Hazen Drive
Health and Welfare Bldg
Concord, NH 03301-6501
Telephone: (603)-271-4576
Contact: Joyce Welch - Program Chief
Contract with health care providers.

New Hampshire AIDS Foundation (NHAF)
PO Box 59
102 Middle Street
Manchester, NH 03105
Telephone: (603)-595-0218
Contact: George V. Mitoulas
Information, support, case management, referrals, support groups, advocacyeducation, buddy referrals

New Hampshire Drug Reimbursement Program

In stqte only (800)-752-2437

New Hampshire STD/HIV Program

Telephone: (603)-271-4576

Belknap County

Home Health Care

Heritage Home Health & Hospice
169 Daniel Webster Highway
Suite 7
Meredith, NH 03253
Telephone: (603)-744-5421
Contact: Linda Roberts
Home health care, hospice, chemo., contracted infusion therapy, sharedhousing, MSW on staff.

Hospice-Laconia Area
P.O. Box 578
780 North Main Street
Laconia, NH 03246
Telephone: (603)-524-8588
Contact: Alicia Milham
Hospice, home care services

Meredith Public Health Nursing Association
Box 176
73 Main Street
Meredith, NH 03253-0176
Telephone: (603)-279-6611
Home Health Care Agencies

Testing Sites

Family Planning/Belknap-Merrimack County
426 Union Ave.
Laconia, NH 03246-2812
Telephone: (603)-271-4490 Fax: (603)-524-5453
HIV/Diagnosis, treatment, testing, counseling

Carroll County

Home Health Care

Carroll County Health and Home Care
Carrol County Complex
Ossipee, NH 03864
Telephone: (603)-539-4171 Fax: (603)-539-2160
Home Health Care Agencies

Hospice of Northern Carroll County
P.O. Box 401
North Conway, NH 03860-0401
Telephone: (603)-356-2324
Contact: Elizabeth George
AIDS support group for HIV patients & their families

V & A Hospice of Southern Carroll County Vicinity
P.O. Box 1162
Wolfeboro, NH 03894-1162
Telephone: (603)-569-1590 Fax: (603)-569-2409
Home Health Care, Hospice

VNA of Wolfeboro & Vicinity
Box 141
South Main Street
Wolfeboro, NH 03894-0141
Telephone: (603)-569-2729
Contact: Nyoka Babbitt - Acting Administrator
Home Health Care Agencies

VNS of Northern Carroll County
PO Box 432
North Conway, NH 03860
Telephone: (603)-356-7006 Fax: (603)-447-6370
Home Health Care Agencies

Cheshire County

Home Health Care

Hospice of Cheshire County, Inc.
7 Center Street
Keene, NH 03431-3351
Telephone: (603)-357-1314
Contact: Teri Riddle - Coordinator
Home Health Care, Hospice

Coos County

Home Health Care

Berlin Home Hospice Volunteers
Christian Life Center
P.O. Box 354
Berlin, NH 03570
Telephone: (603)-752-7883
Contact: Sister Monique Therriaull
Home Health Care, Hospice

North Country Home Health
Town Hall
Park Street
Gorham, NH 03581
Telephone: (603)-466-5021 Fax: (603)-444-0980
Home Health Care Agencies

Northern Coos Community Health Association
9 Monadnock Street
Box 37
Colebrook, NH 03576-1011
Telephone: (603)-237-8083 Fax: (603)-237-4452
Contact: Elaina Johnson
Home Health Care Agencies

Weeks Home Health Service
Middle Street
Lancaster, NH 03584
Telephone: (603)-788-2366
Home health care, HIV testing, counseling

Grafton County

Community Services

HIV Support Group
Dartmouth Hitchook
1 Medical Center
Lebanon, NH 03756
Telephone: (603)-646-5789
Contact: Maris Noble; Allen Hood
Support group for families, friends and partners of HIV+

Home Health Care

Dartmouth-Hitchkock Home Health Center
One Medical Center Drive
Infectious Disease Section, 3D
Lebannon, NH 03756
Telephone: (603)-646-7076
Contact: Kristen Rose; Donna Gibson
Home Health Care Agencies

Home and Community Health Care of Upper Valley Inc.
325 Mount Support Rd.
Lebanon, NH 03766-2813
Telephone: (603)-448-1597
Contact: Mary Hastings - Facility Coordinator
Home Health Care Agencies

Hospice of the Upper Valley
325 Mount Support Rd.
Lebanon, NH 03766-2813
Telephone: (603)-448-5182 Fax: (603)-448-1599
Contact: Karren DeWolf Richard - Administrative Assistant
Hospice care; volunteer respite & support; bereavement counseling

Hospice-NANA
P.O. Box 96
Bristol, NH 03222
Telephone: (603)-744-2733
Contact: Jennie Martin - Executive Director
Home Health Care, Hospice

Newfound Area Nursing Association
Lake Street
Bristol, NH 03222
Telephone: (603)-744-2733
Contact: Janine Martin
Home Health Care Agencies

North Country Home Health Agency
4 Mt. Eustis Road
Littleton, NH 03561
Telephone: (603)-444-5317 Fax: (603)-444-0980
Home health care agencies; nursing services, homemakers & adult in homecare

Pemi-Baker Home Health Agency
79 Highland Street
Plymouth, NH 03264-1237
Telephone: (603)-536-2232
Contact: Elaine Vieira
Home Health Care Agencies

Visiting Nurse Alliance of Vermont/New Hampshire
Box 118
Main Street
Canaan, NH 03741-0118
Telephone: (603)-523-4382
Contact: 603-523-4382 - Bev Brock
Home Health Care Agencies

Medical Services

Dartmouth-Hitchcock Medical Center, Infectious Disease Section, 3D
1 Medical Center Drive
Lebanon, NH 03756
Telephone: (603)-650-6060 Fax: (603)-650-4437
Toll-Free: (800)-458-2437
Contact: Betsy Eccles
Diagnosis, treatment, testing, counseling, NH hotline 800-752-2437, postiveaction-800-540-2352, teen AIDS 800-234-8336 hotline.

Hillsborough County

Home Health Care

Deaconess Home Health Care
915 Holt Avenue
Suite 2
Manchester, NH 03109
Telephone: (603)-625-2133
Home Health Care Agencies

Elliot Hospital and Community Hospice
1 Elliot Way
Manchester, NH 03103-3599
Telephone: (603)-669-5300
Home Health Care, Hospice, Medical Services

Home Health and Hospice Care
79 Camp Sargent Road
PO Box 216
Merrimack, NH 03054-0216
Telephone: (603)-424-3822
Home health care, hospice care

Home Health and Hospice Care
22 Prospect Street
Nashua, NH 03060-3939
Telephone: (603)-882-2941
Home Health Care Agencies

Hospice of Monadnock Regional
P.O. Box 571
20 Grove Street
Peterborough, NH 03458
Telephone: (603)-924-4343
Home Health Care, Hospice

Interim Health Care
PO Box 1780
608 Chestnut Street
Manchester, NH 03105-1780
Telephone: (603)-668-6956
Home Health Care Agencies

Souhegan Nursing Association
24 North River Road
Milford, NH 03055
Telephone: (603)-673-3460
Contact: Betsy White
Home Health Care Agencies

St. Joseph Hospital, Palliative Care Unit
172 Kingsley Street
Nashua, NH 03060
Telephone: (603)-882-3000
Contact: Gloria Dionne, R.N.
Home Health Care, Hospice, Medical Services

Visiting Nurse Association of Manchester & S. New Hampshire Inc.
1850 Elm Street
Manchester, NH 03104-2911
Telephone: (603)-622-3781 Fax: (603)-622-3781
Toll-Free: (800)-624-6084
Home Health Care, Hospice

Visiting Nurse Association of Manchester & Southern New Hampton Inc.
1850 Elm Street
Manchester, NH 03104-4832
Telephone: (603)-622-3781 Fax: (603)-622-3781
Contact: Stacey Vaillantcourt - Director of Division
Home Health Care, Hospice

Visiting Nurse Associaton of Manchester & Southern New Hampshire
1850 Elm Street
Manchester, NH 03104-2911
Telephone: (603)-622-3721
Contact: Mary McKillop, RN
Home health care & hospice services

Testing Sites

Manchester Health Department
795 Elm Street
Manchester, NH 03101-4832
Telephone: (603)-624-6467 Fax: (603)-628-6004
Toll-Free: (800)-852-3345
Contact: Carolynne Shinn
HIV, diagnosis, referral, testing, counseling, NH hotline 800-852-3345

Merrimack County

Home Health Care

Concord Regional Visiting Nurse Association
P.O. Box 1797
250 Pleasant Street
Concord, NH 03302-0797
Telephone: (603)-224-4093
Home health care, hospice, HIV counseling and testing

Concord Regional Visiting Nurse Association
250 Pleasant Street
Yeaple Building
Concord, NH 03301
Telephone: (603)-324-4093
Home Health Care, Hospice

Home Care Association of New Hampshire
8 Green Street
Concord, NH 03301-5141
Telephone: (603)-225-5597 Fax: (603)-225-5817
Toll-Free: (800)-639-1949
Membership association for home health care agencies

Lake Sunapee Region Visiting Nurse Association
County Road
PO Box 2209
New London, NH 03257
Telephone: (603)-526-4077 Fax: (603)-526-4272
Contact: Allison Conlon
Home Health Care Agencies

Lake Sunatee Region Visiting Nurse Association
P.O. Box 2209
New London, NH 03257
Telephone: (603)-526-6544 Fax: (603)-526-4272
Toll-Free: (800)-310-4077
Home health care, hospice, & nursing assessments, infusion therapy,pediatric care, counseling & support

Visiting Nurse Association of Franklin, Inc.
75 Chestnut Stteet
Franklin, NH 03235-1306
Telephone: (603)-934-3454 Fax: (603)-934-2222
Home Health Care Agencies

Rockingham County

Community Services

AIDS Response of the Seacoast (ARS)

Portsmouth, NH 03801-4047
Telephone: (603)-433-5377 Fax: (603)-431-8520
Contact: Jeffrey Jensen - Client Services
Information, support

HIV Counseling
Exeter Area
PO Box 227
New Fields, NH 03856
Telephone: (603)-778-3011
Contact: Tessa Storne-Lyon
AIDS/HIV counseling

HIV Support Group
Regional Hospital
Portsmouth, NH 03801
Telephone: (603)-433-8447
For HIV+ partners, family and friends; 7:00 pm Friday

St. Joseph's School
Main Street
Salem, NH 03079
Telephone: (603)-898-7065
Contact: Paul Donavon
Support group for families and friends of HIV+

Home Health Care

Area Homemaker Home Health Service
1320 Woodbury Avenue
Portsmouth, NH 03801-3222
Telephone: (603)-436-9059
Homemaker services, hospice care

Hillside Hospice
P.O. Box 125
Deerfield, NH 03037-0125
Telephone: (603)-942-7016
Contact: Priscilla Merrill
Home Health Care, Hospice

Portsmouth Regional Visiting Nurse Association
127 Parrott Avenue
Portsmouth, NH 03801-4402
Telephone: (603)-436-0815 Fax: (603)-431-5457
Home health care, hospice care

PRN Home Health Service, Inc.
14 Front Street
Box 1096
Exeter, NH 03833-2747
Telephone: (603)-772-2420
Home Health Care Agencies

Rockingham V.N.A & Hospice
11 Wall Street
Derry, NH 03038-6341
Telephone: (603)-432-7776 Fax: (603)-432-0068
Contact: Simon Paquette - Director
Home health care, hospice, nursing services

Rockingham Visiting Nurse & Hospice Association
11 Wall Street
Derry, NH 03038-0262
Telephone: (603)-432-7776 Fax: (603)-432-0068
Toll-Free: (800)-675-9241
Contact: Barbara Leake - Director
Home health care agencies; chemo., infusion

Rockingham Visiting Nurse Association
137 Epping Rd.
Exeter, NH 03833-2223
Telephone: (603)-772-2981 Fax: (603)-772-0931
Home health care agencies, hospice

Salem District Nurse Association
Court Building
125 Stiles Road, Suite 105
Salem, NH 03079
Telephone: (603)-898-4737 Fax: (603)-890-3622
Home Health Care Agencies

Seacoast Hospice
9 Hampton Road
Exeter, NH 03833-4807
Telephone: (603)-778-7391
Contact: Nancy Chase
Home health care, in-home hospice

Seacoast Visiting Nurse Association
29 Lafayette Road
North Hampton, NH 03862-2436
Telephone: (603)-926-2066
Home Health Care Agencies

Strafford County

Home Health Care

Homedco Infusion
652 Central Avenue "C"
Dover, NH 03820
Telephone: (603)-749-6100 Fax: (603)-749-0128
Nationwide experience in providing home infusion therapy to AIDS patients

Homemakers of Strafford County
97 Rochester Hill Road
Rochester, NH 03867-3322
Telephone: (603)-692-4663 Fax: (603)-335-1773
Contact: Phyllis Goodhue
Home Health Care Agencies

Rural District Home IV Infusion Therapy
PO Box 667
Farmington, NH 03835-1615
Telephone: (603)-755-2202 Fax: (603)-755-3760
Home health care, infusion therpay

Squamscott Visiting Nurses & Hospice Care
89 Old Rochester Road
Dover, NH 03820-2100
Telephone: (603)-742-7921 Fax: (603)-742-3835
Contact: Nancy Boyle - Executive Director
Home health care, visiting nurses, hospice care

Strafford Hospice Care, Inc.
P.O. Box 339
Rollinsford, NH 03869-0339
Telephone: (603)-749-4300
Contact: Susan E. Cole
Home Health Care, Hospice-(no AIDS program specifically)

Tri-Area Visiting Nurse Association
301 High St.
Sommersworth, NH 03878
Telephone: (603)-692-2112 Fax: (603)-692-9940
Home Health Care Agencies

Sullivan County

Home Health Care

Connecticut Valley Home Care
244 Elm Street
Claremont, NH 03743-2000
Telephone: (603)-543-0164 Fax: (603)-542-1812
Home Health Care Agencies

NEW JERSEY

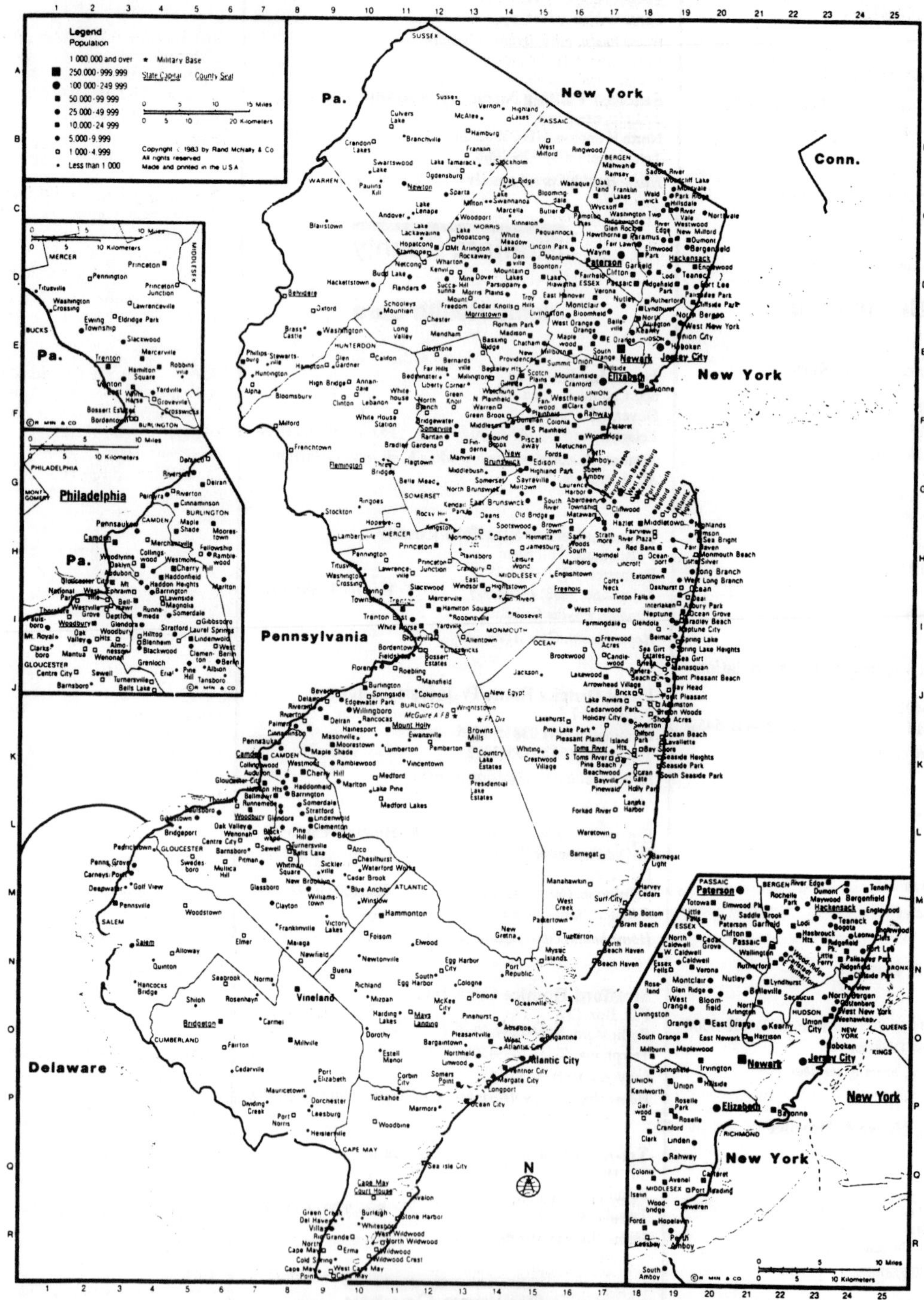

From City/County Planning Atlas Copyright 1989 by Reed McNally & Company, R.L. 90-S-28

New Jersey

General Services

Education

Academy of Medicine of New Jersey
14 Washington Road
Suite 101
Princeton Junction, NJ 08550
Telephone: (609)-896-0486
Contact: SaraJane Garten
Referrals to Education Programs and Speakers for Health Care Providers

American Red Cross
169 Chestnut Street
Nutley, NJ 07110-2311
Telephone: (201)-667-3818
AIDS education prevention

American Red Cross
63 Park Street
Montclair, NJ 07042
Telephone: (201)-746-1800 Fax: (201)-744-2091
Contact: Susan Schwei
Education, Literature, Programs

American Red Cross
29 Elm Street
Morristown, NJ 07960-4101
Telephone: (201)-538-2160
Education, Literature, Programs

American Red Cross
112 North Broad Street
Woodbury, NJ 08096-0592
Telephone: (609)-845-8500
Education, Literature, Programs

American Red Cross
1650 Pennington Road
Trenton, NJ 08618
Telephone: (609)-538-8133 Fax: (609)-538-8154
Education, Literature, Programs

American Red Cross
34 E. Mechanic St.
CM Court House, NJ 08210
Telephone: (609)-465-7382
Contact: Kevin Koknar
Education, Literature, Programs

American Red Cross
205 Madison Avenue
P.O. Box 4123
Burlington, NJ 08060
Telephone: (609)-386-0557
Contact: Joe Blazejewski
Education, Literature, Programs

American Red Cross
389 Millburn Avenue
Millburn, NJ 07041-1369
Telephone: (201)-379-4198
Education, Literature, Programs

American Red Cross - Essex Chapter
P.O. Box 838
106 Washington Street
East Orange, NJ 07019-0838
Telephone: (201)-676-0800 Fax: (201)-676-6267
Contact: Ann Chambers
Education, literature, videos, outreach programs, school curricula

American Red Cross and Middlesex County AIDS Task Force
900 A Woodbridge Center Drive
Woodbridge, NJ 07095
Telephone: (908)-247-9100
Contact: Dolores Nolan
Education, Literature, Programs; County AIDS Task Force, Resource Directory

American Red Cross Bergen Crossroads Chapter
74 Godwin Avenue
Ridgewood, NJ 07450-3788
Telephone: (201)-652-3210
Contact: Sandy Vanhogan
Educational services, transportation

American Red Cross Jersey Coast Chapter
830 Broad Street
PO Box 7101
Shrewsbury, NJ 07701-4291
Telephone: (908)-741-3443
Contact: Valerie Rodgers
Education, Literature, Programs

American Red Cross Worth Hudson Chapter
410 Sixth Street
Union City, NJ 07087
Telephone: (201)-865-5000
Contact: John Huffman
Education, Programs, Literature

American Red Cross, Central New Jersey Chapter
900-A Woodbridge Center
Woodbridge, NJ 07095
Telephone: (908)-634-6500
Educational Services

American Red Cross, New Jersey Capitol Area Chapter
182 North Harrison Street
Princeton, NJ 08540-3852
Telephone: (609)-924-2404 Fax: (609)-683-9025
Education, Literature, Programs

American Red Cross, Rutherford/Wood-Ridge Chapter
176 Park Avenue
Rutherford, NJ 07070-2310
Telephone: (201)-939-2455
Contact: Ruth Decker
Educational Services

Area Health Education Center (AHEC)
Nothgate Plaza I
7th and Linden Streets
Camden, NJ 08102
Telephone: (609)-963-2432 Fax: (609)-541-1342
Education, Spanish Speaking

Center for AIDS Education
Univ. of Medicine & Dentistry of NJ
30 Bergen Street
Newark, NJ 07103
Telephone: (201)-456-6640 Fax: (201)-982-6640
Contact: Charles McKinney, Ed.D.
AIDS/HIV training for health care professionals

Center for Home Health Development, Home Health Agency of NJ
760 Alexander Road
Princeton, NJ 08543
Telephone: (609)-452-8855
Contact: Madalyne Anson
In-service Educational Program for Home-Care Workers, Agency Employees Only

East Orange AIDS Education Advisory Committee
143 New Street
East Orange, NJ 07017-4110
Telephone: (201)-266-5109
Taskforce

The Family Place at St. Barnabas Church
505 West Narket Street
Newark, NJ 07107
Telephone: (201)-481-0955
Contact: Gretchen MacBry, MA, MSW - Program Director
Counseling, education, advocacy, training for care-givers and families.

Garden Area Health Education Center
c/o Bridgeton Hospital
333 Irving Avenue
Bridgeton, NJ 08302-2100
Telephone: (609)-451-6600 Fax: (609)-451-6600
Contact: Shelley Cohen
Education

Gloucester County College
Deptford Township
Sewell, NJ 08080
Telephone: (609)-468-5000
Contact: Phyllis Stafford - College Nurse Ext.219
Education

Greater Northern New Jersey
575 Main Street
Hackensack, NJ 07601-5987
Telephone: (201)-489-1140 Fax: (201)-489-8389
Contact: Ruth Goldman
Women's Services, Education

Head Start for Children
Baby Land IV
563 Orange Street
Newark, NJ 07106-1534
Telephone: (201)-482-0982 Fax: (201)-482-2893
Contact: Sister Susan Janes
Children's Services, Education

Juvenile Resource Center, Inc.
315 Cooper Street
Camden, NJ 08102-1519
Telephone: (609)-963-4060
Contact: Dr. Stella Horton
Education, School Curriculum

MCOSS Foundation, Inc.
141 Bodman Place
Red Bank, NJ 07701
Telephone: (908)-224-6892 Fax: (908)-224-0028
Contact: Pat Buckley, - Adult ACCAP
AIDS resource center

New Jersey AIDS Education and Training Center
Univ. of Medicine & Dentistry of NJ
30 Bergen Street, ADMC 710
Newark, NJ 07107-3000
Telephone: (201)-982-3690 Fax: (201)-982-7128
Contact: Charles McKinney, Ed.D.

General information referrals, on-site clinical training and educationprograms

Planned Parenthood
40 N Van Brunt Street
Englewood, NJ 07631
Telephone: (201)-894-0966
Contact: Pam Bradford
HIV risk assessment & education

Planned Parenthood of Essex County
151 Washington Street
Newark, NJ 07102-3099
Telephone: (201)-622-3900
Contact: Michelle Anderson
Women's Services: Education

Planned Parenthood of Greater Northern New Jersey Inc.
196 Speedwell Avenue
Morristown, NJ 07960-2934
Telephone: (201)-539-9580
Contact: Cathy Mulvihill
Women's Services: Education, Testing and Counseling

Reality House, Inc.
Ashland Office Center
1 Alpha Ave. Suite # 43
Voorhees, NJ 08043
Telephone: (609)-428-5688
Counseling, Education, Referrals

Univ. of Medicine and Dentistry of NJ/Continuing Education
AIDS Program
30 Bergen Street, Rm 710
Newark, NJ 07107
Telephone: (201)-456-4267
Contact: Dr. Robert Moutrie
Training for Physicians, Nurses, Service Providers Focusing on Substance Abuse

West New York Family Planning Center
5305 Hudson Avenue
West New York, NJ 07093-2615
Telephone: (201)-866-8071
AIDS education & referrals

Hotlines

CONTACT 609
1050 North Kings Highway
Cherry Hill, NJ 08034-1909
Telephone: (609)-428-2900
Contact: 609-667-0432
Helpline, Listeners also Provide Referrals

State Health Departments

New Jersey Department of Health, AIDS Division
363 West State Street
Trenton, NJ 08625
Telephone: (609)-984-5874
Contact: Douglas H. Morgan - Assistant Commissioner; Ronald Altman - Medical Director
Research, education and training support, testing, counseling, medicalinformation

New Jersey Department of Health, Special Child Health, CN364
Service for HIV Children
50 East State Street CN 364
Trenton, NJ 08625
Telephone: (609)-292-5676 Fax: (609)-292-3580
Contact: Diane Di Donato
Network of family care centers for children

New Jersey State Department of Health
Division of AIDS Prevention and Control
363 West State Street, CN 363
Trenton, NJ 08625
Telephone: (609)-984-5888
Contact: Carmine Grasso - Active Service Director

NJ Dept. of Health, Div. of AIDS Notification Program (NAP)
153 Halsey Street
7th Floor P.O. Box 47007
Newark, NJ 07101
Telephone: (201)-414-4428
Contact Tracing, Prevention of Spread of HIV, Field Investigations

Statewide Services

A.D.D.P AIDS Drug Distribution Program
CN 722
Trenton, NJ 08625-0722
Telephone: (609)-588-7038 Fax: (609)-588-7037
Contact: Cheryl Mills
Accepts Applications for Retrovir, Pentamadine and Interferon

Aid for AIDS Sake Fund, The Episcopal Diocese of New Jersey
c/o 246 Pearl Street
Trenton, NJ 08618
Telephone: (609)-392-1368
Provides NJ PWAs with $100 Grant for Emergency Non-Medical Use

American Lung Association of Mid-New Jersey
P.O. Box 2006
29 Emmons Drive
Princeton, NJ 08543-2006
Telephone: (908)-452-2112
Contact: Elaine Fisher - Executive Director
Information and Referrals

New Jersey Dept. of Public Advocate
Hughes Justice Complex
25 Market Street, CN-850
Trenton, NJ 08625
Telephone: (609)-292-7087
Legal Class Actions, Public Advocacy and Mental Health Advocacy

New Jersey Dept. of Public Advocate
Hughes Justice Complex
25 Market Street, CN-850
Trenton, NJ 08625
Telephone: (800)-792-8600
Contact: Zulima Farber
Mental health advocacy

New Jersey Dept. of Public Advocate, Law Guardian
210 S. Broad Street
4th Floor, CN 850
Trenton, NJ 08625-2402
Telephone: (609)-292-0220
Advocacy Unit, Legal representation for children

New Jersey Division on Civil Rights
383 West State Street
Trenton, NJ 08625-1809
Telephone: (609)-292-4605
Accepts Complaints about Discrimination

New Jersey State Medicaid District Office
10 Park Place, Room 430
Morristown, NJ 07960-7111
Telephone: (201)-267-1700
Contact: Marie Grubin - Director
Medicaid

New Jersey State Medicaid District Office
153 Halsey Street
4th Floor
Newark, NJ 07101
Telephone: (201)-648-2470
Medicaid

New Jersey State Medicaid District Office
25 S. Main St.
Edison, NJ 08837-3448
Telephone: (909)-603-3151
Medicaid

NJ Department of Community Affairs, Office of Legal Services
101 S. Broad Street
WM-Ashby Building
Trenton, NJ 08625-2401
Telephone: (609)-292-6392
Information on Free Legal Aid

NJ Dept of Insurance, Div of Enforcement & Consumer Protection.
Life and Health Division
CN-329
Trenton, NJ 08625
Telephone: (609)-292-8863
Questions and Complaints about Insurance Coverage, Cancellations, Denials

NJ Dept of Labor, Div of Unemployment & Disability Insurance
Disability Insurance Serv
CN 387
Trenton, NJ 08625-0387
Telephone: (609)-292-2680
Contact: William Schwartz - Assistant Director
Temporary Disability Benefits

NJ Dept. of Health, Division of AIDS, Partner Notification Program
Southern Regional Office
Trenton, NJ
Telephone: (609)-984-6125
Contact: Mike Shumsky
Contact Tracing, Prevention of the Spread of HIV, Field Investigations

NJ Public Advocate, Advocacy for Developmentally Disabled
Hughes Justice Complex
CN 850
Trenton, NJ 08625
Telephone: (609)-292-9742
Legal Resources, General AIDS Discrimination Issues

Atlantic County

Community Services

American Red Cross
850 North Franklin Avenue
Pleasantville, NJ 08232-1446
Telephone: (609)-646-2010 Fax: (609)-646-7004
Contact: Carol Harney
Literature and programs, training

South Jersey AIDS Alliance
1301 Atlantic Avenue
Atlantic City, NJ 08401
Telephone: (609)-348-2437 Fax: (609)-348-8775
Contact: William Mattle; Ira Shaffer - Executive Director
Testing, food bank, case management, outreach, transportation andpharmaceutical assistance, non-medical emergency funding

County Health Depts

Atlantic County Health Department
201 South Shore Road
Northfield, NJ 08225-2370
Telephone: (609)-645-7700 Fax: (609)-645-5931
Contact: Ingrid Hickman - Manager; Nancy Park - Manager
AIDS Community Care Assistance Program, Special Child Health Services

Home Health Care

Homedco Infusion
Rural Delivery 3, Box 2
Fire Road
Pleasantville, NJ 08232
Telephone: (609)-641-8000
Nationwide experience inproviding home infusion therapy to AIDS patients

Shore Care, Shore Memorial Hospital
P.O. Box 150
Somers Point, NJ 08244
Telephone: (609)-646-1776
Contact: Joseph Aiello
Home health care agency

Medical Services

Atlantic City Medical Center, Clinic
19 S. Ohio Avenue
Atlantic City, NJ 08401-6720
Telephone: (609)-441-2104
Contact: Roberta Connors
Women's Services, Education, Testing and Counseling by Appointment for Clients

Atlantic City Medical Center, Clinic
Amubulatory Care Center
16 S. Ohio Avenue 2nd Floor
Pomona, NJ 08401
Telephone: (609)-441-2104 Fax: (609)-441-2140
Contact: Rita Purdy
Women's Services, Education, Testing and Counseling by appointment, HIV treatment and care

Testing Sites

Atlantic City Health Department
1325 Baltic Avenue
Atlantic City, NJ 08401-4516
Telephone: (609)-347-6456
HIV testing & counseling

Atlantic City Medical Center
16 South Ohio Avenue
Atlantic City, NJ 08401
Telephone: (609)-344-4081
Contact: Catherine Forrester
HIV testing, counseling, medical care

Sencit-Baltic Family Practice Center
1325 Baltic Avenue
Atlantic City, NJ 08401-4516
Telephone: (609)-347-6456 Fax: (609)-347-5662
Free HIV Testing/Counseling Site

Bergen County

Community Services

American Cancer Society
20 Mercer Street
Hackensack, NJ 07601-5600
Telephone: (201)-343-2222 Fax: (201)-343-1839
Free Transportation for Kaposi's Sarcoma Patients to Med. Treatment in County

American Lung Association of NJ, Northern Regional Office
14-25 Plaza Road
Fair Lawn, NJ 07410
Telephone: (201)-791-6600 Fax: (201)-791-2939
Contact: Melissa Zanjini
Information and Referrals

Bergen County Board of Social Services
216 Route 17 North
Rochelle Pk, NJ 07662-3300
Telephone: (201)-368-4355
Contact: Edward Testa
Food stamp program, social services

Bergen County Board of Social Services
216 Route 17 North
Rochelle Pk, NJ 07662-3300
Telephone: (201)-368-4200 Fax: (201)-368-8721
Aid for dependent children, adult protective services

Bergen County Community Action Program
214 State Street
Hackensack, NJ 07601-5500
Telephone: (201)-488-5100 Fax: (201)-488-4533
Contact: Robert Hagson
Food services, shelter

Community Action Program
21 East Kansas Street
Hackensack, NJ 07601
Telephone: (800)-624-1489
Contact: Dr. Lillian Ramos
Shelter; drug & alcohol counseling

Family Services of Bergen County
10 Banta Place
Hackensack, NJ 07601-5680
Telephone: (201)-342-9200 Fax: (201)-342-2075
Contact: Natalie Webb
Counseling; HIV & AIDS; patients & family

New Jersey Buddies
P.O. Box 413
Teaneck, NJ 07666-0413
Telephone: (201)-837-8125
Buddies, Education, Advocacy, Financial Aid, Referrals, Support Group, Speakers

Office of Special Transportation
70 Zabriskie Street
Hackensack, NJ 07601-6820
Telephone: (201)-646-3227 Fax: (201)-343-2512
Contact: Margaret Cook
Transportation, medical, HIV & AIDS patients

County Health Depts

Bergen County Health Department
327 Ridgewood Avenue
Paramus, NJ 07652-4899
Telephone: (201)-599-6100 Fax: (201)-986-1068
Contact: Nancy Mc Glade
Confidential and Anonymous HIV Testing, Counseling, Partner Notification

Home Health Care

Hackensack Medical Center Hospice
385 Prospect Avenue
Hackensack, NJ 07601-2570
Telephone: (201)-342-7766 Fax: (201)-342-8104
Contact: Maryann Collins
Hospice Care

Home Care America
131 Main Street
Suite 180
Hackensack, NJ 07601-7140
Telephone: (201)-488-6151 Fax: (201)-488-6165
Contact: JoAnn Marshall - Norell Health Care
Home Health Care

Valley Homecare Inc.
505 Goffle Road
Ridgewood, NJ 07450
Telephone: (201)-444-0040 Fax: (201)-444-1304
Contact: Kathy Kirn; Joan Shafer - Project Outreach
AIDS Community Care Assistance Program Case Management Site, Home Health Care

Medical Services

Englewood Hospital
350 Engle Street
Englewood, NJ 07631-1898
Telephone: (201)-894-3000
Contact: Pat Bain, RN - Infection Control
Medical Services

Hackensack Medical Center
30 Prospect Avenue
Hackensack, NJ 07601-1991
Telephone: (201)-996-2065 Fax: (201)-996-2169
Contact: Mary Ann Michelis - Director of Special Immunology
Medical Services

Hackensack Medical Center Dental Clinic
30 Prospect Avenue
Hackensack, NJ 07601-1991
Telephone: (201)-996-2111
Contact: Dr. Kevin Heaney - Director
Dental Services

Burlington County

Community Services

Burlington Comprehensive Counseling, Inc.
75 Washington Street
Mount Holly, NJ 08060
Telephone: (609)-267-9553
Substance Abuse Outpatient Services: Maintenance, Detox, Drug Free; Counseling

County Board of Social Services
795 Woodlane Road
Mount Holly, NJ 08060
Telephone: (609)-267-7757
Contact: James Suszynski
Social Services

Department of Military and Veterans Affairs
50 Rancocas Rd.
Mount Holly, NJ 08060-1349
Telephone: (609)-871-1900
Contact: David Waltner
Veteran's Services

Home Health Care

Caremark
525 Fellowship Road
Ste 355
Mount Laurel, NJ 08054
Telephone: (609)-235-3332 Fax: (609)-235-6044
Toll-Free: (800)-628-2477
Contact: Kerry Levy - Pharmacy Manager
Clinical Support and Infusion Therapy: Nutrition, Antimicrobials, enteral

Caremark Connection Network
525 Fellowship Road
Route 355
Mount Laurel, NJ 08054
Telephone: (609)-625-1600
Contact: Craig Gardenerr - Nurse Manager
Clinical Support and Infusion Therapy: Nutrition, Antimicrobials, Chemo.,Hematopoeti

Community Nursing Services
Raphael Meadow Health Ctr
P.O. Box 287, Woodlane Rd
Mount Holly, NJ 08060
Telephone: (609)-267-1950 Fax: (609)-261-4974
Toll-Free: (800)-232-0165
Contact: Sharon Goodman
HIV counseling & testing, case management

Moorestown Visiting Nurse Association
907 Pleasant Valley Avenue
Mount Laurel, NJ 08054
Telephone: (609)-235-0462 Fax: (609)-235-0349
Contact: Maryann Flatley
Home Care, Case Mgmt., Home Health Aide, Homemaker/Companion, InfusionTherapies

Moorestown Visiting Nurse Association
907 Pleasant Valley Avenue
Mount Laurel, NJ 08054
Telephone: (609)-235-0221
Contact: Terri Milner, RN - Intake Nurse
Case Management, Home Health Aides, Homemaker/Companions, Various Therapies

Samaritan Hospice
214 West 2nd Street
Moorestown, NJ 08057
Telephone: (609)-778-8181 Fax: (609)-778-0237
Contact: Evelyn McNamara - Assist Director
Hospice Care. Including Burlington, Mercer & Gloucester

Samaritan Hospice
214 West 2nd Street
Moorestown, NJ 08057-2372
Telephone: (609)-778-8181 Fax: (609)-778-0237
Toll-Free: (800)-229-8183
Contact: Clark Dingman - Director
Hospice Care

Medical Services

Brachfield Medical Associates, Rancocas Valley Hospital
Division of Graduate Health Systems
218 C Sunset Road
Willingboro, NJ 08046
Telephone: (609)-877-0400 Fax: (609)-877-1682
Contact: Roy Levinson - MD
Medical Services

Memorial Hospital of Burlington County
175 Madison Avenue
Mount Holly, NJ 08060-2099
Telephone: (609)-267-0700 Fax: (609)-265-8362
Contact: Chester Kaletkowski - President
Medical services

Rancocas Valley Hospital, Div. of Graduate Health Systems
218 A. Sunset Road
Willingboro, NJ 08046-1162
Telephone: (609)-835-3042 Fax: (609)-835-5441
Contact: Patricia A. Douglas
Counseling, Discharge Planning, Education, Inpatient Care, Therapy

Camden County

Community Services

Hispanic Family Center
'La Esperanza'
425 Broadway
Camden, NJ 08103
Telephone: (609)-541-6985 Fax: (609)-963-2663
Contact: Mario Gonzales
Hispanic Substance Abuse Organiz.; Outpatient: Drug Free; Education, Referrals

Mental Health Association of Southwestern New Jersey
505 Cooper Street
Camden, NJ 08102-1210
Telephone: (609)-966-6767
Counseling, Education, Information, Library, Referrals

New Jersey State Medicaid District Office
101 Haddon Ave. #9
Camden, NJ 08103-1477
Telephone: (609)-757-2870 Fax: (609)-757-4626
Contact: Daniel Cooperson
Medicaid

Our Lady of Lourdes Medical Center
1600 Haddon Avenue
Camden, NJ 08103-3117
Telephone: (609)-757-3853
Contact: Donna Gaber
Medical Services, Education, Inpatient and Outpatient Care, Referrals, Testing

Volunteers of America
235 White Horse Pike, 2nd Floor
Collingswood, NJ 08107
Telephone: (609)-757-7285
Shelter for Adult Males

County Health Depts

Camden County Health Department
1800 Pavilion West
2101 Ferry Avenue, Rm 219
Camden, NJ 08104
Telephone: (609)-757-8606 Fax: (609)-757-8737
Contact: Sharon O'Leary - Coordinator
Free Confidential and Anonymous HIV Testing, Counseling, Partner Notification

Camden County Health Department
2101 Ferry Avenue
Room 219
Camden, NJ 08104
Telephone: (609)-757-8606
Free Confidential and Anonymous HIV Testing, Counseling, Partner Notification

Gloucester County Health Department
160 Fries Mill Road
Turnersville, NJ 08012
Telephone: (609)-374-4100 Fax: (609)-629-0469
Contact: Lawrence Devlin - Director
Women's Services: Education

Gloucester County Health Department, Testing Site
160 Fries Mill Road
Turnersville, NJ 08012
Telephone: (609)-374-4100
Free Anonymous and Confidential HIV Testing, Counseling, Partner Notification

Home Health Care

Camden County Board of Social Services
745 Market Street
Camden, NJ 08102-1161
Telephone: (609)-757-8249 Fax: (609)-757-4552
Contact: Marlene McIntyre
Case management, assistance for home care, food stamps, SSI; referrals & treatment assessment programs

Cherry Hill Supportive Care, Inc.
383 North Kings Highway
Suite 213
Cherry Hill, NJ 08034
Telephone: (609)-482-6630
Home Health Care

Curaflex Infusion Services
729 Hylton Road
Pennsauken, NJ 08110-1332
Telephone: (609)-662-3110 Fax: (609)-662-2422
Toll-Free: (800)-825-8493
Contact: Sharrod Madison - Center Manager
Home IV therapy: TPN, Enteral, IV Antibiotics, Aerosolized/IV Pentamidine

Jewish Family and Children Services
100 Park Boulevard
Cherry Hill, NJ 08002-3481
Telephone: (609)-662-8611
Contact: Lisa Field
Counseling, emergency homemaker health aides, community chaplain, special friends, support groups for family & friends, speakers

Olsten Kimberly Quality Care
1909 Route 70 East
3rd Floor
Cherry Hill, NJ 08003-4511
Telephone: (609)-424-6524

Contact: Marie Margot
Home Health Care

Olsten Kimberly Quality Home Care
35 Kings Highway
Suite 203
Haddonfield, NJ 08033
Telephone: (609)-795-7070 Fax: (609)-795-6220
Home health care, hospice

Southern New Jersey Visiting Nurse Service System, Inc.
P.O. Box 250
Runnemede, NJ 08078-0250
Telephone: (609)-845-0460
Contact: Maryann Czoch
AIDS community care assistance program case management site; infusiontherapy

Visiting Nurse and Health Association of Camden County
2201 Route 38 #500
Cherry Hill, NJ 08002-4309
Telephone: (609)-321-0200 Fax: (603)-321-0022
AIDS Community Care Assistance Program, Case Management, Home Health Care

Medical Services

Alcove West Jersey Hospital
1000 Atlantic Avenue
Camden, NJ 08104
Telephone: (609)-342-4505 Fax: (609)-342-4002
Contact: Patricia Saldick - Director
Substance Abuse Inpatient: Detox, 21-day Rehab; Outpatient: Aftercare, Therapy

East Camden Health Center
2631 Federal Street
Camden, NJ 08105-1991
Telephone: (609)-757-0470
TB chest clinic, STD/HIV counseling & testing

J.F. Kennedy Hospital, Washington Township Division
Huffville & Cross Keys Rd
Turnersville, NJ 08012
Telephone: (609)-582-2500
HIV Testing under Doctor's order, Fee Charged

Kennedy Memorial Hospitals, University Medical Center
Chapel Avenue and
Cooper Landing Road
Cherry Hill, NJ 08002
Telephone: (609)-488-6126
Contact: Karen Hickey
Medical Services, Education, Inpatient and Outpatient Care, Referrals, Testing

Kennedy Prenatal Care Center
2 Regulus Drive, Suite A
Turnersville, NJ 08012-2456
Telephone: (609)-589-6168
Contact: Maryanne Mancini
Community Care Assistance Prog., Special Child Health Services, Case Management

North Camden Health Center
801 State Street
Camden, NJ 08102
Telephone: (609)-541-2255
Contact: Dr. Krachman
Women's Services, Clinic, Education

St. Luke's Catholic Medical Services
511 State Street
Camden, NJ 08102-1918
Telephone: (609)-365-4642
Medical Services

Substance Abuse Center of South Jersey
417 Broadway
Camden, NJ 08103
Telephone: (609)-757-9190 Fax: (609)-338-1892
Contact: Roxanne Fletcher - Coordinator
Substance Abuse Outpatient Services: Maintenance, Detox, Drug Free

Substance Abuse Center of South Jersey
417 Broadway
Camden, NJ 08103-1200
Telephone: (609)-757-9190 Fax: (609)-338-1892
Substance Abuse Outpatient Services: Maintenance, Detox, Drug Free

Cape May County

County Health Depts

Cape May County Department of Health & Visiting Nurse Svc.
6 Moore Road
CM Court House, NJ 08210
Telephone: (609)-465-7911 Fax: (609)-465-6564
Contact: Suzanne Towey - Visiting Nurse Service
Community Care Assistance Program, Child Health Services, Home Health Care

Cumberland County

Community Services

Family Planning
6 South Laurel Street
Bridgeton, NJ 08302-1945
Telephone: (609)-451-3339 Fax: (609)-453-0056
Contact: Kimberly McKown'Strait
Task Force; Women's Services: Education

County Health Depts

City of Vineland Dept. of Health, Community Nursing Services
111 North 6th Street
Vineland, NJ 08360
Telephone: (609)-794-4261
Contact: Diane McDaniels
Case management site for home-care expansion, referrals.

Essex County

Community Services

AIDS Resource Foundation for Children
182 Roseville Avenue
Newark, NJ 07107-1619
Telephone: (201)-483-4250 Fax: (201)-483-1998
Contact: Terrence P. Zealand - Executive Director
Fundraising, Family Support Services, Foster Care Facility

AIDS Resource Foundation for Children
182 Roseville Avenue
Newark, NJ 07107
Telephone: (201)-483-4250 Fax: (201)-483-1998
Pediatric Group Homes, Foster Placement & Training, Support Group

American Red Cross
219 Ridgewood Avenue
Glen Ridge, NJ 07028
Telephone: (201)-748-5433
Contact: Carolyn Smith
Education, Literature, Programs

American Rescue Workers
82-84 Magazine Street
Newark, NJ 07105
Telephone: (201)-589-5772
Contact: George Gossett
Shelter, food, clothing

Apostle House
16-24 Grant Street
Newark, NJ 07104-3708
Telephone: (201)-482-0625 Fax: (201)-483-4106
Contact: Sandy Accomande
Transitional housing, referrals for HIV patients

Community Mental Health Center, UMDNJ
Extended Care Unit Outpatient
215 South Orange Avenue
Newark, NJ 07102-2700
Telephone: (201)-983-5430 Fax: (201)-982-6594
Contact: Dr. Lintott
AIDS/HIV counseling

Community United for the Rehabilitation of the Addicted
35 Lincoln Park
P.O. Box 180
Newark, NJ 07101-0180
Telephone: (201)-622-3570 Fax: (201)-621-8330
Contact: Alvaro Vargas
Counseling, Education, Outreach, Publication Dissemination

Essex Soul House
P.O. Box 3278
178 Prince Street
Newark, NJ 07103-0278
Telephone: (201)-643-3888
Toll-Free: (800)-540-7685
Contact: Shirley Coles
Educational services, counseling.

Essex-Newark Legal Services
439 Main Street
Orange, NJ 07050
Telephone: (201)-672-3838 Fax: (201)-678-8241
Contact: Nancy Ahmed
Legal services

Goodwill Home and Mission, Inc.
79 University Avenue
Newark, NJ 07102-2197
Telephone: (201)-621-9560 Fax: (201)-621-1924
Contact: Kent Thomas
Shelter

Missionaries of Charity
60 J Street
Newark, NJ 07103-3234
Telephone: (201)-481-9056
Contact: Sister Ann Francis
Shelter for women, soup kitchen

Newark Community Project for People with AIDS
International Youth Org.
P.O. Box 1241
Newark, NJ 07114
Telephone: (201)-824-5900
Contact: Derek Winans
Fund-raising organization, recruits volunteers, some financial assistance

Newark Emergency Services for Families
303 Washington Street
Newark, NJ 07102-2795
Telephone: (201)-596-6801 Fax: (201)-624-3024
Contact: James Keith
Shelter for Families

Planned Parenthood of Essex County
151 Washington Street
Newark, NJ 07102-3099
Telephone: (201)-622-3900 Fax: (201)-242-3609
Contact: Blanche Duke
Women's Services: Education, HIV Testing, Counseling

County Health Depts

Essex County Department of Health and Rehabilitation
160 Fairview Avenue
Building 37
Cedar Grove, NJ 07009-1399
Telephone: (201)-857-4663 Fax: (201)-857-5163
Contact: Carol Mendalski
Special child health services, case management

Home Health Care

Caring Touch
470 Prospect Avenue
Suite 200
West Orange, NJ 07052
Telephone: (201)-675-6565
Home Health Care

Curaflex Infusion Services
70 New Dutch Lane
Fairfield, NJ 07004
Telephone: (201)-227-0222 Fax: (201)-227-0064
Contact: June Mayer
Home Infusion Therapy

Patient Care Medical Service
59 Main Street
West Orange, NJ 07052-5393
Telephone: (201)-325-3330
Contact: Lucille Richards
Home Health Care

Visiting Nurse Assn of Essex Valley
33 Evergreen Place
East Orange, NJ 07018
Telephone: (201)-414-6743 Fax: (201)-673-0168
Contact: Dorothy Scull - Vice President/Program Develop
AIDS Community Care Assistance Program, Case Management Site, Home Health Care

Medical Services

City of East Orange Substance Abuse Program
160 Halsted Street
East Orange, NJ 07018-2663
Telephone: (201)-266-5200
Contact: Debra Nagler
Substance Abuse; Outpatient: Drug Free/Methadone Maintenance

Dept. of Veterans Affairs Medical Center
37 Central Avenue
Newark, NJ 07102-1920
Telephone: (201)-645-2420 Fax: (201)-643-3032
Contact: Catherine Gilhooley - Assistant Chief
Substance Abuse; Outpatient: Maintenance, Drug Free; methadone maintenanceprogram

Family Service and Child Guidance Center
395 South Center Street
Orange, NJ 07050
Telephone: (201)-675-3817 Fax: (201)-673-5782
Contact: Trina Lewin - Director
Substance Abuse; Outpatient: Drug Free, Detox

Integrity, Inc.
103 Lincoln Park
Newark, NJ 07102-2314
Telephone: (201)-623-0600
Contact: Pat Moses - Coordinator
Substance Abuse; Outpatient and Residential: Drug Free, 24 Hours, 7 Days

The Irvington Bridge
54 Mt. Vernon Avenue
Irvington, NJ 07111-3055
Telephone: (201)-372-2624
Contact: Ellen Heerwig - Site Manager
Substance Abuse; Outpatient: Drug Free

Jersey GYN/North Jersey
22 Ball Street, Suite 100
Irvington, NJ 07111-3521
Telephone: (201)-373-2600
Women's Services

L & L Clinics
57-59 New Street
Irvington, NJ 07111
Telephone: (201)-373-2010 Fax: (201)-373-2205
Contact: Ronald La Morgese - Director
Substance Abuse; Outpatient: Maintenance, Detox, Drug Free

NEDAC--Community Counseling Center
104 Bloomfield Avenue
Montclair, NJ 07042-4723
Telephone: (201)-783-6322 Fax: (201)-783-1658
Contact: Michael Trabucco - Coordinator
Substance Abuse; Outpatient: Drug Free

Newark Beth Israel Medical Center
201 Lyons Avenue
Newark, NJ 07112-2027
Telephone: (201)-926-7328 Fax: (201)-926-6452
Contact: Jeremlas Murillo - MD
Medical Services, HIV Testing, Counseling

Newark Renaissance House, Inc.
P.O.Box 7057
80 Norfolk Street
Newark, NJ 07103-0057
Telephone: (201)-623-3386
Contact: Sylvia Black - Director
Substance Abuse; Residential: Drug Free, 24 Hours, 7 Days

Orange Drug & Alcohol Abuse Program
301 Main Street
Orange, NJ 07050
Telephone: (201)-266-4173
Contact: Nora Williams - Coordinator
Substance Abuse; Outpatient: Drug Free

Spectrum Health Care
461 Frelinghuysen Avenue
Newark, NJ 07114-1426
Telephone: (201)-596-2850 Fax: (201)-596-8180
Contact: Karen Kania - Clinic Supervisor
Substance Abuse; Outpatient: Maintenance, Detox, Drug Free

The Bridge
14 Park Avenue
Caldwell, NJ 07006-4902
Telephone: (201)-228-3000
Substance treatment; Outpatient: counseling for families & HIVpatients

United Hospitals Medical Center, Family Planning
15 South Ninth Street
Newark, NJ 07017
Telephone: (201)-268-8180 Fax: (201)-485-7769
Contact: Mary Boland - Director
HIV positive program for women, social worker

Univ. of Medicine and Dentistry of NJ Dental School-Special Dentistry
Martland Building, GB 138
65 Bergen Street
Newark, NJ 07103
Telephone: (201)-982-6613
Contact: Dr. David Sirois - Director
Special Services Dental Clinic by Referral

University Hospital, Department of Pediatrics
Med. Sciences Bldg F-570A
185 South Orange Avenue
Newark, NJ 07103
Telephone: (201)-982-5066 Fax: (201)-982-6443
Contact: James Oleske, MD - Div of Infectious Disease
Medical Services for Children

University of Medicine & Dentistry of NJ, Univ. Hosp. Family
Martland Bldg., G-A Level
65 Bergen Street
Newark, NJ 07107
Telephone: (301)-982-6350 Fax: (201)-982-6378
Contact: Marilyn Torre - Administrator
Women's Services: Education, Medical Services, HIV Testing by Request

University of Medicine and Dentistry of NJ Medical School
University Hospital
100 Bergen Street
Newark, NJ 07103
Telephone: (201)-456-6000 Fax: (201)-982-6943
Contact: Dr. Eric Munoz - MD; Patricia Kloser, MD - Rm H-240; Phone 456-7188; Robert Palinkas, MD - CHAP, Rm I-248, 456-6061
Medical Services; Other Doctors: J. Oleske, D. Lourta, R. Pallukus, S. Sathe

West Orange Family Youth Service
4 Charles Street
West Orange, NJ 07052
Telephone: (201)-325-4141 Fax: (201)-325-5126
Contact: Debra Matrick - Director
Substance abuse; outpatient: drug free, family service programs

Testing Sites

East Orange Health Department
143 New Street
East Orange, NJ 07017-4110
Telephone: (201)-266-5454
Contact: Arlene Luster

Free Confidential and Anonymous HIV Testing, Counseling, Partner Notification

Newark Municipal Council Task Force-Eligible Met. Area
920 Broad Street
Newark, NJ 07102-2609
Telephone: (201)-733-6427
Contact: Bobi Ruffin
Confidential testing and counseling

St. Michael's Medical Center, Infectious Disease Department
306 M.L King Boulevard
Newark, NJ 07102
Telephone: (201)-877-5649 Fax: (201)-877-2823
Contact: Israel Lamboy
HIV Testing, Counseling

Gloucester County

Community Services

C.A.T.A. Farmworkers Support Committee
P.O. Box F
4 South Delsea Drive
Glassboro, NJ 08028-0458
Telephone: (609)-757-9190
Contact: Tom Silva
Information on HIV testing, educational materials

Home Health Care

Homedco Infusion
301 Hollydell Drive
Sewell, NJ 08080-9196
Telephone: (609)-589-1616
Contact: Cathy Curley
Nationwide experience in providing home infusion therapy to AIDS patients

Medical Services

Reality House, Inc., Mellish Center
490 Black Horse Pike
Williamstown, NJ 08094
Telephone: (609)-728-0404 Fax: (609)-728-5384
Contact: Anthony Comito - Executive Director
Program for children with AIDS & their families

SODAT, Inc.
124 North Broad Street
Woodbury, NJ 08096-1700
Telephone: (609)-845-6363 Fax: (609)-848-3022
Contact: Jeffrey Clayton - Executive Director
Substance Abuse; Outpatient: Drug Free

Wenonah Medical Association
107 East Mantua Avenue
Wenonah, NJ 08090-1999
Telephone: (609)-468-6868 Fax: (609)-464-1855
Contact: Churchill L. Blakely - President
Medical Services

Hudson County

Community Services

Bayonne Economic Opportunity Foundation and Family Planning
555 Kennedy Boulevard
Bayonne, NJ 07002-2627
Telephone: (201)-437-7222 Fax: (201)-437-2810
Contact: Anne Mahan
Food; Women's Services: Education, HIV Testing, Counseling

Catholic Community Services, St. Lucy's Shelter
619 Grove Street
Jersey City, NJ 07302-1237
Telephone: (201)-656-7201 Fax: (201)-656-0412
Contact: Christopher Doscano
Shelter for Adult Males and Females

Hyacinth AIDS Foundation
83 Wayne Street
Jersey City, NJ 07302
Telephone: (201)-944-0346
Toll-Free: (800)-533-0204
Contact: Anthony Salandra - Project Director
Counseling, referrals, support groups

North Hudson Community Action Corp.
507 26th Street
Union City, NJ 07087-3798
Telephone: (201)-866-2255 Fax: (201)-330-3803
Women's Services: Education, HIV Testing, Counseling, Food, Shelter

North Hudson Community Action Corp.
5918 Bergenline Avenue
West New York, NJ 07093-1316
Telephone: (201)-868-8920 Fax: (201)-868-5518
Women's Services: Education, HIV Testing, Counseling, Food, Shelter

Home Health Care

Olston Kimberly Quality Care
601 Pavonia
3rd Floor
Jersey City, NJ 07306
Telephone: (201)-798-1600 Fax: (201)-659-2692
Contact: Xenia Flores
Home Health Care, IV therapy

Medical Services

Intercounty Council on Drug and Alcohol Abuse
416 Kearny Avenue
Kearny, NJ 07032
Telephone: (201)-997-4000
Contact: Harry Bachler - Director
Substance Abuse Services: Outpatient maintenance, detox, alcoholcounseling, outpatient, drug free counseling, juvenile counseling

Jersey City Medical Center, Dental Services
50 Baldwin Avenue
Jersey City, NJ 07304-3154
Telephone: (201)-915-2265
Contact: Dr. Arthur Aria - Director
Dental Services; oral & naturalization surgery

Jersey City Medical Center, Department of Medicine
50 Baldwin Avenue
Jersey City, NJ 07304
Telephone: (201)-915-2433 Fax: (201)-915-2002
Contact: Allen Lin Greenberg - Chief of Infectious Diseases
Medical Services

Testing Sites

Jersey City Medical Center
114 Clifton Place
11th Floor
Jersey City, NJ 07304-3154
Telephone: (201)-451-2607 Fax: (201)-915-2002
Contact: Nora Holmquist - Coordinator
HIV counseling & testing, medical services, support groups

Hunterdon County

Community Services

County Board of Social Services, Community Service Center
6 Gauntt Place
Flemington, NJ 08822-9056
Telephone: (908)-788-1300
Social Services

Planned Parenthood of Flemington
14 Court Street
Flemington, NJ 08822
Telephone: (908)-782-7727
Women's services: education; referrals

County Health Depts

Department of Health of Hunterdon County, AIDS Task Force
71 Main Street
Administration Building
Flemington, NJ 08822
Telephone: (908)-788-1351 Fax: (908)-806-4739
Contact: Julie Newman
Task force on AIDS, testing

Medical Services

Hunterdon Drug Awareness Program
8 Main Street, Suite 7
Flemington, NJ 08822-1468
Telephone: (908)-788-1900 Fax: (908)-788-3836
Contact: Adrienne Peck - Executive Director
Substance Abuse Services: Outpatient Drug Free

Hunterdon Medical Center
2100 Wescott Drive
Flemington, NJ 08822
Telephone: (908)-788-6398 Fax: (908)-788-6370
Contact: Debra Williams-Baumann - Manager
Special Child Hlth Srvcs, Case Mgt for Children, AIDS Comm. Care

Mercer County

Community Services

American Cancer Society
3076 Princeton Pike
Lawrenceville, NJ 08648-2304
Telephone: (609)-394-5000
Contact: Kathy Elberson - Patient Service Director
Free Transportation for Kaposi's Sarcoma Patients to Med. Treatment in County

Mercer County Special Services, Project Child
1068 Old Trenton Road
Trenton, NJ 08690
Telephone: (609)-588-8501 Fax: (609)-588-8411
Special Child Health Services, Case Management for Children

United Progress Emergency Shelter
541 East State Street
Trenton, NJ 08609-1101
Telephone: (609)-392-5815
Shelter for families

Home Health Care

Caremark Connection Network.
525 Fellowship Road
Mount Laurel, NJ 08619
Telephone: (609)-890-2000
Contact: Office Management
CLINICAL SUPPORT AND INFUSION THERAPY: Nutrition, Antimicrobials, Chemo., Hematopoeti

Friends Adult Service
1550 Edgewood Avenue
Trenton, NJ 08618
Telephone: (609)-394-3232
Home Health Care, Companions, Homemakers, Medical Daycare

Friends Home Health Care
223 North Hermitage Ave.
Trenton, NJ 08618-5511
Telephone: (609)-396-1507 Fax: (609)-989-7157
Contact: Receptionist
Home Health Care, Medicare/Medicaid Certified

Medical Services

Corner House, Township of Princeton
Valley Road Building
369 Witherspoon Street
Princeton, NJ 08540
Telephone: (609)-924-8018 Fax: (609)-497-9101
Contact: Linda Meisel - Director
Substance Abuse Services: Outpatient Drug Free

Family Guidance Center
Substance Abuse Program
Klockner Rd & Hamilton Avenue
Trenton, NJ 08619
Telephone: (609)-587-7044 Fax: (609)-587-6765
Contact: Jeff Robbins - Director
Substance Abuse Services: Outpatient Drug Free; Mental Health Services

Hightstown Planned Parenthood Association Mercer Area
268 Academy Street
Hightstown, NJ 08520-3803
Telephone: (609)-448-3439 Fax: (609)-448-8206
Contact: Sandra Gregg - Supervisor
Women's services: education, HIV counseling & testing

Planned Parenthood Association of Mercer Area
Mercerville Road
Mercerville Road; Suite #5
Trenton, NJ 08610-1407
Telephone: (609)-585-4747 Fax: (609)-585-7084
Contact: Lisa Shelby - Director of Community Services
Women's Services: HIV education, counseling & testing

Planned Parenthood Association of Mercer Area, Inc.
437 East State Street
Trenton, NJ 08608-1597
Telephone: (609)-599-3736 Fax: (609)-989-4846
Contact: Lesley Davis Potter
Women's Services: Education, Testing, Counseling

St. Francis Medical Center
601 Hamilton Avenue
Trenton, NJ 08629-1986
Telephone: (609)-599-5000 Fax: (609)-984-9088
Contact: Richard Porwancher - MD
Medical Services

Testing Sites

Henry J. Austin Health Center
321 North Warren Street
Trenton, NJ 08618-4794
Telephone: (609)-989-3335 Fax: (609)-695-3532
HIV Testing, Counseling

Middlesex County

Community Services

Hemophilia Association of New Jersey
37 West Prospect Street
East Brunswick, NJ 08816
Telephone: (908)-238-5250 Fax: (908)-238-7039
Contact: Elena Bostick
Counseling, Education, Referral, Support Groups, Alternative & Holistic Project

Presbyterian Church of New Brunswick
100 Livingston Avenue
New Brunswick, NJ 08901-2412
Telephone: (908)-545-2111
Pastoral Care

County Health Depts

Middlesex County Department of Health
51 Bayard Street
New Brunswick, NJ 08901
Telephone: (908)-745-3157
Contact: Rowena Carowick
Community Care Assistance Program, Special Child Health Services, Case Mgmt.

Middlesex County Public Health Department
841 Georges Road
North Brunswick, NJ 08902-3378
Telephone: (908)-745-4100
Contact: Teri Manes
Primary medical care, transportation, supplementary support services

Home Health Care

Robert Wood Johnson University Hospital
154 Somerset Street
New Brunswick, NJ 08901
Telephone: (908)-828-8884
Contact: Mary Henberman - Director
Home health care, visiting nurses, home health aide, physical, occupationaland speech therapy

Robert Wood Johnson University Hospital, Home Care Dept.
154 Somerset Street
New Brunswick, NJ 08901
Telephone: (908)-828-8884
Home Health Care, Special Child Health Services, Case Management for Children

Medical Services

JFK Center for Drugs and Alcohol
1152 St. George Avenue
Avenel, NJ 07001
Telephone: (908)-634-7910 Fax: (908)-855-7866
Contact: Carolann Kane Cavaiola
Substance Abuse Services: Outpatient Drug Free, Day Care Drug Free

New Brunswick Counseling Center
84 New Street
New Brunswick, NJ 08903-2550
Telephone: (908)-246-4025
Substance Abuse Services: Outpatient Maintenance, Detox, Drug Free

Old Bridge Regional Hospital, Div of Raritan Bay Medical Center
3 Hospital Plaza
Suite 208
Old Bridge, NJ 08857-3087
Telephone: (908)-324-5007 Fax: (908)-360-2703
Contact: John R. Middleton - MD
Medical Services

Planned Parenthood League of Middlesex County
211 Livingston Avenue
New Brunswick, NJ 08901-2931
Telephone: (908)-246-2404 Fax: (908)-246-0173
Contact: Ellen Samuel
Women's services: education, Spanish speaking, testing & referrals

Raritan Bay Mental Health Center, AIDS Project
570 Lee Street
Perth Amboy, NJ 08861-1716
Telephone: (908)-442-1666
Contact: Gladys Cardona, MSW, BCD - HIV Counselor; 908-442-6634 (messages) -
State certified HIV counseling

Rutgers University Health Services
301 Van Nest Hall
New Brunswick, NJ 08903
Telephone: (908)-932-7710
Contact: Fern Goodhart
AIDS Service Organization Limited to Students, Faculty, Staff

St. Peter's Medical Center
254 Easton Avenue
New Brunswick, NJ 08901-1780
Telephone: (908)-745-8528
Education, Pastoral Care

Strathmore Treatment Associates
1 Lower Main St
PO Box 125
South Amboy, NJ 08879
Telephone: (908)-727-2555 Fax: (908)-727-0255
Contact: Christopher Bass
Blood tests, pulmonary function tests, medicines, counseling, testing

University Hospital
1 Robert Wood Johnson Place
New Brunswick, NJ 08901-1947
Telephone: (908)-937-7713 Fax: (908)-235-7951
Contact: Robert Wood Johnson
Medical Services

University of Medicine and Dentistry Medical School
1 Robert Wood Johnson Pl.
CN 19
New Brunswick, NJ 08903-1969
Telephone: (908)-937-7708 Fax: (908)-235-7951
Contact: Ann Brennan - HIV Coord.
Medical services, counseling

Monmouth County

Community Services

Check Mate, Inc.
550 Cookman Avenue
Asbury Park, NJ 07712
Telephone: (908)-502-0011
Contact: Zelma Jones Pennington - Planner
Education, referral, outreach, mobile HIV/AIDS testing

Legal Aid Society of Monmouth County
PO Box 86
1301 Main Street
Asbury Park, NJ 07712-0086
Telephone: (908)-776-7733
Contact: George Wright
Legal Resources, Legal Aid

MCOSS Foundation, Inc.
141 Bodman Place
Redbank, NJ 07701
Telephone: (908)-747-0020
Contact: MaryAnn Vitiello-Taylor, R.N. - Supervisor
Community Care Assistance Program, Special Child Health Svcs, Case Management

Ocean-Monmouth Legal Services, Inc.
25 Broad Street
Freehold, NJ 077281993
Telephone: (908)-747-7400
Legal Resources, Legal Aid

Home Health Care

Greater Monmouth Visiting Nurse Association
111 Union Avenue
Long Branch, NJ 07740-7145
Telephone: (908)-229-0816 Fax: (908)-229-0561
Contact: Susan R. Magyar
Home Health Care

MCOSS Nursing Service, Inc.
141 Bodman Place
Red Bank, NJ 07701
Telephone: (908)-821-9500 Fax: (908)-224-0843
Contact: Theresa Beck - Director of Planning Program
AIDS Community Care Assistance Program, Case Management Site

MCOSS Nursing Services
141 Bodman Place
Red Bank, NJ 07701
Telephone: (908)-224-6894 Fax: (908)-224-0228
Contact: Maryann Vitiello-Taylor
AIDS Community Care Assistance Program, Case Management Site

Medical Services

Addiction Recovery CPC Behavior Health Care
270 Highway #35
Red Bank, NJ 07721
Telephone: (908)-842-2000 Fax: (908)-219-0474
Contact: Virginia Dickenson
Substance Abuse Services

Centra State Medical Center
West Main Street
Freehold, NJ 07728-2551
Telephone: (908)-780-6023 Fax: (908)-294-2805
Contact: Adele Reo
Mental Health Services

Central Jersey Blood Center
494 Sycamore Avenue
Shrewsbury, NJ 07702
Telephone: (908)-842-5750 Fax: (908)-842-1617
Contact: Lydia Blancato
Blood Services, Self-exclusion Program, Testing of Donated Blood

Jersey Shore Addiction Services, Inc.
1200 Memorial Drive
Asbury Park, NJ 07712-5008
Telephone: (908)-988-8877 Fax: (908)-988-2572
Contact: Edward J. Higgins
Substance abuse services, methadone clinic

Jersey Shore Medical Center
1945 Corlies Avenue
(Route 33)
Neptune, NJ 07754-4889
Telephone: (908)-775-5500 Fax: (908)-776-4619
Contact: Elliot Frank - MD
Women's services education, HIV testing, primary care, AIDS clinic

Testing Sites

Monmouth Regional Screening Center
71 Davis Avenue
Neptune, NJ 07753-4401
Telephone: (908)-775-5500
Contact: Ben Cenerino
Free Confidential and Anonymous HIV Testing, Counseling, Partner Notification

Morris County

Community Services

AIDS Center at Hope House
19-21 Belmont Avenue
P.O. Box 851
Dover, NJ 07802-0851
Telephone: (201)-361-5555
Contact: Mike David-Wilson
AIDS Service Organization; Substance Abuse Services: Outpatient Drug Free

Legal Aid Society of Morris County
P.O. Box CN900
Morristown, NJ 07963-0900
Telephone: (201)-361-9386
Legal Resources, Legal Aid

Morris County Bar Association
10 Park Place, Room 308
Morristown, NJ 07960-4700
Telephone: (201)-267-6089 Fax: (201)-605-8325
Contact: Nancy Gardner Green
Legal Resources, Lawyer Referral

Morristown Division of Health
38 Dumont Place
Morristown, NJ 07963-0914
Telephone: (201)-292-6701
Contact: Health Officer Steinberg
Support Groups

New Jersey Self Help Clearing House
St Clare-Riverside Medical Center
Pocono Road
Denville, NJ 07834
Telephone: (800)-367-6274
Support Groups

Home Health Care

HNS Med Teck
10 Bloomfield Avenue
Pinebrook, NJ 07058
Telephone: (201)-227-5623 Fax: (201)-227-0511
Contact: Mike Nestico
Home Infusion Therapy, In-home Nursing and Attendant Care, PhysicalTherapy Services, Pentamidine

Morris Home Care Nursing Alternatives
58 Maple Avenue
Morristown, NJ 07960-5218
Telephone: (201)-540-9000 Fax: (201)-540-8816
Toll-Free: (800)-371-8890
Contact: Carole Hires - Owner
Certified home health care

nmc HOMECARE
23 Vreeland Road
Florham Park, NJ 07932
Telephone: (201)-301-0089
Fax: (201)-301-0299
Contact: Eric Zwick
National JCAHO-Accredited company providing a full range of Infusion and Respiratory therapies and specializing in the care of HIV/AIDS patients. National Case Manager is also available at 800-445-1188

Visiting Nurse Association of Morris County, Inc.
38 Elm Street
Morristown, NJ 07960-4192
Telephone: (201)-539-1216 Fax: (201)-539-8371
Contact: Susan David
Community Care Assistance Program, Special Child Health Services, CaseManagement

Ocean County

Home Health Care

Homedco Infusion
170 Oberlin Avenue North
Lakewood, NJ 08701
Telephone: (908)-905-1400 Fax: (908)-905-3313
Toll-Free: (800)-628-6400
Contact: Carole Meier - Manager
Home care services to AIDS patients: beds, respitory equipment, infusiontherapy, etc.

Passaic County

Community Services

New Jersey Division on Civil Rights
100 Hamilton Plaza
Room 800
Paterson, NJ 07505
Telephone: (201)-977-4500
Accepts Complaints about Discrimination

Home Health Care

Caremark Connection Network
11 H Commerce Way
Totowa, NJ 07512
Telephone: (201)-812-9100 Fax: (201)-812-9110
Contact: Candido Barreto - Operations Manager
CLINICAL SUPPORT AND INFUSION THERAPY: Nutrition, Antimicrobials, Chemo., Hematopoeti, mursing, delivery of pharmaceuticals, case management

Caremark Health Care Services
11 H Commerce Way
Totowa, NJ 07512
Telephone: (800)-524-0319
Contact: Richard Epstein - Pharmacy/Ops Manager
Clinical Support & Infusion Therapy: nutrition, antimicrobials, chemo.,Hematopoeti

Critical Care America
60E Commerce Way
Totowa, NJ 07512
Telephone: (201)-812-9400 Fax: (201)-812-9670
Contact: Phyllis McKiernan
Coordinate & integrate all clinical & psychosocial services for HIV+

Tri-Hospital Home Health and Hospice Program
Beth Israel Hospital
70 Parker Avenue
Passaic, NJ 07055
Telephone: (201)-365-3200
Contact: Billie Jean O'Brien, RN
Home health care, hospice care, Hospice ACAP

Tri-Hospital Home Health and Hospice Program
Beth Israel Hospital
70 Parker Avenue
Passaic, NJ 07055
Telephone: (201)-365-5200
Contact: Billie Jean
Hospice Care, Home Health Care

Medical Services

Wanaque Convalescent Center
1433 Ringwood Avenue
Haskell, NJ 07420
Telephone: (201)-839-2119
Contact: Sid Schiff
Adult Skilled Nursing Care on a 24-hour Basis

Somerset County

Testing Sites

Planned Parenthood of Union County
203 Park Avenue
Plainfield, NJ 07060
Telephone: (908)-756-3736 Fax: (908)-756-3060
Contact: Mary Blatt
HIV Counseling, testing and education

Union County

Community Services

American Lung Association of New Jersey
1600 Route 22 E
Union, NJ 07083-3410
Telephone: (201)-388-4556
Contact: Robert S. Corso - Managing Director
Information and Referrals

Testing Sites

Planned Parenthood
208 Commerce Place
Elizabeth, NJ 07201-2306
Telephone: (908)-351-5384
HIV Counseling & Testing

NEW MEXICO

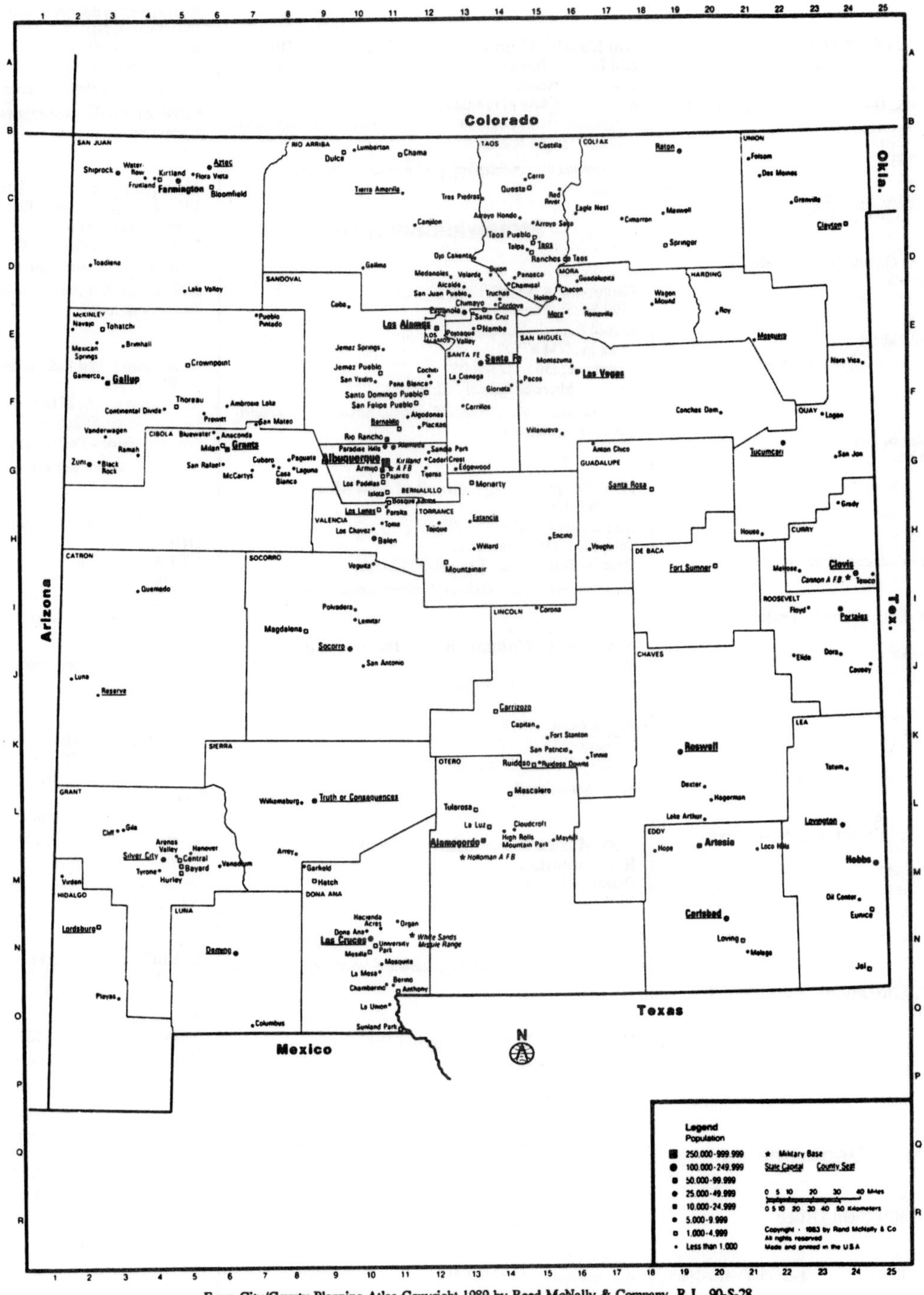

From City/County Planning Atlas Copyright 1989 by Reed McNally & Company, R.L. 90-S-28

New Mexico

General Services

Education

American Red Cross, Dona Ana County Chapter
1301 East Griggs
Las Cruces, NM 88001-2905
Telephone: (505)-526-2631
Contact: Susan Chambers
Lead chapter for AIDS/HIV education

Catholic Center - Archdiocese of Santa Fe
4000 St. Josephs Place NW
Albuquerque, NM 87120-1704
Telephone: (505)-831-8100
Contact: Sister Michelle Micek
HIV/AIDS education to elementry/high school students, distribution ofliterature

Minnick & Associates, Inc.
2403 San Mateo Blvd NE
Suite P-4
Albuquerque, NM 87110
Telephone: (505)-889-9358 Fax: (505)-889-9374
Contact: Kirk Minnick
Needs assessment & evaluations for service providers

New Mexico AIDS Education & Training Center (NMAETC)
UNM School of Medicine
HSSB 302, Box 608
Albuquerque, NM 87131-5271
Telephone: (505)-272-8207
Contact: Greg Mertz, MD - Director; Lucy Bradley-Springer, RN, PhD -
Educational training for health care givers

Planned Parenthood of Southern New Mexico
1882 S. Espina
Las Cruces, NM 88001-5479
Telephone: (505)-524-4471
Contact: Marsha Drapala
AIDS education to public, groups, schools; Counseling

UNM Area Health Education Center (AHEC)
University of New Mexico
Box 712
Albuquerque, NM 87131-0001
Telephone: (505)-277-2442
Contact: Alan Leavitt
Education program

State Health Departments

Anthony Public Health Field Office
865 North Main Street
Anthony, NM 88021-9325
Telephone: (505)-882-5858 Fax: (505)-882-3063
HIV testing & counseling

New Mexico Department of Health
Indian Health Service
P.O. Box 130
San Fidel, NM 87049-0130
Telephone: (505)-552-6634 Fax: (505)-552-7363
Acoma, Cononcito and Laguna Pueblo susbtance abuse & medical treatment,HIVtesting & education

New Mexico Department of Health HIV/AIDS Prev. & Services Bureau
1190 St. Francis Drive
P.O. Box 26110
Santa Fe, NM 87502
Telephone: (505)-827-0086
Contact: Francesca Estrada - Administrator for Bur. Chief

Rio Rancho Field Office, NM Dept. of Health
NM Dept. of Health
224-A 20th Street
Rio Rancho, NM 87124-2470
Telephone: (505)-892-0990 Fax: (505)-892-1844
Contact: Jacque Katsch
Anonymous or confidential HIV testing, counseling and referrals.

Statewide Services

Governor's AIDS Task Force
1190 So. St. Francis Drive
Harold Runnels Building
Santa Fe, NM 87502
Telephone: (505)-827-0006
Contact: Michael Samuel - Chairman
Reviews Statewide HIV/AIDS policy; advocates appropriaterecommendations.

HIV Coordinating Council of New Mexico
4200 B Silver SE
Albuquerque, NM 87108-2623
Telephone: (505)-266-0342
Contact: Bill Jordan - Executive Director
Statewide HIV/AIDS planning/referral consortium

New Mexico Commission on the Status of Women
4001 Indian School Rd. NE
Suite # 220
Albuquerque, NM 87110-3833
Telephone: (505)-841-4662
Contact: Rebecca Vigil-Giron - Director
Advocacy referral

New Mexico Department of Vocational Rehabilitation
Disability Determination Services
3301 Juan Tabo Blvd NE
Albuquerque, NM 87122
Telephone: (505)-292-6711 Fax: (505)-841-8899
Determines if individual is disabled & qualifies for Social Security

New Mexico Income Support Division
Dept. of Human Services
1096 Mechem Drive
Ruidoso, NM 88345
Telephone: (505)-258-3548 Fax: (505)-258-3910
Entitlement programs; food stamps; refferals for medical care and HIV testing.

New Mexico Nurses Association
909 Virginia NE
Suite # 101
Albuquerque, NM 87108-2578
Telephone: (505)-268-7744
Contact: Marie McMillian

Bernalillo County

Community Services

Albuquerque Community Foundation
3301 Menual NE
Albuquerque, NM 87176
Telephone: (505)-883-6420
Contact: Laura Bass - Executive Director
Funding for HIV/AIDS-related projects by grant application process only.

Albuquerque Service Unit, Indian Health Service
801 Vassar Drive, North East
Albuquerque, NM 87106-2952
Telephone: (505)-256-4000 Fax: (505)-256-4088
Contact: Chuck North, MD - Director
STD and HIV testing, counseling, education, outreach to Native Americans.

American Civil Liberties Union
PO Box 80915
Albuquerque, NM 87198-0915
Telephone: (505)-266-5915
Contact: Shirley Pedler - Director
Handles legal matters involving HIV discrimination

Bernalillo County Income Support Div. SE Area Offices (ISD)
1401 Williams SE
P.O. Box 543
Albuquerque, NM 87103
Telephone: (505)-841-2600
Contact: Paul Baca
Entitlement programs, limited emergency assistance, referral service forAIDS

Bernalillo County Income Support Div. SW Area Office (ISD)
1720-C Bridge Blvd SW
P.O. Box 12355
Albuquerque, NM 87198
Telephone: (505)-841-2300
Contact: Sylvia Garcia
Entitlement programs, limited emergency assistance, medical & financialassistance; energy assistance

Catholic Social Services of Albuquerque
Archdiocese of Santa Fe
801 Mountain Road NE
Albuquerque, NM 87102
Telephone: (505)-247-9521 Fax: (505)-247-9523
Community-based outreach, services, education and counseling

Legal Aid Society - Pro Bono Project
121 Tijeras NE, # 3100
Albuquerque, NM 87102-3400
Telephone: (505)-243-7871
Contact: Karen Myers
Simple wills. entitlement, ADC, SSI & food stamp denials after initialappeal

Metropolitan Community Church of Albuquerque
2404 San Mateo Place NE
Albuquerque, NM 87110-4057
Telephone: (505)-881-9088
Contact: Rev. Judy K. Davenport - Pastor
Community outreach and education, physical support for HIV+/PWA's, counseling

New Mexico AIDS Services-Services and Administrative Office
4200 Silver SE
Suite D
Albuquerque, NM 87108
Telephone: (505)-266-0911 Fax: (505)-266-5104
Contact: Keith Smith - Executive Director; Gregg Ferran - Director, Client Services
HIV prevention education, crisis management, referrals, emotional support food bank, travel/reimbursement; clinical grant program

New Mexico Association of People Living with AIDS
N.M.A.P.L.A.
111 Montclaire Dr. SE
Albuquerque, NM 87108-2623
Telephone: (505)-266-0342 Fax: (505)-256-7739
Contact: Maria Snyder
Advocacy, education, support groups, AIDS library, state-wide database,referrals

New Mexico Department of Vocational Rehabilitation

3311 Candelaria Road NE
Albuquerque, NM 87107
Telephone: (505)-841-8800 Fax: (505)-841-8889
Develops & administers individual plans for Vocational Rehab for HIVdisabled

New Mexico Department of Vocational Rehabilitation
Coors District (ALBQ West)
2929 Coor Blvd NW, Suite 102
Albuquerque, NM 87120
Telephone: (505)-841-8752 Fax: (505)-841-8764
Develops & administers individual plans for vocational rehab for HIVdisabled

New Mexico Dept of Human Services Dept. of Children & Families
Income Support Division
10601 Lomas Blvd NE
Albuquerque, NM 87125
Telephone: (505)-841-4478
Administration, operations and entitlement programs.

New Mexico Dept.of Human Services Dept.of Children & Families)
North Bernalillo
1011 Lamberton Pl NE
Albuquerque, NM 87125
Telephone: (505)-841-7700
Contact: ; Paul Baca - Area Director
Entitlement program applications, assistance, referrals or call Santa Fe 800-632-4217

NMAS Food Bank
106 Girard SE
4200 Silver SE STE D
Albuquerque, NM 87106-2228
Telephone: (505)-266-0911 Fax: (505)-266-0911
Contact: Greig Ferran - Director of Client Services
Food bank for referred HIV/AIDS clients only.

Protection and Advocacy System
1720 Louisiana NE
Suite 204
Albuquerque, NM 87110
Telephone: (505)-256-3100 Fax: (505)-256-3184
Contact: James Jackson

Rio Grande Plannd Parenthood Clinic
9809 Candelaria Road NE
Albuquerque, NM 87110
Telephone: (505)-294-1577
Contact: Loretta Sandoval - Manager
Testing and counseling; HIV pre & post, referral service

Social Security Administration
1816 Carlisle Blvd NE
Albuquerque, NM 87110-4998
Telephone: (505)-262-6122 Fax: (505)-262-6005
Contact: Carol Clar - SS AIDS Administrator
Contact person for current procedures, assistance in filing SSI, SSdisability

Southwest Valley (Albuquerque Area) Health Office
Children's Medical Services
2001 Centro Familiar SW
Albuquerque, NM 87105
Telephone: (505)-841-8056 Fax: (505)-841-8201
Children's medical clinic, HIV testing, sliding scale.

Sunrise Cremation Society
P.O.Box 10262
Albuquerque, NM 87184-0262
Telephone: (505)-891-8200 Fax: (505)-892-8407
Contact: Marion deVries - Director
Cremation and burial information, 24 hours.

University of New Mexico Hospitals, Mental Health Center
2600 Marble NE
Albuquerque, NM 87131-0001
Telephone: (505)-843-2800 Fax: (505)-843-2016
24 hr suicide crisis line 505-265-7557

Youth Development, Inc.
1710 Centro Familiar SW
Albuquerque, NM 87105-4520
Telephone: (505)-873-1604 Fax: (505)-873-1602
Contact: Louis F. Carillo
AIDS education targeted to high risk youth, Hispanic AIDS outreach.

County Health Depts

Bernalillo County Health Office/Sexually Transmitted Disease
Central Office
1111 Stanford Drive NE
Albuquerque, NM 87125-3721
Telephone: (505)-841-4780 Fax: (505)-841-4826
Toll-Free: (800)-545-2437
Contact: Nick Keller
Anonymous HIV testing, counseling, medical services, education,referrals, STD clinic.

Home Health Care

Albuquerque Health Care Nurses
Skilled Nursing Services
4545 McCleod NE
Albuquerque, NM 87109
Telephone: (505)-888-3232
Skilled private-duty nursing, home making, shift care nursing & hospiceprogram

Albuquerque Homecare Homemaker Resources
4545 McCleod NE
Albuquerque, NM 87109-2202
Telephone: (505)-883-1222
Comprehensive homemaker services

Care Team
2201 San Pedro NE
Building 1, Suite # 210
Albuquerque, NM 87110-4100
Telephone: (505)-888-3883
Contact: Denise Blake, RN - Field Case Mgr.
Home and nursing care, physical support for CCIC (Medicaid) AIDS clients

Caremark Homecare Branch Network
4421 McLeod NE
Suite B
Albuquerque, NM 87109-2217
Telephone: (505)-884-4444
Contact: Cheryl Kroll - Nurse Manager
Home care, home IV

Hospital Home Care
405 Grand NE
Albuquerque, NM 87102-3541
Telephone: (505)-842-7100
Comprehensive and intermittent care for homebound. CCIC(Medicaid) licensed.

Interim Health Care
1720 Louisiana Blvd NE
Suite # 110
Albuquerque, NM 87110-7063
Telephone: (505)-268-7853
Contact: T K Owens - Branch Manager
Primary home health care and private-duty nursing, CCIC (Medicaid) casemanagement

Western Medical Services
2900 Louisiana NE
Suite D
Albuquerque, NM 87110
Telephone: (505)-880-0171
Contact: Caroline Fisher
Comprehensive skilled private-duty nurses and physical home care.

Medical Services

Albuquerque Area Indian Health Service
505 Marquette NW
Suite # 1502
Albuquerque, NM 87102-3221
Telephone: (505)-766-1053 Fax: (505)-766-2157
Contact: Rachel Chicharello
Education for Native American populations and pueblos. Testing and referrals.

Ted R. Montoya Hemophilia Program
UNM Dept of Pediatrics
3rd Floor Pediatrics
Albuquerque, NM 87131-0001
Telephone: (505)-272-5551
Contact: Connie Gould, MA
Comprehensive Care, Support

University of New Mexico Hospitals
2211 Lomas Blvd NE
Dept. of Clinical Social Work
Albuquerque, NM 87106-2745
Telephone: (505)-843-2328 Fax: (505)-272-1893
Contact: Melissa Stockton - Partners-in-Care Program

Special work and counseling for AIDS, and HIV patients

Testing Sites

AIDS Prevention Program, Health and Environment Department
District 1 Health Office
1111 Stanford NE
Albuquerque, NM 87106
Telephone: (505)-841-4780 Fax: (505)-841-4826
Contact: Nick Keller - Agency Director
Free anonymous or confidential testing; pre and post counseling

Albuquerque Family Health Center (Centro Familiar de Salud)
Clinic & Administration
2001 N. Centro Familiar SW
Albuquerque, NM 87105-4556
Telephone: (505)-768-5440 Fax: (505)-877-8198
Contact: Lynn Nauman
AIDS education testing & counseling

Health and Environment Department/Testing and Counseling
P.O. Box 25846
1111 Stanford Drive NE
Albuquerque, NM 87125-0846
Telephone: (505)-841-4780
Contact: Nick Keller
Confidential and anonymous HIV testing, pre and post counseling, referrals

Rio Grande Planned Parenthood Administration
1804 Carlisle North East
Albuquerque, NM 87110
Telephone: (505)-265-5976
Contact: Carol Tucker
Education, HIV testing and counseling

Scientific Laboratory Division-University of New Mexico
New Mexico Department of Health Virology
PO Box 4700
Albuquerque, NM 87196-4700
Telephone: (505)-841-2535 Fax: (505)-841-2543
HIV testing

SW Valley Health Office
2001 Centro Familar Blvd. SW
Albuquerque, NM 87105-4556
Telephone: (505)-841-8050 Fax: (505)-841-4826
Testing & Counseling

Veterans Administration Medical Center
Dept. of Infectious Disease
2100 Ridgecrest Drive SE
Albuquerque, NM 87108-5138
Telephone: (505)-265-1711 Fax: (505)-256-2803
Contact: Dr. Darwin Palmer, MD - Chief, Infectious Disease
Anonymous or confidential HIV testing & counseling

Cibola County

County Health Depts

Los Lunas Public Health Office
NM Dept. of Health
P.O. Box 177
Los Lunas, NM 87031-0177
Telephone: (505)-865-9616 Fax: (505)-866-1189
Contact: Lupe R Nichols - Nurse Manager
Anonymous or confidential HIV testing, referrrals. Early AZT drug intervention.

Testing Sites

Albuquerque Family Health Centers, Inc.
125 Highway Street
Los Lunas, NM 87031
Telephone: (505)-865-4618 Fax: (505)-865-1062
HIV testing, counseling & risk-prevention education; medical & STDreferrals

Dona Ana County

Community Services

Alliance Hospital of Santa Theresa
P.O. Box 6
Santa Theresa, NM 88001
Telephone: (505)-523-8581 Fax: (505)-589-2860
Medicare licensed substance abuse therapy, counseling, inpatient andoutpatient treatment

Southern AHEC
P.O. Box 30001, Dept. 3TG
1001 Geo Thermal Drive
Las Cruces, NM 88003-8001
Telephone: (505)-646-3441
Contact: Doreen Alexander Garay
Research, referrals

Home Health Care

Casa Arriba, Inc.
165 West Lucero
Las Cruces, NM 88005
Telephone: (505)-525-2545
Contact: Pat Landschoot
Adult & development, disability day care with activities

Coordinated Home Health Care
1100 South Main Street
Suite # 21
Las Cruces, NM 88005
Telephone: (505)-523-8885
Contact: Margaret Pedreny
Comprehensive respite care.

Desert Care (CCIC)
121 Wyatt Drive, #9
Las Cruces, NM 88005
Telephone: (505)-525-1969 Fax: (505)-525-9567
Contact: Irene Evans - Case Manager
CCIC (Medicaid) home health care, case management

Desert States CCIC Case Management
2211 North Main Street
Las Cruces, NM 88001-1136
Telephone: (505)-527-2081
Contact: Atmon Bone - Case Managment Intake
Primary home health care, 24 hr nursing, CCIC (Medicaid) case management

Mesilla Valley Hospice, Inc.
125 Wyatt Drive
Las Cruces, NM 88005-3242
Telephone: (505)-523-4700
Contact: Kay McClain, RN - Clinical Director; Margaret Connealy, RN -
Visiting nurses, counseling, spiritual & social workers, educationalservices

nmc HOMECARE
2801 E. Mission Ave, Suite 36
Las Cruces, NM 88001
Telephone: (800)-525-5603
Contact: Jimmie Lorenz
National JCAHO-Accredited company providing a full range of Infusion and Respiratory therapies and specializing in the care of HIV/AIDS patients. National Case Manager is also available at 800-445-1188

Grant County

Testing Sites

Planned Parenthood of Southern New Mexico
910 East 32nd Street
Silver City, NM 88061-7299
Telephone: (505)-388-1553
Counseling, HIV testing

Hidalgo County

County Health Depts

Hidalgo Field Health Office
500 East 13th Street
Lordsburg, NM 88045-2626
Telephone: (505)-542-9391
Contact: Jan Hopkins, RN
Anonymous or confidential HIV testing, counseling and referrals

Lea County

County Health Depts

Lea County Health Office
1923 N Dal Paso St
Suite B
Hobbs, NM 88240-3044
Telephone: (505)-397-2463
Contact: Claudia Moon
HIV testing and counseling. Mental health professionals and social workers.

Lincoln County

Community Services

Contel Low-Income Telephone Assistance Program
2700 Sudderth Drive
Ruidoso, NM 88345
Telephone: (505)-257-4644
Contact: Espanol: 257-4641 y tambien - 1-800-635-6471 (gratis)
Client must have current Medicaid Card (CCIC-Medicaid Waiver) to qualify,

Medical Services

Lincoln County Medical Center
211 Sudderth Drive
Ruidoso, NM 88345
Telephone: (505)-257-7381
Contact: Betty Testerman
Limited private-pay rural hospital; HIV testing and counseling

Los Alamos County

Testing Sites

Los Alamos Medical Center Visiting Nurses Service
2101 Trinity Drive
Suite T
Los Alamos, NM 87544
Telephone: (505)-662-2525
Anonymous or confidential HIV testing and referrals. Skilled in-home

Luna County

County Health Depts

Luna County Public Health Office
108 East Poplar Street
Deming, NM 88030-4732
Telephone: (505)-546-2771 Fax: (505)-546-9427
Contact: Jean Brown Wadriski, PhN
Testing & counseling

Mc Kinley County

County Health Depts

McKinley County Health Office
1919 College Drive
Gallup, NM 87301-7010
Telephone: (505)-722-4391 Fax: (505)-722-3034
Anonymous or confidential HIV testing, counseling and referrals.

Home Health Care

Innovative Health at Home
111 South 1st Street
Gallup, NM 87301
Telephone: (505)-722-7853
Contact: Rick Zamora, LBSW - Case Manager
CCIC-Medicaid waiver, comprehensive in-home nursingCty

Medical Services

Navajo Indian Health Service
P.O. Box 358
Crownpoint, NM 87313-0328
Telephone: (505)-786-5291 Fax: (505)-786-5840
Contact: Dr. Susie John, MD - AIDS Coordinator
Comprehensive Navajo medical care; HIV testing and counseling.

Testing Sites

Navajo Indian Health Service
P.O. Box 1337
Gallup, NM 87301
Telephone: (505)-722-1000 Fax: (505)-722-1554
Contact: Dr. Thompson - AIDS Coordinator
Comprehensive Navajo medical care; HIV testing and counseling.

Zuni Indian Health Service
P.O. Box 467
Zuni, NM 87327
Telephone: (505)-782-4431 Fax: (505)-782-5723
Contact: David Kessler - AIDS Coordinator
Zuni Native American medical care, HIV/AIDS testing, counseling, referrls

Quay County

County Health Depts

Quay County Health Office
300 S 3rd Street
Drawer I
Tucumcari, NM 88401-2731
Telephone: (505)-461-2610
Contact: Caroline Flores
Anonymous or confidential HIV testing, counseling and referrals.

Rio Arriba County

Medical Services

Jicarilla Apache Community Health Program

P.O. Box 609
Dulce, NM 87528
Telephone: (505)-759-3690 Fax: (505)-759-3005
Contact: Derwin Velarde
Also call 759-3522.

Santa Clara Pueblo Community Health Program
Indian Health Service
P.O. Box 580
Espanola, NM 87532-0580
Telephone: (505)-753-7326 Fax: (505)-753-8988
Contact: Barbara Tafoya
Pueblo medical care in a clinic setting, counseling

Roosevelt County

County Health Depts

Portales Health Office/Public Health Division
214 South Avenue A
Portales, NM 88130
Telephone: (505)-356-4453
Contact: Veronica Adcock
Testing & counseling

San Juan County

Home Health Care

Presbyterian Medical Services (CCIC)
P.O. Box 3336
Farmington, NM 87499
Telephone: (505)-327-0288 Fax: (505)-325-2477
Contact: Dawn Brooks; Carol Tookey -
Private nursing, case management, homemaker services

Medical Services

Indian Health Service
P.O. Box 160
Shiprock, NM 87420-0160
Telephone: (505)-368-4971 Fax: (505)-368-5209
Contact: Chris Percy - Dir. Community Health Services

Testing Sites

Columbia Rodriguez-Irwin
744 West Animas
Farmington, NM 87401-5617
Telephone: (505)-327-4461 Fax: (505)-326-1762
Contact: Joe Treat
Anonymous or confidential HIV testing, counseling and referrals.

San Miguel County

County Health Depts

Las Vegas Field Health Office
San Miguel Health Dept.
P.O. Box 1506
Las Vegas, NM 87701
Telephone: (505)-454-1474
Contact: Ruth Torres Clancy, RN
Anonymous or confidential HIV testing, counseling and referrals.

Sandoval County

Community Services

San Felipe Pueblo Community Health Program
Indian Health Service
P.O. Box A
San Felipe, NM 87001
Telephone: (505)-867-5385 Fax: (505)-867-3383
Education, speakers, counseling

Home Health Care

nmc HOMECARE
6421 Main St Highway 14
Cuba, NM 87013
Telephone: (505)-289-3348
Contact: Mary Pat Romero
National JCAHO-Accredited company providing a full range of Infusion and Respiratory therapies and specializing in the care

of HIV/AIDS patients. National Case Manager is also available at 800-445-1188

Medical Services

Presbyterian Medical Services
Checkerboard Area System
P.O. Box 638
Cuba, NM 87013-0638
Telephone: (505)-289-3291 Fax: (505)-289-3648
Contact: Tom Montoya
HIV/AIDS testing & counseling, education & comprehensive health care forHIV/PWA

Pueblo of Jemez Community Health Program
P.O. Box 100
Jemez Pueblo, NM 87024-0100
Telephone: (505)-834-7521 Fax: (505)-834-7331
Contact: Marianna Kennedy - Director
Comprehensive medical care; HIV/AIDS testing, counseling and referrals,education

Zia Pueblo Indian Health Program
Indian Health Service
155 B. Capital Square Drive
Zia Pueblo, NM 87053
Telephone: (505)-867-5258
Comprehensive health care for Zia Pueblo, clinic setting, HIV testing,counseling

Santa Fe County

Community Services

New Mexico Dept. of Labor, Human Rights Division
1596 Pacheco Street
Santa Fe, NM 87501
Telephone: (505)-827-6838 Fax: (505)-827-6878
Handles labor, civil and ADA discrimination disputes

County Health Depts

Santa Fe County Health Office
605 Letrado
Suite B
Santa Fe, NM 87501
Telephone: (505)-827-3560
Contact: Linda Daniels
Anonymous or confidential HIV testing, counseling, referrals. AZT referrals.

Home Health Care

AIDS/ARC Medicaid Waiver Home Care Program - CCIC
1190 St. Francis Drive
P.O. Box 26110
Santa Fe, NM 87502
Telephone: (505)-827-4483
Contact: Pat Cleveland
Counseling, Medical and Hospice Information and Referrals. HIV Hotline Services

nmc HOMECARE
1589 San Mateo Lane
Santa Fe, NM 87501
Telephone: (505)-983-9680
Fax: (505)-983-7226
Contact: Mary PAt Romero
National JCAHO-Accredited company providing a full range of Infusion and Respiratory therapies and specializing in the care of HIV/AIDS patients. National Case Manager is also available at 800-445-1188

Northern Home Care
826 Camino Del Monte Rey
Santa Fe, NM 87501
Telephone: (505)-983-5408 Fax: (505)-983-2800
Contact: Kathy Boyle
CCIC-Medicaid home health care and physical support provider.

Professional Home Health Care
1345 Pacheco Street
Santa Fe, NM 87501
Telephone: (505)-982-8581 Fax: (505)-982-0457
Private-duty nursing and home health care

Santa Fe Visiting Nurse Service/AIDS Wellness Program/Clinic
811 St. Michael's Drive
Santa Fe, NM 87501-5607
Telephone: (505)-983-1822 Fax: (505)-988-3781
Contact: Alice Sisnemos
HIV/AIDS Clinic, testing & counseling, hospice, referrals, bereavement &emotional support

Medical Services

AIDS Wellness Clinic
811 St. Michael's Drive
Santa Fe, NM 87501
Telephone: (505)-983-1822 Fax: (505)-988-3781
Contact: Alice Sisneros
Medical

La Familia Dental Clinic
1121 Alto Street
Santa Fe, NM 87501
Telephone: (505)-982-4425 Fax: (505)-982-8440
Contact: Dr. Raymond Annaya
HIV disclosure required to obtain dental care.

Pueblo of Pojoaque Community Health Program
Route 11, Box 71
Santa Fe, NM 87501
Telephone: (505)-455-2278 Fax: (505)-455-2950
Limited medical care; HIV/AIDS testing, counseling and referrals.

Santa Fe Indian Hospital
1700 Cerrillos Road
Santa Fe, NM 87501
Telephone: (505)-988-9821 Fax: (505)-983-6243
Contact: Dr. David Gregory, MD - AIDS Coordinator
Comprehensive medical services; HIV testing and counseling.

Women's Health Services/Family Care and Counseling Cente
500 West San Francisco
Santa Fe, NM 87505
Telephone: (505)-988-8869 Fax: (505)-982-7321
Contact: Ernstein Lawrence - Executive Director
HIV testing & counseling, mental health counseling,acupuncture, massage therapy

Sierra County

County Health Depts

NM Department of Health, Public Health Field Office
201 E 4th Street
Truth or
Consequences, NM 87901
Telephone: (505)-894-2716
Contact: Majorie E. Powey, PHN - HIV/AIDS Program
Confidential and anonymous testing, counseling, referrals, earlyintervention support group

Socorro County

Testing Sites

Socorro County Public Health Office
Public Health Department
214 Neel Avenue NW
Socorro, NM 87801-4649
Telephone: (505)-835-0971
Contact: Tammy Ireland,PHN - Case-manager
Confidential and anonymous testing, counseling, referrals, earlyintervention support group

Taos County

Home Health Care

Mountain Home Health Care, Inc.
P.O. Box 2566
Taos, NM 87571-2566
Telephone: (505)-758-1024
Contact: Debra Williams
Case Management, Private Nursing and Home Care

nmc HOMECARE
Box 5757 212A Paseo Del Canyon
Taos, NM 87571
Telephone: (505)-758-3075
Fax: (505)-758-8525
Contact: Mary Pat Romero
National JCAHO-Accredited company providing a full range of Infusion and Respiratory therapies and specializing in the care of HIV/AIDS patients. National Case Manager is also available at 800-445-1188

Testing Sites

Taos County Field Health Office
Dept. of Pubic Health
P.O. Box 1923
Taos, NM 87571-1923
Telephone: (505)-758-2073 Fax: (505)-751-3031
Contact: Faustina Vigil
Confidential and anonymous testing, counseling, referrals earlyintervention support group

Valencia County

Community Services

Living Water Family Ministries
84 Molina Road
Peralta, NM 87042
Telephone: (505)-869-0900
Contact: Niven Dryborough - Minister

Psychosocial and emotional support service provider. Service for newcounceling, disfunctional families, also FWA, disadvantaged children

Presbyterian Family Health Care
Family Practice Pediatrcs
609 S.Christopher Road
Belen, NM 87002
Telephone: (505)-864-5454 Fax: (505)-864-5459
Contact: Dr. Steven Cohen, MD

Family practice and pediatric medical service providers.

Valencia County Income Support Division
Fifth and Becker
P.O. Box 259
Belen, NM 87002-0259
Telephone: (505)-864-5200 Fax: (505)-864-5247
Contact: Albert Delgado

Food stamps and other entitlement benefit programs. 1-800-624-8434

Testing Sites

Belen Public Health Department
855 West Castillo Office
Belen, NM 87002-3123
Telephone: (505)-864-7744
Contact: Rosalie Kercheval - PH Nurse

HIV test(anon/confid),counseling,referrals.AIDS & AZT early intervention progrm

NEW YORK

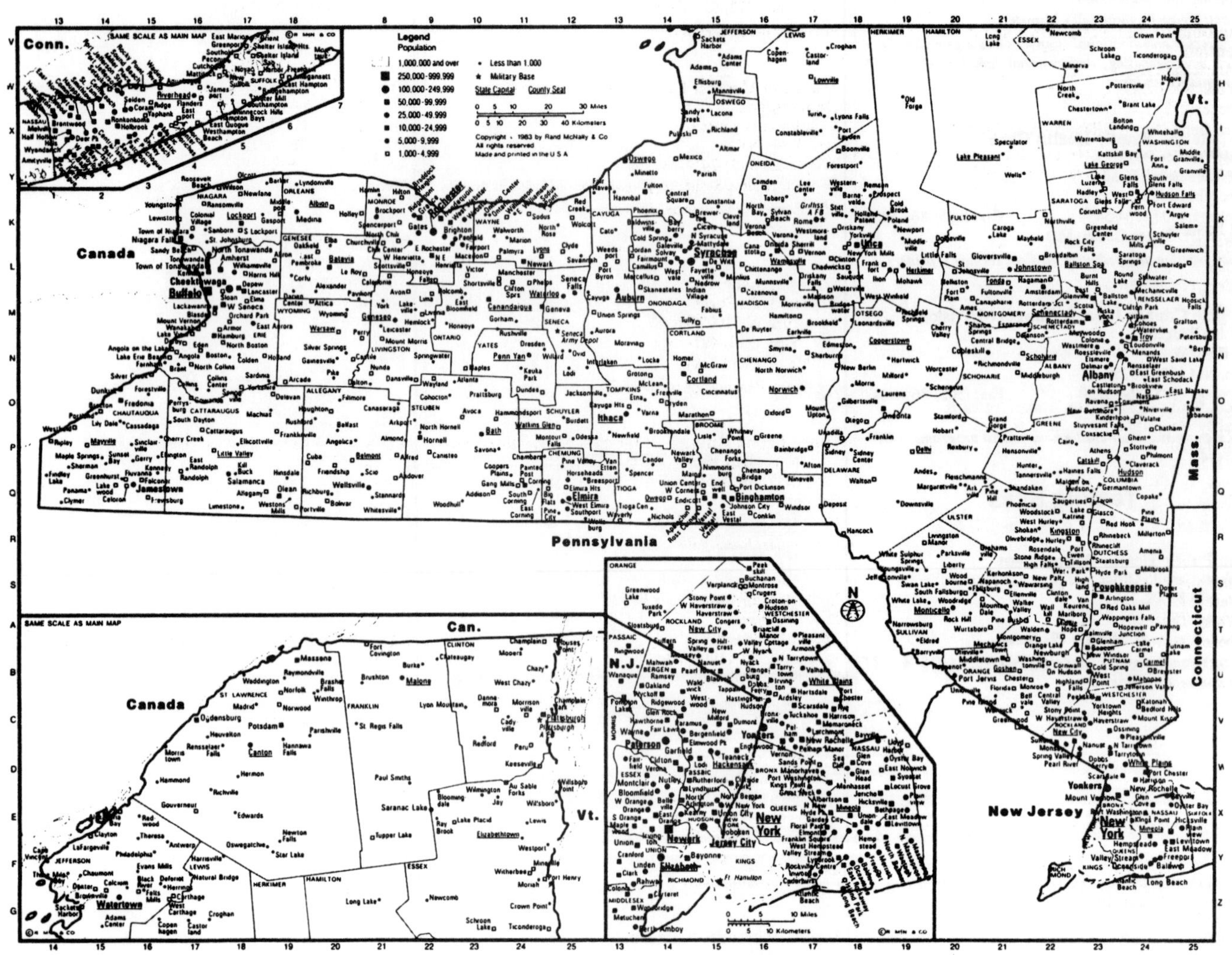

From City/County Planning Atlas Copyright 1989 by Reed McNally & Company, R.L. 90-S-28

New York

General Services

Education

Alianc Dominicana AIDS Outreach & Prevention
2340 Amsterdam Avenue
New York, NY 10033
Telephone: (212)-368-4500
Contact: Gulio Dicent Taillpiers - AIDS Director
Boroughwide: education, outreach, social, support, human services; forhigh risk; AIDS hotline 212-740-3737

Body Positive
2095 Broadway
Suite 306
New York, NY 10023-2895
Telephone: (212)-721-1346 Fax: (212)-787-9633
Contact: Bruce Kernek
Social programs, monthly newsletters, education programs

Clinical Communications, Inc., Human Sexuality Database
132 Hutchin Hill Road
Shady, NY 12479
Telephone: (914)-679-2217
Contact: Howard R. Lewis - President
Living with HIV/AIDS, AIDS information database

Community League of West 159th Street
508 West 159th Street
New York, NY 10032
Telephone: (212)-781-8210 Fax: (212)-781-0732
Contact: Yvonne Stennet
Citywide: Education/Outreach

Focus International
1160 East Jericho Turnpike
Huntington Sta., NY 11743
Telephone: (516)-549-5320 Fax: (516)-549-2066
Produces films for sex education

General Board of Global Ministries of the United Methodist Church
475 Riverside Drive
Room 350
New York, NY 10115
Telephone: (212)-870-3871 Fax: (212)-870-3873
Contact: Rev. Charles Carnahan - Exec. for AIDS/HIV Ministries
Coordinates AIDS education and service programs; publications with AIDSfocus

The Greater Harlem Comprehensive Guidance Center Inc.
127 West 127th Street
New York, NY 10027
Telephone: (212)-862-2440
Contact: Dr. Olivia Pearl
Education, outreach, social, support, human services for community

Hastings Center
255 Elm Road
Briarcliff Mnr., NY 10510-2255
Telephone: (914)-762-8500
Contact: Daniel Callahan - Director
Education, Training, Publication Production, Research, Policy Analysis

Human Relations Media
175 Tompkins Ave
Pleasantville, NY 10570-3156
Educational videos

Montefiore Medical Center, Patient Education Department
111 East 210th Street
Bronx, NY 10467-2490
Telephone: (212)-920-6058
Publisher of AIDS Handbook

Mt. Sinai Medical Center, Health Education Department
1 Gustave Levy Place
New York, NY
Telephone: (212)-241-7389
Contact: Andrea Rothenberg - Director of Health Education
AIDS prevention programs for schools, adolescents, parents in East Harlem

OZ Pharmacy
155 East 116th Street
New York, NY 10029-1302
Telephone: (212)-427-4922
Contact: Robert Litsky
Citywide: Pharmacy Assistance Service

South Bronx Human Development Organization
1 Fordham Plaza, #900
Bronx, NY 10458-5871
Telephone: (212)-295-5501
Contact: Carolyn Gould
Independent living skills

Suffolk Community College
Eastern Campus
Speonk Riverhead Rd
Riverhead, NY 11901-3499
Telephone: (516)-548-2500
Education, information

Suffolk Community College
Ammerman Campus
533 College Rd
Seldon, NY 11784-2899
Telephone: (516)-451-4110
Contact: Pat Foege
Education, information

United Methodist Church, New York Conference
88-40 80th Street
Woodhaven, NY 11421
Telephone: (718)-296-8572
Contact: William T Young
Tri-state area: education/outreach to churches, ministries, clergy, HIVcounseling

Hotlines

NYS AIDS Information Hotline
In state only (800) 542--2437

NYS DOH HIV Confidentiality Law Hotline
In state only (800) 962-5062

Western New York AIDS Program
121 West Tupper Street
Bufflao, NY 14201-2142
Telephone: (716)-847-2441 Fax: (716)-847-0418
Contact: Ronald T. Silverio - Executive Director
Hotline (716) 847-AIDS, newsletter, support group, client services

State Health Departments

New York State Department of Health
AIDS Institute
Corning Tower, Room 342, Empire State Plaza
Albany, NY 12237
Telephone: (518)-473-7542
Contact: Dennis Whelan - Acting Director

New York State Department of Health
227 A Fifth Avenue
Brooklyn, NY 11215
Telephone: (718)-638-2074
Toll-Free: (800)-462-6788
Free Anonymous HIV Testing and Counseling

New York State Department of Health, Office of Public Health
AIDS Institute
Corning Tower
Albany, NY
Contact: Dr. Lloyd Novick - Director

Statewide Services

AIDS Drug Assistance Program (ADAP)
Empire Station
PO Box 2052
Albany, NY 12220
Telephone: (800)-289-1957
Contact: Lanny Cross
Provides free medication for treatment of HIV/AIDS and opportunisticinfections

AIDS Drug Assistance Program Plus (ADAP+)
Empire Station
PO Box 2052
Albany, NY 12220
Telephone: (518)-459-1649
Toll-Free: (800)-542-2437
Contact: Lanny Cross
Provides free primary care services at selected clinics and hospitaloutpatient departments

HIV Home Care Uninsured Fund
Empire Station
PO Box 2052
Albany, NY 12220
Telephone: (518)-459-1641
Contact: Lanny Cross
Provides coverage for home care services to chronically dependentindividuals as offered by their physician

Albany County

Home Health Care

Critical Care America
2 Access Road
Albany, NY 12205
Telephone: (518)-456-8192 Fax: (518)-456-8810
Toll-Free: (800)-666-8192
Contact: Barbara Manzione
Coordinate & integrate all clinical & psychosocial services for HIV+

Equicare - Homedco Infusion
19 Walker Way
Albany, NY 12205
Telephone: (518)-452-4951 Fax: (518)-452-9934
Toll-Free: (800)-342-4004

Respiratory, HME, Infusion Therapy, Nursing Services, also Pharmacy servingKingston,

nmc HOMECARE
16 Walker Way
Albany, NY 12205
Telephone: (518)-456-1011
Fax: (518)-869-4414
Contact: Tom Markert
National JCAHO-Accredited company providing a full range of Infusion and Respiratory therapies and specializing in the care of HIV/AIDS patients. National Case Manager is also available at 800-445-1188

Medical Services

AIDS Treatment Center Albany Medical Center Hospital
47 New Scotland Avenue
Room A-167
Albany, NY 12208
Telephone: (518)-262-4439 Fax: (518)-262-4756
Contact: Dr. Steven Szebenyi
Community based AIDS Research

Allegany County

County Health Depts

Allegany County Health Department
County Office Bldg
Ground Floor
Belmont, NY 14813
Telephone: (716)-268-9250
Contact: Christine Johnson, RN - Director/Patient Services
Anonymous, Confidential HIV Testing & counseling.Callfor apptmnt

Bronx County

Community Services

Bronx AIDS Services
One Fordham Plaza
Suite 903
Bronx, NY 10458
Telephone: (718)-295-5690
New York State Dept. of Health AIDS Institute community service program

Medical Services

Adolescent AIDS Program at Montefiore Medical Center
111 East 210th Street
Bronx, NY 10467
Telephone: (212)-882-0232
Contact: Martha Aleman - Outreach Coordinator
For children ages 13-21 HIV+ or at risk; medical & psychosocial support,case management

Montefiore Medical Center, NW 674
Department of Pediatrics
111 East 210th Street
Bronx, NY 10467
Telephone: (718)-882-0023 Fax: (718)-882-0432
Contact: Karen Hein, M.D., Director - Adolescent AIDS
Primary care for HIV or at risk adolescents, case management, HIV testing &counseling

Veterans Administration Medical Center
130 West Kingsbridge Road
Bronx, NY 10468-3904
Telephone: (718)-584-9000
Medical Services for Veterans with AIDS

Broome County

Community Services

Southern Tier AIDS Program
122 Baldwin Street
Johnson City, NY 13790
Telephone: (607)-798-1706
Contact: Dianne Brown - Executive Director
New York State Department of Health AIDS Institute Community Service Program

Home Health Care

Homedco Infusion
3116 Watson Blvd.
Endwell, NY 13760
Telephone: (607)-754-3511
Contact: Jane Frate - Branch Manager
Respiratory, HME

Cattaraugus County

County Health Depts

Cattaraugus County Health Department
1701 Lincoln Avenue
Olean, NY 14760-1100
Telephone: (716)-373-8050 Fax: (716)-375-5994
Contact: Mary Ann Powers - Supervising Public Health RN; James A. Garvey, MD - Commissioner of Health
AIDS/STD testing clinic

Chautauqua County

Community Services

Family Services of Jamestown
332 East Fourth Street
Jamestown, NY 14701-5598
Telephone: (716)-488-1971
Counseling

County Health Depts

Chautauqua County Department of Health
110 E Fourth Street
Jamestown, NY 14701-5334
Telephone: (716)-661-8123 Fax: (716)-661-8101
Contact: Patricia Johnson - State/Public Health Rep.
HIV Testing, STD clinic, counseling, referrals, & partner notification

Chautauqua County Department of Health
Hall R Clothier Bldg
7 N Erie St, 4th Fl
Mayville, NY 14757
Telephone: (716)-753-4312
HIV Testing, STD clinic, counseling, referrals, & partner notification

Chautauqua County Department of Health
15 Lucas Avenue
Dunkirk, NY 14048-3340
Telephone: (716)-366-8805
HIV Testing, STD clinic, counseling, referrals, & partner notification

Chautauqua County Health Department
Hall R. Clothier Blvd.
2 North Erie Street
Mayville, NY 14757
Telephone: (716)-753-4312 Fax: (716)-753-4794
Contact: Robert Burke, MD - HIV Counselor
County AIDS task force, confidential HIV testing

Genesee County Health Department
3837 West Main Street
Batavia, NY 14720-9406
Telephone: (716)-344-8506
Anonymous, confidential HIV Testing and Counseling

Chemung County

Home Health Care

Homedco Infusion
200 South Main Street
Elmira, NY 14904
Telephone: (607)-734-7220 Fax: (607)-732-5225
Contact: Jane Frate - Branch Manager
Respiratory, HME

nmc HOMECARE
452 E. Water St.
Elmira, NY 14901
Telephone: (607)-733-8635
Fax: (607)-734-1761
Contact: Leah Sperbeck
National JCAHO-Accredited company providing a full range of Infusion and Respiratory therapies and specializing in the care of HIV/AIDS patients. National Case Manager is also available at 800-445-1188

Clinton County

Home Health Care

nmc HOMECARE
785 Cornelia St.
Plattsburg, NY 12901
Telephone: (518)-561-1420
Fax: (518)-561-1593
Contact: Tom Markert
National JCAHO-Accredited company providing a full range of Infusion and Respiratory therapies and specializing in the care

of HIV/AIDS patients. National Case Manager is also available at 800-445-1188

Cortland County

Home Health Care

Homedco Infusion
24 Corporate Circle
East Syracuse, NY 13056
Telephone: (315)-463-8887
Contact: Barbara Verraco - Branch Manager
Respiratory, HME

Erie County

Community Services

Benedict House of Western New York, Inc.
124 Plymouth Avenue
Buffalo, NY 14201-1212
Telephone: (716)-881-3082
Contact: Sister Mary McCarrick - Executive Director
Residence for AIDS patients, in-house counseling

County Health Depts

Erie County Health Department
95 Franklin Street
Buffalo, NY 14202-3959
Telephone: (716)-858-6463
Contact: Patrick Pruski - Coord. AIDS Education
Pre/post HIV counseling, educational inservice for professionals

Home Health Care

Critical Care America
25 Hazelwood Drive
Suite 100
Amherst, NY 14228
Telephone: (716)-691-5751 Fax: (716)-691-5779
Toll-Free: (800)-843-7401
Contact: Paula Karaszewski
Coordinate & integrate all clinical & psychosocial services for HIV+

HNS, Inc.
15 Hazelwood Drive
Suite 100
Amherst, NY 14228
Telephone: (716)-691-1291 Fax: (716)-691-1296
Toll-Free: (800)-872-4467
Contact: Vic Lucci
Home Infusion Therapy, In-home Nursing and Attendant Care

Homedco
1975 Wehrle Drive
Williamsville, NY 14221
Telephone: (716)-631-1192 Fax: (716)-637-1198
Toll-Free: (800)-848-4092
Contact: Eric Forsman, CRTT - Branch Manager
Respiratory, HME

Hospice Buffalo, Inc.
4226 Ridge Lea Rd.
Buffalo, NY 14226-1068
Telephone: (716)-838-4438
Contact: J. Donald Schmacher - Executive Director

nmc HOMECARE
305 Cayuga Road
Buffalo, NY 14225
Telephone: (716)-634-8779
Fax: (716)-634-2614
Contact: Michele Sinclair
National JCAHO-Accredited company providing a full range of Infusion and Respiratory therapies and specializing in the care of HIV/AIDS patients. National Case Manager is also available at 800-445-1188

nmc HOMECARE
550 Orchard Park Road
West Seneca, NY 14224
Telephone: (716)-677-6805
Fax: (716)-677-6807
Contact: Michele Sinclair
National JCAHO-Accredited company providing a full range of Infusion and Respiratory therapies and specializing in the care of HIV/AIDS patients. National Case Manager is also available at 800-445-1188

Medical Services

Erie County Medical Center, AIDS Services
462 Grider Street
Tunnel
Buffalo, NY 14215-3098
Telephone: (716)-898-4119 Fax: (716)-898-3187
Contact: Ross Hewitt, M.D. - Director; Sandra Fundalinski, RN - Nurse Clinician; Beatrice Cross, RN - Case Manager
Full service outpatient clinic prescribing AZT, DDI & experimental therapies

Hemophilia Center of Western New York Inc.
462 Grider Street
Buffalo, NY 14215
Telephone: (716)-896-2470 Fax: (716)-896-3119
Contact: Kathleen Walter, BSN - Executive Director
Serves only clients with hereditary bleeding

Nursing Home Company, Inc.
24 Rhode Island Street
Buffalo, NY 14213-2142
Telephone: (716)-883-7911 Fax: (716)-884-6116
Contact: Janet Thomas - Director of Patient Srvcs; Elfrida Russel - Administrator
Medically eligible for skilled nursing or health related facility care

Testing Sites

New York State Health Departments., Anonymous HIV Counseling & Testing Progra
NY State Health Depart.
Erie, NY 14202
Telephone: (716)-847-4520
Pre-and post counseling, hotline accepts collect calls, M-F (8 am - 5pm),call for appointment

Project Reach of Buffalo Columbus Hospital
228 Franklin Street
Buffalo, NY 14202
Telephone: (716)-842-0555 Fax: (716)-847-1394
Contact: Valerie Eastman - Director
Counseling, HIV testing, support services for substance abusers, & mobiletesting unit.

Jefferson County

Home Health Care

nmc HOMECARE
6 Fisher Drive
Watertown, NY 13601
Telephone: (315)-788-8078
Fax: (315)-782-2005
Contact: Jim O'Hanlon
National JCAHO-Accredited company providing a full range of Infusion and Respiratory therapies and specializing in the care of HIV/AIDS patients. National Case Manager is also available at 800-445-1188

Kings County

Community Services

Brooklyn Legal Services
260 Broadway
Brooklyn, NY 11211
Telephone: (718)-782-6195
Free Legal Representation and Assistance in Housing, Benefits, Immigration

Community Action for Legal Services
1368 Fulton Street
Brooklyn, NY 11226
Telephone: (718)-636-1155
Contact: Cherie Gaines
Free Legal Representation and Assistance in Housing, Benefits,

Community Action for Legal Services
East New York Office
80 Jamaica Avenue
Brooklyn, NY 11207
Telephone: (718)-345-6200 Fax: (718)-342-1780
Free Legal Representation and Assistance in Housing, Benefits

The Division of AIDS Services (DAS), Brooklyn Office
94 Flatbush Avenue
Brooklyn, NY 11217-1412
Telephone: (718)-237-4817
Contact: Peter Connolly
Referrals, Benefits Applications Assistance, Housing, Financial Management

Haitian Coalition on AIDS
50 Court Street
Suite 605
Brooklyn, NY 11201-4859
Telephone: (718)-855-0972 Fax: (718)-852-5377
Contact: Marie Pierre-Louis - Coordinator
Advocacy, Counseling, Referrals, Education, Workshops

Jewish Board of Family and Children's Services
26 Court Street
8th Floor
Brooklyn, NY 11242-1102
Telephone: (718)-855-6900 Fax: (718)-802-1298
Contact: Adina Shapiro
Counseling for Individuals, Couples, Parents of PWAs, PWARCs, HIV+

Southside Community Mission
280 Marcy Avenue
Brooklyn, NY 11211-7921
Telephone: (718)-388-3784 Fax: (718)-384-3739
Contact: Carmen Calderon - Director of Homeless
Services for the Homeless, Temporary Winter Shelter, Counseling, Referrals

The Legal Aid Society, Immigration
166 Montage Street
Brooklyn, NY 11201
Telephone: (718)-722-3120 Fax: (718)-722-3093
Contact: Jean Schneider
Citywide: Legal Assistance for Undocumented Aliens/Residents

Medical Services

Addiction Research & Treatment, Brownsville Clinic
564 Hopkinson Avenue
Brooklyn, NY 11212
Telephone: (718)-385-4233 Fax: (718)-345-1009
Contact: Robert Coleman
Methadone Programs Including Individual and Group Counseling

Addiction Research & Treatment, Bushwick Clinic
1149-55 Myrtle Avenue
Brooklyn, NY 11206
Telephone: (718)-574-1801
Contact: Feli Reyes
Methadone Programs Including Individual and Group Counseling

Addiction Research & Treatment, Ft. Greene Clinic
937 Fulton Street
Brooklyn, NY 11238
Telephone: (718)-789-1214 Fax: (718)-399-6585
Contact: Gene Tomlinson
Methadone Programs Including Individual and Group Counseling

Brooklyn Center for Families in Crisis
535 E. 17th Street
Brooklyn, NY 11226-6607
Telephone: (718)-282-0010 Fax: (718)-693-4490
Contact: Jennifer Hall
Individual and Family Psychotherapy, with Special AIDS Program; Support Groups

Brooklyn Hospital Center
290 Willoughby St. 5th Floor
mailing: 121 Dekalb
Brooklyn, NY 11201-5463
Telephone: (718)-250-6922 Fax: (718)-250-8886
Contact: Dr. Alan Stein
HIV Testing, AIDS Assessment, Medical Treatment

Coney Island Community Health Center
2201 Neptune Avenue
Brooklyn, NY 11224-2311
Telephone: (718)-946-3400 Fax: (718)-996-5644
Contact: Richard Chieco - Administratortor
Pre & post test counseling, medical & dental treatment for AIDS patients

Coney Island Hospital
2601 Ocean Parkway
Brooklyn, NY 11235-7791
Telephone: (718)-615-4143 Fax: (718)-743-5266
Contact: Michele Iesu Rn. - HIV Coordinator
HIV testing & women health programs, AIDS Assessment, AZT, medical services

Damon House
310 South 1st Street
Brooklyn, NY 11211-4604
Telephone: (718)-387-9100 Fax: (718)-387-4016
Contact: David Rivera - Intake
Residential Drug Free Therapeutic Community Offering Treatment for All Drugs

Long Island College Hospital
340 Henry Street
Brooklyn, NY 11201-5591
Telephone: (718)-780-1436
Contact: Dr. Berkowitz
Inpatient/Outpatient Medical Treatment, HIV Testing for Patients/Partners

Manhattan Bowery Corporation/Project Renewal
121 Ft. Greene Place
Brooklyn, NY 11217
Telephone: (718)-643-0407 Fax: (718)-643-5775
Contact: Elsie Campbell
Residential Alcohol and Drug Rehabilitation Program for Men

Phoenix House
55 Flatbush Avenue
Brooklyn, NY 11217
Telephone: (718)-858-2462
Residential Programs for Drug Rehabilitation, School/Drug Rehab for Adolescents

State University of N.Y. Health Science Center at Brooklyn
450 Clarkson Avenue
Box 43
Brooklyn, NY 11203-2012
Telephone: (718)-270-2690 Fax: (718)-270-3386
Contact: Ellen Honey
HIV studies, support programs, education, Pediatric, clinical care

Woodhill Hospital
1420 Bushwick Avenue
Brooklyn, NY 11207-1422
Telephone: (718)-919-1200 Fax: (718)-919-1070
Contact: Sherry Potter
HIV Testing, AIDS Assessment, Medical Treatment, Outpatient Care

Testing Sites

Downstate HIV Testing Program
470 Clarkson Avenue
Brooklyn, NY 11203-2012
Telephone: (718)-270-3745 Fax: (718)-270-2440
Contact: Marcia George
Confidential HIV Testing

NY City Dept. of Health, ACT III, Ft. Greene Health Center
295 Flatbush Avenue
Room 415
Brooklyn, NY 11201
Telephone: (718)-643-2602
Free Anonymous HIV Testing and Counseling

Monroe County

Community Services

AIDS Rochester, Inc.
1350 University Ave.
Rochester, NY 14607-1622
Telephone: (716)-232-3580 Fax: (716)-442-2220
Contact: Annie Long - Acting Director
New York State Department of Health AIDS Institute Community Service Programcase management, education, speakers, fund raising, buddies, meals

Community Health Network
758 South Avenue
Rochester, NY 14620-2237
Telephone: (716)-244-9000
Contact: Craig R. Sellers, MS, RN, C - Nurse Practitioner
HIV testing, counseling, support groups, case management, treatment &pharmacy service

County Health Depts

Caremark Inc.
395 Summit Point Drive
Suite 3A
Henrietta, NY 14467-9609
Telephone: (716)-359-4740 Fax: (716)-359-4587
Toll-Free: (800)-624-8142
Contact: Lou Zambelli - Branch Manager
Clinical support and infusion therapies: nutrition, antimicrobials, chemo.,hematopoeti

Home Health Care

Homedco
395 Summit Point Drive
Suite 1
Henrietta, NY 14467
Telephone: (716)-359-4590 Fax: (716)-359-9809
Contact: Linda Akey - Billing Center Manager
Billing center

Homedco
1250 Scottsville Road
Suite 80
Rochester, NY 14624
Telephone: (716)-436-4910 Fax: (716)-436-6356
Toll-Free: (800)-724-2570
Contact: Mary Rowe,LPN - District Sales Manager
Respiratory, HME

Olsten Kimberly Quality Care
311 Alexander Street
Suite #100
Rochester, NY 14604
Telephone: (716)-232-2800 Fax: (716)-323-7302
Contact: Tracy Kuhn
Home care & nursing services

Medical Services

Community Health Network
758 South Avenue
Rochester, NY 14620
Telephone: (716)-244-9000
American Foundation for AIDS Research & health care center for HIV

Nassau County

County Health Depts

Nassau County Dept. of Health
270 Lawrence Avenue
Lawrence, NY 11559
Telephone: (516)-571-7874
Contact: Brian Harper - MD
Ryan White Title II

Home Health Care

Caremark, Inc.
45 S. Service Rd.
Plainview, NY 11803-4101
Telephone: (516)-753-5330 Fax: (516)-753-5482
Toll-Free: (800)-522-0556
Contact: Lance Adair - Operations Manager; John White - Branch Manager
Clinical support & infusion therapies

nmc HOMECARE
5 Dakota Drive, Suite #306
Lake Success, NY 11042
Telephone: (516)-437-3390
Fax: (516)-437-3696
Contact: Dennis Mahoney; Marion Ratkewitch
National JCAHO-Accredited company providing a full range of Infusion and Respiratory therapies and specializing in the care of HIV/AIDS patients. National Case Manager is also available at 800-445-1188

Medical Services

Long Island Jewish Medical Center
Sect. of Hematology Research
269-11 76th Ave
New Hyde Park, NY 11042
Telephone: (718)-470-8930 Fax: (718)-470-0169
Contact: Dr. F. Siegel

New York County

Community Services

Addiction Research and Treatment Corporation
Harlem Kaleidoscope
132 West 125th Street
New York, NY 10027
Telephone: (212)-932-2810
Contact: Ren'ee Sumpter - Clinical Director
Comm Dists 7/9/10, Boroughwide: Med Svcs; Soc/Supp/Human Svcs; Confid HIV Test

AIDS Resource Center
275 7th Avenue
12th Floor
New York, NY 10001-4410
Telephone: (212)-481-1270
Contact: Gina Quattrachi - Executive Director
Citywide: information, education, outreach; social, support, humanservices; home care housing for homeless people with AIDS

AIDS Resource Center, Inc.
275 7th Avenue
12th Floor
New York, NY 10001
Telephone: (212)-481-1270
Housing for homeless with AIDS

Alianza Dominicana, Inc.
2340 Amsterdam Avenue
New York, NY 10033-7326
Telephone: (212)-927-6810
Contact: Julio Dicent-Taillepierre - AIDS Prevention Director
Comm. Dist. 12: Information, Education, Outreach; Social, Support, HumanServices

American Civil Liberties Union
132 West 43rd Street
2nd Floor
New York, NY 10036
Telephone: (212)-382-0557
Publisher of Fact Sheet on AIDS and Civil Liberties

Catholic Charities, Family and Children Services
1011 1st Avenue
New York, NY 10022
Telephone: (212)-371-1000
Contact: Gilda Morales
Comm. Dist. 11: Social/Support/Human Services; Public Policy Education

Community Service Council of Greater Harlem, Inc.
207 West 133rd Street
New York, NY 10030-3201
Telephone: (212)-926-0281 Fax: (212)-368-9314
Contact: William K. Wolf - Director
Outreach for the community

The Correctional Assoc. of New York, Health Support Network
135 East 15th Street
New York, NY 10003-3596
Telephone: (212)-254-5700
Contact: Aleah Long
Statewide: Education, Outreach; Social, Support, Human Services for GeneralPublic

Covenant House, Housing for Homeless Youth
460 W. 41st Street
New York, NY 10036-6898
Telephone: (212)-613-0300
Contact: George Junco - Unit Manager
Crisis Counseling, Housing Services, Education, Hotline for Homeless Youth,HIV testing & counseling

East Harlem Maternal Infant Care Clinic
158 East 115th Street
New York, NY 10029-2096
Telephone: (212)-369-9500
Citywide: Information, Education/Outreach

Emmaus House
2027 Lexington Avenue
New York, NY 10035-2233
Telephone: (212)-360-7194 Fax: (212)-360-7245
Contact: Susan Salazar
HIV support, education

The Fifth Avenue Community Center of Harlem
173 East 111th Street
New York, NY 10029-2823
Telephone: (212)-410-4315
Contact: Sr. Leotine O'Gorman
Comm Dists 9-11: Education, Outreach; Social, Support, Human Services for Children and Adolescents

Gay & Lesiban Project Two
722 West 168th Street
New York, NY 10032-2603
Telephone: (212)-740-7324
Contact: Margaret Rosario, PhD
Citywide: education, outreach; social, support, human services; forrunaways and gays

God's Love We Deliver, Inc.
895 Amsterdam Avenue
New York, NY 10025
Telephone: (212)-865-4900 Fax: (212)-865-4901
Contact: J. Daniel Stricker
Hot meals delivered to PWA's in 5 boroughs of NYC, newsletters

Graham Windham Services, Manhattan Center
151 West 136th Street
New York, NY 10030-2606
Telephone: (212)-368-4100 Fax: (212)-281-5041
Contact: Judy Lind
Comm. Dists. 9/10: social, support, human services; education, counseling,referrals

Harlem Hospital Center, Volunteer Division
506 Lenox Avenue
New York, NY 10037
Telephone: (212)-491-1234
Contact: Nettie Richards
Citywide: Social, Support, Human Services (Buddies)

Harlem YMCA, Program Development
180 West 135th Street
New York, NY 10030-2902
Telephone: (212)-281-4100
Contact: Marc Martinez - AIDS Program Director
Crisis intervention, case management, individual & group counseling for HIV infected; counseling for friends & family

Hispanic AIDS Forum
121 Avenue America
Suite 505
New York, NY 10013-1510
Telephone: (212)-966-6336 Fax: (212)-966-7890
Contact: Miguelina Maldonado
Boroughwide: Info, Educ/Outreach; Soc/Supp/Human Svcs; For Public, Hispanics

Human Resources Administration, Division of AIDS Services
241 Church Street
New York, NY 10013
Telephone: (212)-966-8127 Fax: (212)-966-8214
Contact: Stephen Fisher
Housing for HIV infected persons

Incarnation Church and School
1290 St. Nicholas Avenue
New York, NY 10033-7204
Telephone: (212)-927-7474 Fax: (212)-928-0315
Contact: Monsignor Walsh - Pastor; Father John Paddock - Incarnation School
Comm. Dist. 12, Parish: Education/Outreach; Social/Support/Human Services

Inwood Community Service, Mental Health/Alcoholism
651 Academy Street
New York, NY 10034-5003
Telephone: (212)-942-0043 Fax: (212)-567-9476
Contact: Charlie Corliss
Community District 12: Social/Support/Human Services; Education

Jewish Board of Families and Children Services
120 West 57th Street
New York, NY 10019-3371
Telephone: (212)-582-9100 Fax: (212)-245-2096
Contact: Toni Mufson - Manhattan/Queens AIDS Pro; Florence Rabinowitz - Volunteer AIDS Services
Boroughwide: Social/Support/Human Services; Education/Outreach

LUCHA, Substance Abuse Services
127 East 105th Street
New York, NY 10029-4917
Telephone: (212)-289-1004 Fax: (212)-427-3433
Contact: MArlene Cruz
Boroughwide: education, outreach; social, support, human services

MFY Legal Services, Inc.
45 Avenue A
New York, NY 10029-1322
Telephone: (212)-427-0693 Fax: (212)-475-1043
Contact: Jill Boskey
Community District 11: Social/Support/Human Services (Legal Assistance)

Minority Task Force on AIDS, Inc.
505 8th Avenue
16th Floor
New York, NY 10018
Telephone: (212)-749-2816
Contact: Linda Campbell - Executive Director
Citywide: Education, Outreach; Social, Support, Human Services

Network
259 West 30th Street
9th Floor
New York, NY 10001
Telephone: (212)-268-4196 Fax: (212)-268-4199
Contact: Kenneth Fornataro
HIV/AIDS treatment, Counseling and Referrals

New York/Virgin Island AIDS ETC
Columbia Univ, PH School
600 W 168th St
New York, NY 10032
Telephone: (212)-305-3616 Fax: (212)-305-6832
Contact: Cheryl Healton, Ed.D.
New York City/Long Island, Puerto Rico, Virgin Islands

NYS Div. of Human Rights, Off. of AIDS Discrimination Issues
55 West 125th Street
12th Floor
New York, NY 10027-4516
Telephone: (212)-870-8624 Fax: (212)-870-5883
Contact: Armando Martinez
Statewide: Legal Assistance, Human Rights for General Public, HIV+; Advocacy

Pentecostal Faith Church, InterCouncil Community Fellowship
60 West 130th Street
New York, NY 10037
Telephone: (212)-534-2437 Fax: (212)-534-5420
Contact: Bishop Betty Middleton
Hospital discharge program, Ryan White grants

Pet Owners with AIDS/ARC Resource Service, Inc.
P.O. Box 1116 Madison Square Station
New York, NY 10159
Telephone: (212)-744-0842
Contact: Steve Kohn
Citywide: Animal Pet-sitting for PWAs, PWARCs, HIV+

Phoenix House
164 West 74th Street
New York, NY 10023-2301
Telephone: (212)-595-5810 Fax: (212)-496-6035
Contact: Isidoro Gonzales, M.D.
Citywide: Educ.; Med. Svcs.; Confid HIV Test; Soc/Supp/Human Svcs for High-Risk

Presbyterian Hospital in the City of NY, Pastoral Care
622 West 168th Street
New York, NY 10032-3702
Telephone: (212)-305-5817 Fax: (212)-305-8008
Contact: Fred Carrigan
Spiritual/Pastoral Counseling for Hospital Patients

Reality House, Inc.
637 West 125th Street
New York, NY 10027-2319
Telephone: (212)-666-8000 Fax: (212)-666-8290
Contact: Cameron Thornhill - Community AIDS Program
HIV testing, HIV support group

Social Security Admin. Washington Heights District
4292 Broadway
New York, NY 10033
Telephone: (212)-923-2545
Contact: Stephen De Lisie
Community District 12: Entitlements and Benefits Assistance

Social Security Admin., Upper Westside, Upper Eastside
55 West 125th Street
New York, NY 10027-4592
Telephone: (212)-560-6140
Contact: Andrew Haviland
Community District 12: Entitlements/Benefits Assistance

St. John the Divine, Cathedral AIDS Ministry
1047 Amsterdam Avenue
New York, NY 10025-1798
Telephone: (212)-316-7541 Fax: (212)-932-7348
Contact: Canon-Aston Brooks
Citywide: Social, Support, Human Services for Public, High-Risk

The Tamarand Foundation, Inc.
202 Riverside Drive
Apt. 7D
New York, NY 10025-7251
Telephone: (212)-864-4245
Contact: Bruce Detrick
Recreation and social programs for PWAs, Volunteers bring roof gardens andchildren's music & art to AIDS care facilities

The Legal Aid Society, Community Law Offices
230 East 106th Street
New York, NY 10029-4000
Telephone: (212)-722-2000 Fax: (212)-876-5365
Contact: Elizabeth Hay
Comm Dists 9-12: education, outreach; legal assistance for low incomeresidents and parents with HIV & AIDS

The Patriarch Inc.
128, West 36th Street
2nd Floor
New York, NY 10018-6901
Telephone: (301)-624-6844 Fax: (201)-624-2623
Contact: Lucien J. Engelmajer - Founder
Counseling - drug rehab, detox program, vocational training

Unitarian Church of All Souls
1157 Lexington Avenue
New York, NY 10021-0440
Telephone: (212)-924-9287 Fax: (212)-535-5641
Contact: Joe Miller
Citywide: Social/Support/Human Services, HIV counseling

United Families of East Harlem
104 East 107th Street
4th Floor
New York, NY 10029-3904
Telephone: (212)-876-0367 Fax: (212)-410-4345
Contact: Paula Martin - '
Family/individual counseling

United Welfare League
20 West 104th Street
New York, NY 10025-2646
Telephone: (212)-865-4040
Contact: Mildred Dweck
Community District 7:legal assistance/human rights, adovacy, HIV assistance with benefits

Upper Room AIDS Ministry
207 West 133rd Street
New York, NY 10030
Telephone: (212)-234-3771
Contact: John Mesta
Housing, pastoral care, support, case management

Veritas Inc.
68 West 106th Street
New York, NY 10025-3855
Telephone: (212)-666-1411 Fax: (212)-666-9193
Contact: Mike Loydpeiser
Citywide: social, support, human services, AIDS counseling

Westpark Presbyterian Church
168 West 86th Street
New York, NY 10024
Telephone: (212)-362-4890
Contact: Rev Phillip Newell - Pastor
Citywide: Social/Support/Human Services for community residents

Home Health Care

Access Nursing Services
160 E. 56th Street
2nd floor
New York, NY 10022-3609
Telephone: (212)-754-4333 Fax: (212)-754-5898
Toll-Free: (800)-645-6877
Contact: Vivian Badami
Citywide: Home Nursing; infusion therapy, home health aides

Caremark
205 E. 85th Street
3rd Floor
New York, NY 10028-3046
Telephone: (212)-517-7822 Fax: (516)-753-5480
Toll-Free: (800)-522-0556
Contact: Karen Morris
Clinical Support and Infusion Therapies: Nutrition, Antimicrobials, Chemo.,Hematopoeti, home health aides, physical therapy, occupational therapy,social work, skilled nursing

Curaflex Infusion Services
200 Varick Street
6th Floor
New York, NY 10014
Telephone: (212)-627-0116
Toll-Free: (800)-677-0116
Contact: Phyllis Tarallo - General Manager
Most forms of home IV therapy connected with any HIV/AIDS related illnesses, cancer and other diseases

Harlem Hospital Center, Home Health Agency
506 Lenox Avenue, W-P 126
New York, NY 10037
Telephone: (212)-491-1639
Contact: Jolene Connor R.N.
Community Districts 9/10/11: Medical Services (Home Nursing Care)

Human Resources Administration-Home Care Services Program
109 East 16th Street
New York, NY 10003
Telephone: (212)-420-7490
Contact: Ann Gregg McIver - Deputy Commissioner

Little Sisters of the Assumption, Family Health Services
426 East 119th Street
New York, NY 10035-3626
Telephone: (212)-289-6484 Fax: (212)-348-8284
Contact: Sr. Susanne Lachapelle
Comm Dist 11: Home Nursing, Physical Therapy, Social/Support/Human Services

Salem Home Care Services, Inc.
211 West 129th Street
3rd Floor
New York, NY 10027-1902
Telephone: (212)-678-2721 Fax: (212)-316-5849
Contact: Sam Egbe
W100th/5th Ave to 228th/Broadway: Home Care Services for Elderly, Handicapped

Settlement Home Care, Inc.
219 East 115th Street
New York, NY 10029
Telephone: (212)-427-7005 Fax: (212)-996-4084
Contact: George Cortez
Home care for homebound, elderly & handicapped

Washington Heights Home Care Program, Inc.
1802 - 4 Amsterdam Avenue
New York, NY 10031-6818
Telephone: (212)-690-4830
Contact: Nkeonyelu Ebo
North of East and West 100th Street: Home Care Attendants

Medical Services

Addiction Research and Treatment Corporation
2195 Third Avenue
New York, NY 10035-3529
Telephone: (212)-348-5788
Contact: Doris Hammond
East 96-132 St./Fifth-Madison Ave.: Medical Services; Social,Support, Human Services; Confidential HIV Test

Addicts Rehabilitation Center
1881 Park Avenue
New York, NY 10035-1128
Telephone: (212)-427-1342 Fax: (212)-534-2494
Contact: Phalathia Hall
Citywide: Info, Education/Outreach; Medical Svcs; Social/Support/Human Services

Association to Benefit Children
404 East 91st Street
New York, NY 10128-6807
Telephone: (212)-996-4166 Fax: (212)-369-2107
Contact: Gretchen Buchenholz
Citywide: Med. Svcs; Confid. HIV Test; Soc/Supp/Human Svcs; Info/Educ/Outreach

Beth Israel Medical Center MMTP
250 East 25th Street
New York, NY 10010
Telephone: (212)-576-1810 Fax: (212)-213-5693
Contact: Glorice Sanders
Citywide: Med. Svcs; Confid. HIV Test; Soc/Supp/Human Svcs; Info/Educ/Outreach

Boriken Neighborhood Health Center
2253 Third Avenue, 3rd Fl
New York, NY 10035-2206
Telephone: (212)-289-6650 Fax: (212)-360-6149
Contact: Mildred Colon
Comm Dist 11: Med Svcs; Confid. HIV Test; Soc/Support/Human Svcs; Educ/Outreach, primary care center

Community League Health Clinic, Community Family Planning Council
1996 Amsterdam Avenue
New York, NY 10032
Telephone: (212)-781-7979
Contact: Lois McCartney
Citywide: Education, Outreach; Medical Services, Confidential HIV Test;Social, Support, Human Services

Day Top Village, Inc.
54 West 40th Street
Medical Dept. 4th Floor
New York, NY 10018
Telephone: (212)-354-6000
Contact: Dr. Azimah Ehr
HIV primary care

Harlem Hospital Center, Harlem MMTPIII
500 West 180th Street
New York, NY 10033
Telephone: (212)-923-4338
Contact: Leonard Ampy
Citywide: Education; Medical Svcs; Confid HIV Test; Social/Support/Human Svcs.

Incarnation Children's Center of Catholic Home Bureau
142 Audubon Avenue
New York, NY 10032-2102
Telephone: (212)-928-2590 Fax: (212)-928-5077
Contact: Sr. Bridget Kinily
Transitional residence for HIV+ children under 5. Med Svcs; Soc/Supp/Human Svcs

Lenox Clinic Renaissance Health Care
34 West 118th Street
New York, NY 10026-1904
Telephone: (212)-860-4400
Contact: Iria Miller, Eleanor Low
Citywide: Medical Services; Anonymous and Confidential HIV Testing

Metropolitan Hospital, Consultation Liaison Psychiatry
1900 2nd Avenue
Room 9M29
New York, NY 10029
Telephone: (212)-230-6262
Contact: Dr. Mary Ann Adler Cohen
Citywide: Educ/Outreach; Med Svcs; Anon. HIV Test; Social/Support/Human Svcs.

Metropolitan Hospital, Family Planning Clinic
1901 First Avenue
New York, NY 10029-7496
Telephone: (212)-230-7670 Fax: (212)-230-8050
Contact: Mairiam Kreytak
Citywide: Educ/Outreach; Med Svcs; Confid HIV Test; Social/Support/Human Svcs, referrals

Metropolitan Hospital, Youth Health Services
1918 1st Avenue
Draper Hall 14F
New York, NY 10029
Telephone: (212)-230-7408 Fax: (212)-230-8050
Contact: Merian Kreytak
Comm Dist 11: Educ/Outreach; Med Svcs; Confid HIV Test; Soc/Support/Human Svcs

Mt. Sinai Hemophilia Treatment Center
19 East 98th Street-Suite 9D
New York, NY 10029-6501
Telephone: (212)-241-5089 Fax: (212)-722-6079
Contact: Dr. Louis Aledort - Director
International: Medical Svcs; Social/Support/Human Svcs; Information/Education, orthopedics, hematology adults, pediatrics

Mt. Sinai Medical Center
1 Gustave Levy Place
P.O. Box 1009
New York, NY 10029
Telephone: (212)-241-1897 Fax: (212)-831-1127
Contact: Dr. David Rose - Director
Community District 11: Medical Services; Confid HIV Test; Human Svcs; Education

Mt. Sinai Medical Center, Narcotics Rehabilitation Center
17 East 102nd Street
New York, NY 10029-5204
Telephone: (212)-241-6646 Fax: (212)-410-6318
Contact: Dr. Vic Sturiano - Director
Boroughwide: Med Svcs; Confid HIV Test; Educ/Outreach; Soc/Supp/Human Svcs,cocaine neurobehavioral service

National Expert Care Consultation, National Recovery Institute
455 West 50th Street
New York, NY 10019
Telephone: (212)-262-6000 Fax: (212)-262-9378
Contact: Dr. Daniel Crane
Citywide: medical services; social, support, human services;education, referrals for testing, counseling

New Amsterdam Drug Mart
739 Amsterdam Avenue
New York, NY 10025-6309
Telephone: (212)-865-9700
Contact: David Ruben
Citywide: Medical Services (Pharmacy Assistance Service), no specialservice for AIDS

Polo Grounds Medical Services Renaissance Health Care
2987 8th Avenue
New York, NY 10039-1324
Telephone: (212)-281-9005
Contact: Hyacinth Kerby
Citywide: Medical Services; Anonymous and Confidential HIV Testing;Education

Presbyterian Hosp in the City of NY, HIV/AIDS Mental Health
513 West 166th Street
New York, NY 10032-4207
Telephone: (212)-305-5977 Fax: (212)-305-6440
Contact: Dr. Lucy Wicks
Citywide: Educ./Outreach; Med. Svcs.; Confid. HIV Test; Soc./Supp./Human Svcs.

Presbyterian Hospital in the City of New York, Womens & Childrens Ctr.
622 West 168th Street
New York, NY 10032-3702
Telephone: (212)-305-5000 Fax: (212)-305-4739
Contact: Alice Higgins
Citywide; Outreach; Med Svcs; Confid HIV Test; Human Svcs for Women/Children

Presbyterian Hospital in the City of NY, Family Planning
Pregnant & Young Adult Clinic
622 W. 168th St, VC-4
New York, NY 10032-3702
Telephone: (212)-305-5000 Fax: (212)-305-4739
Contact: Nancy Arceley
Citywide: Education, Outreach; Medical Services; Confidential HIV Test; ForWomen and Adolescents

Presbyterian Hospital in the City of NY, Infectious Disease
622 West 168th Street
New York, NY 10032-3702
Telephone: (212)-305-2544
Contact: Dr. Jay Dobkin
Community District 12: Medical Services; Confidential HIV Testing

Settlement House & Med Svcs, E. Harlem Settlement AIDS Program
314 East 104th Street
New York, NY 10029
Telephone: (212)-860-0401
Contact: Rick Plaisancn - Executive Director
Comm. Dist. 11: Education, Outreach; Med.,Soc.,Supp., and Human Svcs;Confidential HIV Testing

St Clare's Hospital and Health Center
Spellman Center
415 West 51st Street
New York, NY 10019
Telephone: (212)-459-8130 Fax: (212)-459-8061
Contact: Stephen Abel, DDS - Director of Dentistry
Medical services & dentistry - HIV related disease

Upper Harlem Health Community Clinic
2348 7th Avenue
New York, NY 10030-2301
Telephone: (212)-234-5800 Fax: (212)-234-6402
Contact: Dorothy McCauley
Citywide: Medical Services for General Public

William F. Ryan Community Health Center
110 West 97th Street
New York, NY 10025-6450
Telephone: (212)-749-1820 Fax: (212)-932-8323
Contact: Dean LaBate
Comm. Dists. 7, 9-10: Medical Svcs.; Confid HIV Test; Social/Support/Human Svcs

Women in Need: Alcoholism and Drug Free Outpatient Treatment
406 W. 40th Street
New York, NY 10018
Telephone: (212)-695-7330 Fax: (212)-564-2091
Contact: Noreen Legall - Intake
Outpatient Substance Abuse Treatment, Counseling, Client Childcare, Shelters

Testing Sites

Central Harlem Group, Diagnostic and Treatment Center
159 West 127th Street
New York, NY 10027-3797
Telephone: (212)-749-3507
Contact: Pat Garcia
Citywide: Medical Svcs., Confid. HIV Test; Soc./Support/Human Svcs.; Education

East Harlem Council for Human Services, Health Services
2253 3rd Avenue
New York, NY 10035-2298
Telephone: (212)-289-5651
Contact: Evelyn Gonzales
Comm. Dist. 11: Educ/Outreach; Anon HIV Test; Soc/Supp/Human Svcs for High Risk

New York City Department of Health, Community Development
125 Worth Street
P.O. Box A-1
New York, NY 10013
Telephone: (212)-285-4627
Contact: Elliott Rivera
HIV testing and counseling

New York City Dept. of Health
158 East 115th Street
Room 153
New York, NY 10029-2031
Telephone: (212)-360-5962
Citywide: Anonymous and Confidential HIV Testing; Education/Outreach

New York City Dept. of Health, Bureau of STD Control/Education
158 East 115th Street
Room 413
New York, NY 10029
Telephone: (212)-427-5120
Contact: John Thacker
Citywide: Education and Outreach; Confidential HIV Testing

Niagara County

County Health Depts

Niagara County Health Department
5467 Upper Mountain Road
Lockport, NY 14094
Telephone: (716)-439-7430 Fax: (716)-439-7440
Contact: Marie Karamanski RN
Anonymous, confidential HIV testing and counseling, for appt.(716) 847-4520

Home Health Care

Niagara Hospice
460 Wheatfield St, #201
North Tonawanda, NY 14120-7035
Telephone: (716)-731-5840
Contact: Carolyn Richel
Care for individuals facing life threatening disease, family support counseling, MSW on staff

Testing Sites

Planned Parenthood of Niagara County
Haeberle Plaza
Pine & Portage Avenues
Niagara Falls, NY 14301
Telephone: (716)-282-2501 Fax: (716)-282-2558
Contact: Mary St. Onge - Community Educator; Susan Gatley - Community Educator
HIV testing, Primary care for HIV and AIDS patients, Counseling

Oneida County

County Health Depts

Oneida County Health Dept.
800 Park Avenue
Utica, NY 13501
Telephone: (315)-798-5220
Contact: Jeane Brennan - Director

Home Health Care

Homedco Infusion
Arterial at Chenango Road
New Hartford, NY 13413
Telephone: (315)-733-5865
Contact: Michael Vicik
Respiratory, HME, equipment where necessary

Onondaga County

Home Health Care

nmc HOMECARE
6700 Thompson Rd.
Mattydale, NY 13211
Telephone: (315)-434-9393
Fax: (315)-437-7037
Contact: Jim O'Hanlon
National JCAHO-Accredited company providing a full range of Infusion and Respiratory therapies and specializing in the care of HIV/AIDS patients. National Case Manager is also available at 800-445-1188

Ontario County

County Health Depts

Ontario County Dept. of Health
3907 County Road 46
RD 2
Canandaigua, NY 14424
Telephone: (716)-396-4343
Contact: Barbara Kommer - Director

Home Health Care

nmc HOMECARE
6300 Collett West
Farmington, NY 14425
Telephone: (716)-294-0280
Fax: (716)-924-0291

Contact: Leah Sperbeck
National JCAHO-Accredited company providing a full range of Infusion and Respiratory therapies and specializing in the care of HIV/AIDS patients. National Case Manager is also available at 800-445-1188

Orange County

County Health Depts

Orange County Dept. of Health
124 Main Street
Goshen, NY 10924
Telephone: (914)-294-5151
Contact: Linda DeStefano - Coord.
Services fund for primary care and support to medically indigent personswith HIV/AIDS

Orange County Dept. of Health, HIV Prevention
72 Broadway
Newburgh, NY 10924
Telephone: (914)-569-1571
Contact: Sally Dorfman - MD

Orleans County

Community Services

AIDS Task Force of Orleans County
Human Service Council
14012 Rout 31 West
Albion, NY 14411
Telephone: (716)-589-7004 Fax: (716)-589-6647
Contact: Kerry Perese
HIV counseling, testing, TB testing, education

County Health Depts

Orleans County Health Department
14012 Route 31 West
Albion, NY 14411
Telephone: (716)-589-7004 Fax: (716)-589-6647
Contact: Andrew Lucyszyn - Public Health Director
HIV education and counseling

Testing Sites

Planned Parenthood - Orleans
168 S Main Street
Albion, NY 14411
Telephone: (716)-589-5681 Fax: (716)-589-1613
Anonymous, confidential HIV testing & counseling

Queens County

Home Health Care

Homedco Infusion
60-71 Metropolitan Avenue
Ridgewood, NY 11385
Telephone: (800)-422-5545
Contact: Ellen Scharaga - 718-456-2010
TPN, Antibiotic Therapy, Chemotherapy, Enteral, Hydration, Pain Management, Aerosolized Penta

Rockland County

County Health Depts

Rockland County Dept. of Health
Robert L. Yeager Health Center
Sanatorium Road, Bldg. D
Pomona, NY 10970
Telephone: (914)-364-2500
Contact: Angela Usobiaga - Public Health Coord.; Scott Sullam - Case Manager
Case management, primary care

Saint Lawrence County

Home Health Care

nmc HOMECARE
900 Champlain St.
Ogdensburg, NY 13669
Telephone: (315)-393-4879
Fax: (315)-393-9404
Contact: Jim O'Hanlon
National JCAHO-Accredited company providing a full range of Infusion and Respiratory therapies and specializing in the care of HIV/AIDS patients. National Case Manager is also available at 800-445-1188

Suffolk County

Community Services

Olsten Kimberly Quality Care
90 West Main Street
Smithtown, NY 11787
Telephone: (516)-366-1900 Fax: (516)-366-1904
Contact: Doreen Gargano
Leading provider in home health care and staffing services.

County Health Depts

Suffolk County Health Department, Division of Patient Care
225 Rabro Drive East
Hauppauge, NY 11788
Telephone: (516)-853-2905
Contact: Mary J. Finnin, MS,RN - Primary Care AIDS Nurse
9 clinics HIV testing (confidental), primary care services, home care

Ulster County

Home Health Care

Homedco Infusion
625 Sawkill Road
Kingston, NY 12401-1710
Telephone: (914)-336-3333
Toll-Free: (800)-831-9398
Contact: Joan Tenchar - Branch Manager
Respiratory, HME, Infusion Therapy

Westchester County

Community Services

AIDS Related Community Services
2269 Saw Mill River Road
Building 1
Elmsford, NY 10523
Telephone: (914)-345-8888 Fax: (914)-785-8227
Toll-Free: (800)-992-1442
Contact: Barbara Shannon
NY State Dept of Health AIDS Institute Community Service Provider

Home Health Care

Critical Care America
100 Corporate Dr
Yonkers, NY 10701
Telephone: (914)-376-6510 Fax: (914)-379-6540
Toll-Free: (800)-284-6510
Contact: Nancy Vincent
Coordinate & integrate all clinical & psychosocial services for HIV+

Homedco Infusion
8 Westchester Plaza
Elmsford, NY 10523
Telephone: (914)-592-1410
Contact: Barbara Fiori - Branch Manager
Respiratory, HME, Infusion Therapy

Olsten Kimberly Quality HealthCare
213 Main Street
Mount Kisco, NY 10549
Telephone: (914)-241-3033 Fax: (914)-241-2835
Contact: Phyllis Danello - Coordinator
Home care & nursing services

Medical Services

Westchester County Medical Center
Grasslands Reservation
Valhalia, NY 10595
Telephone: (914)-285-7700 Fax: (914)-285-7289
Contact: Nadine H. Latterman, MPH - Dir. Patient Care Services
In-patient & outpatient, dental referrals; education, testing, mobilemedical unit

Wyoming County

County Health Depts

Wyoming County Health Department
338 North Main Street
Warsaw, NY 14569-1025
Telephone: (716)-786-8890
Contact: Audrey Parmele, RN - Public Health Director
Anonymous, confidential HIV testing, counseling & home care

NORTH CAROLINA

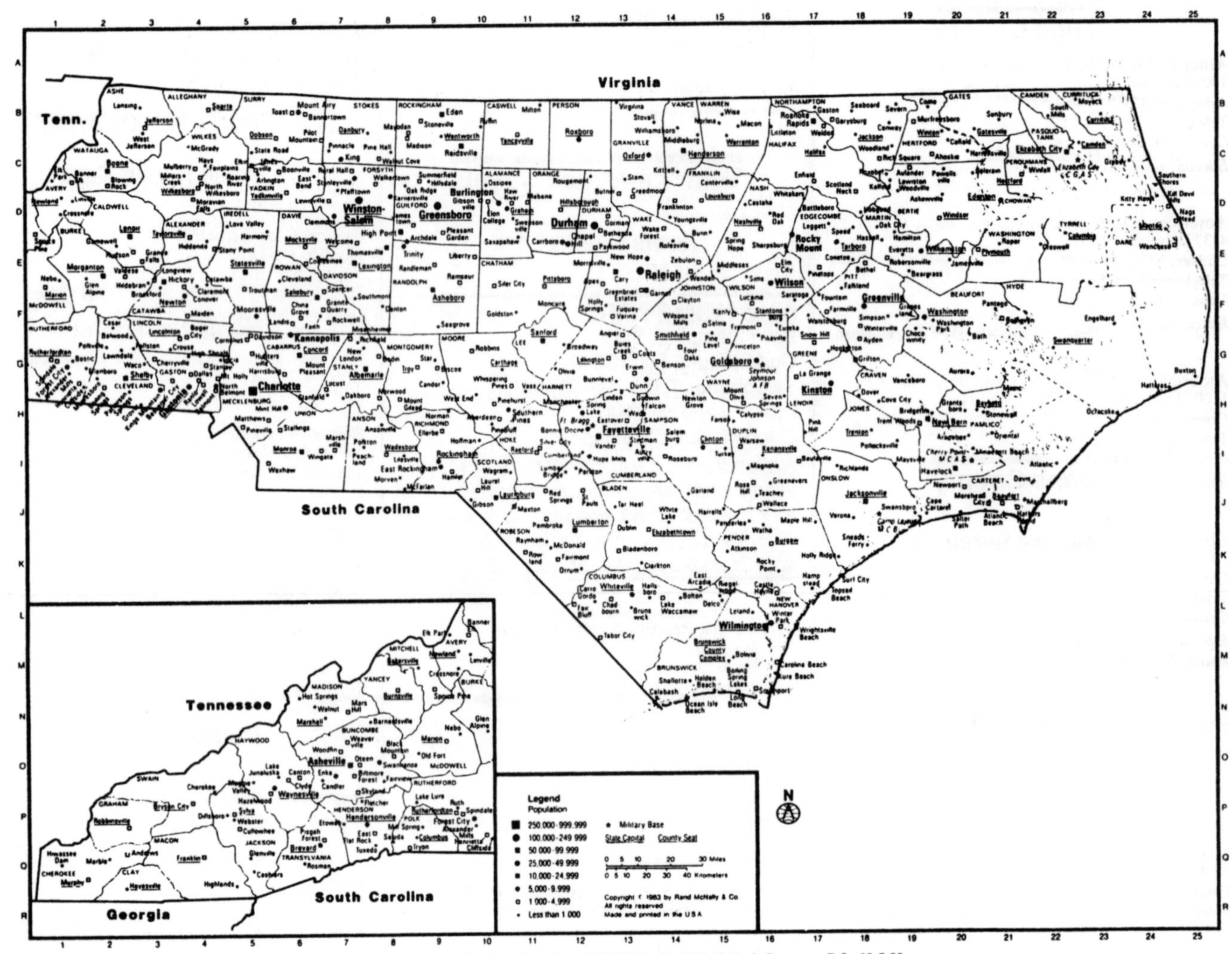

From City/County Planning Atlas Copyright 1989 by Reed McNally & Company, R.L. 90-S-28

North Carolina

General Services

Education

American Red Cross, Asheville Area Chapter
100 Edgewood Road
Asheville, NC 28804-3597
Telephone: (704)-258-3888
Contact: Harriet Williams
Education, Community Services

American Red Cross, Durham County Chapter
4737 University Drive
Durham, NC 27707-1806
Telephone: (919)-489-6541
Contact: Sherron Williams
Education, Community Services

American Red Cross, Greensboro Chapter
1100 Church Street
Greensboro, NC 27401-1008
Telephone: (919)-273-4481
Contact: Kim Mroski
Education, Community Services

Charlotte Area Health Education Center
P.O. Box 32861
Charlotte, NC 28232
Telephone: (704)-338-3120
Contact: Dr. William Williams - Director
Education for health care providers, medical, mental health,pharmaceutical, home care

Fayetteville Area Health Education Center
1601-B Owen Drive
Fayetteville, NC 28304-3425
Telephone: (919)-323-1152
Contact: Dr. Charles Ellenbogen

Greensboro Area Health Education Center
1200 N. Elm Street
Greensboro, NC 27401-1004
Telephone: (919)-379-4025

Lee-Harnett MH/MR/SAS
P.O. Box 457
Buies Creek, NC 27605-0457
Telephone: (919)-892-5008
Residential Detoxification Program, For South Central Region

Mountain Area Health Education Center
501 Biltmore Avenue
Asheville, NC 28801-4601
Telephone: (704)-257-4440

Northwest Area Health Education Center
Medical Center Blvd.
Winston-Salem, NC 27157
Telephone: (919)-777-3000
Contact: Ann Graves
Health education

Opportunities Industrialization Center, Inc.
P.O. Box 2723
402 E Virginia
Rocky Mount, NC 27801-2723
Telephone: (919)-977-3731
Contact: Pat Hunter
Projects for AIDS Risk Reducation and Minority Education

Southlight
2500 Blue Ridge Road
Suite 400
Raleigh, NC 27607
Telephone: (919)-832-4453
Contact: Trudy Harris
Projects for AIDS Risk Reduction among Intravenous Drug Users, Education

Step One, AIDS Task Force of Winston-Salem
5445 North Trade Street
Winston-Salem, NC 27101
Telephone: (919)-732-5031
Contact: Sandra Smith
Projects for AIDS Risk Reducation among Intravenous Drug Users, Education

Teens Against AIDS
St. Augustine's College
Robinson Library, Rm 207
Raleigh, NC 27602-9299
Telephone: (919)-828-4451
Contact: Angela Cloud
Projects for AIDS risk reduction and minority education

Tuscarora Tribe of North Carolina, Inc.
P.O. Box 8
106 Main Street
Pembroke, NC 28372-1455
Telephone: (919)-521-3231
Contact: Barbara Graham
Projects for AIDS risk reduction and minority education

Wake Area Health Education Center
300 New Bern Avenue
Raleigh, NC 27610-1418
Telephone: (919)-755-8548
Medical seminars

Wilmington Area Health Education Center
2131 S. 17th Street
Wilmington, NC 28402-7407
Telephone: (919)-343-0161
Education

State Health Departments

North Carolina Dept. of Environment, Health and Natural Resources
Education & Training
PO Box 27867
Raleigh, NC 27611-7687
Telephone: (919)-733-7081 Fax: (919)-715-3144
Contact: Claudia Egelhoff - Training Coordinator

North Carolina Dept.of Environment, Health & Nat'l.Resources
Division of Adult Health, HIV Service Unit
P.O. Box 27687
Raleigh, NC 27611-7687
Telephone: (919)-733-7081
Contact: Hope K. Lucas - Program Manager
Ryan White Program & Housing Program.

Statewide Services

Health Education Foundation of Eastern North Carolina
P.O. Box 7368
Rocky Mount, NC 27804-0368
Telephone: (919)-972-6958

Alamance County

Community Services

Salvation Army
P.O. Box 2581
2345 La Vista Drive
Burlington, NC 27215-2581
Telephone: (919)-227-5529
Food assistance, emergencies

County Health Depts

Alamance County Health Department and Home Health Agency
209 N. Graham-Hopedale Rd
Burlington, NC 27217
Telephone: (919)-227-0101
AIDS/HIV Education, Counseling and Testing

Home Health Care

Community Care, Inc.
Eric Lane
Burlington, NC 27215-5757
Telephone: (919)-229-6919
In-Home Aides and Private Duty Services

Home Care Providers
421 Alamance Road
Burlington, NC 27215
Telephone: (919)-228-1307
Contact: Dorothy Moseley
Home care

MedVisit, Inc.
1111 Huffman Mill Road
Burlington, NC 27215
Telephone: (919)-229-7110
Contact: Sue Cliffton
Home care

MedVisit, Inc.
1111 Huffman Mill Rd
Burlington, NC 27215-8862
Telephone: (919)-538-0670 Fax: (919)-538-0980
Home Care and Hospice Services

Medical Services

Alamance Cares
2501 South Mebane Street
Burlington, NC 27215-2965
Telephone: (910)-570-5325 Fax: (910)-570-4477
Contact: David Atkins
Case management, support groups, AIDS education, transportation, buddyprogram

Alexander County

Community Services

Alexander County Department of Social Services
322 1st Avenue, SW
Taylorsville, NC 28681
Telephone: (704)-632-9723
Medical, Financial, Social, Psychological Services

County Health Depts

Alexander County Health Department and Home Health Agency
322 First Avenue, SW
Taylorsville, NC 28681-2493
Telephone: (704)-632-9704
Medical Services, Education, Counseling and Testing, Home Health Care

Home Health Care

Hospice of Alexander County, Inc.
412 3rd Street SW
Taylorsville, NC 28681-3004
Telephone: (704)-632-5026
Contact: Lynn Chambera, R.N. - Patient Care Coordinator
Home Care and Hospice Services for AIDS patients: nursing, emotionalsupport

Alleghany County

Community Services

Alleghany County Department of Social Services
Doctor's Street
Sparta, NC 28675
Telephone: (910)-372-2411 Fax: (910)-372-2635
Contact: Sandra Ashley
Medical, Financial, Social, Psychological Services

Community Action Mission
P.O. Box 116
Laurel Springs, NC 28644
Telephone: (919)-359-2246
Emergency Shelter and Food Assistance

County Health Depts

Alleghany County Health Department (Appalachian Health Dist)
Route 2, Box 36
Hospital Street
Sparta, NC 28675-9616
Telephone: (919)-372-5641
Medical Services, Education, Free Counseling and Testing, Home Health Care

Amelia County

Home Health Care

Interim Health Care
2401 Robison Street
Fayetteville, NC 23105
Telephone: (919)-483-6144 Fax: (919)-483-6049
Home Care and Hospice Services includes AIDS services

Anson County

Community Services

Anson County Department of Social Services
118 N. Washington Street
Wadesboro, NC 28170-2235
Telephone: (704)-694-9351
Contact: Jeanete Brown
Medical, Financial, Social, Psychological Services

County Health Depts

Anson County Health Department
110 Ashe Street
Wadesboro, NC 28170
Telephone: (704)-694-5188
Medical Services, Education, Counseling and Testing

Home Health Care

St Joseph Hospital Home Health Agency
Hospice of Anson County
P.O. Box 974
Wadesboro, NC 28170-0974
Telephone: (704)-694-5992 Fax: (704)-694-6419
Contact: Kathy Appenzeller - Director of Operations
Home care visits & hospice care for AIDS patients, family counseling

St. Joseph Hospital Home Health Agency
117 Wortham Street
PO Box 974
Wadesboro, NC 28170-0974
Telephone: (704)-692-2212
Home Care and Hospice Services

Ashe County

County Health Depts

Ashe County Health Department (Appalachian Health District)
McConnell Street
PO Box 208
Jefferson, NC 28640-0208
Telephone: (919)-246-9449
Medical Services, Education, Counseling and Testing, Home Health Care

Home Health Care

Ashe County Council on Aging
P.O. Box 190
McConnell Street
Jefferson, NC 28640-0181
Telephone: (919)-246-2461
In-Home Aides and Private Duty Services

Avery County

County Health Depts

Avery County Health Department
P.O. Box 325
Newland, NC 28657-0325
Telephone: (704)-733-6031
Medical Services, Education, Counseling and Testing

Home Health Care

Hospice of Avery County, Inc.
P.O. Box 221
Newland, NC 28657-0221
Telephone: (704)-898-8581
Home Care and Hospice Services

Beaufort County

Community Services

Emergency Management
P.O. Box 124
Washington, NC 27889-0124
Telephone: (919)-946-2046
Contact: Daden Wolfe
Emergency Shelter and Food Assistance

Salvation Army
P.O. Box 877
Washington, NC 27889-0877
Telephone: (919)-946-2523 Fax: (919)-946-1048
Contact: Major Floyd Langley
Emergency Shelter and Food Assistance

County Health Depts

Beaufort County Health Department
P.O. Box 579
Washington, NC 27889-0579
Telephone: (919)-946-1902
Contact: Al Gerard - Minority Education
Medical Services, Counseling and Testing, Minority Education Project

Home Health Care

Aurora Home Health Agency
Highway 33
PO Box 40
Aurora, NC 27806
Telephone: (919)-322-7181 Fax: (919)-322-7219
Toll-Free: (800)-682-0019
Contact: Ed Wilder
Home Care and Hospice Services

Medical Services

Tideland Mental Health Center
1308 Highland Drive
Washington, NC 27889-3494
Telephone: (919)-946-8061 Fax: (919)-946-8078
Toll-Free: (800)-682-0767
Contact: Lynda Watkins; Janice Wynne -
Mental health services, education, substance abuse counseling

Bertie County

Community Services

Bertie County Department of Social Services
Wayland Street
Windsor, NC 27983
Telephone: (919)-794-4841
Medical,Financial,Social, and Psychological Services

County Health Depts

Bertie County Health Department and Home Health Agency
P.O. Box 586
Barringer & Wayland Sts.
Windsor, NC 27983-0586
Telephone: (919)-794-2057
Contact: Joanne Jordan
Medical Services, Education, Counseling and Testing, Home Health Care

Bladen County

Community Services

Bladen County Department of Social Services
PO Box 365
Elizabethtown, NC 28337
Telephone: (919)-862-4181
Medical,Financial,Social and Psychological Services

County Health Depts

Bladen County Health Department
300 Mercer Road
PO Box 188
Elizabethtown, NC 28337-0188
Telephone: (910)-862-6900 Fax: (910)-862-6859
Contact: Debbie Long
Medical Services, Education, Counseling and Testing

Home Health Care

Lower Cape Fear Hospice, Inc.-Bladen
PO Box 2452
103 North Morehead
Elizabethtown, NC 28337-2452
Telephone: (919)-862-3111
Home Care and Hospice Services

Brunswick County

County Health Depts

Brunswick County Health Department
P.O. Box 9
Bolivia, NC 28422-0009
Telephone: (919)-253-4381
Contact: Michael Rhodes
Medical Services, Education, Counseling and HIV testing

Buncombe County

Community Services

Pisgah Legal Services
89 Montford Avenue
Asheville, NC 28802-2529
Telephone: (919)-483-0400
Legal Services

County Health Depts

Buncombe County Health Department and Home Health Agency
35 Woodfin Street
Asheville, NC 28801-3072
Telephone: (704)-255-5671
Medical Services, Education, Counseling and Testing, Home Health Care

Home Health Care

Interim Health Care
168 Patton Avenue
Asheville, NC 28801
Telephone: (704)-253-0301 Fax: (704)-252-1909
Contact: Margaret White - Administrator
Home Care and Hospice Services for AIDS patients in terminal phase; skilled nursing; physical therapy

Medical Services

Blue Ridge Center for MH/MR/SA
356 Biltmore Avenue
Asheville, NC 28801-4594
Telephone: (704)-258-3500 Fax: (704)-258-1225
Contact: Charlie Schoenheit
Mental health services, substance abuse, development disabilities

Burke County

Community Services

Catawba Valley Legal Services, Inc.
200 Avery Avenue
Morganton, NC 28655-3100
Telephone: (704)-437-8280 Fax: (704)-437-9397
Contact: John Vail
Legal Services

County Health Depts

Burke County Health Department and Home Health Agency
700 East Parker Road
PO Box 1266
Morganton, NC 28655-1266
Telephone: (704)-433-4250
Medical Services, Education, Counseling and Testing, Home Health Care

Cabarrus County

County Health Depts

Cabarrus County Health Department
715 Cabarrus Avenue W
PO Box 1149
Concord, NC 28025-1149
Telephone: (704)-786-8121
Contact: Huey Garvin - AIDS Task Force
Medical Services, Counseling, Testing, Information, Education, AIDS TaskForce

Home Health Care

Cabarrus County Home Health Agency
P.O. Box 707
46 McCachem Boulevard SE
Concord, NC 28026-0707
Telephone: (704)-788-8180 Fax: (704)-788-9876
Home Care and Hospice Services

CMH Home Care
487 Lake Concord Road
PO Box 3374
Concord, NC 28025-3374
Telephone: (704)-788-5919
Contact: Carolyn Sherril
Home Care and Hospice Services

Hospice of Cabarrus County, Inc.
P.O. Box 1235
60 Diploma Place Southeast
Concord, NC 28026
Telephone: (704)-788-9434 Fax: (704)-788-6013
Home Care and Hospice Services

Medical Personnel Pool of Metrolina, Inc.
141 Providence Road
Charolette, NC 28027
Telephone: (704)-372-8230
Home Care and Hospice Services

Caldwell County

County Health Depts

Caldwell County Health Department
321 Mulberry Street, SW
Lenoir, NC 28645-5720
Telephone: (704)-758-8451
Medical Services, Education, Counseling and Testing

Home Health Care

Caldwell County Health Department Home Health Agency
1966 B Morganton Blvd.
Lenoir, NC 28645-4523
Telephone: (704)-758-8451
Contact: Ann Allen
Home care

Caldwell County Hospice, Inc.
902 Kirkwood Street
Lenoir, NC 28645-5121
Telephone: (704)-754-0101 Fax: (704)-757-3335
Home care and hospice services, ALFA, in patient care

Caldwell County Mental Health Center
606 College Avenue S.W.
Lenoir, NC 28645
Telephone: (704)-754-4551 Fax: (704)-563-0911
Mental Health Services

Camden County

County Health Depts

Camden County Health Department
P.O. Box 72
Camden, NC 27921-0072
Telephone: (919)-335-4486
Medical Services, Education, Counseling and Testing

Carteret County

County Health Depts

Carteret County Health Department
402 Broad Street
Beaufort, NC 28516
Telephone: (919)-728-8550
Medical Services, Education, Counseling and Testing

Home Health Care

Hospice of Carteret County, Inc.
P.O. Box 3598
107 South 9th Street
Morehead City, NC 28557-5598
Telephone: (919)-247-4800 Fax: (919)-247-2808
Home Care and Hospice Services

Tar Heel Home Health Care
1410 Arendell Street
Morehead City, NC 28557
Telephone: (919)-726-9300
Home Care and Hospice Services

Caswell County

County Health Depts

Caswell County Health Department
P.O. Drawer H
Yanceyville, NC 27379-2002
Telephone: (919)-694-4129
Contact: Sharon Kupit - Physician's Asst.
Medical Services, Education, Counseling and Testing

Home Health Care

Community Care, Inc.
P.O. Box 400
Yanceyville, NC 27379-0400
Telephone: (919)-694-9905
In-Home Aids and Private Duty Services, casual care, support groups

Catawba County

Community Services

AIDS Leadership/Foothills Area Alliance
P.O. Box 2987
Hickory, NC 28603
Telephone: (704)-433-4295
Contact: Michele Francois
Support Groups, Buddy Program, Speakers, Educational Workshops, Referrals

County Health Depts

Catawba County Health Department and Home Health Agency
Route 3, Box 338
Hickory, NC 28601-0338
Telephone: (704)-328-2561
Medical Services, Education, Counseling and Testing, Home Health Care

Home Health Care

Frye Home Health Services
420 N. Center Street
Hickory, NC 28601-5033
Telephone: (704)-324-3025 Fax: (704)-327-8741
Home Care and Hospice Services

Chatham County

Community Services

Chatham County Department of Social Services
Graham Road
Pittsboro, NC 27312
Telephone: (919)-542-2759 Fax: (919)-542-6355
Contact: Robert E. Hall
Medical,Financial,Social and Psychological Services

Joint Orange-Chatham Community Action
P.O. Box 27
Pittsboro, NC 27312-0027
Telephone: (919)-542-4781 Fax: (919)-542-0563
Contact: Gloria Williams
Comprehensive homeless services, nutrition assistance, job training,information and referrals

Salvation Army
P.O. Box 752
Pittsboro, NC 27312-0752
Telephone: (919)-542-4781 Fax: (919)-542-0563
Contact: Shiela Crump
Emergency Shelter and Food Assistance

County Health Depts

Chatham County Health Department
P.O. Box 126
Pittsboro, NC 27312-0126
Telephone: (919)-542-8220
Contact: Brenda Truitt - RN, Nursing Supervisor
Medical Services, Education, Counseling and Testing for HIV

Chatham County Health Department
Chatham Co. Office Bldg.
Pittsboro, NC 27312
Telephone: (919)-742-5641
Medical Services, Education, Counseling and Testing

Home Health Care

Chatham County Council on Aging
P.O. Box 212
Pittsboro, NC 27312-0212
Telephone: (919)-542-4512
In-Home Aides and Private Duty Services

Hospice of Chatham County
P.O.Box 1077
Pittsboro, NC 27312-1077
Telephone: (919)-542-5545
Home Care and Hospice Services

Cherokee County

County Health Depts

Cherokee County Health Department
206 Hilton Street
Murphy, NC 28906-2899
Telephone: (704)-837-7486
Medical services, education, counseling and testing, HIV/STD testing &counseling

Chowan County

Community Services

Chowan County Department of Social Services
P.O. Box # 296
Edenton, NC 27932
Telephone: (919)-482-7441 Fax: (919)-482-4925
Contact: Ben Rose
Medical, Financial, Social and Psychological Services

Community Action
P.O. Box 549
Edenton, NC 27932-0549
Telephone: (919)-482-4458 Fax: (919)-482-7564
Contact: Fentress Morris
Emergency Shelter and Food Assistance

Emergency Management Office
208 West Hicks Street
Edenton, NC 27932-1030
Telephone: (919)-482-4365 Fax: (919)-482-7940
Contact: Douglas Belch
Emergency medical, AIDS awareness

County Health Depts

Chowan County Health Department
County Office Building
PO Box 808
Edenton, NC 27932-0808
Telephone: (919)-482-2511
Medical services, education, counseling, HIV/STD testing

Clay County

Community Services

Clay County Department of Social Services
Community Services Bldg.
PO Box 147
Hayesville, NC 28904
Telephone: (704)-389-6301
Contact: Sandra Henderson
Medical, Financial, Social, and Psychological Services

County Health Depts

Clay County Health Department
PO Box 55
Hayesville, NC 28904-0055
Telephone: (704)-389-8052
Medical services, education, counseling and testing, STD/HIV testing &counseling

Home Health Care

Good Shepherd Home Health Agency
P.O. Box 465
Main Street
Hayesville, NC 28904-0465
Telephone: (704)-389-6311
Home Care and Hospice Services

Mountain Home Nursing Services, Inc.
P.O. Box 1306
US Highway 64 Bypass
Hayesville, NC 28904-0306
Telephone: (704)-389-8106
Home Care and Hospice Services

Cleveland County

Community Services

Cleveland County Department of Social Services
County Office Building
Shelby, NC 28150
Telephone: (704)-487-0661 Fax: (704)-484-1051
Contact: Andrea Moss
Medical, Financial, Social, and Psychological Services

Salvation Army
P.O. Box 1764
Shelby, NC 28151-1764
Telephone: (704)-482-0375 Fax: (704)-482-8710
Contact: Major Simmons
Emergency Shelter and Food Assistance

United Way
P.O. Box 2242
Shelby, NC 28151-2242
Telephone: (704)-482-7344 Fax: (704)-482-9662
Contact: Barbara Long
Emergency shelter and food assistance; information & referrals

County Health Depts

Cleveland County Health Department
315 Grover Street
Shelby, NC 28150-3998
Telephone: (704)-484-5200
Education, counseling, anonymous and confidential testing with outappointment

Home Health Care

Cleveland Home Health Agency, Inc.
P.O. Box 2247
719 Grover Street
Shelby, NC 28151-2247
Telephone: (704)-487-5225 Fax: (704)-484-7235
Contact: Katherine Ramsey, R.N. - Nursing Supervisor
Home care and hospice services, terminal phase patient services, skillednursing and therapy

Cleveland Home Health Agency, Inc.
719 Grover Street
PO Box 2247
Shelby, NC 28151-2247
Telephone: (704)-487-5225
Home Care and Hospice Services

Hospice of Cleveland County, Inc.
201 West Marion Street
Suite 306
Shelby, NC 28150-5361
Telephone: (704)-487-4677
Home Care and Hospice Services

Columbus County

Community Services

Emergency Management
111 Washington Street
Room 27
Whiteville, NC 28472-3323
Telephone: (910)-642-4728 Fax: (910)-640-1241
Contact: John H. Moore, Jr.
Emergency Shelter and Food Assistance

County Health Depts

Columbus County Health Department and Home Health Agency
P.O. Box 810
Miller Building
Whiteville, NC 28472-0810
Telephone: (919)-642-5700
Home health care

Home Health Care

Columbus County Hospice, Inc.
121 West Main Street
Whiteville, NC 28472-3602
Telephone: (919)-642-9051
Home Care and Hospice Services

Comprehensive Home Health Care I, Inc.
P.O. Box 366
902 Jefferson Street
Whiteville, NC 28472-0366
Telephone: (919)-642-5808 Fax: (919)-640-1374
Home Care and Hospice Services

Comprehensive Home Health Care I, Inc.
902 Jefferson Street
PO Box 366
Whiteville, NC 28472-0366
Telephone: (919)-642-5808
Home Care and Hospice Services

Lower Cape Fear Hospice, Inc.-Columbus
P.O.Box 636
Whiteville, NC 28472-0636
Telephone: (919)-762-0200
Home Care and Hospice Services

Medical Personnel Pool--Whiteville
1402 Liberty Street
PO Box 1557
Whiteville, NC 28472-1595
Telephone: (919)-642-2106
Home Care and Hospice Services

Medical Personnel Pool-Whiteville
P.O. Box 1595
1402 Liberty Street
Whiteville, NC 28472-1595
Telephone: (919)-642-2106
Home Care and Hospice Services

Craven County

Community Services

Craven County Department of Social Services
2818 Neuse Blvd.
PO Box 12039
New Bern, NC 28561
Telephone: (919)-633-0131
Medical, Financial, and Social Services

County Health Depts

Craven County Health Department and Home Health-Hospice
2100 Neuse Blvd
PO Box 1390
New Bern, NC 28560-1390
Telephone: (919)-633-4121
Medical services, education, counseling, testing and home health care

Home Health Care

Craven County Health Department Home Health-Hospice Agency
2102 Neuse Blvd
PO Box 12610
New Bern, NC 28560-1390
Telephone: (919)-633-4121
Contact: Wanda Sandle - Director
Home care and hospice services, HIV testing, counselingand educational services

Craven Regional Medical Center
2500 Trent Road, #36
New Bern, NC 28562-2007
Telephone: (919)-633-8186 Fax: (919)-633-8144
Contact: Kathryn Krauss
Home Care and Hospice Services

Medical Services

Neuse Center for MH/MR/SA
2102 Neuse Boulevard
New Bern, NC 28560
Telephone: (919)-633-4171 Fax: (919)-633-3930
Contact: Millard Godwin - Director
Mental health services counseling, referrals

Cumberland County

Community Services

Cumberland County Department of Social Services
P.O. Box 2429
Fayetteville, NC 28302-2429
Telephone: (910)-323-4292
Contact: Marvin Rouse
Emergency Shelter and Food Assistance; in-home aide, transportation, carecenter, protective services.

Cumberland Emergency Management Agency
131 Dick Street
Fayetteville, NC 28301-5750
Telephone: (910)-483-3903
Contact: John McInnius
Coordinates emergency shelter and food assistance, 24 hour dispatch

Salvation Army
P.O. Box 514
Fayetteville, NC 28302-0514
Telephone: (919)-483-8119
Contact: Major Robert Melton
Emergency Shelter and Food Assistance

County Health Depts

Cumberland County Health Department
227 Fountainhead Lane
Fayetteville, NC 28301-5417
Telephone: (919)-433-3783
Medical services, education, HIV/STD counseling and testing

Home Health Care

Cape Fear Valley Home Health Care
P.O. Box 2000
Owen Drive
Fayetteville, NC 28302-2000
Telephone: (910)-323-6740 Fax: (910)-609-6573
Contact: Patricia Prescott - Director
Home Care and Hospice Services for AIDS patients: nursing & emotionalsupport

Cape Fear Valley Home Health Care
3357 Village Drive
Fayetteville, NC 28304
Telephone: (919)-323-6740
Home Care and Hospice Services

Cape Fear Valley Home Health Care
3358 Village Drive
Suite 100
Fayetteville, NC 28304
Telephone: (919)-323-6740
Contact: Pat Prescott
Home Care and Hospice Services includes AIDS

Comprehensive Home Health Care II, Inc.
1800 Ski Bo
Suite 228
Fayetteville, NC 28303
Telephone: (919)-323-2423
Home Care and Hospice Services

Comprehensive Home Health Care II, Inc.
1800 Skibo
Suite 228
Fayetteville, NC 28303
Telephone: (919)-323-2423
Home Care and Hospice Services

Hospice of Harnett County, Inc.
111-A North Ellis Avenue
Dunn, NC 28344-3804
Telephone: (910)-892-1213
Contact: Grace Tart - Administrator
Home Care and Hospice Services for AIDS patients in terminal phase, skillednursing, andfamily support

Currituck County

Community Services

Currituck County Department of Social Services
1 Court House
P.O. Box 99
Currituck, NC 27929-9998
Telephone: (919)-232-3083 Fax: (919)-232-2167
Medical, Financial, Social and Psychological Services

County Health Depts

Currituck County Health Department
P.O.Box 26
Currituck, NC 27929-0026
Telephone: (919)-232-2271
Medical Services, Education, Counseling and Testing

Dare County

Home Health Care

Dare County Home Health Services
P.O. Box 1000
Main Highway
Manteo, NC 27954
Telephone: (919)-473-1101
Home care, AIDS support group

Davidson County

Community Services

Community Action
P.O. Box 389
Lexington, NC 27293-0389
Telephone: (704)-249-0234 Fax: (704)-294-2078
Contact: Sandra Sanchez
Self sufficiency programs & some emergency money

Davidson County Department of Social Services
915 North Main Street
Lexington, NC 27292
Telephone: (704)-249-9134
Medical, Financial, Social and Psychological Services

Meals-on-Wheels
106 East Dale Drive
Lexington, NC 27292
Telephone: (704)-246-5456
Contact: Charlotte Fulp
Food assistance

Salvation Army
P.O. Box 770
Lexington, NC 27293-0770
Telephone: (704)-249-0336
Contact: Rena Thore
Emergency shelter, food, medical, rent and utilities assistance

Home Health Care

Home Health Professionals
1501 Winston Road
Lexington, NC 27292-1450
Telephone: (704)-249-0382
Home Care Services

Hospice of Davidson County, Inc.
524 South State Street
PO Box 1941
Lexington, NC 27292-1941
Telephone: (704)-246-6185
Home Care and Hospice Services

Davie County

Community Services

Yadkin Valley Economic Development Dist
622 North Main Street
Mocksville, NC 27028-2122
Telephone: (704)-634-2188
Emergency Shelter and Food Assistance

Duplin County

Community Services

Duplin County Department of Social Services
Welfare Building
P.O. Box 439
Kenansville, NC 28349
Telephone: (919)-296-1457
Medical, Financial, Social and Psycological Services

Home Health Care

Duplin County Services for the Aged
Seminary Street
PO Box 367
Kenansville, NC 28349-0367
Telephone: (919)-296-2140
In-Home Aides and Private Duty Services

Duplin Home Care and Hospice, Inc.
Duplin St, Duplin Gen Hos
PO Box 887
Kenansville, NC 28349-0235
Telephone: (919)-296-0819
Contact: Lynn Hardy
Home Care and Hospice Services

Durham County

Community Services

Community Kitchen
112 North Queen Street
Durham, NC 27701-3751
Telephone: (919)-688-7378
Contact: Betsy Rollins
Food assistance

Durham AIDS Network, Durham Health Department
414 E. Main Street
Durham, NC 27701-3720
Telephone: (919)-560-7768 Fax: (919)-560-7664
Contact: Kathy Kerr - Health Educator
HIV early interview treatment, HIV testing and counseling, training,technical assistance, policy development and case management

Durham County Department of Social Services
220 East Main Street
PO Box 810
Durham, NC 27702-0810
Telephone: (919)-683-3500
Contact: Gale Hallenbeck - Assistant Director
Medical, financial, social, psychological services and home care

Meals-on-Wheels
112 N. Queen Street
Durham, NC 27701-3751
Telephone: (919)-682-7255
Contact: Dorothy Scott
Food assistance

North Central Legal Assistance Program
301 West Main Street
Durham, NC 27702-3227
Telephone: (919)-688-6396
Contact: Judith E. Washington
Legal Services

County Health Depts

Durham County Health Department
414 East Main Street
Durham, NC 27701
Telephone: (919)-560-7600
STD services, HIV counseling and testing, case management, early intervention, information and family planning.

Home Health Care

Coordinating Council for Senior Citizens, Durham
519 East Main Street
Durham, NC 27701-3701
Telephone: (919)-682-8104
In-Home aides and private duty services

Durham Health Department, Visiting Nurse Service
414 East Main Street
Durham, NC 27701
Telephone: (919)-560-7700
Home care and hospice services, STD division, HIV counsel testing

Interim Health Care
3326 Chapel Hill Blvd.
Suite 230, Building A
Durham, NC 27707-2646
Telephone: (919)-929-4396 Fax: (919)-493-0454
Home Care and Hospice Services

Medical Personnel Pool of Raleigh/Durham
3326 Chapel Hill Blvd.
Suite 230, Building A
Durham, NC 27707-2646
Telephone: (919)-493-7575
Home Care and Hospice Services

MedVisit, Inc.
411 Andrews Road
Suite 240
Durham, NC 27705
Telephone: (919)-383-4444
Home Care and Hospice Services

MedVisit, Inc.
411 Andrews Road
Suite 142
Durham, NC 27705-2993
Telephone: (919)-383-0305
Contact: Jack Pleasant
Home Care and Hospice Services

New England Critical Care
4020 Stirrup Crk Road
Suite 111
Durham, NC 27703
Telephone: (919)-544-7747 Fax: (919)-544-7769
Superior, quality, traditional and innovative infusion therapies in home

Olsten Kimberly Quality Care
3622 Lyckan Parkway
Suite 6008
Durham, NC 27707-3939
Telephone: (919)-419-1700 Fax: (919)-419-1750
Toll-Free: (800)-695-0373
Contact: Craig Ballard
Private duty services & staff relief

Triangle Home Health Care, Inc.
1318 Broad Street
Durham, NC 27707
Telephone: (919)-286-0121
In-Home Aides and Private Duty Services

Triangle Home Health Care, Inc.
1318 Broad Street
Durham, NC 27705
Telephone: (919)-286-0121
In-Home Aides and Private Duty Services

Triangle Hospice, Inc.
1804 West Southern parkway
Suite #112
Durham, NC 27707
Telephone: (919)-942-8597 Fax: (919)-493-0242
Toll-Free: (800)-849-2053
Contact: Gail Kelly
Home Care and Hospice Services

Medical Services

Duke University Medical Center
Dept.of Medicine, Div.of Infectious Dis.
Box 3238, Room 0207, Hospital South
Durham, NC 27710
Telephone: (919)-684-5260 Fax: (919)-681-8474
Contact: John A. Bartlett, M.D. - Principal Investigator
Adult AIDS Clinical Trial Unit

Duke University Medical Center, Department of Pediatrics
P.O. Box 5499
Durham, NC 27710
Telephone: (919)-684-6335 Fax: (919)-681-8934
Contact: Dr. McKinney - MD
Children's Services: medical, treatment, education, and drug research

Edgecombe County

Community Services

Meals-on-Wheels
1501 Sunset Avenue
Rocky Mount, NC 27801-5014
Telephone: (919)-446-4336
Emergency Shelter and Food Assistance

Salvation Army
P.O. Box 1977
Rocky Mount, NC 27802-1977
Telephone: (919)-446-4496
Emergency Shelter and Food Assistance

County Health Depts

Edgecombe County Health Department
2909 Main Street
Tarboro, NC 27886-1920
Telephone: (919)-641-7511
Contact: Janet Gardner
Medical Services, Education, Counseling and Testing.

Home Health Care

Edgecombe Home Care
2909 Main Street
Tarboro, NC 27886-1920
Telephone: (919)-641-7521 Fax: (919)-641-7565
Contact: Betty Lewis
Home care and hospice services, private duty AIDS

Forsyth County

Community Services

The Legal Aid Society of Northwest North Carolina, Inc.
216 W.Fourth Street
Winston-Salem, NC 27101-2896
Telephone: (910)-725-9166 Fax: (910)-723-9140
Contact: Kay House
Legal Services

County Health Depts

Forsyth County Health Department
741 Highland Avenue
Winston-Salem, NC 27102
Telephone: (919)-727-8172
Contact: Marie Bivens
Medical Services, Education, Counseling and Testing

Home Health Care

Forsyth County Health Department, Home Health
799 North Highland Avenue
PO Box 686
Winston-Salem, NC 27102
Telephone: (919)-727-8297 Fax: (919)-727-8135
Testing and counseling for HIV/AIDS patients

Hospice of Winston-Salem/Forsyth County, Inc.
1100-C South Stratford Rd
Winston-Salem, NC 27103-3212
Telephone: (919)-768-3972
Home Care and Hospice Services

nmc HOMECARE
150 South Streford Rd, Suite 280
Winston, NC 27104
Telephone: (919)-727-0690
Contact: Gayle Beatty
National JCAHO-Accredited company providing a full range of Infusion and Respiratory therapies and specializing in the care of HIV/AIDS patients. National Case Manager is also available at 800-445-1188

Olston/Upjohn Healthcare Services
2990 Bethesda Place
Suite 603 D
Winston-Salem, NC 27103
Telephone: (919)-768-9330 Fax: (919)-768-6174
Home Care and Hospice Services

Medical Services

Wake Forest Univ. Medical Center, Bowman Gray Medical School
Infectious Disease Clinic
300 S. Hawthorne Road
Winston-Salem, NC 27103
Telephone: (919)-716-4152
Contact: P. Samuel Pegram, Jr., MD - Assoc. Prof. of Medicine
Medical Services, AIDS Treatment, Evaluation Services

Testing Sites

Forsyth County Health Department
741 Highland Avenue
STD Clinic
Winston-Salem, NC 27102
Telephone: (910)-727-8271 Fax: (910)-727-8135
Contact: Jennifer Brown
HIV testing & counseling

Franklin County

County Health Depts

Franklin County Health Department and Home Health Agency
107 Industrial Drive
Suite C
Louisburg, NC 27549
Telephone: (919)-496-2533
Contact: Keith Patton
Medical Services, Education, Counseling and Testing, Home Health Care, HIV testing

Home Health Care

Community Care, Inc.
P.O. Box 188
Louisburg, NC 27549
Telephone: (919)-496-3612 Fax: (919)-496-2967
Contact: Patricia Dement
In-Home Aides and Private Duty Services

Gaston County

Home Health Care

Gaston Memorial Home Health Care/Med, Inc.
469 Hospital Drive
PO Box 2568
Gastonia, NC 28053
Telephone: (704)-868-3561 Fax: (704)-834-2038
Toll-Free: (800)-962-5132
Home Care and Hospice Services

Home Health Care of Gaston County, Inc.
2923 Rousseau Court
Gastonia, NC 28054-5155
Telephone: (704)-867-1141
Contact: Ann Scruggs - Director of Nursing
Home Care

Home Health Professionals
2949 Reality Court
Gastonia, NC 28054-0413
Telephone: (704)-864-1131
Home care

Total Care, Inc.
2550 Court Drive
Suite 103
Gastonia, NC 28054
Telephone: (704)-861-8542
Home Care and Hospice Services; home care for HIV

Total Care, Inc.
802 North LaFayette
Shelby, NC 28054
Telephone: (704)-484-3294
Home Care and Hospice Services

Medical Services

Gaston-Lincoln Mental Health Center and Detox Unit
401 North Highland Street
Gastonia, NC 28052-2198
Telephone: (704)-867-2361 Fax: (704)-854-4809
Contact: Nilima Shukla - MD; Dr. Peter Adler - PHD
Residential Detoxification Program for Western Region, Mental Health Services

Gates County

County Health Depts

Gates County Health Department
RR # 1 Box 112-A
Gates, NC 27937
Telephone: (919)-357-1380
Medical service, education, HIV counseling and testing

Graham County

County Health Depts

Graham/Sawin Health Dist.
P.O. Box 546
Robbinsville, NC 28771-0546
Telephone: (704)-479-7900 Fax: (704)-479-6956
Education, Counseling and Testing

Granville County

County Health Depts

Granville County Health Department
P.O. Box 367
101 Hunt Drive
Oxford, NC 27565-0367
Telephone: (919)-693-2141
Medical Services, Education, Counseling and Testing

Greene County

County Health Depts

Greene County Health Department
106 Hines Street
Snow Hill, NC 28580-1608
Telephone: (919)-747-8181
Medical Services, Education, Counseling and Testing

Medical Services

Greene County Mental Health Center
P.O. Box 661
Snow Hill, NC 28580-0661
Telephone: (919)-747-5919
Contact: Glenn Bunch
Mental Health Services

Guilford County

Community Services

Guilford County Department of Social Services
300 S. Centennial Street
P.O. Box 1142
High Point, NC 27261-1142
Telephone: (919)-884-7771 Fax: (919)-884-3004
Medical, financial, social and psychological services

Central Carolina Legal Services, Inc.
107 N. Murrow Boulevard
1st Floor Suite 100
Greensboro, NC 27402
Telephone: (919)-272-0148 Fax: (910)-333-9825
Contact: Ronald Halpern
Legal Services

Central Carolina Legal Services, Inc.
107 N. Murrow Boulevard
Suite 100
Greensboro, NC 27402
Telephone: (910)-272-0148 Fax: (910)-333-9825
Legal Services

High Point Drug Action Council
119 Chestnut Drive
High Point, NC 27262
Telephone: (919)-882-2125
Contact: Stephanie Blake - AIDS Director
AIDS counseling & prevention

Triad Health Project
P.O. Box 5716
Greensboro, NC 27435-0716
Telephone: (910)-275-1654 Fax: (910)-275-2209
Support Group, Budies, Medical Referral, Financial/Housing Help

County Health Depts

Guilford County Health Department
301 North Eugene Street
Greensboro, NC 27401
Telephone: (919)-373-3725
Contact: Sue Lamberth, RN - HIV Counselor
Medical Services, Education, Free HIV Counseling and Testing

Guilford County Health Department
501 East Green Drive
High Point, NC 27260-6707
Telephone: (919)-884-7699
Contact: Rita Jennings
Medical Services, Education, Counseling and Testing

Home Health Care

Home Care of Central Carolina, Inc.
11 Oak Branch Drive
Greensboro, NC 27402
Telephone: (919)-852-3033 Fax: (919)-632-1750
Home Care and Hospice Services; no AIDS treatment program

Hospice at Greensboro, Inc.
2500 Summit Avenue
Greensboro, NC 27405-4522
Telephone: (919)-621-2100
Contact: Marion Taylor
Home Care and Hospice Services. Adult services for terminally ill.

Hospice of the Piedmont, Inc.
213 North Lindsey Avenue
High Point, NC 27262
Telephone: (919)-884-3450
Home Care and Hospice Services

Hospice of the Piedmont, Inc.
213 North Lindsay
Suite 110
High Point, NC 27262
Telephone: (919)-889-8446
Home Care and Hospice Services

Medical Personnel Pool of Metrolina,Inc.
706 Green Valley Road
Suite 105
Greensboro, NC 27408
Telephone: (919)-294-2900
Home Care

Medical Services

Substance Abuse Service of Gilford
P.O. Box 36180
Greensboro, NC 27416-6180
Telephone: (919)-373-5800 Fax: (919)-373-5814
Alcohol, drug and residential detox treatment program for central region

Halifax County

Community Services

Community Action
1015 Roanoke Avenue
Roanoke Rapids, NC 27870-3701
Telephone: (919)-537-1111
Emergency Shelter and Food Assistance

Halifax County Department of Social Services
Highway 301 North
Halifax, NC 27839
Telephone: (919)-536-2511
Medical/Financial/Social/Psycological Services

Harnett County

Community Services

Harnett County Department of Social Services
P.O. Box 669
Lillington, NC 27546-0669
Telephone: (919)-893-7500
Medical, financial, social and psychological services

County Health Depts

Harnett County Health Department
P.O. Box 491
Dunn, NC 28334-0491
Telephone: (919)-892-2424
Medical Services, Education, Counseling and Testing

Harnett County Health Department
904 West Edgerton Street
Dunn, NC 28334
Telephone: (910)-892-2424 Fax: (910)-891-4171
Contact: Belinda Pettiford
Medical Services, Education, Counseling and Testing

Home Health Care

Harnett County Home Health Agency
308 Front Street
PO Box 400
Lillington, NC 27546-0400
Telephone: (919)-893-7544 Fax: (910)-893-9109
Contact: Sharon Pollard - Home Health Supervisor
Home Care and Hospice Services for AIDS patients: skilled nursing,emotional support, physical & speech therapy

St. Joseph Home Health Agency
504 West Broad Street
Dunn, NC 28334
Telephone: (910)-892-6427 Fax: (910)-892-1592
Contact: Gina Sasser - Clinical Coordinator
At home service for AIDS patients: skilled nursing, emotional support,physical & occupational therapy, home health aides

Haywood County

Community Services

Haywood County Department of Social Services
514 East Marshall Street
Waynesville, NC 28786
Telephone: (704)-452-6620
Contact: Judy Sutton - Adult Service Supervisor
Medical, financial, social and psychological services

Salvation Army
P.O. Box 358
Waynesville, NC 28786-0358
Telephone: (704)-452-7054
HIV counseling

County Health Depts

Haywood County Health Department
2216 Asheville Road
Waynesville, NC 28786-3142
Telephone: (704)-452-6675
Medical Services, Education, Counseling and Testing

Henderson County

Community Services

Community Action
P.O. Box 685
Hendersonville, NC 28739-0685
Telephone: (704)-692-2255
Emergency Shelter and Food Assistance

County Health Depts

Henderson County Health Dept.
1347 Spartanburg Highway
Hendersonville, NC 28792
Telephone: (704)-692-2215
HIV testing, counseling

Home Health Care

Pardee Home Care
2029 A Ashville Highway
Hendersonville, NC 28739-3525
Telephone: (704)-692-6702
Home Care

Visiting Health Professionals, Inc.
30 Francis Raod
Hendersonville, NC 28739
Telephone: (704)-697-6908
Contact: Pam Tidwell
Home Care and Hospice Services; general, includes AIDS

Medical Services

Trend Community Mental Health Services
800 N. Fleming Street
Hendersonville, NC 28739-3528
Telephone: (704)-692-7790 Fax: (704)-693-9566
Contact: Ronald Metzger
Mental health services, referrals to in-patient and counseling

Hertford County

Community Services

Community Action
P.O. Box 280
Murfreesboro, NC 27855-0280
Telephone: (919)-398-4131
Emergency Shelter and Food Assistance

Hertford County Department of Social Services
County Office Building
King Street
Winton, NC 27986
Telephone: (919)-358-7830
Medical, financial, social and psychological services

Legal Services of the Coastal Plains
5 West Hargett
Suite 600
Ahoskie, NC 27910
Telephone: (919)-828-4647 Fax: (919)-839-8370
Civil cases, domestic problems, food stamps, medicaid, and wills, nocriminal cases

County Health Depts

Hertford County Health Department
King Street
PO Box 246
Winton, NC 27986-0246
Telephone: (919)-358-7833
Medical services, education, counseling and HIV & STD testing

Home Health Care

Hertford-Gates Home Health Agency
King Street
PO Box 246
Winton, NC 27986-0246
Telephone: (919)-358-7833
Home care, hospice, task force

Hertford-Gates Home Health Agency
P.O. Box 246 King Street
Winton, NC 27986-0246
Telephone: (919)-358-7833
Contact: Ann Evans
Home Care and general includes AIDS

Roanoke-Chowan Hospice, Inc.
P.O. Box 272
521 Myers Street
Ahoskie, NC 27910-0272
Telephone: (919)-332-8121
Home care and hospice, task force, support group

Hoke County

County Health Depts

Hoke County Health Department
429 East Central Avenue
Raeford, NC 28376-2911
Telephone: (919)-875-3717
Medical Services, Education, Counseling and Testing for HIV & STD conseling

Home Health Care

Hospice of Hoke County
108 Dickson Street
PO Box 879
Raeford, NC 28376-0879
Telephone: (919)-692-2212 Fax: (919)-692-7629
Contact: Judy Ferguson
Home Care and Hospice Services AIDS included

St. Joseph Hospital Home Health Agency
336 South Main Street
Raeford, NC 28376
Telephone: (919)-875-5132
Home Care and Hospice Services for hoke counties, In-state 800-682-2246

Iredell County

Community Services

Community Action
P.O. Box 349
Statesville, NC 28677-0349
Telephone: (704)-872-8141 Fax: (704)-871-1299
Contact: Paul Wilson
Emergency Shelter and Food Assistance

Crisis Intervention
906 Fifth Street
Statesville, NC 28677-6676
Telephone: (704)-872-3403
Contact: Gary West
Emergency Shelter and Food Assistance

Iredell County Department of Social Services
P.O. Box 1146
Statesville, NC 28677-1146
Telephone: (704)-873-5631 Fax: (704)-878-5419
Medical, financial, social and psychological services

Salvation Army
P.O. Box 91
Statesville, NC 28687
Telephone: (704)-872-5623
Contact: Major Pete Costas
Food, medication and emergency assistance

County Health Depts

Iredell County Health Department
735 Hartness Road
PO Box 1268
Statesville, NC 28687
Telephone: (704)-873-7291
Contact: Mary Etheridge - AIDS Task Force
Medical Services, Education, Counseling, Testing, Community AIDS Task Force

Home Health Care

Hospice of Iredell County, Inc.
P.O. Box 822
2347 Simonton Road
Statesville, NC 28677-0822
Telephone: (704)-873-4719 Fax: (704)-872-1810
Contact: Annette Kiser
Hospice Services

Total Care, Inc.
615 Sullivan Street
Statesville, NC 28677
Telephone: (704)-667-3389
Home Care and Hospice Services

Total Care, Inc.
615 Sullivan Road
Statesville, NC 28677
Telephone: (704)-872-3606
Home care and hospice services

Total Care, Inc.
615 Sullivan Road
Statesville, NC 28677
Telephone: (704)-872-3606
Contact: Gayle Gibson
Home Care and Hospice Services

Veterans Service Office
412 East Center Avenue
Mooresville, NC 28115
Telephone: (704)-663-1163
Financial assistance

Medical Services

Tri-County Area MH/MR/SAS
1419 Wilson-Lee Boulevard
Statesville, NC 28677-7021
Telephone: (704)-872-5502
Contact: Karen McCoy
Residential Detoxification Program, For Western Region Day Treatment &night program HIV & AIDS Education.

Jackson County

Community Services

Jackson County Department of Social Services
102 Scotts Creek Road
Sylva, NC 28779-2629
Telephone: (704)-586-5546
Medical, financial, social and psychological services

Western North Carolina Legal Services, Inc.
134 W. Main Street
Sylva, NC 28779-2928
Telephone: (704)-586-8931
Legal Services-to low income people

Western North Carolina Legal Services, Inc.
134 W. Main Street
Sylva, NC 28779-2928
Telephone: (704)-586-8931 Fax: (704)-586-4082
Contact: Jim Holloway - Director
Legal Services

Western North Carolina Legal Services, Inc.
134 W. Main Street
Sylva, NC 28779-2928
Telephone: (704)-586-8931 Fax: (704)-586-4085
Toll-Free: (800)-458-6817
Contact: Perry Eury
Legal Services

County Health Depts

Jackson County Health Department
102 Scotts Creek Road
Sylva, NC 28779-2799
Telephone: (704)-586-8994
Medical Services, Education, Counseling and TestingSTD HIV testing

Home Health Care

Hospice, Home Health Service Agency, C.J. Harris Community Hospital
59 Hospital Road
Sylva, NC 28779-2732
Telephone: (704)-586-7414 Fax: (704)-586-7467
Contact: Jane Perry - Director
Home Care and Hospice Services

Johnston County

County Health Depts

Johnston County Health Dept., Home Health and Hospice Prog.
618 North 8th Street
Smithfield, NC 27577-4194
Telephone: (919)-989-5200
Contact: Joey Olive - HIV Coordinator
AIDS testing

Jones County

Community Services

Jones County Department of Social Services
Jones Street
Trenton, NC 28585
Telephone: (919)-448-2581
Medical/Financial/Social/Services

County Health Depts

Jones County Health Department
P.O. Box 216
Trenton, NC 28585-0216
Telephone: (919)-448-9111
Medical Services, Education, Counseling and Testing, HIV STD testing

Lee County

Community Services

Lee County Department of Social Services
530 Carthage Street
Sanford, NC 27330
Telephone: (919)-774-4955
Medical, financial, and social services

County Health Depts

Lee County Health Department
PO Box 1528
Sanford, NC 27331-1528
Telephone: (919)-775-3603
Medical Services, Education, Counseling and Testing

Home Health Care

St. Joseph Home Health Agency
P.O. Box 66
Sanford, NC 27330
Telephone: (919)-774-9522
Contact: Lorrena Moree - V.P. Home Health Service
Home Health nursing care, physical & occupational therapy, hospice AIDStreatment

St. Joseph Hospital Home Health Agency
P.O.Box 66
216 Hawkins Avenue
Sanford, NC 27330
Telephone: (919)-692-2049
Home Care and Hospice Services; HIV health care

Lenoir County

Community Services

Lenoir County Department of Social Services
130 W. King Street
Kinston, NC 28501-4830
Telephone: (919)-559-6400 Fax: (919)-527-3854
Contact: Jack Jones
Medical, financial, social and psychological services

County Health Depts

Lenoir County Health Department
201 North McLewean Street
Kinston, NC 28501-4997
Telephone: (919)-527-7116
Medical Services, Education, Counseling and Testing for HIV & STD

Home Health Care

Britthaven Home Health, Inc.
P.O. Box 190
1304 S.E. Second Street
Hookerton, NC 28572
Telephone: (919)-747-8126 Fax: (919)-747-8851
Contact: Joe Doby
In-Home Aides and Private Duty Services

Frye Home Health Services
420 North Center Street
Hickory, NC 28501-5033
Telephone: (704)-324-3375
Home Care and Hospice Services

Home Health and Hospice Care, Inc.
115 Airport Road
Kinston, NC 28501
Telephone: (919)-658-5083
Home Care and Hospice Services

Home Health and Hospice Care, Inc.
744 Airport Road
Kinston, NC 28501
Telephone: (919)-527-9561 Fax: (919)-527-6617
Contact: Kay Boykin
Home Care and Hospice Services

Tar Heel Health Care Services
P.O. Box 1464
Kinston, NC 28503-1499
Telephone: (919)-522-1458
Home Care and Hospice Services

Tar Heel Health Care Services, Inc.
1305 North Queen Street
Kinston, NC 28503
Telephone: (919)-522-1458
Contact: Retha Ginn - Agency Administrator
Home Care and Hospice Services

Tar Heel Health Care Services, Inc.
1305 North Queen Street
Kinston, NC 28503
Telephone: (919)-522-1458 Fax: (919)-522-5940
Toll-Free: (800)-541-9986
Contact: Retha Ginn, R.N.
Home Care and Hospice Services

Tar Heel Health Care Services, Inc., Wayne Home Health
1305 North Queen Street
Kinston, NC 28501
Telephone: (919)-731-7254 Fax: (919)-522-5940
Home Care and Hospice Services

Medical Services

Lenoir County MH & MR Center
2901 North Herritage Street
Kinston, NC 28501-3805
Telephone: (919)-527-7086 Fax: (919)-523-3262
Contact: James H. Waller
Mental health services, information, counseling, referrals for AIDSpatients

Lincoln County

Community Services

Christian Ministry
P.O. Box 423
Lincoln, NC 28092-0423
Telephone: (704)-732-0383
Food assistance

Lincoln County Department of Social Services
Sigmon Road
Lincolnton, NC 28092
Telephone: (704)-732-0738 Fax: (704)-736-8692
Medical/Financial/Social/food stamps, child protection medicaid & adult services

Home Health Care

Hospice of Lincoln County, Inc.
P.O Box 1526
Lincolnton, NC 28093-1526
Telephone: (704)-732-6146 Fax: (704)-732-9808
Contact: Debbie Barringer, R.N. - Director of Nursing
Hospice Services for AIDS patients in terminal phase skilled nursing ;social work; chaplains; physical & occupational therapy

Macon County

Community Services

Macon County Department of Social Services
5 West Main Street
Franklin, NC 28734-3098
Telephone: (904)-524-6421
Contact: Jane C. Kimsey
Medical, Financial, Social and Psychological Services

Home Health Care

Hospice of Macon County, Inc.
P.O. Box 1594
Roller Mill Road
Franklin, NC 28734-1594
Telephone: (704)-369-6641
Contact: Ruby Shaheen - Director
Home Care and Hospice Services for AIDS patients in terminal phase; skilled nursing; bereavement services.

Madison County

Community Services

Madison County Department of Social Services
Old REA Building
Marshall, NC 28753
Telephone: (704)-649-2711 Fax: (704)-649-3687
Medical, Financial, Social, Psychological Services

Home Health Care

Madison Home Care and Hospice
P.O. Box 909
170 Carl Eller Road
Mars Hill, NC 28754-0909
Telephone: (704)-689-3491 Fax: (704)-689-3496
Contact: Mary Palmer - Patient Care Coordinator
Home Care and Hospice Services for AIDS patients, nursing care, emotional support

Martin County

Community Services

Martin County Department of Social Services
305 East Main Street
Williamston, NC 27892
Telephone: (919)-792-2133 Fax: (919)-792-5186
Medical, Financial, Social, and Psychological Services

Home Health Care

Roanoke Home Care (M-T-W District)
Liberty Street
Williamston, NC 27892-0596
Telephone: (919)-792-7811
Contact: Social Worker
Home Care and Hospice Services

Mc Dowell County

Community Services

McDowell County Department of Social Services
207 East Court Street
P.O. Drawer 338
Marion, NC 28752
Telephone: (704)-652-3355 Fax: (704)-652-9167
Medical, Financial, Social, Psychological Services

Home Health Care

McDowell Home Health Care Program
515 North Main Street
Marion, NC 28752
Telephone: (704)-659-6901 Fax: (704)-659-6401
Home Care Services

Mecklenburg County

Community Services

Equal Opportunity Commission
5500 Central Avenue
Charlotte, NC 28212
Telephone: (704)-567-7100 Fax: (704)-567-7155
AIDS-Related Employment Discrimination in Federal Contracts and Agencies

Legal Services of Southern Piedmont
1431 Elizabeth Avenue
Charlotte, NC 28204
Telephone: (704)-376-1608 Fax: (704)-376-8627
Contact: Kenneth Shorr
Legal service and civil cases

Mecklenburg County Department of Social Services
301 Billingsley Road
Charlotte, NC 28211-1005
Telephone: (704)-336-3150 Fax: (704)-336-4816
Medical, Financial, Social and Psychological Services

Metrolina AIDS Project
P.O. Box 32662
Charlotte, NC 28232-2662
Telephone: (704)-333-2437 Fax: (704)-376-8794
Contact: Barbara Rein
Support group, medical and financial aid, legal referral, minorityeducation project

Salvation Army Area Command
P.O. Box 31443
Charlotte, NC 28231
Telephone: (704)-334-4731 Fax: (704)-333-4351
Contact: Major Marshall Clary
Emergency Shelter and Food Assistance

Southern Piedmont
1431 Elizabeth Avenue
Charlotte, NC 28204
Telephone: (704)-376-1608 Fax: (704)-376-8627
Legal Services

St. Peter's Soup Kitchen
115 W. 7th Street
Charlotte, NC 28202-1227
Telephone: (704)-332-7746 Fax: (704)-332-7747
Contact: Oleen McLeod
Emergency Shelter and Food Assistance

Home Health Care

Care Team Health Services
5821 Park Road to Fairvw
Suite 104
Charlotte, NC 28209
Telephone: (704)-552-2273 Fax: (704)-552-1944
In-Home Aides and Private Duty Services

Caremark Connection Network
9401-J Southern Pine Blvd
Charlotte, NC 28273
Telephone: (704)-523-7731 Fax: (704)-523-8001
Contact: Tom Piasecny; Larry Burnette
CLINICAL SUPPORT AND INFUSION THERAPIES: Nutrition, Antimicrobials, Chemo.,Hematopoe

HNS, Inc.
9771-D Southern Pines Blv
Charlotte, NC 28273
Telephone: (704)-525-6392 Fax: (704)-525-6394
Contact: Charles Wiggins
Home Infusion Therapy, In-home Nursing and Attendant Care, P.T. Services, Penta

Home Health Professionals, Inc.
6101 Idlewild Road
Suite 230
Charlotte, NC 28212-0517
Telephone: (704)-536-4930 Fax: (704)-563-0911
Contact: Karen Johnson
Home Care and Hospice Services

Hospice at Charlotte, Inc.
1420 East 7th Street
Charlotte, NC 28204
Telephone: (704)-375-0100 Fax: (704)-375-8623
Home Care and Hospice Services

Interim Health Care
PO Box 36699
Charlotte, NC 28236-6699
Telephone: (704)-372-8230 Fax: (704)-348-2665
Toll-Free: (800)-234-8230
Home Care and Hospice Services

Interim Health Care
P.O. Box 36699
141 Providence Road
Charlotte, NC 28236
Telephone: (704)-372-8230
Contact: Cynthia Debias - Director
Home Care for AIDS patients in terminal phase: nursing care physicaltherapy, emotional support

Interim Health Care
P.O. Box 36699
Page Road
Charlotte, NC 28236
Telephone: (704)-372-8230
Home Care and Hospice Services; HIV testing, counseling

Mecklenburg County Department of Social Services
301 Billingsley Road
Charlotte, NC 28211-1005
Telephone: (704)-336-3171 Fax: (704)-336-7965
Adult in-take unit for all kind of services, referrals

Medical Personnel Pool of Metrolina, Inc.
141 Providence Road
PO Box 36699
Charlotte, NC 28236
Telephone: (704)-372-8230 Fax: (704)-348-2665
Home Care and Hospice Services

Mercy Home Care, Inc.
2001 Vail Avenue
Charlotte, NC 28207
Telephone: (704)-379-5200 Fax: (704)-379-6103
Contact: Wynetta Hasty
Home Care and Hospice Services

Mercy Home Care, Inc.
2001 Vail Avenue
Charlotte, NC 28207-1289
Telephone: (704)-379-5200 Fax: (704)-379-6103
Home Care and Hospice Services

Mercy Home Care, Inc.
2001 Vail Avenue
Charlotte, NC 28207
Telephone: (704)-379-5200
Home Care and skilled nurses, general, includes AIDS

nmc HOMECARE
834 Tyvola Rd, Suite 114
Charlotte, NC 28217
Telephone: (704)-522-8213
Fax: (704)-522-7862
Contact: Gayle Beatty
National JCAHO-Accredited company providing a full range of Infusion and Respiratory therapies and specializing in the care of HIV/AIDS patients. National Case Manager is also available at 800-445-1188

Nursefinders of Charlotte
1900 Randolph Road
Charlotte, NC 28207-1106
Telephone: (704)-335-7241 Fax: (704)-335-8434
In-Home Aides and Private Duty Services

Olsten Kimberly Quality Care
3325 Washburn Ave, #3
Suite A
Charlotte, NC 28205-7024
Telephone: (704)-332-8141 Fax: (704)-332-2248
Toll-Free: (800)-753-0402
Contact: Lavonne Kerr
Home Care and Hospice Services

Partners Home Health of Charlotte
1012 S King Drive
Suite 100
Charlotte, NC 28207
Telephone: (704)-342-4223 Fax: (704)-358-8928
Contact: Terry White - Administrator
Home Care

Presbyterian Home Care
P.O.Box 33549
1710 East Fourth Street
Charlotte, NC 28233-3208
Telephone: (704)-342-2565
Home Care and Hospice Services

Presbyterian Home Care
P.O. Box 33549
1710 East Fourth Street
Charlotte, NC 28233-3549
Telephone: (704)-342-2565
Contact: Audrey Belk - Director
Home Care and Hospice Services; infusion care, child therapy

Presbyterian Home Care
1710 East Fourth Street
PO Box 33549
Charlotte, NC 28233
Telephone: (704)-384-4130 Fax: (704)-384-4838
Home Care and Hospice Services

Total Care, Inc.
1200 East Morehead Street
Suite 190
Charlotte, NC 28204
Telephone: (704)-332-1121 Fax: (704)-334-9428
Contact: Marsha Buraglio
Home Care and Hospice Services

Medical Services

Amethyst Treatment Center
1715 Sharon Road, West
Charlotte, NC 28224-5663
Telephone: (704)-554-8373
Contact: Bill Brown
Substance Abuse Inpatient Facility, For Western Region

CPC Cedar Spring Hospital
9600 Pineville-Matthew Rd
Charlotte, NC 28134
Telephone: (704)-541-6676 Fax: (704)-541-7194
Contact: Sherley Ward
Substance Abuse Inpatient Facility, For Western Region

Mecklenburg County Mental Health Authority
429 Billingsly Roadd
2nd Floor
Charlotte, NC 28211-1009
Telephone: (704)-336-2023 Fax: (704)-336-4383
Contact: Peter Safir
Mental Health Services

Open House, Inc., Jonnie McLeod Treatment Center
145 Remount Road
Charlotte, NC 28203-5039
Telephone: (704)-332-9001 Fax: (704)-332-0124
Contact: Gene Hall - Director
Methadone Detox/Maintenance, Residential Treatment Program, For Western Region

Mitchell County

County Health Depts

Toe River Health District
P.O. Box 98
Spruce Pine, NC 28777
Telephone: (704)-765-2239
Contact: Sonie Sullins
Information & education, community AIDS task force, HIV testing

Montgomery County

Community Services

Community Action
South Main Street
Troy, NC 27371
Telephone: (919)-576-9071 Fax: (919)-576-3490
Contact: David Richardson
Emergency Shelter and Food Assistance

Montgomery County Department of Social Services
Community Services Bldg.
117 South Main Street
Troy, NC 27371
Telephone: (919)-057-6653 Fax: (919)-057-6220
Medical, Financial, Social and Psychological Services

Medical Services

Sandhills Center for MH/MR/SA Services
227 North Main Street
Troy, NC 27371-3015
Telephone: (919)-572-3681 Fax: (919)-572-5579
Contact: Edward Vito
Mental health services, mental retardation & substance abuse

Moore County

Community Services

Community Action
P.O. Box 937
Carthage, NC 28327-0937
Telephone: (919)-947-5675
Emergency Shelter and Food Assistance

Moore County Department of Social Services
P.O. Box 938
Currie Building
Carthage, NC 28327-0938
Telephone: (919)-947-2436 Fax: (919)-947-1618
Medical, Financial, Social, Psychological Services, and in-home healthaides

Home Health Care

Medical Personnel Pool of Metrolina, Inc.
30 Page Drive
Suite #3
Pinehurst, NC 28374
Telephone: (910)-295-2211 Fax: (910)-295-3451
Toll-Free: (800)-876-2212
Home Care and Hospice Services

St. Joseph Hospital Home Health Agency
285 Pinehurst Avenue
Southern Pines, NC 28387
Telephone: (919)-692-2049 Fax: (919)-692-4147
Home Care and Hospice Services

Nash County

Community Services

Nash County Department of Social Services
110 Washington Street
Nashville, NC 27856
Telephone: (919)-459-9818 Fax: (919)-459-9833
Medical, Financial, Social and Counseling Services

Home Health Care

Nash County Home Health Agency
301 South Church Street
Station Square Suite 390
Rocky Mount, NC 27804
Telephone: (919)-446-1777 Fax: (919)-446-0026
Contact: Jacrie Pully
Home Care

New Hanover County

Community Services

GROW AIDS Resource Project
P.O. Box 4535
Wilmington, NC 28406-1535
Telephone: (919)-675-9222
Contact: Leo Teachout
Support Groups, Buddy Program, Speakers, Medical/Legal Referrals, For SE NC

Legal Services of the Lower Cape Fear
106 Market Street
Wilmington, NC 28402
Telephone: (910)-763-6207 Fax: (910)-343-8894
Legal services: social services, medicaid, food stamps

Legal Services of the Lower Cape Fear
106 Market Street
Wilmington, NC 28402-4442
Telephone: (910)-763-6207 Fax: (910)-343-8894
Legal services: social security, disability, medicaid

New Hanover County Department of Social Services
1650 Greenfield Street
P.O. Drawer 1559
Wilmington, NC 28402-6456
Telephone: (910)-341-4700 Fax: (910)-341-4747
Medical, social and limited financial services

Salvation Army
820 North 2nd Street
PO Box 637
Wilmington, NC 28406-0637
Telephone: (919)-762-6611
Emergency Shelter and Food Assistance

Home Health Care

Comprehensive Home Health Care I, Inc.
221 North Front Street
PO Box 307
Wilmington, NC 28402-0307
Telephone: (910)-343-0938 Fax: (910)-343-0048
Contact: Carrie Davis
Home Care and Hospice Services

Comprehensive Home Health Care I, Inc.
P.O. Box 307
221 North Front Street
Wilmington, NC 28402-0307
Telephone: (919)-343-0398
Contact: Glen Wells
Home Care and Hospice Services

Lower Cape Fear Hospice, Inc.-Pender
810 Princess Street
Wilmington, NC 28401
Telephone: (919)-762-0200 Fax: (919)-762-9146
Toll-Free: (800)-733-1476
Contact: Eloise Thomas
Home Care and Hospice Services

New Hanover County Health Department Home Health Agency
2029 South 17th Street
Wilmington, NC 28401-6699
Telephone: (910)-341-4180 Fax: (910)-341-4146
Home Care

Norfolk (city) County

Community Services

Tidewater AIDS Crisis Taskforce
740 Duke Street
Suite 520
Norfolk, VA, NC 23501
Telephone: (804)-423-5859
Contact: Giles Nurrington
Support Groups, Buddy Program, Speakers, Medical Referrals

Northampton County

Community Services

Community Action Agency
P.O. Box 530
Rich Square, NC 27869-0503
Telephone: (919)-539-4155 Fax: (919)-539-2048
Emergency Shelter and Food Assistance

Northampton County Department of Social Services
Highway 305
Jackson, NC 27845
Telephone: (919)-534-5811 Fax: (919)-534-0061
Medical/Financial/Social/Psychological Services

Onslow County

Community Services

Community Action Agency
P.O. Drawer 796
Jacksonville, NC 28541-0796
Telephone: (919)-347-2151 Fax: (919)-347-1237
Emergency Shelter and Food Assistance

Onslow County Department of Social Services
PO Box 1379
Jacksonville, NC 28541
Telephone: (919)-455-4145 Fax: (919)-455-2901
Contact: Mr. West Fall - 938-5509
Medical, Financial, Social and Psychological Services

Home Health Care

Comprehensive Home Health Care, Inc.
1039 Western Blvd.
Jacksonville, NC 28540-6270
Telephone: (910)-346-4800 Fax: (910)-346-5870
Toll-Free: (800)-800-0614
Contact: Angela Brooks
Home Care and Hospice Services

Comprehensive Home Health Care I, Inc.
3840 Henderson Drive
Jacksonville, NC 28546
Telephone: (910)-346-4800 Fax: (910)-346-5870
Toll-Free: (800)-800-0614
Contact: Angela Brooks
Home Care and Hospice Services

Onslow Hospice, Inc.
2507-B North Marine Blvd.
Jacksonville, NC 28540-4822
Telephone: (910)-347-6266 Fax: (910)-347-9279
Toll-Free: (800)-735-5734
Contact: Judy Ryan - Patient Care Coordinator
Home Care and Hospice Services

Orange County

Community Services

North State Legal Services, Inc.
102 West King Street
Hillsborough, NC 27278-2541
Telephone: (919)-732-8137 Fax: (919)-644-0694
Contact: Brenda Ford McGhee
Legal Services

County Health Depts

Orange County Health Department
300 West Tryon Street
Hillsborough, NC 27278
Telephone: (919)-732-8181
Contact: Belinda Jones
Medical Services, Testing and Counseling, Minority Education Project

Home Health Care

Home Health Agency of Chapel Hill, Inc.
1101 Weaver Dairy Road
Chapel Hill, NC 27514-2570
Telephone: (919)-929-7149 Fax: (919)-929-1344
Toll-Free: (800)-672-5905
Contact: Charles Milch
Home Care and Hospice Services

Home Health Agency of Chapel Hill, Inc.
1101 Weaver Dairy Road
Chapel Hill, NC 27514
Telephone: (919)-929-7149 Fax: (919)-929-1344
Toll-Free: (800)-672-5905
Contact: Terre Oosterwyk
Home Care and Hospice Services

Pamlico County

County Health Depts

Pamlico County Health Department
P.O. Box 306
Bayboro, NC 28515-0306
Telephone: (919)-745-5111
Medical Services, Education, Counseling and Testing

Home Health Care

Hospice of Pamlico County, Inc.
P.O. box 827
Bayboro, NC 28515-0827
Telephone: (919)-745-5171
Contact: Diane McDaniels
Home Care and Hospice Services

Pasquotank County

County Health Depts

Pasquotank County Health Department
Cedar Street
Elizabeth City, NC 27909
Telephone: (919)-338-2167
Medical Services, Education, Counseling and Testing

Home Health Care

Albemarle Home Care
P.O. Box 189
Elizabeth City, NC 27909-0189
Telephone: (919)-338-4066 Fax: (919)-338-5526
Contact: Robin Temple
Home Care and Hospice Services & transportation

Albemarle Home Care
P.O. Box 189
400 South Road Street
Elizabeth City, NC 27909
Telephone: (919)-338-4066 Fax: (919)-338-5526
Home Care and Hospice Services

Pender County

County Health Depts

Pender County Health Department
803 S. Walker Street
Burgaw, NC 28425
Telephone: (919)-259-1230
Contact: Connie Bell; Irma Simpson -
Medical Services, Education, Counseling and Testing

Home Health Care

Pender County Home Health Agency
803 South Walker Street
PO Box 1209
Burgaw, NC 28425-1317
Telephone: (910)-259-1230 Fax: (910)-259-1258
Contact: Irma Simpson
Home Care and Hospice Services

Senior Citizen Services of Pender, Inc.
312 West Williams Street
Burgaw, NC 28425
Telephone: (919)-259-9119
Contact: Wesley B. Davis
In-Home Aides and Private Duty Services

Perquimans County

Community Services

Open Door
P.O. Box 721
Hertford, NC 27944-0721
Telephone: (919)-426-7776
Contact: Cecil Timms
Food assiatance & utilities

County Health Depts

Perquimans County Health Department
103 Charles Street
Hertford, NC 27944-1503
Telephone: (919)-426-5488
Contact: Virginia Bailey
Medical Services, Education, Counseling and Testing

Person County

County Health Depts

Person County Health Department
325 South Morgan Street
Roxboro, NC 27573
Telephone: (919)-597-2204
Contact: Tom Bridges
Medical Services, Education, Counseling and Testing

Home Health Care

Home Health Professionals
P.O. Box 1084
Roxboro, NC 27573-1084
Telephone: (919)-597-3050 Fax: (919)-597-4703
Toll-Free: (800)-292-5055
Contact: Barbara Bradsher
Home Care and Hospice Services

Person County Council on Aging
121A Depot Street
PO Box 764
Roxboro, NC 27573-0764
Telephone: (919)-599-7484
Contact: Phyllis Bridgeman
In-Home Aides and Private Duty Services

Pitt County

Community Services

Pitt County Department of Social Services
1717 W. Fifth Street
Greenville, NC 27834-1695
Telephone: (919)-413-1101
Medical, Financial, Social and Psychological Services

Salvation Army
P.O. Box 113
Greenville, NC 27835-0113
Telephone: (919)-756-3388
Emergency Shelter and Food Assistance

Shelter
P.O. Box 687
Greenville, NC 27835-0687
Telephone: (919)-752-0829
Emergency Shelter and Food Assistance

Soup Kitchen
1120 W. 5th Street
Greenville, NC 27834-3008
Telephone: (919)-758-1504
Emergency Shelter and Food Assistance

County Health Depts

Pitt County Health Department
1825 West Sixth Street
Greenville, NC 27834-2893
Telephone: (919)-752-4141
Contact: Brenda Respess
Medical Services, Education, Counseling and Testing

Home Health Care

Apple Nursing Services, Inc.
P.O. Box 8402
Greenville, NC 27835-8402
Telephone: (919)-355-7719 Fax: (919)-355-0728
Contact: Margarete Moore
In-Home Aides and Private Duty Services

Health Force/Prime Care of Wake, Orange and Durham Counties
2245 Statonsburg Road
Suite K
Greenville, NC 27834
Telephone: (919)-758-2700
Contact: Tom Harmelink
In-Home Aides and Private Duty Services

Northcare Health Services
640-H Medical Drive
PO Box 8424
Greenville, NC 27835-8424
Telephone: (919)-757-0029 Fax: (919)-757-0034
Toll-Free: (800)-849-0029
Contact: Tom Deimantis
In-Home Aides and Private Duty Services, live-in companions

Tarheel Home Health
104 Staton Court
PO Box 7145
Greenville, NC 27835]
Telephone: (919)-758-5932 Fax: (919)-758-2379
Toll-Free: (800)-932-4429
Home Care and Hospice Services

Polk County

County Health Depts

Polk County Health Department
Walker Street
Columbus, NC 28722
Telephone: (704)-894-8271
Contact: Clifford Fields
Medical Services, Education, Counseling and Testing

Home Health Care

Hospice of Polk County, Inc.
423 Trade Street
PO Box Y
Tryon, NC 28782-0722
Telephone: (704)-859-2270 Fax: (704)-859-2731
Home Care and Hospice Services

Randolph County

Community Services

Randolph County Department of Social Services
PO Box 3239
Asheboro, NC 27204-7368
Telephone: (910)-318-6400
Medical, Financial, Social, Psychological Services

Home Health Care

Hospice of Randolph, Inc.
416 Vision Drive
PO Box 9
Asheboro, NC 27204-0009
Telephone: (919)-629-9300 Fax: (919)-672-0868
Toll-Free: (800)-762-5900
Home Care and Hospice Services, adult day health care

Housecalls Home Health Care
P.O. Box 339
Fayettelle Street
Liberty, NC 27298-0339
Telephone: (919)-622-3071
Home Care and Hospice Services

Housecalls Home Health Care, Inc.
120 West Swannonoa St
PO Box 339
Liberty, NC 27298-0339
Telephone: (919)-622-3071 Fax: (919)-622-4398
Toll-Free: (800)-533-9270
Contact: Tiffany Mathews
Home Care and Hospice Services

Olston/Upjohn Healthcare Services
1200 East North Fayetteville Street
Asheboro, NC 27204-5772
Telephone: (919)-629-3178 Fax: (919)-629-0603
Toll-Free: (800)-835-5749
Contact: Betty Dale
Home Care and Hospice Services

Richmond County

County Health Depts

Richmond County Health Department
P.O. Box 429
Rockingham, NC 28379-0429
Telephone: (919)-997-8300 Fax: (919)-997-8336
Contact: Mary Brigman - Nursing Supervisor
Medical Services, Education, Counseling and Testing

Home Health Care

Richmond County Home Health Agency, Richmond Memorial Hosp.
1000 Long Drive
PO Box 1928
Rockingham, NC 28379-1928
Telephone: (919)-997-2561
Home Care

Robeson County

Community Services

Lumbee River Legal Services
Comer E. Main & 2nd St.
Pembroke, NC 28372
Telephone: (910)-521-2831 Fax: (910)-521-9824
Contact: Dale Deese
Legal Services

Robeson County Department of Social Services
Old Laurinburg Road
Lumberton, NC 28359
Telephone: (919)-738-9351
Medical, Financial, Social and Psychological Services

County Health Depts

Robeson County Health Department and Home Health Agency
Route 4, Box 388
Lumberton, NC 28358-0388
Telephone: (919)-671-3200 Fax: (919)-671-3484
Contact: Enice Inman
Medical Services, Education, Counseling and Testing, Home Health Care

Home Health Care

Health Horizons, Inc., Home Health Agency
2002 North Cedar Street
Suite B
Lumberton, NC 28358
Telephone: (919)-739-5433
Home Care and Hospice Services

Health Horizons, Inc., Home Health Agency
20002 North Cedar Street
PO Box 1408
Lumberton, NC 28359-1408
Telephone: (919)-739-5433
Contact: Meriam Edwards
Home Care and Hospice Services

Hospice of Robeson/Health Horizons, Inc.
2002 North Cedar Street
Lumberton, NC 28358-1408
Telephone: (919)-738-1905 Fax: (919)-739-3551
Home Care and Hospice Services; no AIDS treatment program

Medical Services

Southeastern Regional Mental Health Program
207 West 29th Street
Lumberton, NC 28358
Telephone: (910)-738-5261 Fax: (910)-738-8230
Contact: Don McKee
Mental Health Services

Rockingham County

County Health Depts

Rockingham County Health Department
Route 8, Box 204
Wentworth, NC 27320-9808
Telephone: (910)-342-8200
Contact: William Thompson - Health Director
Medical Services, Education, Counseling and Testing

Home Health Care

Annie Penn Memorial Hospital Home Health Agency
618 South Main Street
Riedsville, NC 27320-5094
Telephone: (919)-634-1010
Contact: Linda Lothian
Home Care and Hospice Services

Annie Penn Memorial Hospital Home Health Agency
618 South Main Street
Reidsville, NC 27320-5094
Telephone: (919)-349-8461
Contact: Linda Lothian
Home Care and Hospice Services

Rockingham County Home Health Agency
Governmental Center P.O. Box 204
Wentworth, NC 27375-8881
Telephone: (910)-342-8100 Fax: (910)-342-8356
Contact: Lydia Patterson Seagrave - Public Health Educator
Home Care and Hospice Services; HIV testing, counseling & referrals toother services

Rowan County

Community Services

Community Action
P.O. Box 631
Salisbury, NC 28145-0631
Telephone: (704)-633-6633
Contact: Diane Fowler
Food assistance, AIDS support, clothing

County Health Depts

Rowan County Health Department
2728 Old Concord Road
Salisbury, NC 28144-8389
Telephone: (704)-633-0411
Contact: John Shaw
Medical Services, Education, Counseling and Testing

Home Health Care

Home Health Professionals
318-320 Mocksville Ave.
Salisbury, NC 28144
Telephone: (704)-633-7213
Contact: Jody Kepley
Home Care and Hospice Services

Home Health Professionals
318-320 Mocksville Ave.
Salisbury, NC 28144
Telephone: (704)-633-7213
Home Care and Hospice Services

Kimberly Olsten Quality Care
650 Statesville Blvd
Suite # 5
Salisbury, NC 28144
Telephone: (704)-637-2598
Contact: Tammi Pendetalton
Home Care

Total Care, Inc.
216 State Seville Blvd.
Salisbury, NC 28144-2723
Telephone: (704)-636-3334 Fax: (704)-639-0070
Home Care and Hospice Services

Total Care, Inc.
216 Statesville Blvd.
Salisbury, NC 28144-2314
Telephone: (704)-636-3334
Home Care and Hospice Services

Rutherford County

County Health Depts

Rutherford County Health Department
203 Koone Road
Spindale, NC 28160
Telephone: (704)-287-2211
Contact: Clifford Field
Medical Services, Education, Counseling and Testing

Home Health Care

Carolina Home Care
121 Tryon Road, Suite 3
Rutherfordton, NC 28139-3036
Telephone: (704)-287-2267 Fax: (704)-286-5594
Home Care, companion services, cap DA program

Carolina Home Care, Inc.
121 Tryon Road, Suite 3
Rutherfordton, NC 28139
Telephone: (704)-287-2267 Fax: (704)-286-5594
Contact: Marsha Baker
Home Care

McDowell Home Health Care Program
203 Callaham-Koone Road
Spindale, NC 28160-2207
Telephone: (704)-287-6220 Fax: (704)-287-6059
Contact: Cliff Fields
Home Care

Sampson County

County Health Depts

Sampson County Health Department and Home Health Agency
Rowan Road
County Complex
Clinton, NC 28328
Telephone: (919)-592-1131
Contact: Kenneth Jones
Medical Services, Education, Counseling and Testing, Home Health Care

Home Health Care

Home Health and Hospice Care, Inc.
1023 Beaman Street Street
Clinton, NC 28328-2858
Telephone: (919)-658-5083
Home Care and Hospice Services

Home Health Care and Hospice Care, Inc.
313 H Roland Road
Clinton, NC 28328-0852
Telephone: (919)-592-1131

Contact: Kenneth Jones
Home Care and Hospice Services

Scotland County

County Health Depts

Scotland County Health Department
1405 West Boulevard
P.O. Box 69
Laurinburg, NC 28353
Telephone: (919)-277-2440
Contact: Richard Steeves
Medical Services, Education, Counseling and Testing

Stanly County

Community Services

Stanly County Department of Social Services
201 South Second Street
Albemarle, NC 28001-5747
Telephone: (704)-983-7300 Fax: (704)-983-3133
Contact: Barbara Whitley
Medical, Financial, Social and Psychological Services

County Health Depts

Stanly County Health Department
945 North Fifth Street
Albemarle, NC 28001-3417
Telephone: (704)-982-9171
Contact: Mary Jensen - AIDS Task Force
Medical Services, Education, Counseling/Testing, Community AIDS Task Force

Home Health Care

Home Care of the Carolinas
P.O. Box 837
907 North Second Street
Albemarle, NC 28002
Telephone: (704)-982-2273 Fax: (704)-983-2963
Home Care and Hospice Services

Home Care of the Carolinas, Inc.
907 North Second Street
PO Box 837
Albemarle, NC 28002-0837
Telephone: (704)-982-2273 Fax: (704)-983-2963
Contact: Keith Arbuckle
Home Care and Hospice Services

Medical Services

Stanly County Mental Health Center
P.O. Box 1396
Albemarle, NC 28001-1396
Telephone: (704)-983-2117 Fax: (704)-983-2636
Mental Health Services

Stokes County

Community Services

Ministry Outreach
P.O. Box 1450
King, NC 27021-1450
Telephone: (919)-983-4357
Emergency Shelter and Food Assistance

County Health Depts

Stokes County Health Department and Home Health Agency
Highway 89
PO Box 187
Danbury, NC 27016-0089
Telephone: (919)-593-2811
Contact: Bill Johnson
Medical Services, Education, Counseling and Testing, Home Health Care

Home Health Care

Hospice of Stokes County
Stokes-Reynolds Mem. Hosp
Highway & Highway 89
Danbury, NC 27016
Telephone: (919)-593-2831
Home Care and Hospice Services

Surry County

Community Services

Salvation Army
P.O. Box 443
Mt. Airy, NC 27030-0443
Telephone: (910)-786-4075 Fax: (910)-786-5881
Emergency Shelter and Food Assistance

Surry County Department of Social Services
Cooper and Blessing Sts.
Dobson, NC 27017
Telephone: (919)-386-9244
Aid for families with children, medicaid

County Health Depts

Surry County Health Department and Home Health Agency
118 Hamby Rd
PO Box 1062
Dobson, NC 27017-1062
Telephone: (919)-374-2131
Contact: Claubia Bryant
Medical Services, Education, Counseling and Testing, Home Health Care

Home Health Care

Hospice of Surry County, Inc.
1326 North Main Street
PO Box 1034
Mount Airy, NC 27030-1034
Telephone: (919)-789-7844 Fax: (919)-789-0856
Home Care and Hospice Services

Northern Surry Home Care
834 Rockford St
PO Box 1605
Mount Airy, NC 27030-0605
Telephone: (919)-786-3415
Home Care and Hospice Services

Medical Services

Crossroads, The Surry-Yadkin Area MH/MR/SA Authority
P.O. Box 1428
150 Franklin Street
Mount Airy, NC 27030-1428
Telephone: (919)-789-5011 Fax: (919)-719-3215
Mental Health Services, includes HIV

Hope Valley, Inc. (Men)
P.O. Box 467
Dobson, NC 27017-0467
Telephone: (919)-386-8511 Fax: (919)-386-9181
Substance Abuse, Residential Treatment and Group Living For North Central Region

Hope Valley, Inc.--Women Division
Route 3, Box 112
Pilot Mountain, NC 27041-0112
Telephone: (919)-368-2427
Recovery Model Alcohol and Other Drug Treatment, For Western Region

The Surry-Yadkin Mental Developmental Disabilities & Substance Service
P.O. Box 1428
Mount Airy, NC 27030
Telephone: (910)-789-5011 Fax: (910)-719-3215
Mental Health Services

Swain County

Home Health Care

Cherokee Home Health Services, Cherokee Indian Reservation
P.O. Box 365
Sequoyah Tr., Old Clinic
Cherokee, NC 28719-0365
Telephone: (704)-497-7599 Fax: (704)-497-7380
Home Care and Hospice Services

Transylvania County

Community Services

Christian Ministry--Sharing House
P.O. Box 958
Brevard, NC 28712-0958
Telephone: (704)-884-2866
Assistance with food, utilities & prescriptions

County Health Depts

Transylvania County Health Department
Community Services Bldg.
Brevard, NC 28712
Telephone: (704)-884-3135
Contact: Terry Pierce
Education, Counseling and Testing

Home Health Care

Carolina Health Professionals, Inc.
206 Cooper Street
Statesville, NC 28766-5856
Telephone: (704)-872-2388 Fax: (704)-873-9112
Contact: Virginia Stewart
In-Home Aides and Private Duty Services, nurses

Medical Services

Trans Community Mental Health Services
Morgan and Gaston Street
18 Hospital Drive
Brevard, NC 28712
Telephone: (704)-884-2027 Fax: (704)-884-2099
Mental Health Services

Tyrrell County

Community Services

Tyrrell County Department of Social Services
408 Bridge Street
Columbia, NC 27925
Telephone: (919)-796-3421
Medical, Financial, Social and Psychological Services

County Health Depts

Tyrrell County Health Department
408 Bridge Street
Columbia, NC 27925-9998
Telephone: (919)-796-2681
Contact: Judy Wright
Medical Services, Education, Counseling and Testing

Home Health Care

Roanoke Home Care (M-T-W District)
P.O. Box 238
Bridge Street
Columbia, NC 27925-0238
Telephone: (919)-796-2681
Home Care and Hospice Services

Union County

Community Services

Union County Department of Social Services
P.O. Box 489
Union County Courthouse
Monroe, NC 28111
Telephone: (704)-289-6581
Contact: Drake McCain - AIDS Task Force
Medical, Financial, Social, Psychological, Education Services and AIDS TaskForce

County Health Depts

Union County Health Department
500 North Main Street
Courthouse
Monroe, NC 28112-4799
Telephone: (704)-283-3792
Contact: Lorey White
Medical services, education, counseling and testing

Vance County

Community Services

Salvation Army
P.O. Box 2510
Henderson, NC 27536-0793
Telephone: (919)-438-7107
Toll-Free: (800)-922-9728
Emergency Shelter and Food Assistance 1-800-922-9728 North Carolina only

Vance County Department of Social Services
2035 Ruin Creek Road
Henderson, NC 27536-4202
Telephone: (919)-492-5001
Medical/financial/social

County Health Depts

Vance County Health Department
115 Emergency Road
Henderson, NC 27536-2939
Telephone: (919)-492-7915
Contact: Robert Mc Ilwain
Medical Services, Education and HIV Counseling and Testing

Home Health Care

Community Care, Inc.
P.O. Box 1262
Henderson, NC 27536-1262
Telephone: (919)-492-6028
In-Home Aides and Private Duty Services

MedVisit, Inc.
P.O. Box 265
Henderson, NC 27536
Telephone: (919)-492-6046 Fax: (919)-492-9967
Contact: Tammy Winston
Home health agency

Medical Services

Area MH/MR/SA Program of Vance, Granville, Franklin & Warren
125 Emergency Road
Henderson, NC 27536
Telephone: (919)-492-4011 Fax: (919)-492-9453
Mental Health Services

Wake County

Community Services

AIDS Service Agency of Wake County
P.O. Box 12583
Raleigh, NC 27605-2583
Telephone: (919)-833-9521
Contact: Beth McAllister
Support Group, Buddies, Speakers, Legal and Financial Help, Referrals, TempHousing

East Central Community Legal Services
5 W. Hargett Street
Suite 600
Raleigh, NC 27601
Telephone: (919)-828-4647
Legal Services

East Central Community Legal Services
5 W. Hargett Street
Suite 600
Raleigh, NC 27602
Telephone: (919)-828-4647
Contact: Victor Boone
Legal services, housing, handle problems with SSI, food stamps for AIDSpatients as well

East Central Community Legal Services
5 W. Hargett Street
Suite 600
Raleigh, NC 27602
Telephone: (919)-828-4647
Housing employment to low income people, legal services

Governor's Advocacy Council for Persons with Disabilities
Dept. of Administration
1318 Dale Street, Suite #100
Raleigh, NC 27605
Telephone: (919)-733-9250
Contact: Brenda Carter - Case Intake Analyst
AIDS-Related Discrimination Assistance (Does Not Deal with Housing)

Human Relations Council
Department of Administrat
121 West Jones Street
Raleigh, NC 27603
Telephone: (919)-733-7996
Mediation of AIDS-Related Job and Housing Discrimination

Planned Parenthood of Greater Raleigh, Inc.
100 S. Boylan Avenue
Raleigh, NC 27603-1802
Telephone: (919)-833-7534 Fax: (919)-833-0730
Contact: Pam Kohl - Executive Director
Safer Sex Counseling, Pamphlet Dissemination

Salvation Army
P.O. Box 27584
Raleigh, NC 27611-8024
Telephone: (919)-834-6733 Fax: (919)-828-0911
Emergency shelter & food assistance, works with AIDS patients-don't know towhat extent

Wrenn House
605 W. North Street
Raleigh, NC 27603-1416
Telephone: (919)-832-7866 Fax: (919)-856-6369
Emergency Shelter and Food Assistance - runaway care

County Health Depts

Wake County Health Department
P.O Box 14049
10 Sunnybrook Road
Raleigh, NC 27620-1049
Telephone: (919)-250-4510
Contact: Gibbie Harris
Case Management, Medical Services, Education, Counseling and Testing

Home Health Care

Alpha-Omega Health Inc.
7406 J. Chapel Hill Road
Raleigh, NC 27605
Telephone: (919)-233-0042
Contact: Jeff Jenkins
In-Home Aides and Private Duty Services

Caremark Connection Network
1100 Perimeter Park Dr
Suite 114
Morrisville, NC 27560-9119
Telephone: (919)-481-2885
Toll-Free: (800)-245-2463
Contact: Alan Knight
Clinical Support and Infusion Therapies: Nutrition, Antimicrovirals,Chemo., Hematopoeti

Children's Healthcare, Inc.
4601 Six Forks Road
Suite # 524C
Ralliegh, NC 27609
Telephone: (919)-783-6063 Fax: (919)-783-5974
Contact: Mary Rollins
In-Home Aides and Private Duty Services

Easter Seal Home Health Services
2315 Myron Drive
Raleigh, NC 27607-3357
Telephone: (919)-881-9492 Fax: (919)-881-9539
Contact: Joan Hoffman
Home Care and Hospice Services

Easter Seal Home Health Services
2315 Myron Drive
Raleigh, NC 27607-3357
Telephone: (919)-783-8898 Fax: (919)-782-5486
Home Care and Hospice Services

Health Force of Wake and Durham Counties
4009 Barrett Drive
Suite 103
Raleigh, NC 27609-6616
Telephone: (919)-787-2137
Contact: Debra Szuba - Manager
In-Home Aides and Private Duty Services; no AIDS treatment program

Health Force of Wake and Durham Counties
4009 Barrett Drive
Suite 103
Raleigh, NC 27609-6616
Telephone: (919)-787-2137 Fax: (919)-787-2139
In-Home Aides and Private Duty Services

Nursefinders of Raleigh-Durham
5974 Six Forks Road
Raleigh, NC 27609
Telephone: (800)-768-4422
In-Home Aides and Private Duty Services

Nursefinders of Raleigh-Durham
5974 Six Forks Road
Raleigh, NC 27609
Telephone: (919)-846-1018 Fax: (919)-846-5954
Toll-Free: (800)-849-4800
Contact: Margret Rice - RN
In-Home Aides and Private Duty Services, infusion therapy, chemo therapy

Nursefinders of Raleigh-Durham
5974 Six Forks Road
Raleigh, NC 27609
Telephone: (800)-768-4422
In-Home Aides and Private Duty Services

Nursefinders of Raleigh-Durham
5974 Six Forks Road
Raleigh, NC 27609
Telephone: (800)-768-4422
In-Home Aides and Private Duty Services

Nursefinders of Raleigh-Durham
5974 Six Forks Road
Raleigh, NC 27609
Telephone: (919)-846-1018
Contact: Margeret Rice
In-Home Aides and Private Duty Services

Rehab Home Care, Inc.
3004 New Bern Avenue
Raleigh, NC 27610-1215
Telephone: (919)-832-8111
Contact: Alan Silver
Home Care and Hospice Services

Rehab Home Care, Inc.
2660-Q Yonkers Road
Raleigh, NC 27604
Telephone: (919)-832-8111
Home Care and Hospice Services

Rehab Home Care, Inc.
2660-Q Yonkers Road
Raleigh, NC 27604
Telephone: (919)-832-8111
Home Care

Medical Services

Charter Northridge Hospital
400 Newton Road
Raleigh, NC 27615
Telephone: (919)-847-0008 Fax: (919)-870-6739
Contact: Andy Delbridge
Substance abuse inpatient facility, psychiatric patients-adult teens,substance abuse

Warren County

Home Health Care

Warren County Health Department and Home Health Agency
544 W. Ridgeway Street
Warrenton, NC 27589-1797
Telephone: (919)-257-1185 Fax: (919)-257-2897
Contact: Dennis Retz Laff
Medical Svcs, Education, Testing/Counseling, Home Health Care, AIDS Task Force

Washington County

Community Services

Washington County Department of Social Services
209 East Main Street
Plymouth, NC 27962-1321
Telephone: (919)-793-4041 Fax: (919)-793-3195
Medical, Financial, Social, Psychological Services and Child Support

County Health Depts

Washington County Health Department
Route 2 Box 78 R
Plymouth, NC 27962
Telephone: (919)-793-3023
Contact: Judy Wright
Medical Services, Education, Counseling and Testing

Home Health Care

Roanoke Home Care-Hospice (M-T-W District)
Rt. 2 Box 78
Plymouth, NC 27962-0396
Telephone: (919)-793-3023 Fax: (919)-793-3417
Contact: Judith Wright
Home Care and Hospice Services

Watauga County

Community Services

Hospitality House
302 West King Street
Boone, NC 28607-4172
Telephone: (704)-264-1237
Emergency Shelter and Food Assistance

Legal Services of the Blue Ridge
171 Grand Boulevard
Boone, NC 28607-3617
Telephone: (704)-264-5640 Fax: (704)-264-5667
Legal Services (Low income)

Watauga County Department of Social Services
769 West King Street
Boone, NC 28607-3519
Telephone: (704)-265-8100
Medical, Financial, Social and Psychological Services - AFDC

Home Health Care

Watauga County Health Department-Hospice
Route 5, Box 199
Bamboo Road
Boone, NC 28607-9312
Telephone: (704)-264-4995 Fax: (704)-264-4997
Contact: Sue Sweeting, F.N.P.
Medical Services, Education, Counseling and Testing, Home Health Care

Watauga County Project on Aging
783 West King Street
Boone, NC 28607-3519
Telephone: (704)-265-8090 Fax: (704)-265-8018
Contact: Robert E Nelson
In-Home Aides and Private Duty Services

Medical Services

Watauga County Mental Health
Route 5, Box 20-A
Boone, NC 28607-9308
Telephone: (704)-264-9007 Fax: (704)-262-5860
Contact: Dorothy Beamon
Mental Health Services

Wayne County

County Health Depts

Wayne County Health Department
301 North Herman Street
Goldsboro, NC 27530-2973
Telephone: (919)-731-1000
Contact: Carolyn King
Education, Counseling and Testing

Home Health Care

Home Health and Hospice Care, Inc.
P.O. Box 88
Goldsboro, NC 27533-1025
Telephone: (919)-658-5083
Home Care and Hospice Services

Salvation Army
P.O. Box 264
Goldsboro, NC 27533-0793
Telephone: (919)-735-4811 Fax: (919)-735-8460
Contact: Barbara Neff
Emergency Shelter and Food Assistance

Wayne County Services on Aging
P.O. Box 227
Goldsboro, NC 27530-0277
Telephone: (919)-731-1591 Fax: (919)-731-1446
Contact: Louise Phillips
In-Home Aides and Private Duty Services

Medical Services

Wayne County Area MH/MR/SA Program
301 North Herman Street
Goldsboro, NC 27530
Telephone: (919)-731-1133 Fax: (919)-731-1333
Contact: Listen Edwards
Mental Health Services

Wilkes County

County Health Depts

Wilkes County Health Department
West College Street
Wilkesboro, NC 28697
Telephone: (919)-651-7450
Contact: Judy Sturgill
Medical Services, Education, Counseling and Testing

Home Health Care

Hospice of Wilkes, Inc.
P.O. Box 609
West D Street
N. Wilkesboro, NC 28659-0609
Telephone: (919)-651-8107
Contact: Terrye Walsh
Home Care and Hospice Services

Wilkes County Home Health Agency
P.O. Box 609
North Wilkesboro, NC 28659
Telephone: (910)-651-8491 Fax: (910)-651-8449
Home Care and Hospice Services

Medical Services

Detox Center
Route 2, Box 26
Old 421 Highway
Wilkesboro, NC 28697-9203
Telephone: (919)-667-7191 Fax: (919)-667-6859
Contact: Geraldine Call
Substance Abuse Residential Treatment and Group Living, For Western RegionAids Program

Wilkes County Mental Health Center
P.O. box 831
Wilkesboro, NC 28697-0831
Telephone: (919)-667-5151 Fax: (919)-667-5048
Contact: Dr. NIta Bogart
Mental Health Services

Wilson County

Community Services

Eastern Carolina Legal Services
P.O. Box 2688
Wilson, NC 27894
Telephone: (919)-291-6851
Legal Services

Eastern Carolina Legal Services
P.O. Box 2688
Wilson, NC 27894
Telephone: (919)-291-6851 Fax: (919)-291-6407
Legal Services - low income families

Salvation Army
316 South Tarboro Street
Wilson, NC 27894-0096
Telephone: (919)-243-2696 Fax: (919)-243-6744
Emergency Shelter and Food Assistance

Soup Kitchen
202 North Goldsbora Street
Wilson, NC 27894-1527
Telephone: (919)-243-6208
Contact: Brock Plauche
Emergency Shelter and Food Assistance

Wilson County Department of Social Services
100 Gold Street North East
Wilson, NC 27894
Telephone: (919)-206-4000 Fax: (919)-237-1544
Medical, Financial, Social and Psychological Services

Home Health Care

Interim Health Care
103 North Ward Boulevard
Wilson, NC 27893
Telephone: (919)-243-7665 Fax: (919)-243-4966
Toll-Free: (800)-476-7665
In-Home Aides and Private Duty Services

Medical Personnel Pool--Wilson
103 North Ward Boulevard
Wilson, NC 27893
Telephone: (919)-243-7665 Fax: (919)-243-4966
In-Home Aides and Private Duty Services

Medical Services

Wilson County Mental Health Center
1709 South Tarboro
Wilson, NC 27893
Telephone: (919)-399-8021
Contact: John White
Mental Health Services

Yadkin County

Community Services

Yadkin County Department of Social Services
County Office Building
PO Box 548
Yadkinville, NC 27055
Telephone: (919)-679-2081
Medical, Financial, Social and Psychological Services

Home Health Care

O.P.T.I.O.N Care
103 Valley Drive
Jonesville, NC 28642-2620
Telephone: (919)-526-4140 Fax: (919)-526-8329
Toll-Free: (800)-745-8348
Contact: David Morrison
Home IV and Nutritional Services

Yadkin County Hospice
P.O. Box 457
Yadkinville, NC 27055
Telephone: (919)-679-4207 Fax: (919)-679-6005
Yadkin county home health and hospice

Yancey County

Community Services

Yancey County Department of Social Services
P.O. Box 67
Burnsville, NC 28714-0067
Telephone: (704)-682-6148 Fax: (704)-682-6712
Medical, Financial, Social and Psychological Services

County Health Depts

Yancey County Health Department
10 Swiss Avenue
Burnsville, NC 28714-2819
Telephone: (704)-682-6118
Medical Services, Education, Counseling and Testing

Home Health Care

Hospice of Yancey County, Inc.
P.O. Box 471
314 West Main Street
Burnsville, NC 28714-0471
Telephone: (704)-682-9675
Hospice Services

NORTH DAKOTA

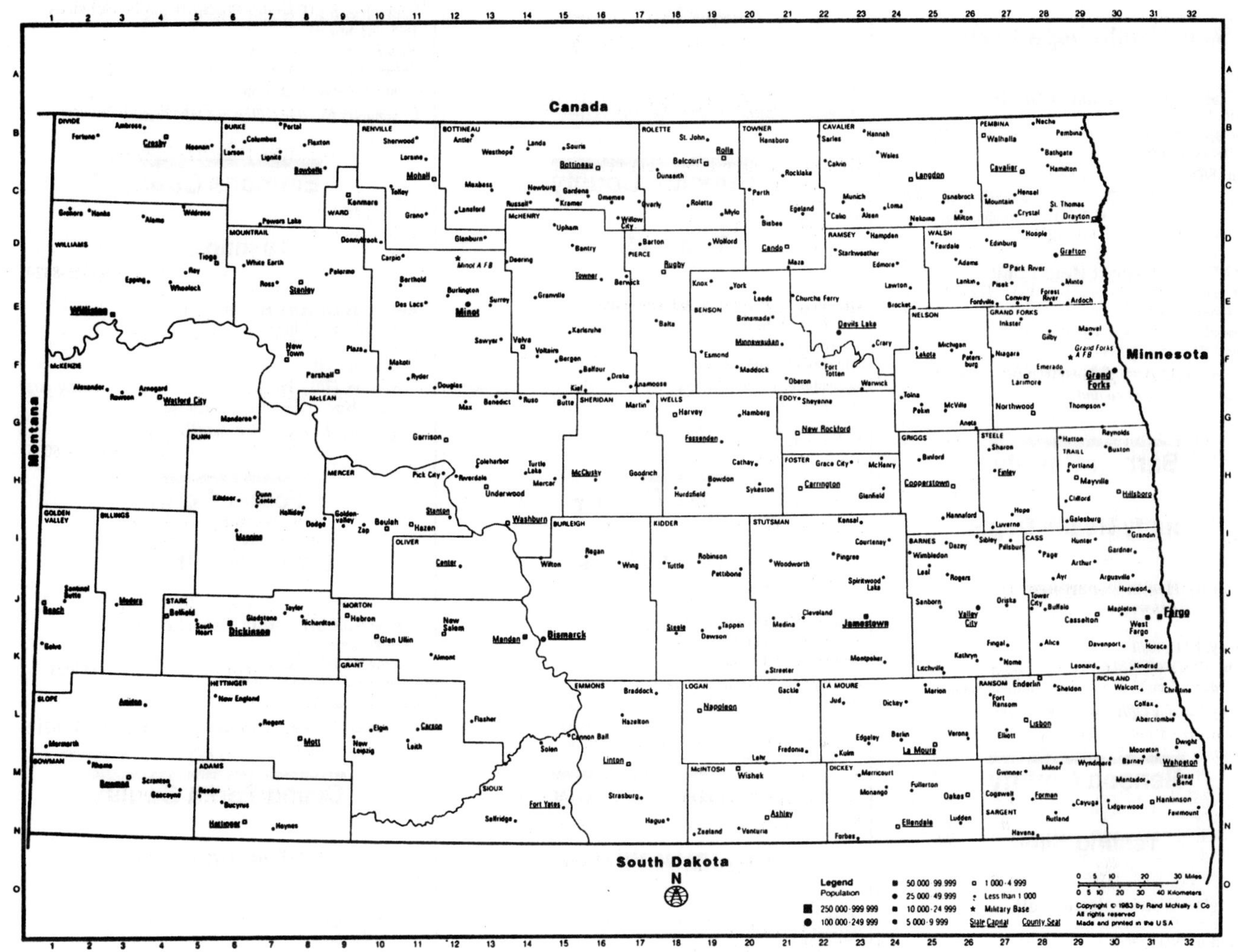

From City/County Planning Atlas Copyright 1989 by Reed McNally & Company, R.L. 90-S-28

North Dakota

General Services

State Health Departments

North Dakota Department of Health, AIDS Project
600 East Blvd. Avenue
Judicial Wing, 2nd Floor
Bismarck, ND 58505
Telephone: (701)-224-2378 Fax: (701)-224-4727
Contact: Susan Pederson - HIV/AIDS Program Mgr.

Upper Missouri District Health Unit
507 University Avenue
512 4th Avenue East
Williston, ND 58801
Telephone: (701)-572-3763
Contact: Janice Trimmer - Department Administrator
Community Nursing Office and HIV Testing

Barnes County

County Health Depts

City-County Health Department
230 4th Street Northwest
Room 102
Valley City, ND 58072
Telephone: (701)-845-8518
Contact: Marcy Grant - Department Administrator
Community Nursing Office and HIV Testing

Benson County

Testing Sites

Lake Region District Health Unit
Benson County Courthouse
Minnewaukan, ND 58351
Telephone: (701)-473-5444
Contact: Darlene Alderston
Community Nursing Office and HIV Testing

Bottineau County

Testing Sites

First District Health Unit
Courthouse
Bottineau, ND 58318
Telephone: (701)-228-3101
Contact: Theresa Delikat
Community Nursing Office and HIV Testing

Burke County

Testing Sites

First District Health Unit
Courthouse
Bowbells, ND 58721
Telephone: (701)-377-2316
Contact: Nancy Deslauriers
Community Nursing Office and HIV Testing

Burleigh County

Testing Sites

Bismarck-Burleigh Nursing Service
221 N. 5th Street
Box 5503
Bismarck, ND 58502
Telephone: (701)-222-6525 Fax: (701)-222-6606
Contact: Doris Fischer - Director of Nursing
Community Nursing Office and HIV Testing

Cass County

Testing Sites

Fargo Community Health Center
401 3rd Avenue North
Fargo, ND 58102
Telephone: (701)-241-1360
Contact: Mary Kay Herman - Director of Nursing
Community Nursing Office and HIV Testing

Cavalier County

County Health Depts

Cavalier County Health District
901 3rd Street
Langdon, ND 58249
Telephone: (701)-256-2402 Fax: (701)-256-2566
Contact: Terri Gustafson
Community Nursing Office and HIV Testing

Divide County

Testing Sites

Upper Missouri District Health Unit
Box 69
Crosby, ND 58730
Telephone: (701)-965-6813
Contact: Barbara Andrist
Community Nursing Office and HIV Testing

Eddy County

Testing Sites

Lake Region District Health Unit
16 S. 8th Street
New Rockford, ND 58356
Telephone: (701)-947-5311
Contact: Arlyss Lesmeister
Community Nursing Office and HIV Testing

Emmons County

Testing Sites

Emmons District Health Unit
Linton Medical Clinic
Box 636
Linton, ND 58552
Telephone: (701)-254-4027 Fax: (701)-254-4027
Contact: Bev Voller - Department Administrator
Community Nursing Office and HIV Testing

Foster County

County Health Depts

Foster County Health Department
Courthouse
Carrington, ND 58421
Telephone: (701)-652-3087
Contact: Jean Kulla
Community Nursing Office and HIV Testing

Grand Forks County

Testing Sites

Grand Forks Public Health Department
122 S. 5th Street
Box 1518
Grand Forks, ND 58206-1518
Telephone: (701)-746-2525 Fax: (701)-746-2534
Contact: Pam Engle - Director of Nursing
Community Nursing Office and HIV Testing

Hettinger County

County Health Depts

Southwestern District Health Department
Box 575
Mott, ND 58646
Telephone: (701)-824-3215
Contact: Jodi Olson
Community Nursing Office and HIV Testing

Kidder County

Home Health Care

Kidder District Health Unit
Box 52
Steele, ND 58482
Telephone: (701)-475-2582
Toll-Free: (800)-475-8483
Contact: Ann Iszler; Kathy Johnson
Community Nursing Office, homecare, referrals

La Moure County

Testing Sites

Central Valley Health Unit
LaMoure Clinic
Box 692
LaMoure, ND 58458
Telephone: (701)-883-4359
Contact: Sharon Unruh - Health Maintenance
HIV testing & counseling; community nursing

Mc Henry County

County Health Depts

First District Health Unit
Box 517
Towner, ND 58788
Telephone: (701)-537-5732
Contact: A. Pauline Bold
Community nursing office & HIV testing

Mercer County

County Health Depts

Custer District Health Unit
Box 39
Stanton, ND 58571
Telephone: (701)-745-3599
Contact: Sharon Huber
Community nursing office & HIV testing

Morton County

County Health Depts

Custer District Health Unit
210 2nd Avenue NW
Box 185
Mandan, ND 58554
Telephone: (701)-667-3370
Contact: Jocelyn Koch
Community Nursing Office and HIV Testing

Pembina County

County Health Depts

Pembina County Health Department
Box 369
Cavalier, ND 58220
Telephone: (701)-265-4248
Contact: Mary Sandison - Administrator
Community Nursing Office

Pierce County

County Health Depts

Lake Region District Health Unit
Courthouse
Rugby, ND 58368
Telephone: (701)-776-6783
Community Nursing Office and HIV Testing

Ransom County

County Health Depts

Ransom County Health Department
PO Box 89
Lisbon, ND 58054
Telephone: (701)-683-5823
Contact: Deb Bergestorm - Administrator
Community nursing office & counseling

Richland County

County Health Depts

Richland County Health Department
413 3rd Avenue North
Wahpeton, ND 58075
Telephone: (701)-642-7735
Contact: Peggy Heartling - Department Administrator
Community Nursing Office and HIV Testing

OHIO

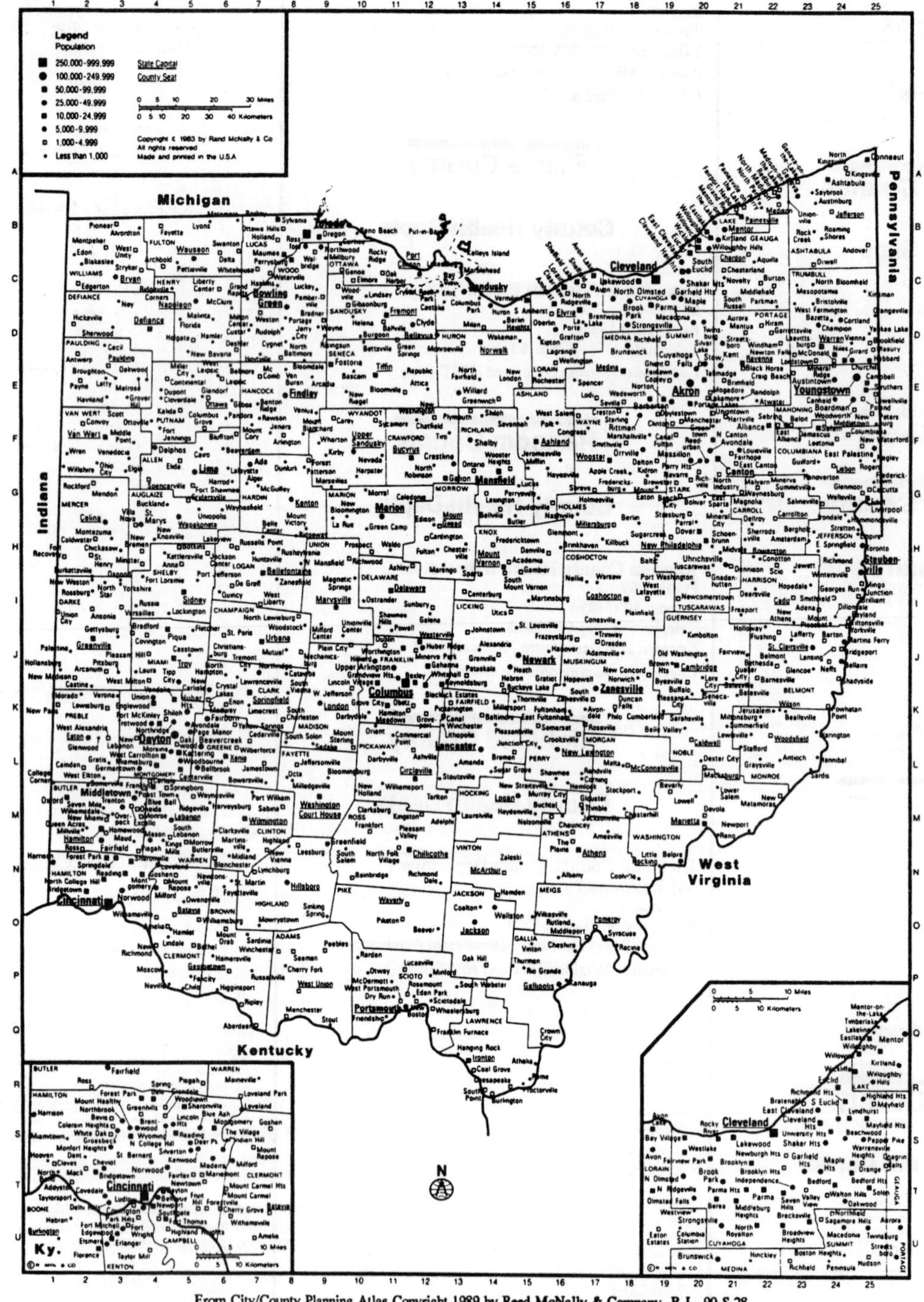

From City/County Planning Atlas Copyright 1989 by Reed McNally & Company, R.L. 90-S-28

Ohio

General Services

Education

AIDS Volunteers of Cincinnati
2183 Central Parkway
Cincinnati, OH 45214
Telephone: (513)-421-2437
Contact: Karer Johnson
Producer of: Directory of AIDS-Related Services in Cincinnati, casemanagers

American Red Cross
39 North Park Street
Mansfield, OH 44902-1711
Telephone: (419)-524-0311
Contact: S. Douglas Skroback - Exec.
Education, Blood bank, Support, referral.

American Red Cross - Allen County Chapter
610 S. Collett Street
Lima, OH 45805
Telephone: (419)-227-5121
Contact: Jed E. Metzger - Executive Director
Education

American Red Cross - Ashland County Chapter
432 Center Street
Ashland, OH 44805-3247
Telephone: (419)-289-3535
Contact: Glorene Shenberger - Exec.
AIDS education materials

American Red Cross - Ashtabula County Chapter
433 Center Street
Ashtabula, OH 44004-6996
Telephone: (416)-998-1020
Contact: Mary Ellen Coneglio - Exec.
HIV education program

American Red Cross - Athens County Chapter
132 North Congress Street
Athens, OH 45701-1623
Telephone: (614)-593-5273
Contact: Sandra Shirey - Exec.
Blood bank, AIDS education programs

American Red Cross - Barberton Chapter
600 West Park Avenue
Barberton, OH 44203
Telephone: (216)-753-7766
Contact: Beverly Synder
Blood bank, educational program

American Red Cross - Canton Chapter
618 Second Street, NW
Canton, OH 44703-2756
Telephone: (216)-453-0146
Blood bank, education

American Red Cross - Canton, Ohio Chapter
618 2nd Street NW
Canton, OH 44703
Telephone: (519)-673-5159
Contact: Lisa Martin
AIDS education

American Red Cross - Central Ohio Chapter
995 East Broad Street
Columbus, OH 43205-1339
Telephone: (614)-253-7981
Contact: Dr. Ambrose Ng., M.D. - Director Blood Services
Support for HIV+ from blood transfusion, AIDS task force, education, casemanagement

American Red Cross - Champaign County Chapter
P.O. Box 285
1202 North Main Street
Urbana, OH 43078-0285
Telephone: (513)-653-7276
Contact: Tim Settles
Blood bank, HIV instruction

American Red Cross - Cincinnati Area Chapter
720 Sycamore Street
Cincinnati, OH 45202
Telephone: (513)-579-3000
Contact: John Yarcuskon - Exec.
AIDS information

American Red Cross - Cincinnati Area Chapter
720 Sycamore Street
Cincinnati, OH 45202
Telephone: (513)-579-3000
Contact: John Yarcuskon - Exec.
HIV classes & educational materials

American Red Cross - Cincinnati Area Chapter
720 Sycamore Street
Cincinnati, OH 45202-2185
Telephone: (513)-579-3080
Contact: Patti Ettensohn
Blood bank, AIDS education

American Red Cross - Columbus Area Chapter
995 East Broad Street
Columbua, OH 43205
Telephone: (614)-253-7981
Contact: Sheila Nalawadi - AIDS Coordinator
Course on AIDS/HIV for instructors, speakers bureau, case managementwith Ohio Department of Health

American Red Cross - Coshocton County Chapter
245 North 4th Street
P.O. Box 695
Coshocton, OH 43812-1116
Telephone: (614)-622-0228
Contact: Carolyn Snedden - Exec.
Educational material on HIV

American Red Cross - Crestline Area Chapter
907 S. Thoman Street
Crestline, OH 44827-1859
Telephone: (419)-683-3772
Contact: Laura Horning
HIV information

American Red Cross - Dayton Area Chapter
370 West First Street
Dayton, OH 45402
Telephone: (513)-222-6711
AIDS classes

American Red Cross - Dayton Area Chapter
Health Services
370 West First Street
Dayton, OH 45402-3006
Telephone: (513)-222-6711
Contact: Paula Good - Education
HIV education

American Red Cross - E. Liverpool Area Chapter
401 College Street
East Liverpool, OH 43920
Telephone: (216)-386-4144
Contact: Ben Weber - Exec.
Brochures & HIV educational training courses

American Red Cross - Fayette County Chapter
135 North Main Street
P.O. Box 315
Washington C.H., OH 43160
Telephone: (614)-335-3101
Contact: Bob Green - Director
Public awarness education concerning AIDS/HIV

American Red Cross - Firelands Chapter
P.O. Box 835
Sandusky, OH 44870-0835
Telephone: (419)-626-1641
Contact: Ron Rudebel - Exec.
Blood bank, AIDS education

American Red Cross - Galion Chapter
124 N. Union Street
Galion, OH 44833-1736
Telephone: (419)-468-5611 Fax: (419)-468-4673
Contact: Pat Wittelslager - Executive Director
Educational services

American Red Cross - Gallia County Chapter
275 State Street
Gallipolis, OH 45631
Telephone: (216)-871-2175
Contact: Ray Bailey - Exec.
Blood bank.

American Red Cross - Greater Cleveland Chapter
3747 Euclid Avenue
Cleveland, OH 44115-2501
Telephone: (216)-431-3010
Contact: Diane Dunleavy - Director of Health Services
Cousre in AIDS/HIV awareness for instructors & speakers

American Red Cross - Hamilton Area Chapter
112 North 2nd Street
Hamilton, OH 45011-2702
Telephone: (513)-868-7616
Contact: Richard Johnson - Exec.
AIDS education

American Red Cross - Hancock County Chapter
125 Fair Street
Findlay, OH 45840-3501
Telephone: (419)-422-9322
Contact: Stacey Connell - AIDS/HIV Coordinator
Course in HIV awareness for instructors, speakers bureau, buddy system

American Red Cross - Mahoning Chapter
266 West Wood Street
Youngstown, OH 44502-1170
Telephone: (216)-744-0161
Contact: W. Russell Preston
Instructor training, Speakers bureau

American Red Cross - Miami County Chapter
3130 North Dixie Highway
Troy, OH 45373
Telephone: (513)-332-7876
Blood bank, educational materials.

American Red Cross - Miami County-Ohio
3130 North Dixie Highway
Troy, OH 45373
Telephone: (513)-773-7353
Educational materials & speakers

American Red Cross - Middletown Area Chapter
125 South Main Street
Middleton, OH 45044
Telephone: (513)-423-9233
Contact: Jerrie Stover
Education, counseling

American Red Cross - Muskingham Lakes Chapter
1458 Fifth Street
New Philadelphi, OH 44663
Telephone: (216)-343-8633
Contact: Lisa S. Miller - Director
Brochures on AIDS

American Red Cross - Muskingum Valley Chapter
22 South Seventh Street
Zanesville, OH 43701
Telephone: (614)-452-2731
Contact: Nancy Evans - Exec.
Blood bank, AIDS education

American Red Cross - North Columbiana County
667 N. Ellsworth Avenue
Salem, OH 44460-1650
Telephone: (216)-332-0028
HIV classes & printed material

American Red Cross - Northern Ohio Region
3747 Euclid Avenue
Cleveland, OH 44115-2501
Telephone: (216)-431-3010 Fax: (216)-391-3501
Contact: Nora V. Hairsler - Exec.
Educational & information services

American Red Cross - Sandusky County Chapter
701 East State Street
Fremont, OH 43420-4252
Telephone: (419)-332-5574
Blood bank, HIV instructors

American Red Cross - Shelby County Chapter
207 West Water Street
Sidney, OH 45365
Telephone: (513)-492-6151
Contact: Alice Watts - Exec.
AIDS education

American Red Cross - Western Stark County Chapter
325 3rd Street SE
Amherst Centre
Massillon, OH 44646-4182
Telephone: (216)-833-9943
Contact: MaryLou Cooper - Exec.
Educational, literature, community outreach

American Red Cross, Trumbull County Chapter
626 Mahoning Avenue, NW
PO Box 1390
Warren, OH 44482-1390
Telephone: (216)-392-2551
Contact: William Mottice - Executive Director
Blood Bank, education, support group for care givers

American Red Cross, Van Wert County Chapter
208 E. Main Street
Suite J
Van Wert, OH 45891
Telephone: (419)-238-9977
Contact: Lawrence Rockwell
Blood Bank, educational program

Auglaize County AIDS Task Force
214 South Wagner Street
Wapakoneta, OH 45895-1660
Telephone: (419)-738-3410 Fax: (419)-738-7818
Contact: Janet M. Bassitt
Education & referrals

Central State University
Brush Row Road
Wilberforce, OH 45384
Telephone: (513)-376-6011 Fax: (513)-376-6647
Contact: Loraine Glenn, R.N. - Director
AIDS information, educational & referral

Champaign Health District
40 Monument Square
Suite 101
Urbana, OH 43078
Telephone: (513)-653-4444
Contact: Theodore E. Richards, M.D. - Health Commissioner
Pamphlets & referrals

Doctors Hospital of Nelsonville
1950 Mount St. Mary's Dr
Nelsonville, OH 45764
Telephone: (614)-753-1931
Contact: Joel Kaiser
AIDS awareness program

East Central AIDS Education and Training Center
Ohio State University
1314 Kinnear Road, Ar 300
Columbus, OH 43212
Telephone: (614)-292-1400 Fax: (614)-292-4056
Contact: Dr. Lawrence L. Gabel, PhD.
AIDS/HIV education & training for health care professionals

East Liverpool City Health Department
126 West 6th Street
East Liverpool, OH 43920-2960
Telephone: (216)-385-7900
Contact: G. Ryan, R.S. - Health Commissioner; J. Keith Rugh, M.D. - Medical Director
Educational materials, videos, seminars, referrals for testing

Fulton County Chapter-American Red Cross in Wauseon
P.O. Box 156
631 W. Elm Street
Wauseon, OH 43567-0156
Telephone: (419)-335-4636
Contact: Liana Baldwin - Director
Blood bank, educational materials

OSMA AIDS Task Force
1500 West 3rd Avenue
Suite 329
Columbus, OH 43219
Telephone: (614)-228-6971
Contact: Gloria Smith - Executive Director
Information & referral service

Riverside Methodist Hospital
3535 Olentangy River Road
Columbus, OH 43214-3998
Telephone: (614)-261-5000
Contact: Debbie Bingle
Education- for in service & patients

Summit County Medical Society
430 Grant Street
Akron, OH 44311
Telephone: (216)-434-1921 Fax: (216)-253-1330
Contact: Shirley Bee
Referrals, AIDS seminars

Hotlines

Ohio AIDS Hotline

Columbus, OH 43266-0118
Telephone:
Toll-Free: (800)-332-2437

State Health Departments

Ohio Department of Health, AIDS Unit
Bureau of Preventive Medicine
246 North High Street, PO Box 118
Columbus, OH 43266-0118
Telephone: (614)-466-5480

Statewide Services

Ohio Energy Credits Program
P.O. Box 2619
Columbus, OH 43266
Telephone: (000)-614-7810
For elderly and disabled

Adams County

Community Services

Department of Human Services
#482 Rice Drive
P.O. Box 386
West Union, OH 45693-1316
Telephone: (513)-544-2317
Contact: Martha Bennett - Supervisor
Social service referrals.

County Health Depts

Adams County Health Department
116 W. Mulberry Street
West Union, OH 45693-1595
Telephone: (513)-544-5547 Fax: (513)-544-8251
Contact: Bruce M. Ashley, M.D. - Health Commissioner
Nursing services

Medical Services

Adams County Family Planning
51 Logans Lane
West Union, OH 45693
Telephone: (513)-544-3796
Contact: Barbara Chandler
Child-family health clinic

Allen County

Community Services

St. Gerards' Catholic Church
240 West Robb Avenue
Lima, OH 45801-2899
Telephone: (419)-224-3080
Contact: Denis Sweeny
Bereavement support.

County Health Depts

Allen County Health Department
219 E Market Street
PO Box 1503
Lima, OH 45802-1503
Telephone: (419)-228-4457 Fax: (419)-224-4161
Contact: David Rosebrock, M.P.H. - Health Commissioner
Anonymous HIV testing & counseling; education program

Allen County Health Department (Family Planning Project)
72 Town Square
Lima, OH 45801-4932
Telephone: (419)-228-6154 Fax: (419)-229-2082
Parenthood affiliate.

Combined Allen County Health Department
219 Market Street
PO Box 1503
Lima, OH 45802
Telephone: (419)-228-4457
Contact: Jody Willeke
Counseling/testing site.

Combined Allen County Health Department
219 East Market Street
Lima, OH 45802
Telephone: (419)-228-4457
Contact: Ann Purdy; Grace Marshall -
County Health Department, counseling/testing site anonymous

Home Health Care

Homedco Infusion
2010 Spencerville Road
Lima, OH 45805
Telephone: (419)-222-1500 Fax: (419)-224-6026
Contact: Bonnie Waterman
Home infusion therapy for AIDS patients, home medical equipment, homenursing care

Lima Visiting Nurse Association
226 South West Street
Lima, OH 45801-4842
Telephone: (419)-229-9055 Fax: (419)-228-2612
Contact: Richard Locke
Home health services.

Medical Services

Bluffton Community Hospital
139 Garau Street
Bluffton, OH 45817-1028
Telephone: (419)-358-9010 Fax: (419)-358-1532
Contact: Barbara Plaugher
Inpatient care, HIV testing and counseling

Lima Memorial Hospital
1001 Bellefontaine Ave
Lima, OH 45804-2894
Telephone: (419)-228-3335 Fax: (419)-226-5095
Contact: Arlett Pollock-Evans, MS, RN - Clinical Specialist
Hospital blood bank, support groups, home health services, counseling

Northwest Center of Human Resources
529 South Elizabeth St
Lima, OH 45804-1298
Telephone: (419)-228-5508 Fax: (419)-222-0235
Counseling, drug & alcohol treatment

Practice of Clinical Psychology, Inc.
1000 West Market Street
Lima, OH 45805-2730
Telephone: (419)-227-5515 Fax: (419)-222-7103
Contact: Ester Van Dyne, PhD
Mental health services.

St. Rita's Medical Center
730 West Market Street
Lima, OH 45801-4670
Telephone: (419)-227-3361 Fax: (419)-226-9718
Contact: Becky Goecke - Infextious Disease Coordinator
Blood bank, alcohol and drug abuse, social service, support groups,hospice, AIDS testing and education

Ashland County

County Health Depts

Ashland County Health Department
County Office Building
110 Cottage Street
Ashland, OH 44805
Telephone: (419)-289-0000
Contact: Julia Jones, RN - AIDS Educator
AIDS education & counseling

Ashtabula County

Community Services

Ohio Bar Association
Lawyer Referral Service
Ashtabula, OH 44004
Telephone: (800)-282-6500
Contact: William McCarthy
Legal referrals.

St.Joseph's Parish-Interfaith Clergy Representative
3330 Lake Avenue
Ashtabula, OH 44004-5799
Telephone: (216)-997-5666
Contact: Fr. Thomas G. Bishop
Religious support,Counseling

County Health Depts

Ashtabula County Health Department
Old Courthouse
12 West Jefferson Street
Jefferson, OH 44047-1096
Telephone: (216)-576-6010
Contact: Ray Saporito, M.D. - Health Commissioner
Education & referrals

Medical Services

CONTACT Ashtabula County, Inc.

Ashtabula, OH 44004
Telephone: (216)-998-2607
Toll-Free: (800)-474-4357
Mental health services.

Testing Sites

Conneaut City Health Department
327 Mill Street
Conneaut, OH 44030-2439
Telephone: (216)-593-3087
Contact: Sally Kennedy R.N., B.S. - Health Commissioner
Immunization clinics, vital statistics, environmental health

Athens County

Community Services

Open DOor 100%
United Campus Ministry
18 North College Street
Athens, OH 45701
Telephone: (614)-593-7301
Gay/lesbian Association, counseling meetings, support groups

County Health Depts

Athens City/County Health Department
278 West Union Street
Athens, OH 45701-2395
Telephone: (614)-592-4431
Contact: Robert E. Main, M.D. - Health Commissioner
Public Health

Belmont County

County Health Depts

Belmont County Health Department

68501 Bannock Road
St. Clairsville, OH 43950
Telephone: (614)-695-1202
Contact: Matt L. Kirkland, M.D. - Health Commissioner
Cancer screenings, family services, STD & Immunizations.

Medical Services

East Ohio Regional Hospital
90 N. Fourth St
Martins Ferry, OH 43935-1648
Telephone: (614)-633-1100
Contact: Irene Lovell
Hospital blood bank.

Brown County

County Health Depts

Brown County Health Department
204-D East Cherry Street
Georgetown, OH 45121-1314
Telephone: (513)-378-6892

Contact: Kevin McGann, M.D. - Health Commissioner
Education & referrals

Medical Services

Brown and Adams County Substance Abuse Center
200 Green Street
Georgetown, OH 45121-1337
Telephone: (513)-378-6068
Contact: Parker Moore
Substance abuse services.

Butler County

County Health Depts

Butler County Health Department
202 South Monument Street
130 High Street
Hamilton, OH 45011
Telephone: (513)-863-1770 Fax: (513)-863-4372
Contact: Robert J. Lerer, M.D. - Health Commissioner
Child clinic

Medical Services

Middletown Regional Hospital
105 McKnight Drive
Middletown, OH 45044-4898
Telephone: (513)-424-2111 Fax: (513)-420-5171
Contact: Karen Knerr
Hospital blood bank.

Carroll County

County Health Depts

Carrol County Health Department
24 2nd Street, N.E.
Carrollton, OH 44615-1202
Telephone: (216)-627-4866
Contact: Jon H. Marshall, MD - Health Commissioner
Referrals

Clark County

Community Services

American Red Cross - Clark County Chapter
1830 North Limestone Street
Springfield, OH 45503
Telephone: (513)-399-3872
Contact: Karen Henschen
Medical referrals, support groups, food pantries, hospice care, 24hr Hotline

Medical Services

McKinley Hall Inc.
529 East Home Road
Springfield, OH 45503
Telephone: (513)-322-5433 Fax: (513)-390-5615
Substance abuse program.

Mercy Medical Center
1343 N. Fountain Blvd
Springfield, OH 45501
Telephone: (513)-390-5000 Fax: (513)-390-5527
Hospital blood bank, physician referrals.

Neighborhood Church Clinic
23 West Pleasant Street
Springfield, OH 45505-4054
Telephone: (513)-325-0464 Fax: (513)-325-9548
Contact: Gwen Bellamy - Executive Director
Sickle cell program.

Clinton County

Community Services

Public Defender
39 E. Locust Street
Wilmington, OH 45177-2322
Telephone: (513)-382-1316
Contact: Elaine H. File
Legal referrals, criminals

County Health Depts

Clinton County Health Department
Courthouse
S. South and Sugartree
Wilmington, OH 45177
Telephone: (513)-382-3829
Contact: Director of Nursing
Home care agency, general

Medical Services

Clinton County Family Planning
615 W. Main Street
Wilmington, OH 45177-2321
Telephone: (513)-382-0265 Fax: (513)-382-0390
Contact: Dolores Lehr
Planned parenthood affiliate.

Columbiana County

Community Services

Valley, Inc.
15549 State ROute 170
Ogilive Square East, Suite 10
East Liverpool, OH 43920-3130
Telephone: (216)-385-2508 Fax: (216)-385-8484
Contact: Roberta Geidner-Antoniotti
STD testing and treatment, counseling for HIV & AIDS, planned parenthood

County Health Depts

Columbiana County Health Department
321 South Beaver Street
P.O. Box 396
Lisbon, OH 44432-1205
Telephone: (216)-424-0272
Contact: Robert Morehead - Administrator
Referrals for testing, food, clothing and medical assistance, AIDSeducation, support groups

Medical Services

East Liverpool City Hospital
425 West 5th Street
East Liverpool, OH 43920-2498
Telephone: (216)-386-2006 Fax: (216)-386-2028
Hospital blood bank.

Coshocton County

County Health Depts

Coshocton County Health Department
724 South 7th Street
Coshocton, OH 43812-2391
Telephone: (614)-622-1426
Contact: Becky Bider - Director of Nursing
Referral for testing and counseling

Home Health Care

Hospice of Coshocton County
P.O. Box 1284
Coshocton, OH 43812-6284
Telephone: (614)-622-6411
Contact: Barbara Emmons, R.N. - Coordinator
Hospice.

Crawford County

Community Services

Community Counseling Service
1376 State Route 598
Pally, OH 44833
Telephone: (419)-468-3010 Fax: (419)-468-4720
Contact: Bob Moneysmith
Mental health referrals, out-patient services for HIV

County Health Depts

Crawford County Health Department
Courthouse
112 E. Mansfield Street
Bucyrus, OH 44820
Telephone: (419)-562-5871
Contact: Jack B. Lentz, M.P.H. - Health Commissioner
Referrals for testing & counseling

Medical Services

Bucyrus Community Hospital
629 N Sandusky Ave
PO Box 627
Bucyrus, OH 44820-0627
Telephone: (419)-562-4677
Hospital blood bank.

Testing Sites

Planned Parenthood of Crawford County
125 North Columbus Street
Galion, OH 44833
Telephone: (419)-468-9926 Fax: (419)-468-1280
Contact: Beth Stephan
HIV testing

Cuyahoga County

Community Services

Lesiban/Gay Community Service Center of Cleveland
P.O. Box 6177
Cleveland, OH 44101-1177
Telephone: (216)-781-6736 Fax: (216)-522-0025
Contact: Linda Malicki - Administrative Manager
Gay/lesbian association, living room program for AIDS/HIV support froups,library, message therapy

The Cleveland Foundation
1422 Euolid Avenue
Room 437
Cleveland, OH 44115
Telephone: (216)-861-3810 Fax: (216)-861-1729
Contact: Steven Minter - Director
Fund programs for direct services & prevention; provides funding for HIV &AIDS projects

County Health Depts

Cuyahoga County Health Department
1375 Euclid Avenue
5th Floor South 514
Cleveland, OH 44115
Telephone: (216)-443-7520
Contact: Robert O. Walton, M.D. - Health Commissioner

East Cleveland Health Department
14340 Euclid Avenue
East Cleveland, OH 44112-3499
Telephone: (216)-681-2188
Vital statistics

Home Health Care

Caremark
4350 Emery Industrial Prk
Unit P
Warrensville Ht, OH 44128-5758
Telephone: (216)-591-0900 Fax: (216)-591-0664
Toll-Free: (800)-826-2175
Contact: Kitty Ribar
CLINICAL SUPPORT AND INFUSION THERAPIES: Nutrition, Antimicrobials, Chemo.,Hematopoe

Curaflex Fusion Services
4949 Galaxy Parkway
Warrensville Ht, OH 44128-5948
Telephone: (216)-831-5443 Fax: (216)-831-5639
Toll-Free: (800)-752-5938
Contact: Mimi Puro
Home Infusion Therapy

HNS, Inc.
9800 Rockside Road
Suite 500
Valleyview, OH 44125
Telephone: (216)-642-1155 Fax: (216)-642-5693
Contact: Colleen Bedard
Home Infusion Therapy, In-home Nursing and Attendant Care, P.T. Services, Pentamidine

Homedco Infusion
8555 Suite Valley Drive
Valley, OH 44125
Telephone: (216)-573-7500 Fax: (216)-573-7522
Nationwide experience in providing home infusion therapy to AIDS patients

nmc HOMECARE
6801 Engle Rd, Suite C, D, E
Middleburgh Hts, OH 44130
Telephone: (216)-243-8900
Fax: (216)-243-7660
Contact: Wayne Meyer
National JCAHO-Accredited company providing a full range of Infusion and Respiratory therapies and specializing in the care of HIV/AIDS patients. National Case Manager is also available at 800-445-1188

Medical Services

Cleveland Treatment Center, Inc.
1127 Carnegie Avenue
Cleveland, OH 44115-2805
Telephone: (216)-861-4246 Fax: (216)-241-1879
Licensed Ohio methadone treatment program, substance abuse program.

Dept of Veterans Affairs Medical Center
10000 Brecksville Rd
Brecksville, OH 44141
Telephone: (216)-526-3030
Contact: Betty Green
Hospital blood bank.

Health Issue Task Force, University Hospital
University Hospital
2074 Abington Road
Cleveland, OH 44106
Telephone: (216)-621-0766 Fax: (216)-844-5356
Contact: John Carey, M.D.
Out patient clinic

Hough-Norwood Health Care Center
8300 Hough Avenue
Cleveland, OH 44103-1375
Telephone: (216)-231-7700
Contact: Marybeth Mercer

Kaiser Permente Medical Center
12301 Snow Road
Parma, OH 44130-1099
Telephone: (216)-362-2000 Fax: (216)-362-2345
Contact: Ms. Maria Pollard
Hospital blood bank.

Lutheran Medical Center
2609 Franklin Boulevard
Cleveland, OH 44113-2992
Telephone: (216)-696-4300
Contact: Linda Schoolcraft - Infection Control
HIV testing, primary care, dental, hospice, ambulatory clinic

Southwest Community Health Systems & Hospital
18697 East Bagley Road
Middleberg Hts., OH 44130-3497
Telephone: (216)-826-8000 Fax: (216)-826-8063
Contact: Flo Hollenbaugh
Counseling, primary care, medical, nursing, home care, HIV testing,education.

Survivors
Metro Health Medical Center
2500 Metro Health Drive
Cleveland, OH 44109
Telephone: (216)-459-4141
Contact: Michael Anderson
Support group, infectious disease clinic, clinical trails referrals, outpatient & inpatient clinic.

The Free Medical Clinic of Greater Cleveland
12201 Euclid Avenue
Cleveland, OH 44106-4299
Telephone: (216)-721-4010 Fax: (216)-721-2431
Contact: Martin Hiller
Early intervention program, HIV testing, dental referrals

Testing Sites

Cleveland City Health Department
Mural Building
1925 St. Clair Avenue
Cleveland, OH 44114
Telephone: (216)-664-2525
Contact: Jeffrey Comfort - Health Commissioner; Joan Mallick, R.N., Ph.D. - Acting Commissioner
Local AIDS task force.

Lakewood Hospital
14519 Detroit Avenue
Lakewood, OH 44107-4383
Telephone: (216)-521-4200
Contact: Dr. Riebel
HIV testing; social services

Meridia Suburban Hospital
4180 Warrensville Ctr Rd
Warrensville Ht, OH 44122
Telephone: (216)-491-6000 Fax: (216)-561-8379
Contact: Elizabeth Antolik
HIV testing

Metro Health Clement Center
2500 East 79th Street
Cleveland, OH 44104-2164
Telephone: (216)-391-3200
Contact: Dolores Mitchell - Coordinator
HIV testing, counseling, primary & early intervention

Darke County

Community Services

Darke County Blood Bank
240 State Route 503
Arcanum, OH 45304
Telephone: (513)-548-6700
Contact: 513-461-3450
Blood bank, referral services only

County Health Depts

Darke County Health Department
300 Garst Avenue
Greenville, OH 45331
Telephone: (513)-548-4196
Contact: Terrence Holman, D.V.M. - Health Commissioner
Social service referrals, home health care

Medical Services

Darke County Recovery Services
134 West 4th Street
Greenville, OH 45331
Telephone: (513)-548-6842 Fax: (513)-548-8938
Substance abuse program.

Wayne Hospital
835 Sweitzer Street
Greenville, OH 45331-1077
Telephone: (513)-548-1141 Fax: (513)-547-5712
Contact: Emma Dunlap
Hospital blood bank, physician referrals.

Defiance County

Community Services

ABLE
201 East Second Street
Defiance, OH 43512
Telephone: (419)-782-1828 Fax: (419)-782-5830
Toll-Free: (800)-544-7369
Legal referrals.

Catholic Charities
1012 Ralston
Defiance, OH 43512-1335
Telephone: (419)-782-4933
Contact: Sandra Herman
Counseling for HIV

County Health Depts

Defiance County Health Department
197-C Island Park Avenue
Defiance, OH 43512-2551
Telephone: (419)-784-3818 Fax: (419)-782-4979
Contact: Charlotte Parsons, M.S.E.P.H. - Health Commissioner

Medical Services

American Red Cross - Defiance County Chapter
1220 South Clinton Street
Defiance, OH 43512-2735
Telephone: (419)-782-0136
Contact: W. Tom Wiseman - Exec.
Blood bank.

Five County Alcohol/Drug Program
418 Auglaize Street
Defiance, OH 43512-2205
Telephone: (419)-782-9920 Fax: (419)-784-2523
Contact: Miquel L. Gomez
Outpatient substance abuse program.

Testing Sites

Women and Family Services, Inc.
508 Wayne Avenue
Defiance, OH 43512
Telephone: (419)-782-4906 Fax: (419)-782-5941
Contact: Connie Allgire
HIV testing, referrals

Delaware County

County Health Depts

Delaware City-County Health Department
115 N. Sandusky Street
Delaware, OH 43015-1732
Telephone: (614)-368-1700 Fax: (614)-368-1736
Contact: Kay Fale RN - AIDS Educator
AIDS education for schools & communitys

Home Health Care

Delaware City/County Health Department
109 N. Sandusky
Delaware, OH 43015-1770
Telephone: (614)-368-1700 Fax: (614)-368-1736
Contact: Kay Gale, R.N. - AIDS Educator
Education, counseling & referral for AIDS patients, families & the public.

Medical Services

American Red Cross - Delaware County Chapter
5 West Winter Street
Delaware, OH 43015-1918
Telephone: (614)-548-7300
Contact: Richard Snouffer - Exec.
Blood bank.

Erie County

Community Services

Counseling and Growth Center
412 Jackson Street
Sandusky, OH 44870-2735
Telephone: (419)-627-0712 Fax: (419)-627-2826
Contact: Bruce A. Graebner - Executive Director
Mental health services, parent/family, individual counseling

Erie County Department of Human Services
221 West Parish Street
Sandusky, OH 44870-4877
Telephone: (419)-626-6781 Fax: (419)-626-5854
Contact: Judith Englehart
Social services, legal referrals.

Erie County Legal Aid & Public Defenders Association
416 Columbus Avenue
Sandusky, OH 44870-2723
Telephone: (419)-627-8373
Contact: Erich O'Brien
Legal referrals.

Social Security Administration
200 Hancock Street
Sandusky, OH 44870
Telephone: (800)-234-5772
Applications for disablity benefits. Also serves Huron County

County Health Depts

Erie County Health Department
420 Superior Street
PO Box 375
Sandusky, OH 44870-0375
Telephone: (419)-626-5623 Fax: (419)-626-8778
Contact: Stephen Casali
Family planning clinic, speaker's bureau, short-term care, AIDS task force.

Medical Services

Firelands Center (In-Patient)
2020 Hayes Avenue
Sandusky, OH 44870-4738
Telephone: (419)-627-5118 Fax: (419)-627-5169
Toll-Free: (800)-334-3562
Contact: Sister Mary Gregery George
Substance abuse program.

Stein Hospice Service Inc.
1200 Sycamore Lane
Sandusky, OH 44870
Telephone: (419)-625-5269
Contact: Rosalie Gdula - Director
Social services, support groups, short-term care. Also serves Huron County

Tri-County Addiction Center
334 East Washington Street
Sandusky, OH 44870
Telephone: (419)-625-7262 Fax: (419)-621-2361
Contact: A. Lisa Clark
Substance abuse program.

Fairfield County

Community Services

Department of Welfare
121 East Chestnut Street
Lancaster, OH 43130
Telephone: (614)-653-1701 Fax: (614)-687-6810
Contact: Jim Winegardner
Social services, administers Medicare

County Health Depts

Fairfield County Health Department
1587 Granville Pike
Lancaster, OH 43130-3794
Telephone: (614)-653-4489 Fax: (614)-653-6626
Physician referrals, testing

Fairfield County Health Department/AIDS Task Force
1587 Granville Pike
Lancaster, OH 43130
Telephone: (614)-653-4489 Fax: (614)-653-6626
Contact: Laura Holten
Anonymous AIDS testing & referrals for support groups

Testing Sites

Family Health Service
126 East Chestnut Street
Lancaster, OH 43130
Telephone: (614)-654-0985
Contact: Marilyn Moore
STD/HIV testing, well child care

Fayette County

County Health Depts

Fayette County Health Department
317 South Fayette Street
Washington C.H., OH 43160
Telephone: (614)-335-5910
Contact: Robert Vanzant, D.V.M. - Health Commissioner
Counseling, referrals

Medical Services

Choice Recovery Center
133 South Main Street
B-109
Washington C.H., OH 43160
Telephone: (614)-335-8228 Fax: (614)-335-8228
Contact: Michael Mason - Director
Substance abuse program.

Fayette County Memorial Hospital
1430 Columbus Avenue
Washington C.H., OH 43160
Telephone: (614)-335-1210
Contact: Sherry Jacks
Blood bank, social services.

Scioto-Paint Valley Mental Health Center
Fayette County Clinic
1300 East Paint Street
Washington C.H., OH 43160
Telephone: (614)-335-6935 Fax: (614)-335-7423
Mental health services.

Franklin County

Community Services

Al-Anon Alateen of Central Ohio
1561 Old Leonard Avenue
Columbus, OH 43219
Telephone: (614)-253-2701
12 Step non-professional support group

Columbus AIDS Task Force
1500 West 3rd Avenue
Suite 329
Columbus, OH 43212
Telephone: (614)-224-0411
Local AIDS task force, parent/family support groups, hotline

County Department Human Services
80 East Fulton Street
Columbus, OH 43215
Telephone: (614)-462-5335 Fax: (614)-462-4531
Contact: William N. Bugler
Social service assistance.

Legal Aid Society of Columbus
40 W Gay St
Columbus, OH 43215
Telephone: (614)-224-8374
Contact: Marcia Brehmer
Legal referrals.

Lutheran Social Services of Central Ohio
57 E Main St
Columbus, OH 43215
Telephone: (614)-228-5209 Fax: (614)-228-1471
Contact: Nelson Meyer
Social services, chapliancy, thrift stores, food pantries family/individual counseling

Narcotics Anonymous
1561 Old Leonard Avenue
Columbus, OH 43219
Telephone: (614)-252-1700
Substance abuse program.

Ohio State University Affirmative Action
2130 Neil Avenue
Archer House, Room 124
Columbus, OH 43210
Telephone: (614)-292-4207 Fax: (614)-292-4424
Contact: Dr. Robert Ransom
Legal referrals for students & employees of OSU.

Ohio State University College of Law
55 West 12th Street
College of Law
Columbus, OH 43210
Telephone: (614)-229-6818
Contact: Rhonda R. Rivera
Legal referrals

Veterans Administration - Outpatient Clinic and Center
2090 Kenny Rd
Columbus, OH 43221
Telephone: (614)-469-5127 Fax: (614)-469-2420
Contact: Dr. Lillian Thorne
Social service assistance.

County Health Depts

Franklin County Board of Health
410 S High St
Columbus, OH 43215
Telephone: (614)-462-3160
Contact: Dr. Mary-Jo Steiner
AIDS education, HIV home care

Franklin County Health Department
Courthouse Annex, 4th Fl.
410 South High Street
Columbus, OH 43215
Telephone: (614)-462-3160 Fax: (614)-462-3851
Contact: Mary Jo Steiner, MD - Health Commissioner
Home health nursing

Home Health Care

Caremark Connection Network
Brooksedge Corporate Ctr.
691 Greencrest Drive
Westerville, OH 43081-2848
Telephone: (614)-899-7999
Contact: Barbara Fisher - Branch/Ops Manager, Michael Kondik - Pharmacy Manager

Critical Care America
4333 Tuller Road, #A
Dublin, OH 43017
Telephone: (614)-792-9699
Contact: Maggie Wooding-Scott - Director of Nursing
HIV Program - Infusion services with dietitian and social work support

HNS, Inc.
4601 Hilton Corporate Dr
Columbus, OH 43232
Telephone: (614)-575-2200
Contact: Colleen Bedard
Home Infusion Therapy, In-home Nursing and Attendant Care, PhysicalTherapy, Pentamidine

Homedco Infusion
6175 Shamrock Court
Suite W
Dublin, OH 43017
Telephone: (614)-792-7778
Nationwide experience in providing home infusion therapy to AIDS patients

Hospice of Columbus
181 Washington Blvd
Columbus, OH 43215
Telephone: (614)-222-6471
Contact: Eileen Corwin, R.N.
Hospice; home health aide nurses, maternal child health, registered nurse,chaplain, volunteer care, social worker in home setting.

Hospice at Riverside
3595 Olentangy River Rd
Columbus, OH 42314
Telephone: (614)-566-5377 Fax: (614)-566-4391
Contact: Jusith Lebanowski - Executive Director
Help for terminally ill including AIDS

Mt. Carmel Home Health Care
793 W State St
Columbus, OH 43222
Telephone: (614)-486-6063
Contact: Sue Dempsey
Home health care.

nmc HOMECARE
4406 Tuller Road
Dublin, OH 43017
Telephone: (614)-252-3178
Fax: (614)-252-2614
Contact: Jim Schwamburger
National JCAHO-Accredited company providing a full range of Infusion and Respiratory therapies and specializing in the care of HIV/AIDS patients. National Case Manager is also available at 800-445-1188

Medical Services

Children's Hospital
700 Children's Drive
Columbus, OH 43205-2696
Telephone: (614)-461-2000 Fax: (614)-722-3553
Contact: Fredrich B. Ruymann, M.D.
Blood bank, hemophilia center, education, HIV clinic, testing, counseling

Chilren's Hospital HIV Program
700 Children's Drive
Columbus, OH 43205
Telephone: (614)-722-4451
Contact: Dr. Michael Brady

Columbus Area Community Mental Health Center
1515 East Broad Street
Columbus, OH 43205
Telephone: (614)-252-9250
Contact: Denise Ramos Laboy
Mental health services, outreach case management, counseling, home visits,referrals

Harding Hospital
445 E Granville Rd
Columbus, OH 43085
Telephone: (614)-885-5381 Fax: (614)-885-9813
Mental health services, counseling

Ohio State University Hospital
410 West Tenth Ave
Columbus, OH 43210
Telephone: (614)-293-8000
Contact: Stanley P. Balcerzak, M.D. - Hemophilia; Dr. Robert L. Perkins; Dr. Susan Koletar
Blood bank, hemophilia center, physician referrals, testing, counseling

Park Medical Center
1492 East Broad Street
Columbus, OH 43205
Telephone: (614)-251-3000
Contact: Lee Chamberlin
Blood bank, inpatient for AIDS

University Hospital Clinic 4715
456 West Tenth Avenue
Room 4725
Columbus, OH 43210
Telephone: (614)-293-8112
Contact: Dr. Michael Para
Physician referrals.

VITA Treatment Center
Methadone Program
700 Bryden Road

Columbus, OH 43215
Telephone: (614)-224-4506
Contact: Michele Condo
Substance abuse program, testing & counseling

Fulton County

Community Services

Fulton County Department of Human Services
146 South Fulton Street
Wauseon, OH 43567-1390
Telephone: (419)-337-0010 Fax: (419)-335-0337
Contact: Dennis McKay - Director
Social services.

County Health Depts

Fulton County Health Department
734 South Shoop Avenue
Wauseon, OH 43567-1707
Telephone: (419)-337-0915 Fax: (413)-337-0561
Contact: Hans Schmalzried, MSEPH - Health Commissioner
AIDS education in school & in community

Gallia County

County Health Depts

Gallia County Health Department
Gallia County Courthouse
18 Locust Street
Gallipolis, OH 45631
Telephone: (614)-446-4612 Fax: (614)-446-4804
Contact: Gerald E. Valee, M.D. - Health Commissioner
Public health services

Testing Sites

Holzer Medical Center
100 Jackson Pike
Gallipolis, OH 45631
Telephone: (614)-446-5000
Contact: Joyce Knight
HIV testing, counseling

Geauga County

County Health Depts

Geauga County Health Department
219 Main Street
Chardon, OH 44024-1296
Telephone: (216)-285-2222 Fax: (216)-286-1290
Contact: Susan Negron
Public health services.

Greene County

Community Services

Family Services Association
74 North Orange Street
Xenia, OH 45385
Telephone: (800)-762-9538
Contact: Mark Piermann - Executive Director
Referrals, literature

County Health Depts

Greene County Combined Health District
360 Wilson Drive
Xenia, OH 45385
Telephone: (513)-376-9411 Fax: (513)-376-3361
Contact: William P. McCullough, M.S.P.H - Health Commissioner
Public health services.

Medical Services

The Community Network
452 West Market Street
Xenia, OH 45385
Telephone: (513)-376-8700
Contact: Sue Giga - Executive Director
Chemical dependency services

Greene Hall Chemical Dependency Services
Greene Memorial Hospital
1141 North Monroe
Xenia, OH 45385
Telephone: (513)-372-8011
Contact: Dr. John Peter Angelo
Substance abuse program, lectures, testing, counseling

Greene Memorial Hospital
1141 N Monroe Dr
Zenia, OH 45385
Telephone: (513)-372-8011 Fax: (513)-376-6983
Contact: Michael Stephens - President
Medical services

Greene Memorial Hospital Inc.
1141 N Monroe Dr
Xenia, OH 45385
Telephone: (513)-372-8011 Fax: (513)-376-6983
Toll-Free: (800)-456-7362
Contact: Michael R. Stephens - President
Medical services

Guernsey County

Community Services

Guernsey Alcohol and Drug Addiction Treatment Center
60788 South Gate Road
Byesville, OH 43723
Telephone: (614)-439-4532 Fax: (614)-439-1031
Contact: Linda Secrest
Substance abuse program, HIV counseling

County Health Depts

Guernsey County Health Department
326 Highland Avenue
Cambridge, OH 43725-2595
Telephone: (614)-439-3577 Fax: (614)-432-7463
Contact: John R. Bennett, M.S. - Health Commissioner
Referrals

Home Health Care

Hospice of Guernsey, Inc.
1300 Clark Street
P.O. Box 1537
Cambridge, OH 43725-2504
Telephone: (614)-432-7440 Fax: (614)-432-7424
Contact: Patricia Howell - Administrator
Home care, social services, support group for patients and family homehealth aides, referrals, all RNs

Medical Services

Guernsey Counseling Center
2500 John Glen Highway Rd
Cambridge, OH 43725
Telephone: (614)-439-4428 Fax: (614)-439-3389
Contact: Peggy Davis - Manager
Mental health services, pre-hospitalization program

Guernsey Memorial Hospital
1341 Clark Street
PO Box 610
Cambridge, OH 43725-0610
Telephone: (614)-439-3561 Fax: (614)-439-5476
Toll-Free: (800)-544-1234
Contact: Kathy McClure
Physician/social service referrals, patient representatives

Hamilton County

Community Services

Social Security Administration
Federal Building-Rm 8004
550 Main Street
Cincinnati, OH 45202
Telephone: (513)-684-2685
Contact: Kaye Brunne - AIDS Community Liaison
Social service referrals.

County Health Depts

Cincinnati City Health Department
3101 Burnett Avenue
Cincinnati, OH 45229-3014
Telephone: (513)-357-7200 Fax: (513)-357-7290
Counseling/testing site, dental referrals, HIV testing

Cincinnati Department of Health
3101 Burnett Avenue
Cincinnati, OH 45229
Telephone: (513)-352-3100
Contact: Debbie Tripp
Counseling/testing site, local AIDS task force, education

Hamilton District Health Department
11499 Chester Road
138 E.Court St., Room 707
Sharonville, OH 45246
Telephone: (513)-632-8456
Contact: Timothy Ingram - Health Commissioner
HIV testing

Home Health Care

Caremark
Carnegie Center
53 Circle Freeway Drive
Cincinnati, OH 45246
Telephone: (513)-874-1161
Contact: Michele Hacker - Branch Manager
Clinical support and infusion therapies: nutrition, antimicrobials,chemotherapy, hematopoeti

Critical Care America
10234 Alliance Road
Cincinnati, OH 45242
Telephone: (513)-791-3880
Coordinate & integrate all clinical & psychosocial services for HIV+, homeIV therapy service

New England Critical Care America
10234 Alliance Road
Cincinnati, OH 45242-4710
Telephone: (513)-791-3880
Infusion therapies in home

Medical Services

AIDS Treatment Clinic, Holms Hospital Division
Mail Location 560
231 Bethesda Avenue
Cincinnati, OH 45267-0001
Telephone: (513)-558-6977 Fax: (513)-558-6386
Contact: Peter G. Frame, M.D. - Director
Primary care, clinical trials, social services, psychiatric care

Bethesda Hospital-North
10500 Montgomery Road
Cincinnati, OH 45242-4415
Telephone: (513)-745-1111 Fax: (513)-569-5428
Acute care, referrals, testing, education, social services

Central Community Mental Health Board
Drug Services
3020 Vernon Place
Cincinnati, OH 45219
Telephone: (513)-559-2000
Contact: Marilyn Cherry - Program Director
Substance abuse program, testing & counseling

Children's Hospital Medical Center
3333 Burnet Avenue
Elland and Bethesda Ave.
Cincinnati, OH 45229-3039
Telephone: (513)-559-4411
Contact: Ralph A. Gruppo, MD
Hemophilia center, testing; counseling for children, teenagers; servicesfor patients

Christ Hospital
2139 Auburn Avenue
Cincinnati, OH 45219-2989
Telephone: (513)-369-2000
Blood bank, testing & counseling

Cincinnati Sickle Cell Project
Children's Hospital
3333 Byrnet Avenue
Cincinnati, OH 45229
Telephone: (513)-559-4541
Contact: Beatrice C. Lampkin, M.D. - Director
Sickle cell program.

University of Cincinnati
Childrens Hosp. Med. Cntr
33 Burnet Avenue
Cincinnati, OH 45229
Telephone: (513)-559-4200 Fax: (513)-559-7247
Contact: Nancy McOwen
Hemophilia center.

Testing Sites

Clement Health Center
3101 Burnet Avenue
Cincinnati, OH 45229
Telephone: (513)-357-7200
Contact: Marva Anderson - Supervisor
Counseling/testing site.

Jewish Hospital of Cincinnati
3200 Burnet Avenue
Cincinnati, OH 45229-3099
Telephone: (513)-569-2000
Contact: David Krasofsky - Blood Bank Supervisor
Blood bank, HIV testing

Planned Parenthood of Cincinnati
2314 Auburn Avenue
Cincinnati, OH 45219-2802
Telephone: (513)-721-7635
Contact: Shirley Everrett-Clark; Ann Mitchell -
HIV testing (anonymous confidential) pre/post counseling, education,outreach, referrals

Providence Hospital
2446 Kipling Avenue
Cincinnati, OH 45239-6695
Telephone: (513)-853-5249
Contact: Pat Bussard - Manager Infection Control
HIV testing, social services, physician referral service

St. Francis-St. George Hospital
3131 Queen City Avenue
Cincinnati, OH 45238-2396
Telephone: (513)-389-5000
Contact: Pat Bussard - Manager Infection Control
HIV testing, social services, physician referral service

Hancock County

Community Services

Advocates for Basic Legal Equality, Inc.
237 South Main Street
Findlay, OH 45840
Telephone: (419)-422-1500 Fax: (419)-422-1595
Legal referrals for AIDS & HIV

County Health Depts

Findlay City Health Department
Municipal Building
1918 North Main Street
Findlay, OH 45840
Telephone: (419)-424-9768 Fax: (419)-424-7245
Contact: Stuart O. Kerr - Health Commissioner
Positive actsions - testing referrals

Hancock County Health Department
222 Broadway
Findlay, OH 45840-3380
Telephone: (419)-422-9212
Contact: Alice Kagy
Limited medical services & referral

Testing Sites

Planned Parenthood of NW Ohio
1039 North Main Street
Findlay, OH 45840-3671
Telephone: (419)-423-4611
Contact: Beth Stough
HIV testing & education

Hardin County

County Health Depts

Kenton-Hardin County Health Department
175 West Frankline Street
Courthouse Annex Suite 120
Kenton, OH 43326
Telephone: (419)-673-6230
Contact: Jay E. Pfeiffer, M.D. - Health Commissioner
Medical & economic referral service

Harrison County

Community Services

Human Services
521 North Main Street
PO Box 239
Cadiz, OH 43907
Telephone: (614)-942-2171
Child protective services, Medicaid,food stamps

County Health Depts

Harrison County Health Department
943-B East Market St
Cadiz, OH 43907-9799
Telephone: (614)-942-2616
Contact: Isam Tabbah, M.D. - Health Commissioner
Referral service

Henry County

Community Services

First Call For Help
1330-A N. Scott St
Napoleon, OH 43545-1024
Telephone: (419)-599-1660 Fax: (419)-592-8339
Toll-Free: (800)-468-4357
Contact: Joetta Prost
Crisis stablization unit, emergency assesments, information, referrals,free adolescent/adult screenings

Henry County Department of Human Services
104 East Washington St.
Napoleon, OH 43545-1629
Telephone: (419)-592-0896
Contact: Connie Schuette
Social services & referrals

County Health Depts

Henry County Health Department
104 E. Washington
Suite 302
Napoleon, OH 43545-1629
Telephone: (419)-599-5545
Contact: Hans Schmalzried, M.S.E.P.H. - Health Commissioner
Visiting nurses, hospice care

Medical Services

American Red Cross - Henry County Chapter
117 West Washington
Napoleon, OH 43545-1739
Telephone: (419)-592-4806
Blood bank.

Highland County

County Health Depts

Highland County Health Department
135 1/2 North High Street
Hillsboro, OH 45133-1157
Telephone: (513)-393-1941
Contact: Karen Ogleby, RN - Health Commissioner

Hocking County

County Health Depts

Hocking County Health Department
605 S.R. 664
Logan, OH 43138
Telephone: (614)-385-3030
Contact: Sheila Wilson, RN - Health Commissioner
Counseling & referrals

Home Health Care

Buckeye Home Health
525 East Front Street
P.O. Box 964
Logan, OH 43138
Telephone: (614)-385-4761 Fax: (614)-385-3645
Toll-Free: (800)-322-1317
Contact: Patricia Lytle, R.N.
Social service referrals, skilled nursing care, home health aides, physicaltherapy

Testing Sites

Planned Parenthood of Southeast Ohio
63 West Main Street
Logan, OH 43138
Telephone: (614)-385-3476
Contact: Cheryl Kinnison - Clinic Supervisor
HIV/STD testing

Holmes County

County Health Depts

Holmes County Health Department
931 Wooster Drive
Millersburg, OH 44654
Telephone: (216)-674-5035
Contact: Maurice E. Mullet, M.D. - Health Commissioner
Local AIDS task force, social service referrals.

Huron County

Home Health Care

Fisher-Titus Medical Center
272 Benedict Avenue
Norwalk, OH 44857-2399
Telephone: (419)-668-8101 Fax: (419)-663-6036
Toll-Free: (800)-589-3862
Contact: Richard Westhofen - Administrator
Home care, occupational therapy, physical therapy, oncology clinic

Medical Services

Counseling Center of Huron County
292 Benedict Avenue
Norwalk, OH 44857
Telephone: (419)-663-3737 Fax: (419)-663-5096
Toll-Free: (800)-242-5393
Contact: Marsha Mruk - Director
Mental health referrals, parent/family support groups.

Lawrence County

Medical Services

Lawrence County Medical Center
2228 S Ninth St
Ironton, OH 45638
Telephone: (614)-532-3231 Fax: (614)-532-3214
Contact: Ilene Kamap

Licking County

Community Services

Catholic Social Services
417 West Church Street
Newark, OH 43055-4238
Telephone: (614)-345-2565 Fax: (614)-534-0199
Contact: Debbie Nye
Social service referrals.

Home Health Care

Spencer Halfway House
69 Granville Street
Newark, OH 43055-4908
Telephone: (614)-345-7030
Social services (alcohol/drug related problems).

Medical Services

Center for Alternative Resources
35 South Park Place
P.O. Box 77
Newark, OH 43058-0077
Telephone: (614)-345-6166 Fax: (614)-349-9894
Contact: Cynthia Deal - Executive Director
Substance abuse program, 24 hr. crisis line 614-345-4357

Family Health Services of East Central Ohio
843 North 21st Street
Newark, OH 43055-2992
Telephone: (614)-366-3372 Fax: (614)-366-5757
Toll-Free: (800)-688-3266
Contact: Marilyn Moore - Executive Director
HIV testing and counseling

Licking Memorial Hospital
1320 West Main Street
Newark, OH 43055-3699
Telephone: (614)-344-0331 Fax: (614)-366-0449
Toll-Free: (800)-783-4677
Contact: William Andrews - President
Blood bank.

Testing Sites

Newark City Health Department
Newark City Building
40 W. Main Street
Newark, OH 43055
Telephone: (614)-349-6680 Fax: (614)-349-6810
Contact: Judith Carr, RN, RS, MS - Health Commissioner; Michael E. Campolo, D.O. - Medical Director
Anonymous HIV Test site, STD Clinic, medical/dental referrals, home health

Logan County

County Health Depts

Logan County Health Department
310 South Main Street
Bellefontaine, OH 43311-1696
Telephone: (513)-592-9040
Contact: William Verdsky - VMD

Lorain County

Community Services

Elyria City Health Department
202 Chestnut Street
Elyria, OH 44035-5398
Telephone: (216)-323-7595 Fax: (216)-284-1558
Contact: Kathryn Boylan, R.N., M.S.E.D. - Health Commissioner
AIDS task force, community group

Medical Services

Lorain Community Hospital
3700 Kolbe Road
Lorain, OH 44053-1699
Telephone: (216)-960-3000 Fax: (216)-960-4631
Toll-Free: (800)-431-9105
Contact: Paul Balcom - President
Hospital blood bank.

Lucas County

Community Services

David's House Compassion Corp.
501 North Detriot Avenue
Suite 204
Toledo, OH 43607
Telephone: (419)-244-6682 Fax: (419)-249-2741
Contact: Rust Bailey
Social services referrals, parent/family support groups, HIV housing, foodpantry, transportation, buddy support, financial assistance

Dignity
PO Box 1388
Toledo, OH 43603
Telephone: (419)-242-9057

Contact: Paul Kaltenbach
Gay/Lesbian association, religious support, HIV buddy support

County Health Depts

Lucas County Health Department
One Government Center
Suite 470
Toledo, OH 43604-2245
Telephone: (419)-245-4100
Contact: Dan Rutt - Health Commissioner
Education management, needs assessment

Toledo City Health Department
Health Center
635 North Erie Street
Toledo, OH 43624
Telephone: (419)-245-1700 Fax: (419)-245-1720
Contact: George Nowels - Dist. Supervisor
HIV testing (anonymous), pre & post counseling, STD clinic, referrals,partner notification (confidential)

Medical Services

The Academy of Medicine of Toledo & Lucas County
4428 Secor Road
Toledo, OH 43623-4285
Telephone: (419)-473-3200 Fax: (419)-475-6744
Contact: Lee Wealton - Executive Director
Physicians referrals.

Cordelia Martin Health Center
905 Nebraska Avenue
Toledo, OH 43607
Telephone: (419)-255-7883 Fax: (419)-255-6438
Contact: Doni Miller - Director
Sickle cell program.

Mercy Hospital
2200 Jefferson Avenue
Toledo, OH 43624-1181
Telephone: (419)-259-1500 Fax: (419)-259-4116
Contact: Camille A. Karatta, MD - Chairman Infectous Diseases
Hospital blood bank, physician referrals.

St. Charles Hospital
2600 Navarre Avenue
Oregon, OH 43616-3297
Telephone: (419)-698-7200 Fax: (419)-698-7761
Contact: Maryann Bowyer - Coordinator
Hospital blood bank, counseling & testing

St. Luke's Hospital
5901 Monclova Road
Maumee, OH 43537-1889
Telephone: (419)-893-5911 Fax: (419)-893-5996
Contact: Frank Bartell, III - President
Hospital blood bank.

St. Vincent Hospital
2213 Cherry
Toledo, OH 43608
Telephone: (419)-255-5665 Fax: (419)-321-3831
Contact: Fred Jordan
Substance abuse program, counseling.

Toledo Dental Society
4895 Monroe Street
Suite 103
Toledo, OH 43623
Telephone: (419)-474-8611 Fax: (419)-473-0860
Contact: Kathy Cohen
Dental referrals.

Testing Sites

Medical College of Ohio Hospital
3000 Arlington Ave
PO Box 10008
Toledo, OH 43614
Telephone: (419)-381-4172
Contact: Ann Locher R.N.
Hospital blood bank, testing & referrals

Planned Parenthood of NW Ohio
1301 Jefferson Avenue
Toledo, OH 43624
Telephone: (419)-255-1115 Fax: (419)-255-5216
Contact: Betty Marais - Executive Director
Free anonymous HIV testing, pre/post education, community education,gay risk, support group, outreach

Toledo Health Department
Health Center
635 North Erie Street
Toledo, OH 43624
Telephone: (419)-245-1710 Fax: (419)-245-1696
Counseling/testing site.

Mahoning County

Community Services

Mahoning County AIDS Task Force
c/o Neil Altman
P.O. Box 1143
Youngstown, OH 44501
Telephone: (216)-742-8766 Fax: (216)-742-8784
Local AIDS task force.

Mahoning County Drug Programs, Inc.
527 North Meridan
Youngstown, OH 44509
Telephone: (216)-797-0070 Fax: (216)-797-9148
Substance Abuse Program, HIV testing

Parkview Counseling
1350 Fifth Ave
Suite 300
Youngstown, OH 44504
Telephone: (216)-747-2601
Contact: Thomas Racich
Social service referrals, mental health counseling

Planned Parenthood of Mahoning Valley
77 East Midlothian Blvd.
Youngstown, OH 44507-2053
Telephone: (216)-788-6506 Fax: (216)-788-7805
Contact: Roberta Antoniotti - Executive Director
Planned parenthood affiliate, HIV testing, counseling

County Health Depts

Mahoning County Health Department
2801 Market Street
Youngstown, OH 44507-164]
Telephone: (216)-788-7041
Contact: Matthew A. Stefanak, M.P.H. - Health Commissioner
STD clinic, Anonymous HIV testing & counseling

Youngstown City Health Department
City Hall, 7th Floor
Youngstown, OH 44503
Telephone: (216)-742-8766 Fax: (216)-742-8784
Contact: Neil Haltman
Counseling/testing site (HIV)

Home Health Care

O.P.T.I.O.N Care of Northeast Ohio
397 Churchill-Hubbard Rd
Youngstown, OH 44505
Telephone: (216)-759-1332 Fax: (216)-759-1104
Contact: Ralph DiMuccio, RPh - Director of Patient Relat
Home IV and Nutritional Services

Medical Services

Western Reserve Care System, Southside Medical Center
Gypsy Lane and Goleta Ave
Youngstown, OH 44501
Telephone: (216)-744-5558
Contact: Sauna Cianciola - RN
Hemophilia center, HIV testing, dietary assistance, support-groups, referrals, home IV therapy

Testing Sites

Mahoning County AIDS Task Force
City Hall, 7th Floor
Youngstown, OH 44503
Telephone: (216)-742-8700 Fax: (216)-742-8784
Contact: Neil Altman
HIV testing, counseling

Marion County

Community Services

American Red Cross - Marion County Chapter
297 Mt. Vernon Avenue
Marion, OH 43302-4180
Telephone: (614)-387-8685
Contact: Gary Gibson - Chapter Manager
Local AIDS task force.

Marion Area Counseling Center
320 Executive Drive
Marion, OH 43302-6373
Telephone: (614)-387-5210 Fax: (614)-383-3472
Mental health referrals.

Smith Clinic
1040 Delaware Avenue
Marion, OH 43302-6483
Telephone: (614)-387-0850
Social service referrals.

Medina County

County Health Depts

Medina County Health Department
P.O. Box 1033
246 Northland Drive
Medina, OH 44258-1033
Telephone: (216)-723-9688
Contact: Patricia Stevens - Health Commissioner
Referrals, home-health care & testing.

Meigs County

County Health Depts

Meigs County Health Department
Multi-Purpose Health Cntr
112 East Memorial Drive
Pomeroy, OH 45769
Telephone: (614)-992-6626
Contact: Norma Torres - Nursing Director
AIDS/HIV educational materials, referrals for testing, counseling

Welfare Department
175 Race Street
PO Box 191
Middleport, OH 45760
Telephone: (614)-992-2117 Fax: (614)-992-7500
Contact: Cindy Mills - Social Services
Referrals, case work management, social services

Mercer County

County Health Depts

Mercer County Health Department
311 South Main Street
Lower Level
Celina, OH 45822-2295
Telephone: (419)-586-3251
Contact: Dr. Phillip Masser - Health Commissioner

Miami County

County Health Depts

Miami County/Troy City Health Departments
P.O. Box 677
3232 N. County Road 25A
Troy, OH 45373
Telephone: (513)-335-5675
Contact: Dr. R Guy Shake - Health Commissioner
Planned Parenthood affiliate

Medical Services

Miami County Alcoholism Council
423 N. Wayne Street
Piqua, OH 45356
Telephone: (513)-335-4543
Contact: Byron Ewick - Director
Substance abuse program, outpatient counseling

Piqua Memorial Medical Center
624 Park Avenue
Piqua, OH 45356
Telephone: (513)-778-6500
Hospital blood bank.

Monroe County

County Health Depts

Monroe County Health Department
47029 Moore Ridge Road
Woodsfield, OH 43793-9484
Telephone: (614)-472-1677

Immunization

Montgomery County

Community Services

AIDS Foundation Miami Valley
819 Salem Ave
PO Box 3539
Dayton, OH 45406-5822
Telephone: (513)-223-2437 Fax: (513)-277-2437
Local AIDS task force, client care, food pantry, housing, education

Church of Our Savior
HIV+ and Partners
155 East Thruston Blvd.
Dayton, OH 45419
Telephone: (513)-292-4195
Contact: Clark Gosley
Religious support group.

Community Blood Center
349 South Main Street
Dayton, OH 45402
Telephone: (413)-461-3450
Contact: Mary Anne Share - Coordinator
Blood bank.

Dayton Gay/Lesbian Association
445 Forest Avenue
Dayton, OH 45405-4439
Telephone: (513)-274-1776
Social activities, AIDS hotline referral, community support groups

United Health
184 Salem Avenue
Dayton, OH 45406-5803
Telephone: (513)-220-6622
Contact: Amy Dyer
Parent/family support groups; AIDS education, hotline for counseling

County Health Depts

Combined Health District of Montgomery County
451 West Third Street
Dayton, OH 45422
Telephone: (513)-225-4507 Fax: (513)-225-4507
Counseling/testing site.

Montgomery County Health District
P.O. Box 972
451 West 3rd Street
Dayton, OH 45422
Telephone: (513)-225-4395 Fax: (513)-496-3073
Counseling/testing site.

Home Health Care

Homedco Infusion
7740 Washington Villge Dr
Dayton, OH 45459
Telephone: (513)-438-1200 Fax: (513)-438-1281
Nationwide experience in providing home infusion therapy to AIDS patients ,hospital beds & oxygen

Medical Services

Community Blood Center
349 South Main Street
Dayton, OH 45402-2736
Telephone: (513)-461-3450 Fax: (513)-461-9217
Contact: Mary Anne Share
Blood bank.

Grandview Hospital & Medical Center
405 Grand Avenue
Dayton, OH 45405-4796
Telephone: (513)-226-3200
Contact: Sharon Virgallito
Hospital blood bank.

Health Outreach
1944 North main Streetnue
Dayton, OH 45405
Telephone: (513)-262-3500 Fax: (513)-496-7133
Contact: Diana Alexander
Anonymous testing, research project concentrating on IDU & crack & theirsexual partners (confidential), assessment, referrals

St. Elizabeth Medical Center
601 Edwin C Moses Rd
Dayton, OH 45408
Telephone: (513)-229-6000 Fax: (513)-229-7093
Contact: Joan Janning
Infectious control department.

Testing Sites

Miami Valley Planned Parenthood Inc.
224 N. Wilkinson Street
Dayton, OH 45402
Telephone: (513)-226-0164
Contact: Marrion Haines; Cheryl Radeloff
HIV/AIDS testing (anonymous), counseling (pre/post), education, referrals

Paulding County

County Health Depts

Paulding County Health Department
101 West Perry Street
Paulding, OH 45879
Telephone: (419)-399-3921
Contact: Don K. Snyder, M.D. - Health Commissioner

Perry County

County Health Depts

Perry County Health Department
P.O. Box 230
121 West Brown Street
New Lexington, OH 43764-0230
Telephone: (614)-342-5179
Contact: Stephen C. Ulrich, M.D. - Health Commissioner
AIDS education & testing

Pickaway County

County Health Depts

Pickaway County Health Department
110 Island Road
P.O. Box 613
Circleville, OH 43113-9575
Telephone: (614)-474-8861
Contact: Dr. Sharon Stanley
Referral, AIDS education & information

Medical Services

Alcoholism Program - Berger Hospital
210 Sharon Road
Circleville, OH 43113
Telephone: (614)-474-2126 Fax: (614)-477-6070
Toll-Free: (800)-589-2126
Contact: Debbie Wright
Substance abuse program.

Pike County

County Health Depts

Pike County Health Department
229 Valleyview Drive
Waverly, OH 45690
Telephone: (614)-947-7721
Contact: Joan I. Dass, M.D. - Health Commissioner
HIV testing

Portage County

County Health Depts

Portage County Health Department
County Administration Bld
449 South Meridian Street
Ravenna, OH 44266
Telephone: (216)-296-9919
Contact: Kenneth F. Rupp, M.D., FAAFP - Health Commissioner
Tracks communicable diseases; referrals for HIV testing

Home Health Care

Kent Visiting Nurses Association
145 Gougler Avenue
Kent, OH 44240-2401
Telephone: (216)-673-5314 Fax: (216)-673-3819
Contact: Anna French
Home health care.

Ravenna Visiting Nurses Association
145 North Chestnut Street
Ravenna, OH 44266-2287
Telephone: (216)-297-7623 Fax: (216)-297-7457
Contact: Gayle Bentley, BSN - Executive Director
Home health care, hospice

Medical Services

Portage County Alcohol Service and Drug Abuse
127 East Main Street
Ravenna, OH 44266-2214
Telephone: (216)-296-3255 Fax: (216)-296-6865
Contact: Sue Whitehurst
Substance abuse program - AIDS Education

Testing Sites

Planned Parenthood of Portage County
241 South Chestnut Street
Ravenna, OH 44266-3024
Telephone: (216)-296-7526
HIV testing & counseling

Preble County

County Health Depts

Preble County Health Department
County Office Building
119 S. Barron St.-Room 20
Eaton, OH 45320-2395
Telephone: (513)-456-8187
Contact: James Lucas, M.S., E.H. - Health Commissioner

Putnam County

County Health Depts

Putnam County Health Department
336 East Main Street
Ottawa, OH 45875-1946
Telephone: (419)-523-5608
Contact: Dr. John C Biery - D.O.
Referrals

Richland County

Community Services

Planned Parenthood of Mansfield Area
35 North Park Street
Mansfield, OH 44902-1762
Telephone: (419)-525-3075 Fax: (419)-522-3629
Contact: Cindy Biggs
Planned Parenthood affiliate.

Shelby Help Line Ministries
60 1/2 West Main Street
Shelby, OH 44875-1237
Telephone: (419)-347-6307
Social service referrals, financial aid/budgeting, hospital equipment loan

County Health Depts

Mansfield-Richland County Health Department
555 Lexington
Mansfield, OH 44907
Telephone: (419)-524-2333
Contact: Stan Saalman - Health Commissioner
HIV testing, counseling

Mansfield/Richland County Health Department
555 Lexington Avenue
Mansfield, OH 44907
Telephone: (419)-774-4504 Fax: (419)-774-4585
Counseling/testing site.

Testing Sites

Planned Parenthood of Mansfield Area
35 North Park Street
Mansfield, OH 44902
Telephone: (419)-525-3075 Fax: (419)-522-3629
Contact: Cindy Biggs
HIV testing

Ross County

County Health Depts

Ross County General Health District
425 Chestnut Street
Suite 2077
Chillicothe, OH 45601-2306
Telephone: (614)-775-1146
Contact: Sharon Stanley, R.N., M.S. - Health Commissioner
Counseling and testing site

Medical Services

Veterans Administration
Medical Center
17273 S.R. #104
Chillicothe, OH 45601-8603
Telephone: (614)-773-1141 Fax: (614)-772-7023
Contact: Troy E. Page
Hospital blood bank, HIV counseling

Sandusky County

Community Services

Sandusky Human Services
500 West State Street
Fremont, OH 43420-2532
Telephone: (419)-334-3891
Contact: Don Morton - Administrator
Social services referrals.

Sandusky Valley Center
675 Bartson Road
Fremont, OH 43420-2638
Telephone: (419)-332-5524 Fax: (419)-332-7581
Mental health referrals.

Scioto County

Community Services

Catholic Social Services
524 6th Street
Portsmouth, OH 45662-3843
Telephone: (614)-353-3185 Fax: (614)-353-3186
Social service referrals, counseling, emergency transportation & foodpantry

Legal Aid Association
Bank Ohio Building
Suite 700
Portsmouth, OH 45662-9998
Telephone: (614)-354-7563 Fax: (614)-354-2508
Contact: Mark Cardosi
Legal referrals.

Legal Aid Association
800 Gallia Street
Suite 700
Portsmouth, OH 45662
Telephone: (614)-354-7563
Civil legal services

Scioto County Counseling Center, Inc.
1311 2nd Street
Portsmouth, OH 45662-4602
Telephone: (614)-354-6685 Fax: (614)-354-5061
Contact: Ed Hughes
Substance abuse program; counseling.

Southern Ohio Psychological Services
Bank One Plaza
Portsmouth, OH 45662
Telephone: (614)-353-8063
Mental health referrals.

County Health Depts

Scioto County Health Department
Courthouse Room 303
6th Street and Court
Portsmouth, OH 45662
Telephone: (614)-354-3241
Contact: Keith Gaspich, M.D. - Health Commissioner

Medical Services

Shawnee Mental Health Center
2203 25th Street
Portsmouth, OH 45662
Telephone: (614)-354-7702 Fax: (614)-353-6206
Mental health referrals.

Seneca County

County Health Depts

Seneca County Health Department
3140 South State Rte 100
Tiffin, OH 44883-9709
Telephone: (419)-447-9340 Fax: (419)-447-3691
Contact: Ken Kerik, M.P.H. - Health Commissioner
Testing

Medical Services

American Red Cross - Fostoria Chapter
P.O. Box 406
207 Tiffin Street
Fostoria, OH 44830-0406
Telephone: (419)-435-5360
Contact: Fay Sweeney
Blood bank.

Shelby County

County Health Depts

Shelby County Health Department
Courthouse
100 E. Court Street
Sidney, OH 45365
Telephone: (513)-498-7249
Contact: Richard H. Breece, M.D. - Health Commissioner

Home Health Care

Homedco Infusion
4040 State Route 705
Ft Loramie, OH 45845
Telephone: (513)-295-3581
Toll-Free: (800)-456-1986
Contact: Ron Drees
Nationwide experience in providing home infusion therapy to AIDS patients

Wilson Memorial Hospital
915 West Michigan Street
Sidney, OH 45365
Telephone: (513)-498-2311 Fax: (513)-498-1075
Contact: Steve Osterholt, R.N.
Hospital blood bank; home health

Stark County

Community Services

Alcohol and Drug Assistance
724 South Union Avenue
Alliance, OH 44601-2919
Telephone: (216)-821-3846
Substance abuse program.

County Health Depts

Stark County Health Department
3951 Convience Circle Northwest
Canton, OH 44718-2272
Telephone: (216)-493-9904 Fax: (216)-493-9920
Contact: William J. Franks, B.S., M.P.H - Health Commissioner
Counseling

Home Health Care

Visiting Nurses of Stark County
Central Stark County
1445 Harrison Avenue, NW
Canton, OH 44708
Telephone: (216)-452-7955
Home health care therapy, title 3 & 20

Medical Services

American Red Cross - Alliance Chapter
222 South Arch Street
Alliance, OH 44601-2504
Telephone: (216)-823-0660
Blood bank.

Aultman Hospital
2600 South Sixth Street, S.W.
Canton, OH 44710
Telephone: (216)-452-9911 Fax: (216)-588-2607
Contact: Dr. James Oliver
Hospital blood bank, mental health referrals, religious support

Testing Sites

Canton City Health Department
City Hall, 3rd Floor
420 Market Avenue N.
Canton, OH 44702
Telephone: (216)-489-3231 Fax: (216)-489-3335
Counseling/testing site.

Planned Parenthood of Stark County
2663 Cleveland Ave Northwest
Canton, OH 44709
Telephone: (216)-456-7191
Contact: Bonnie Bolitho; Sarah Babb -
HIV testing, pre & post counseling, education prevention

Summit County

County Health Depts

Barberton Health Department
571 West Tuscarawas Avene
Barberton, OH 44203
Telephone: (216)-745-6067
Contact: Majorie Broadhead, RN - Nursing Supervisor

Summit County Health Department
1100 Graham Circle
Cuyahoga Falls, OH 44224-2993
Telephone: (216)-923-4891
Contact: Martha D. Nelson, M.D. - Health Commissioner

Medical Services

Akron General Medical Center
400 Wabash Avenue
Akron, OH 44307-2463
Telephone: (216)-384-6880 Fax: (216)-996-2300
Contact: Jan Susman; Marilyn Henry -
Social service referrals.

Western Reserve Psychiatric Hospital
PO Box 305
Northfield, OH 44067
Telephone: (216)-467-7131 Fax: (216)-467-2420
Inpatient psychiatric hospital

Trumbull County

Community Services

Planned Parenthood of Mahoning Valley
418 South Main Street
Warren, OH 44481
Telephone: (216)-399-5104 Fax: (216)-395-2231
Contact: Holly Hensen
HIV testing

Valley Counseling Services, Inc.
150 East Market Street
Warren, OH 44481
Telephone: (216)-399-6451 Fax: (216)-394-6266
Mental Health Referrals

Medical Services

American Red Cross - Seneca County Chapter
210 East Market Street
Tiffen, OH 44483-2835
Telephone: (419)-447-1424
Contact: Alice Shrode - Exec.
Blood bank.

Union County

Community Services

American Red Cross, Union County Chapter
112 E. Fifth Street
Marysville, OH 43040-1259
Telephone: (513)-642-6651 Fax: (513)-642-4899
Contact: Marge Myers - Executive Director; Deloris Bills, RN, MSN - AIDS Task Force; Judy Kohn, RN, CIC - AIDS Task Force
AIDS Task Force, Blood Bank

County Health Depts

Union County Health Department
621 South Plum Street
Marysville, OH 43040-1697
Telephone: (513)-642-0801
Contact: Dee Dee Houdashelt RN - Health Commissioner
Home care, referral & intake, AIDS task force, education, training for careproviders

Van Wert County

County Health Depts

Van Wert County Health Department
Medical Arts Building
140 Fox Road
Van Wert, OH 45891
Telephone: (419)-238-0808
Contact: Harold C. Smith, MD - Health Commissioner

Warren County

Home Health Care

Curaflex Infusion Services
4700 Duke Drive
Suite 135
Mason, OH 45040
Telephone: (800)-999-2872
Home IV therapy: TPN, Enteral, IV Antibiotics, Aerosolized/IV Pentamidine

Wayne County

Community Services

Wooster/ Wayne Legal Aid Society Inc.
#132 South Market Street
Wooster, OH 44691-2823
Telephone: (216)-264-1927
Contact: Frank G. Avellone - Manager
Legal aid for low income

Wood County

Community Services

Planned Parenthood of NW Ohio
920 North Main Street
Bowling Green, OH 43402-1819
Telephone: (419)-354-3540
Contact: Stephanee Wohler
HIV testing & counseling

Wyandot County

Community Services

American Red Cross, Wyandot County Chapter
206 S. Sandusky
Upper Sandusky, OH 43351-1426
Telephone: (419)-294-1935
Contact: Gloria Estep - Executive Director
Blood bank, HIV support group

Wyandot County Ministerial Association
St. Peter Catholic Church
225 North Eighth Street
Upper Sandusky, OH 43351
Telephone: (419)-294-1268
Contact: Sr. Barbara Jean Miller
Religious Support

County Health Depts

Wyandot County Health Department
127A S. Sandusky Avenue
Upper Sandusky, OH 43351
Telephone: (419)-294-3852
Contact: Kyu Park, MD - Health Commissioner
AIDS task force; educational & community information

OKLAHOMA

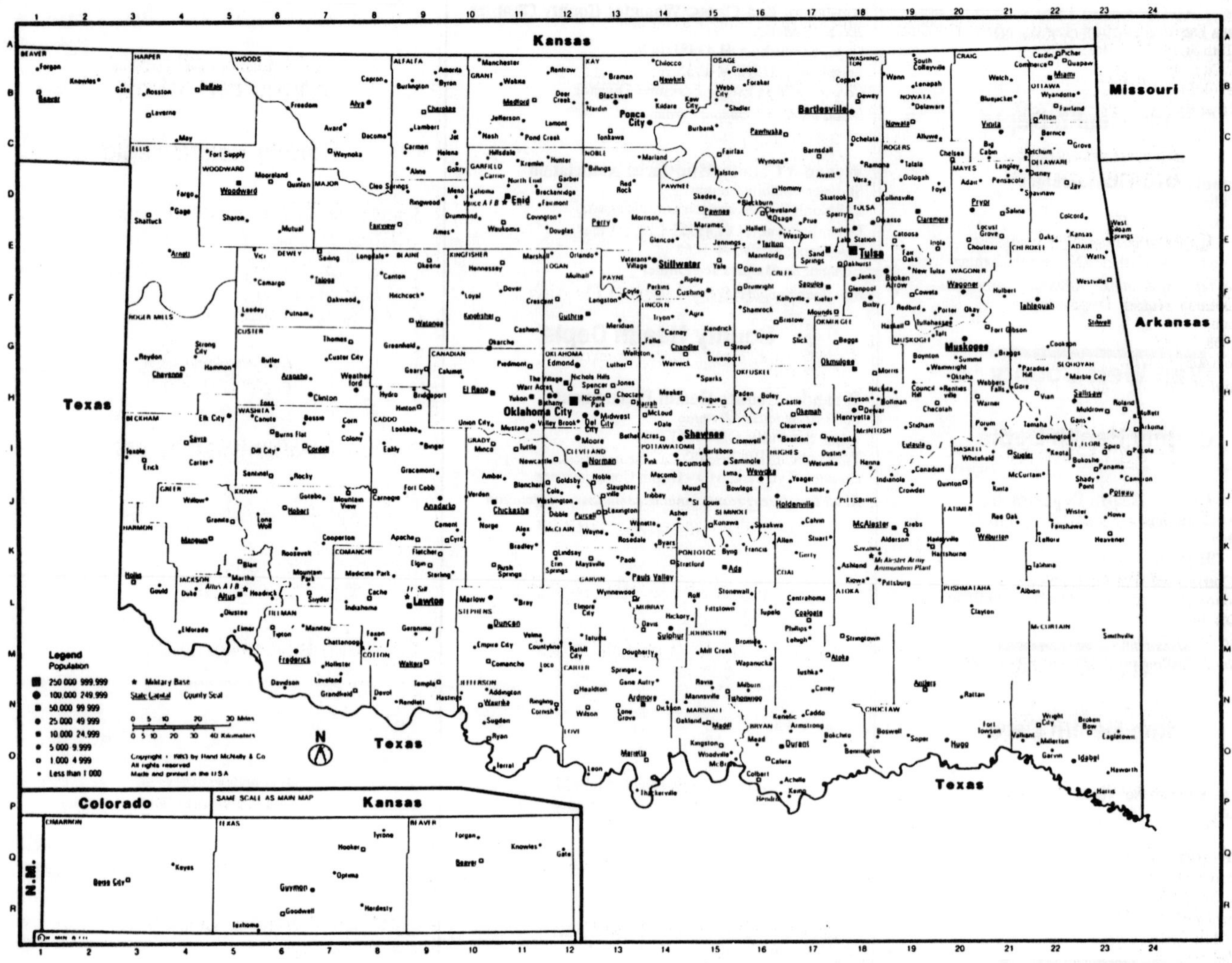

From City/County Planning Atlas Copyright 1989 by Reed McNally & Company, R.L. 90-S-28

Oklahoma

General Services

State Health Departments

Oklahoma Department of Health, AIDS Division
1000 NE 10th Street, Mail Drop 0308
Oklahoma City, OK 73152
Telephone: (405)-271-4636
Contact: Janet Richey - Administrative Dir. AIDS/HIV

Blaine County

County Health Depts

Blaine County Health Department
204 W Main
Watonga, OK 73772
Telephone: (405)-623-7977
Confidential HIV testing. Call for appointment

Bryan County

County Health Depts

Bryan County Health Department
1303 Waco
Durant, OK 74701
Telephone: (405)-924-4285
HIV Antibody Testing, Confidential/Call for Appointment.

Carter County

County Health Depts

Carter County Health Department
101 First Avenue, SW
Ardmore, OK 73401
Telephone: (405)-223-9705
Contact: Mike Clairbourne
HIV Antibody Testing, Confidential

Choctaw County

County Health Depts

Choctaw County Health Department
107 S 3rd
Hugo, OK 74743
Telephone: (405)-326-6106 Fax: (405)-326-5124
Contact: Doyle Carper
Confidential HIV testing. Call for appointment

Cleveland County

County Health Depts

Cleveland County Health Department
641 E. Robinson
Norman, OK 73071
Telephone: (405)-321-4048
HIV Antibody Testing, Confidential

Cleveland County Health Department
224 South Chestnut Ave
Moore, OK 73160
Telephone: (405)-794-1591
HIV Antibody Testing, Confidential

Coal County

County Health Depts

Coal County Health Department
210 N Main
Box 365
Coalgate, OK 74538
Telephone: (405)-927-2367
Confidential HIV testing. Call for appointment

Comanche County

County Health Depts

Comanche County Health Department
1010 South Sheridan Road
Lawton, OK 73501
Telephone: (405)-248-5890
HIV Antibody Testing, Confidential

Garfield County

County Health Depts

Garfield County Health Department
2501 Mercer Drive
Enid, OK 73702-8602
Telephone: (405)-233-0650
HIV Antibody Testing, Confidential/Anonymous

Harper County

County Health Depts

Woodward County Health Department
104 Temple Houston Drive
Woodward, OK 73801
Telephone: (405)-256-6416
Confidential HIV Testing and Information. Call for Appointment.

Jackson County

County Health Depts

Jackson County Health Department
201 S Lee
Altus, OK 73521
Telephone: (405)-482-7308
Confidential HIV testing.

Johnston County

County Health Depts

Johnston County Health Department
1151 S Byrd
Tishomingo, OK 73460
Telephone: (405)-371-2470 Fax: (405)-371-3347
Contact: Marsha Nichols
Confidential HIV testing. Call for appointment

Kay County

County Health Depts

Kay County Health Department
1201 East Hartford
Ponca City, OK 74601
Telephone: (405)-762-1641
HIV Antibody Testing, Confidential

Kay County Health Department
1706 S Main
Blackwell, OK 74631
Telephone: (405)-363-5520
Confidential HIV testing.

Love County

County Health Depts

Love County Health Department
200 CE Colsten Blvd.
Marietta, OK 73448
Telephone: (405)-276-2531
Confidential HIV testing.

Mc Curtain County

County Health Depts

McCurtain Health Department
1300-D SE Adams
Idabel, OK 74745
Telephone: (405)-286-6620
Confidential HIV testing.

Muskogee County

County Health Depts

Muskogee Health Department
530 S 34th Street
Muskogee, OK 74401
Telephone: (918)-683-0321
Confidential HIV testing.

Oklahoma County

Community Services

Other Options
5915 Northwest 23rd Street
Suite 105
Oklahoma City, OK 73127
Telephone: (405)-728-3222
HIV test sites; AIDS education; case management

County Health Depts

Oklahoma City-County Health Department
921 N.E. 23rd Street
Oklahoma City, OK 73105
Telephone: (405)-427-8651
HIV testing-confidential/walk-in Mon-Fri(8am to 11am) & Tues & Thurs (1pmt o 8pm) anonymous.

Home Health Care

Caremark Connection Network
5924 NW 2nd Street
Suite 600
Oklahoma City, OK 73127
Telephone: (405)-495-2273 Fax: (405)-787-6018
Contact: Michael Gold - General Manager, Craig Reno - Pharmacy/Ops Manager
Clinical Support and Infusion Therapy: Nutrition, Antimicrobials, Chemo.,Hematopoeti

Pittsburg County

County Health Depts

Pittsburg County Health Department
620 South Third Street
McAlester, OK 74501
Telephone: (918)-423-1267
Confidential HIV Testing

Pontotoc County

County Health Depts

Pontotoc Health Department
1630 E Beverly
P.O. Box 10
Ada, OK 74820
Telephone: (405)-332-2011
Confidential HIV testing.

Pottawatomie County

County Health Depts

Pottawatomie County Health Department
1904 Gordon Cooper Drive
PO Box 1487
Shawnee, OK 74802
Telephone: (405)-273-2157
Contact: Rod Huffman
Confidential HIV testing

Pushmataha County

County Health Depts

Pushmataha Health Department
211 SW 3rd
Antlers, OK 74523
Telephone: (405)-298-3383
Contact: Doyle Carper
Confidential HIV testing

Texas County

County Health Depts

Texas County Department of Health
1410 North East Street
Guymon, OK 73942
Telephone: (405)-338-8544
Contact: Larry Olmstead
Confidential HIV testing

Tulsa County

Community Services

SHANTI - Tulsa
P.O. Box 4318
Tulsa, OK 74159-0318
Telephone: (918)-749-7898
Contact: Mary Collier
AIDS education, counseling, referrals, support, buddy systems

County Health Depts

Tulsa City Health Department
4616 E 15th
Tulsa, OK 74112
Telephone: (918)-744-1000
Confidential/Anonymous Testing

Tulsa City-County Health Department
4616 East 15th Street
Tulsa, OK 74112
Telephone: (918)-744-1000
Confidential/Anonymous Testing. Mon - Thurs (8am - 3:30pm) and Fri. (8am -10:30am)

Home Health Care

Caremark Connection Network.
3158 S 108th E Avenue
Suite 284
Tulsa, OK 74146
Telephone: (918)-665-2273 Fax: (918)-665-2986
Contact: Michael Gold - General Manager, Thomas Kaye - Operations Manager
CLINICAL SUPPORT AND INFUSION THERAPY: Nutrition, Antimicrobials, Chemo., Hematopoeti

OREGON

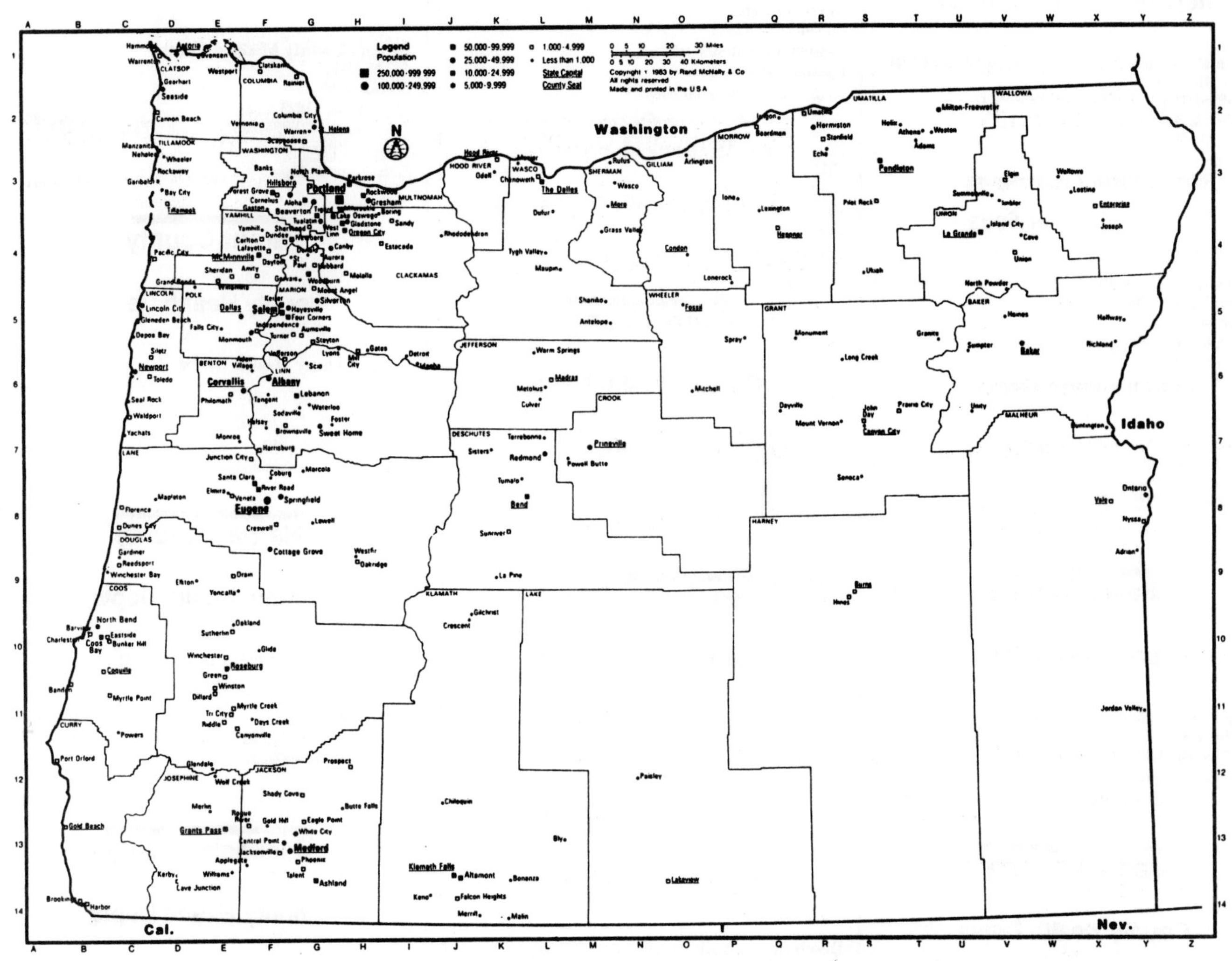

From City/County Planning Atlas Copyright 1989 by Reed McNally & Company, R.L. 90-S-28

Oregon

General Services

State Health Departments

Oregon Department of Human Resources, State Health Division
State Office Bldg.
1400 SW 5th Avenue
Portland, OR 97214
Telephone: (503)-731-4029
Contact: Robert McAlister - HIV Program Mgr.

Statewide Services

Oregon AIDS Task Force
c/o Oregon Health Div.
PO Box 14450
Portland, OR 97214-0450
Telephone: (503)-248-3674
AIDS/HIV Service Organization and Task Force

Oregon Minority AIDS Coalition
3415 NE Broadway
Portland, OR 97232
Telephone: (503)-282-4501
AIDS/HIV Service Organization and Task Force

Baker County

County Health Depts

Baker County Health Department
2610 Grove Street
Baker City, OR 97814
Telephone: (503)-523-8211
Medical, testing & counseling

Benton County

County Health Depts

Benton County Health Department
530 N.W. 27th Street
Corvallis, OR 97330
Telephone: (503)-757-6835
AIDS testing & counseling

Clatsop County

County Health Depts

Clatsop County Health Department
PO Box 206
Astoria, OR 97103-0206
Telephone: (503)-325-8500
Referrals, testing, counseling

Coos County

County Health Depts

Coos County Health Department
Courthouse
240 North Collier
Coquille, OR 97423
Telephone: (503)-396-3121
Contact: Frances Smith
Medical testing & counseling

Coos County Mental Health Department
1975 McPherson
North Bend, OR 97459
Telephone: (503)-756-2020 Fax: (503)-756-5466
Contact: Linda Manous
Counseling, HIV testing, speakers, written information

Curry County

County Health Depts

Curry County Health Department
PO Box 746
Gold Beach, OR 97444
Telephone: (503)-247-7011
Medical services, testing & counseling

Deschutes County

Community Services

Central Oregon AIDS Support Team
PO Box 9184
Bend, OR 97708
Telephone: (503)-389-6391
Contact: Mike Craven
AIDS/HIV Service Organization and Task Force, Ryan White title II

County Health Depts

Deschutes County Health Department
409 N.E. Greenwood Avenue
Bend, OR 97701
Telephone: (503)-388-6616
Contact: David Glassman
Testing, counseling

Douglas County

Community Services

ADAPT
621 W. Madrone
Roseburg, OR 97470
Telephone: (503)-672-2691 Fax: (503)-672-2691
Contact: Bruce Piper
In-patient, out-patient services, drug & alcohol counseling

Medical Services

Veterans Administration Medical Center
913 NW Garden Valley Blvd
Roseburg, OR 97470
Telephone: (503)-440-1000
Contact: Perry C. Norman
Medical & Social Services to Eligible Veterans

Gilliam County

Medical Services

Gilliam County Medical Center
422 N. Main
PO Box 705
Condon, OR 97823
Telephone: (503)-384-2061 Fax: (503)-384-3121
Contact: Bruce Carlson, M.D.
Testing, counseling

Grant County

County Health Depts

Grant County Health Office
PO Box 70
Canyon City, OR 97820
Telephone: (503)-575-0429
Contact: Johnnie Titus
HIV education, counseling

Harney County

County Health Depts

Harney County Health Department
323 North Grand Avenue
PO Box 551
Burns, OR 97720
Telephone: (503)-573-2271
Contact: Michele Davies
HIV, STD testing

Jackson County

County Health Depts

Jackson County Health Department
1005 E. Main Street
Medford, OR 97504-7459
Telephone: (503)-779-7335

Testing Sites

Jackson County Health Department
1005 E. Main Street
Medford, OR 97504-7459
Telephone: (503)-776-7328 Fax: (503)-776-6261
HIV testing

Jefferson County

County Health Depts

Jefferson County Health Department
66 Southeast D Street
Suite D
Madras, OR 97741
Telephone: (503)-475-4456 Fax: (503)-475-4457

Contact: Linda Marlen - Director
HIV testing (anonymous & confidential), pre/post counseling, referrals,education, literature, community outreach

Josephine County

County Health Depts

Josephine County Health Department
714 N.W. A Street
Grants Pass, OR 97526
Telephone: (503)-474-5325 Fax: (503)-774-5353
HIV testing

Klamath County

County Health Depts

Klamath County Department of Health Service
403 Pine Street
Klamath Falls, OR 97601-6035
Telephone: (503)-882-8846
Contact: Gwen Short
Wellness program, testing

Lake County

County Health Depts

Lake County Public Health Department
628 North First Street
Lakeview, OR 97630
Telephone: (503)-947-6045
Contact: Barbara Wheelock
Medical counseling, referrals

Lincoln County

County Health Depts

Lincoln County Health Department
255 S.W. Coast Highway
Newport, OR 97365
Telephone: (503)-265-4179
Contact: Pat Bilodeau RN
HIV testing (anonymous), pre/post counseling, referrals, literature,education, community outreach

Linn County

County Health Depts

Linn County Department of Health Services
Courthouse Annex
PO Box 100
Albany, OR 97321
Telephone: (503)-967-3888
Contact: Mary Henderson
Testing, case management

Malheur County

County Health Depts

Malheur County Health Department
2671 SW 4th Avenue
Ontario, OR 97914
Telephone: (503)-889-7279
Contact: Terry Warrington

Marion County

Community Services

Mid-Oregon AIDS/Health/Education Support Services, Inc.
1410 12th Street S.E.
Salem, OR 97301
Telephone: (503)-363-4963
Contact: Patricia Jackson
AIDS/HIV service organization and task force; support resources, publicspeaking

County Health Depts

Marion County Health Department
3180 Center St. NE
Room 200
Salem, OR 97301-4592
Telephone: (503)-588-5342
Contact: Linda Suza

Multnomah County

Community Services

Cascade AIDS Project
620 SW Fifth Avenue
Suite 300
Portland, OR 97204
Telephone: (503)-223-5907
AIDS/HIV Service Organization and Task Force

Northwest Portland Area Indian Health Board
520 SW Harrison
Suite 440
Portland, OR 97201-5258
Telephone: (503)-228-4185 Fax: (503)-228-8180
Contact: Jillene Joseph
AIDS/HIV and STD prevention project, training for county health departmentsand other AIDS organizations serving the Native American population

County Health Depts

Multnomah County Health Department
426 S.W. Stark Street
2nd Floor
Portland, OR 97204-2394
Telephone: (503)-248-3406 Fax: (503)-248-3407
Contact: Cheryl Hyer
Medical services for HIV+

Polk County

County Health Depts

Polk County Public Health Department
182 SW Academy Street
Suite 302
The Dallas, OR 97338
Telephone: (503)-623-8175
Medical, testing, counseling

Umatilla County

Community Services

Blue Mountain AIDS Task Force
P.O. Box 701
Pendleton, OR 97801
Telephone: (503)-278-1529 Fax: (503)-278-1782
Contact: Mary Kraft
AIDS/HIV service organization and task force, testing counseling, supportreferrals

County Health Depts

Umatilla County Health Department
431 S.E. Third
Pendleton, OR 97801
Telephone: (503)-276-3211
Testing, counseling, wellness program, exam, city testing; Ryan Whiteclient services

Union County

County Health Depts

Union County Health Department
1100 K Avenue
La Grande, OR 97850
Telephone: (503)-963-1013

Wallowa County

County Health Depts

Wallowa County Health Department
PO Box 272
Enterprise, OR 97828
Telephone: (503)-426-3627
Testing, counseling, home nursing, referrals

Wasco County

County Health Depts

Wasco-Sherman County Health Department
400 East Fifth Street
Courthouse A
The Dallas, OR 97058-2676
Telephone: (503)-296-4636
Medical, testing & counseling

Washington County

County Health Depts

Washington County Department of Health & Human Services
155 N 1st Avenue
Hillsboro, OR 97124-3072
Telephone: (503)-648-8889
Contact: Leslie Uebel
Medical, AIDS info and referral

Home Health Care

Caremark Connection Network
7358 SW Durham Road
Portland, OR 97224
Telephone: (503)-684-3046 Fax: (503)-684-6627
Toll-Free: (800)-288-3030
Contact: Kathy Woodall
Clinical Support and Infusion Therapy: Nutrition, Antimicrobials, Chemo.,Hematopoeti

Wheeler County

County Health Depts

Wheeler County Health Department
c/o Asher Clinic
PO Box 307
Fossil, OR 97830
Telephone: (503)-763-2725
Medical testing

Yamhill County

County Health Depts

Yamhill County Health Department
412 North Ford Street
McMinnville, OR 97128-4692
Telephone: (503)-434-7525
Contact: Carole Hanson
Wellness program, counseling, testing

PENNSYLVANIA

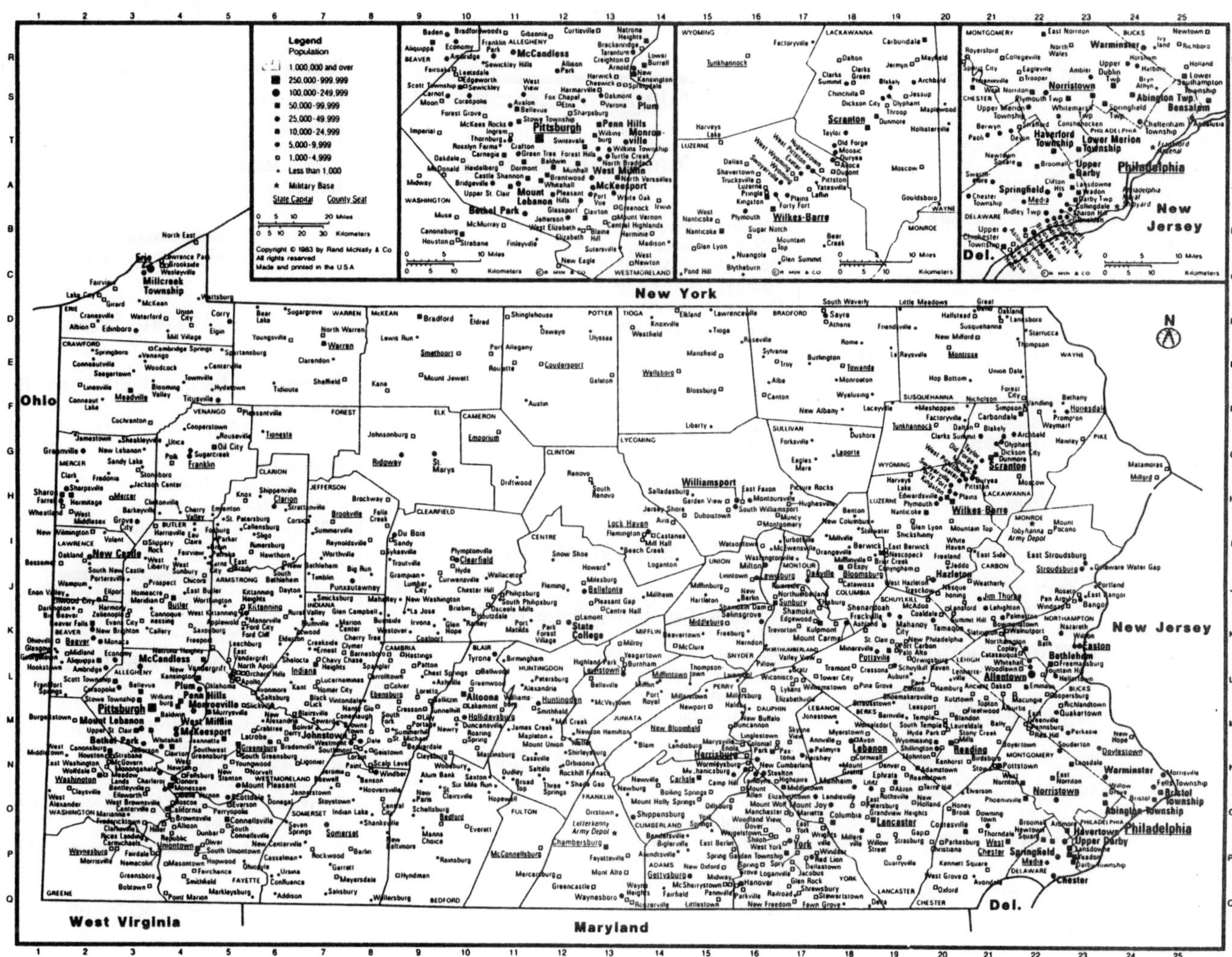

From City/County Planning Atlas Copyright 1989 by Reed McNally & Company, R.L. 90-S-28

Pennsylvania

General Services

Education

Pennsylvania AIDS Education and Training Center
Univ of Pittsburgh
130 DeSoto St, Rm A-425
Pittsburgh, PA 15261
Telephone: (412)-624-1895
Contact: Linda Frank PhD,MS
Training and education, HIV mental health project

South Central Aids Assistance Network (SCAAN)
2A Kline Village
Harrisburg, PA 17104-1528
Telephone: (717)-238-2437 Fax: (717)-238-1709
Contact: Peg Dierkers
Prevention education, support

Hotlines

Berks AIDS Health Crisis
429 Walnut Street
P.O. Box 8626
Reading, PA 19603-8626
Telephone: (215)-375-2242
Hotline, support services, education

State Health Departments

Pennsylvania Department of Health
AIDS Program/Aids Ed. Sec
912 Health & Welfare Bldg
Harrisburg, PA 17120
Telephone: (717)-783-0572
Contact: Joe Pease
AIDS education, testing, support, counseling

Pennsylvania State Department of Health, AIDS Division
912 Health & Welfare Bldg.
Harrisburg, PA 17108
Telephone: (717)-783-0572
Contact: Jack Clock - AIDS Program Admin.; Doris Black - Coordinator

Adams County

Community Services

AIDS Resource Program - Family Planning & Health Center
963 Biglerville Road
P.O. Box 3116
Gettysburg, PA 17325-3116
Telephone: (717)-334-8344 Fax: (717)-334-8906
Contact: Kandy Ferree
Client care, prevention education, case management, video/resource library

Testing Sites

Pennsylvania Dept. of Health, State Health Center
424 East Middle Street
Gettysburg, PA 17325-1926
Telephone: (717)-334-2112
Contact: Nancy Bushey - RN
HIV Counseling and Testing site

Allegheny County

Community Services

Persad Center, Inc.
5150 Penn Avenue
Pittsburgh, PA 15224-1616
Telephone: (412)-441-0857
Contact: Jim Huggins
Clinical, counseling, HIV postive

Pittsburgh AIDS Task Force
905 West Street
4th Floor
Pittsburgh, PA 15221-2833
Telephone: (412)-242-2500
Contact: Michael Neal
HIV testing, case management, counseling

County Health Depts

Allegheny County Department of Health
3441 Forbes Avenue
Pittsburgh, PA 15213-3258
Telephone: (412)-578-8332
Contact: Bill Smith
HIV Counseling and Testing site

Home Health Care

Critical Care America
400 Business Center Dr
Pittsburg, PA 15205-1332
Telephone: (412)-788-4948 Fax: (412)-788-4982
Infusion therapies in home

HNS, Inc.
300 Old Pond Road
Suite 206
Bridgeville, PA 15017
Telephone: (412)-221-9601 Fax: (412)-221-0217
Contact: Deb Vermillion
Home Infusion Therapy, In-home Nursing and Attendant Care, PhysicalTherapy Services, Pentamidine

nmc HOMECARE
500 Business Ctr. Dr, Suite 505
Pittsburgh, PA 15205
Telephone: (412)-788-1280
Fax: (412)-788-4650
Contact: Debi Yakunich
National JCAHO-Accredited company providing a full range of Infusion and Respiratory therapies and specializing in the care of HIV/AIDS patients. National Case Manager is also available at 800-445-1188

Armstrong County

Testing Sites

Pennsylvania Dept. of Health, State Health Center
354 Vine Steet
Kittanning, PA 16201
Telephone: (412)-543-2818
Contact: Melissa Stahlman - RN
Health Care services, HIV Counseling and Testing, Referrals

Berks County

Testing Sites

Pennsylvania Dept. of Health -- State Health Center
625 Cherry Street
Room # 401
Reading, PA 19602-1152
Telephone: (215)-378-4377
Contact: Barbara Allerton - RN
HIV Counseling and Testing site

Blair County

Home Health Care

AIDS Intervention Project
c/o Home Nursing Agency
201 Chestnut Ave, POB 352
Altoona, PA 16603-0352
Telephone: (814)-944-2982 Fax: (814)-941-2482
Contact: Gary Gates
Community education and PWA support services in 8 county region

Testing Sites

Pennsylvania Dept. of Health -- State Health Center
615 Howard Avenue
Altoona, PA 16601-4813
Telephone: (814)-946-7300
Contact: Suzanne Snyder - RN
HIV Counseling and Testing site

Bradford County

Community Services

Valley AIDS Task Force
Robert Packer Mem. Hsptl.
1 Gutherie Square
Sayre, PA 18840
Telephone: (717)-882-4309 Fax: (717)-882-4443
Contact: Chaplain Roy Ansen
AIDS education

Testing Sites

Pennsylvania Dept. of Health -- State Health Center
P.O. Box 29
Towanda, PA 11848
Telephone: (717)-265-2194
HIV Counseling and Tese

Bucks County

Community Services

Bucks Country AIDS Network
P.O. Box 242
Jamison, PA 18929
Telephone: (215)-348-0555
Contact: Magee Boyer
Counseling, seminars, hotline

Project Reach of Bucks County
One Oxford Valley
Suit 717
Langhorne, PA 19047
Telephone: (215)-757-6916
Contact: Susie Birenbaum
Case management, counseling, AIDS project, home visits

County Health Depts

Bucks County Health Department
Building K
Neshaminy Manor Center
Doylestown, PA 18901
Telephone: (215)-345-3894
HIV Counseling and Testing site

Butler County

Home Health Care

Caremark Connection Network
230 Executive Drive
Suite 126
Mars, PA 16046-8304
Telephone: (412)-772-3701 Fax: (412)-772-3970
Contact: Cindy Thomas
Clinical Support and Infusion Therapy: Nutrition, Antimicrobials, Chemo.,Hematopoeti

Caremark Homecare Branch Network
230 Executive Dr
Suite 126
Mars, PA 16046-8304
Telephone: (412)-772-3701
Contact: Cindy Thomas,RN - Nurse Manager
TPN, Antibiotics, Pain Management, Enteral, Nutrition Support, Chemotherapy

Testing Sites

Pennsylvania Dept. of Health, State Health Center
125 Pittsburgh Road
Butler, PA 16001-3259
Telephone: (412)-287-1769
HIV Counseling and Testing site

Cambria County

Testing Sites

Laurel Highland Aids Resource Council
C/O Lee Hospital
320 Main Street
Johnstown, PA 15901
Telephone: (814)-533-0117 Fax: (814)-533-0666
Contact: Bernice Adams
HIV testing & counseling

Pennsylvania Dept. of Health, State Health Center
430 Main Street
Jupiter Bldg., 2nd Floor
Johnstown, PA 15901
Telephone: (814)-533-2205
HIV Counseling and Testing site

Centre County

Community Services

AIDS Project of Centre County
301 South Allen Street
Suite #102
State College, PA 16801
Telephone: (814)-234-7087
Contact: Sally Modi-Robinson - 800-233-AIDS
Services for HIV+ persons on drugs

Chester County

Home Health Care

Caremark Connection Network
6 Spring Mill Drive
Suite One
Malvern, PA 19355
Telephone: (302)-428-0924
Clinical Support and Infusion Therapies: Nutrition, Antimicrobials, Chemo., AIDS infusions

Crawford County

Testing Sites

Pennsylvania Dept. of Health, State Health Center
900 Water Street
Meadville, PA 16335-3485
Telephone: (814)-336-6947 Fax: (814)-332-6947
Health care services, HIV Counseling and Testing site

Cumberland County

Testing Sites

Pennsylvania Dept. of Health, State Health Center
425 East North Street
Carlisle, PA 17013-2620
Telephone: (717)-697-6549
HIV Counseling and Testing

Dauphin County

Community Services

South Central AIDS Assistance Network (SCAAN)
2A Cline Village
Suite A
Harrisburg, PA 17104-1528
Telephone: (717)-238-2437
Contact: Peg Dierkers
Financial assessment, case management, community education, support groups,referrals

Home Health Care

Caremark
6340 Flank Drive
Suite 100
Harrisburg, PA 17112
Telephone: (717)-540-7625 Fax: (717)-540-7694
Toll-Free: (800)-727-1778
Contact: Mark Jeannette - Branch Manager
Clinical Support and Infusion Therapy

Delaware County

Community Services

Chester AIDS Coalition
P.O. Box 253
Chester, PA 19016
Telephone: (215)-344-6243
Contact: Joan H. Sudler - Executive Director
Prevention, risk reduction, education, early intervention for case management

Delaware County AIDS Network
907 Chester Pike
Sharon Hill, PA 19079
Telephone: (215)-891-0805
Contact: Dennis Murphy
Buddy program, education, advocacy, clothing bank, food bank, drop incenter; financial assistance

Home Health Care

Homedco Infusion
800 Primos Avenue
Folcroft, PA 19032-2095
Telephone: (215)-586-2215
Nationwide experience in providing home infusion therapy to AIDS patients

Testing Sites

Pennsylvania Dept. of Health, State Health Center
5th and Penn Streets
Chester, PA 19013
Telephone: (215)-447-3250
HIV Counseling and Testing

Elk County

Testing Sites

Pennsylvania Dept. of Health, State Health Center
778 Washington Road
St. Marys, PA 15857
Telephone: (814)-773-3113
HIV Counseling and Testing

Erie County

County Health Depts

Erie County Health Department
606 West Second Street
Erie, PA 16507-1199
Telephone: (814)-451-6700
HIV Counseling and Testing site

Franklin County

Community Services

Franklin Area Aids Network (FAAN)
P.O. Box 356
Chambersburg, PA 17201-0356
Telephone: (717)-264-7799
Support groups, newsletter, case management, financial assistance, transportation

Testing Sites

Pennsylvania Dept. of Health, State Health Center
518 Cleveland Avenue
Chambersburg, PA 17201-3409
Telephone: (717)-263-4143
HIV Counseling and Testing

Greene County

Testing Sites

Pennsylvania Dept. of Health, State Health Center
33 South Washington St.
Waynesburg, PA 15370-2035
Telephone: (412)-627-3168
HIV Counseling and Testing

Lackawanna County

Testing Sites

Pennsylvania Dept. of Health, State Health Center
100 Lackawanna Avenue
Scranton, PA 18503-1923
Telephone: (717)-963-4567
Contact: Jay Locker - RN
Health care services, HIV Counseling and Testing

Lancaster County

Community Services

Lancaster AIDS Project
44 North Queen Street
P.O. Box 1543
Lancaster, PA 17603-1543
Telephone: (717)-394-9900
Contact: Leanne Gellat
HIV testing, case management, referral

Home Health Care

Homedco Infusion
240 Harrisburg Avenue
Lancaster, PA 17603-2968
Telephone: (717)-397-8000 Fax: (717)-397-8078
Contact: Josie Marsala - Customer Service Supervisor
Nationwide experience in providing home infusion therapy to AIDS patients;other home medical equipment.

Testing Sites

Pennsylvania Dept. of Health, State Health Center
1661 Old Philadelphia Pike
Lancaster, PA 17602
Telephone: (717)-299-7597
Contact: Doris Kolb; Kay Moyer
HIV Counseling and Testing site

Lebanon County

Community Services

Lebanon Family Health Services AIDS Project
1 Cumberland Street
Lebanon, PA 17046
Telephone: (717)-270-9965 Fax: (717)-273-6337
Contact: Sylvia D. Moyer - Aids Educator/Coordinator
HIV education, support groups, buddies, case management, infoservices, bereavement counseling

Testing Sites

Pennsylvania Dept. of Health, State Health Center
201 Cumberland Street
Lebanon, PA 17042-5307
Telephone: (717)-272-2044
Contact: Jean Bennetch - RN
HIV Counseling and Testing

Lehigh County

Community Services

AIDS Outreach
112 North 5th Street
Allentown, PA 18102
Telephone: (908)-813-3058
Contact: Linda Lobach
Transportation, buddy system, hospital visitation

Testing Sites

Allentown Bureau of Health
235 North 6th Street
Allentown, PA 18102-1603
Telephone: (215)-437-7577
Health care services, HIV Counseling and Testing site

Luzerne County

Community Services

Wyoming Valley AIDS Council
P.O. Box 2677
Wilkes-Barre, PA 18703-2677
Telephone: (717)-457-1639
Contact: Alfie Chewning
Support groups for HIV+ persons, education, case management, referrals

Medical Services

Wyoming Valley AIDS Task Force
P.O. Box 2677
Wilkes-Barre, PA 18703
Telephone: (717)-823-5808
Contact: Alfie Chewning
Support, case management, education, buddy system

Testing Sites

Planned Parenthood of Northeast PA
10 West Chestnut Street
Hazelton, PA 18201
Telephone: (717)-454-0876 Fax: (717)-454-0878
Contact: Brenda Long
Health care services, HIV Counseling and Testing site

State Health Center
297 South Main Street
Wilkes-Barre, PA 18701-2201
Telephone: (717)-826-2071
Contact: Carol Yozviak
Health care services, HIV Counseling and Testing site

Lycoming County

Community Services

AIDS Resource Alliance of North Centerl Pennsylvania
507 West 4th Street
Williamsport, PA 17701-4980
Telephone: (717)-327-3440 Fax: (717)-322-8448
Contact: Linda Dieffenbach
Prevention education, case management, support group

Testing Sites

Pennsylvania Department of Health
440 Little League Blvd.
Williamsport, PA 17701-4980
Telephone: (717)-327-3440
Contact: Carol Gray
Health services, HIV Counseling and Testing site

Mc Kean County

Medical Services

Family Planning of McKean County
39 Mechanic Street
Bradford, PA 16701-2028
Telephone: (814)-368-6129 Fax: (814)-368-6174
Health care services, HIV Counseling and Testing site

Mercer County

Medical Services

Grove City Family Planning
408-B Hillcrest Med. Ctr.
Grove City, PA 16127-1708
Telephone: (412)-458-8505
Contact: Barbara Arblaster
Medical services, HIV counseling and testing site, education

Mifflin County

Testing Sites

Pennsylvania Dept. of Health -- State Health Center
21 South Brown Street
Lewistown, PA 17044
Telephone: (717)-242-1452
Contact: Jane Shearer - RN
Health care services, HIV Counseling and Testing site

Monroe County

Medical Services

Planned Parenthood of Northeast PA
28 North 7th Street
Stroudsburg, PA 18360
Telephone: (717)-424-8306 Fax: (717)-476-4580
Medical services, HIV Counseling and Testing site, AIDS education (bothstaff & staff client with confidence), referrals

Montgomery County

County Health Depts

Montgomery County Health Department
Lafayette Pl.
Suite 325
Norristown, PA 19401-3110
Telephone: (610)-278-5117 Fax: (610)-278-5167
Health services, HIV Counseling and Testing site

Home Health Care

Critical Care America
2495 Blvd of the Generals
Norristown, PA 19403
Telephone: (215)-630-0100
Toll-Free: (800)-937-3690
Coordinate & integrate all clinical & psychosocial services for HIV+

HNS, Inc.
1019 West 9th Ave
Suite H
King of Prussia, PA 19406
Telephone: (215)-337-9267 Fax: (215)-337-9436
Toll-Free: (800)-187-2446
Contact: Christime Ledesma
Home Infusion Therapy, In-home Nursing and Attendant Care, Physical Therapy Services, Pentamidine

HNS, Inc.
1019 9th Avenue
Suite H
King of Prussia, PA 19406
Telephone: (717)-737-8226
Home Infusion Therapy, In-home Nursing and Attendant Care, Physical Therapy Services, Pentamidine

Young's O.P.T.I.O.N Care
Cedar Creek Corporate Ctr
125-B Witmer Road
Horsham, PA 19044
Telephone: (215)-957-0844 Fax: (215)-957-0519
Toll-Free: (800)-548-9903
Contact: Judy Dubiansky
Home IV and Nutritional Services

Northampton County

Testing Sites

Planned Parenthood of Northeast PA
2906 William Penn Hghwy
Easton, PA 18042
Telephone: (215)-253-7195
Medical services, HIV Counseling and Testing site

Philadelphia County

Community Services

Action AIDS, Inc.
P.O. Box 1625
1216 Arch Street-4th Floor
Philadelphia, PA 19105-1625
Telephone: (215)-981-0088 Fax: (215)-854-0735
Contact: Joan Curran - Director of Client Services
Advocacy, Buddies, Case Management, Education, Support Groups

Philadelphia Community Health Alternatives, AIDS Testing
1642 Pine Street
Philadelphia, PA 19103-6711
Telephone: (215)-545-8686 Fax: (215)-545-1569
Housing, support fund, minority outreach, support groups, buddies

The Circle of Care
260 South Broad Street
Suite 1510
Philadelphia, PA 19102
Telephone: (215)-985-2657 Fax: (215)-732-1610
Contact: Alicia Beatty-Tee - Project Director; Darlene Harris - Contract Coordinator
HIV testing, AIDS care, clinical and social services

US Public Health Service
P.O. Box 13716
Philadelphia, PA 19101-3716
Telephone: (215)-596-1561 Fax: (215)-596-6660
Contact: Alicia Blessington - Regional AIDS Coordinator
Financial aid, health services, HIV support groups

Home Health Care

Caremark Connection Network
1518 Rodman Street
Philadelphia, PA 19146
Telephone: (215)-985-4042 Fax: (215)-985-4214
Contact: Bruce Marrison - Nursing Supervisor
Clinical Support and Infusion Therapy: Nutrition, Antimicrobials, Chemo.,Hematopoeti

Medical Services

Immunodeficiency Program Clinic Hospital of the Univ. of PA
3400 Spruce Street
Philadelphia, PA 19104-4220
Telephone: (215)-662-6932 Fax: (215)-662-7899
Contact: Dr. Harvey Friedman
HIV testing, out patient

Veterans Administration Medical Center
University & Woodland Avs
Philadelphia, PA 19104
Telephone: (215)-823-5800 Fax: (215)-823-6054
Medical Services for Veterans with AIDS

Washington County

Testing Sites

Pennsylvania Dept. of Health, State Health Center
410 North Main Street
Washington, PA 15301-4328
Telephone: (412)-223-4540
Contact: Barbara Golensky - RN
Health services, HIV counseling and testing site

York County

Home Health Care

Homedco Infusion
1500 North George Street
York, PA 17404
Telephone: (717)-848-8000 Fax: (717)-843-5541
Nationwide experience in providing home infusion therapy to AIDS patients

Testing Sites

Pennsylvania Dept. of Health, State Health Center
1750 North George Street
York, PA 17404-1807
Telephone: (717)-771-1336
Contact: Robert Walter
HIV Counseling and Testing site

Y.H.E.S.S.
101 East Market Street
2nd Floor
York, PA 17401
Telephone: (717)-846-6776 Fax: (717)-854-0377
HIV testing, support group, medical assistance

Puerto Rico

General Services

Education

Puerto Rico AIDS Education and Training Center
Univ of Puerto Rico
GPO 36-5067 Rm 745A
Rio Piedras, PR 00936-5067
Telephone: (809)-759-6528 Fax: (809)-764-2470
Contact: Angel Bravo, MPH - Director
Training for care providers; HIV & AIDS management

Carolina County

Home Health Care

nmc HOMECARE
Via Mirta 3FS #2 Fragoso Ave Villa Fontana
Carolina, PR 00983
Telephone: (305)-427-7200
National JCAHO-Accredited company providing a full range of Infusion and Respiratory therapies and specializing in the care of HIV/AIDS patients. National Case Manager is also available at 800-445-1188

RHODE ISLAND

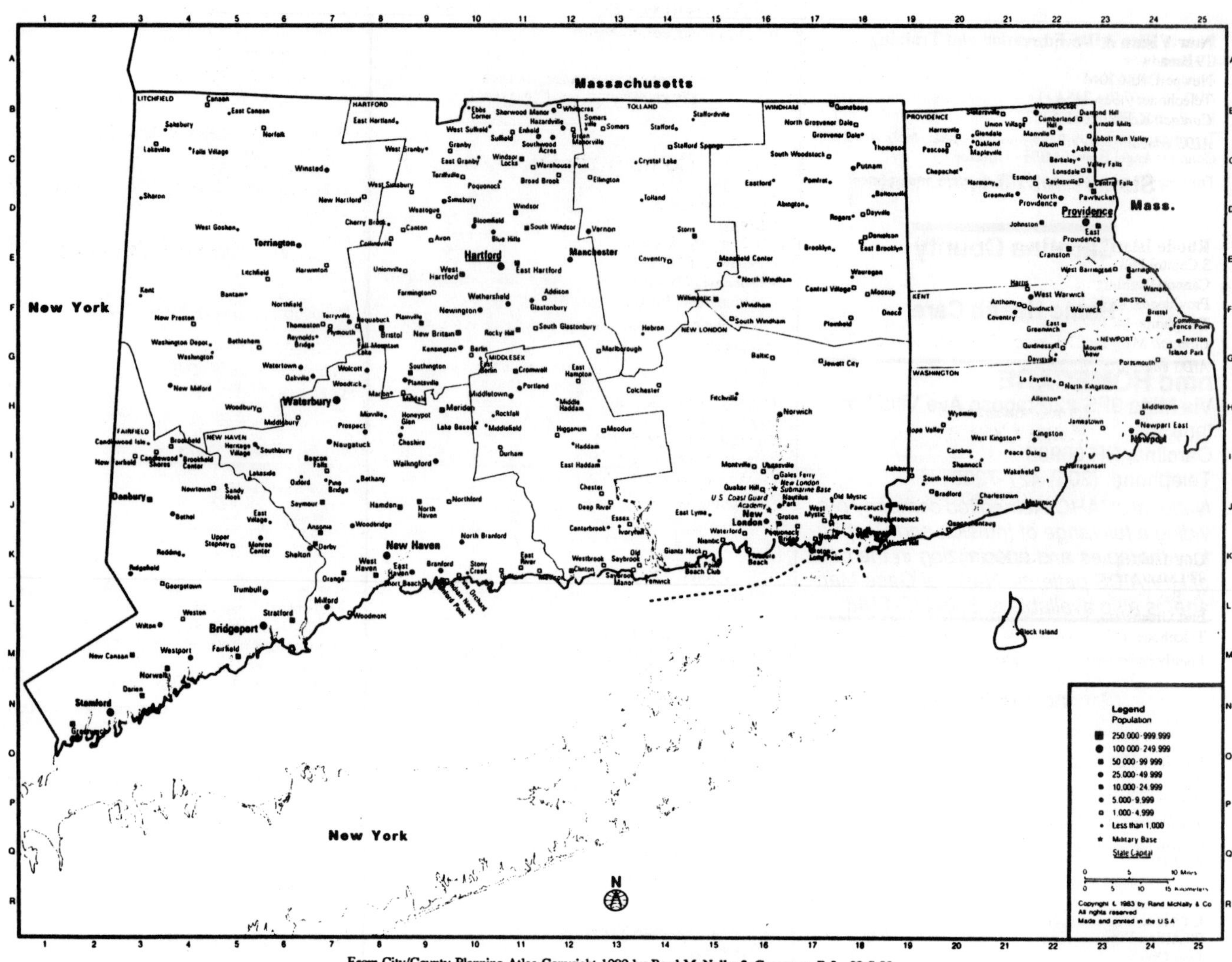

From City/County Planning Atlas Copyright 1989 by Reed McNally & Company, R.L. 90-S-28

Rhode Island

General Services

Education

New Vision of Newport
19 Broadway
Newport, RI 02840
Telephone: (401)-847-7821
Contact: Ken Robertson
AIDS educators for minority populations

State Health Departments

Rhode Island Department of Health
3 Capitol Hill
Cannon Building
Providence, RI 02908
Telephone: (401)-277-2320
Contact: MaryLou DeCiantis - Chief Admin. AIDS/STD
AIDS educators, HIV testing

Kent County

Community Services

Counseling and Mental Health Services, Inc.
990 Main Street
W. Bay Professional Bldg
East Greenwich, RI 02818-3114
Telephone: (401)-884-6880 Fax: (401)-884-8380
Family counseling, stress managment

Home Health Care

Critical Care America
20 Altieri Way
Warwick, RI 02886
Telephone: (401)-732-8200 Fax: (401)-732-8209
Coordinate & integrate all clinical & psychosocial services for HIV+

Critical Care America
20 Altieri Way
Unit One
Warwick, RI 02886-1756
Telephone: (401)-732-8200 Fax: (401)-732-8209
Toll-Free: (800)-955-4502
Contact: Kevin Ronan - General Manager
Infusion therapies in home

Medical Services

Kent County Mental Health Center
50 Health Lane
Warwick, RI 02886
Telephone: (401)-738-4300 Fax: (401)-738-7718
Contact: David Lauterbach
Mental health counseling

Newport County

Community Services

Child & Family Service of Newport County
24 School Street
Newport, RI 02840
Telephone: (401)-849-2300 Fax: (401)-841-8841
Support groups, social services

Providence County

Community Services

Chispa
421 Elmwood Avenue
Providence, RI 02907
Telephone: (401)-467-0111 Fax: (401)-467-2507
Contact: Marta Martinez
Commmunity outreach, education, risk prevention, services in Spanish

Family Services, Inc.
55 Hope Street
Providence, RI 02906-2048
Telephone: (401)-331-1350 Fax: (401)-274-7602
Contact: Karen Cunningham
Counseling for HIV+, support groups for lovers and family friends

Gay Alanon - Providence Center
520 Hope Street
3rd Floor
Providence, RI 02906-2532
Telephone: (401)-274-2500 Fax: (401)-421-3066
Contact: Dr. Michael Silver
Support group, social services, AIDS awarness

Hemophilia Center of Rhode Island
593 Eddy Street
Aldrich Building 511
Providence, RI 02903
Telephone: (401)-277-8250
Contact: Virginia Cerbo
Support groups, social services

Junction Human Services
PO Box 3477
Providence, RI 02909
Telephone: (401)-272-5960 Fax: (401)-454-0195
Drug counseling, AIDS education, referrals

Rhode Island Commission for Human Rights
10 Abbott Park Place
Providence, RI 02903
Telephone: (401)-277-2661 Fax: (401)-277-2616
Contact: Gene Booth
Discrimination, employment, public housing accomodations, credit issues forHIV+ & others

Rhode Island Legal Service
77 Dorrance Street
Providence, RI 02903
Telephone: (401)-274-2652 Fax: (401)-453-0310
Contact: Robert Barge
Housing, HIV legal services

Rhode Island Project AIDS
95 Chestnut St.,3rd Floor
Providence, RI 02903-4110
Telephone: (401)-831-5522 Fax: (401)-454-0299
Toll-Free: (800)-726-3010
Contact: Annie Silvia
AIDS Services and English/Spanish Hotline 1-800-726-3010

Home Health Care

Home Front Health Care
400-6th Street
Providence, RI 02908
Telephone: (401)-751-3152
Contact: Robert Cafferx
Home health aids, RN's LPN's

Hospice Care of Rhode Island
169 George Street
Pawtucket, RI 02860
Telephone: (401)-727-7070 Fax: (401)-727-7080
Contact: Judy Gordon

Medical Services

Allen Barry Health Center
202 Prarie Avenue
Providence, RI 02905
Telephone: (401)-861-6300
Dental care

Capitol Health Center
40 Candace Street
Providence, RI 02908
Telephone: (401)-861-6300
Contact: Uah Perez
Dental services & primary care

Memorial Hospital
111 Brewster Street
Providence, RI 02860
Telephone: (401)-729-2616 Fax: (401)-722-0198
Contact: Marg Eddy
Primary care, research studies, high risk individuals, dental referrals counseling prevention education, HIV testing

Northern RI Community Mental Health Center
P.O. Box 1700
Woonsocket, RI 02895
Telephone: (401)-766-3330 Fax: (401)-769-1810
Contact: Chirstian Stephens
Mental Health Services, for emergencies 401-762-1577

Eleanor Slater Hospital
P.O. Box 8269
Cranston, RI 02920
Telephone: (401)-364-3456 Fax: (401)-464-3466
Contact: Rajnikant Shah - M.D.
Primary care, HIV testing, dental care, AIDS education

Testing Sites

Division of Disease Prevention and Control
3 Capitol Hill
Providence, RI 02908-5097
Telephone: (401)-277-2320 Fax: (401)-272-3771
Contact: Dr. Marylou Deciantis - Case Manager; Bela T. Matjas -
HIV/STD testing

SOUTH CAROLINA

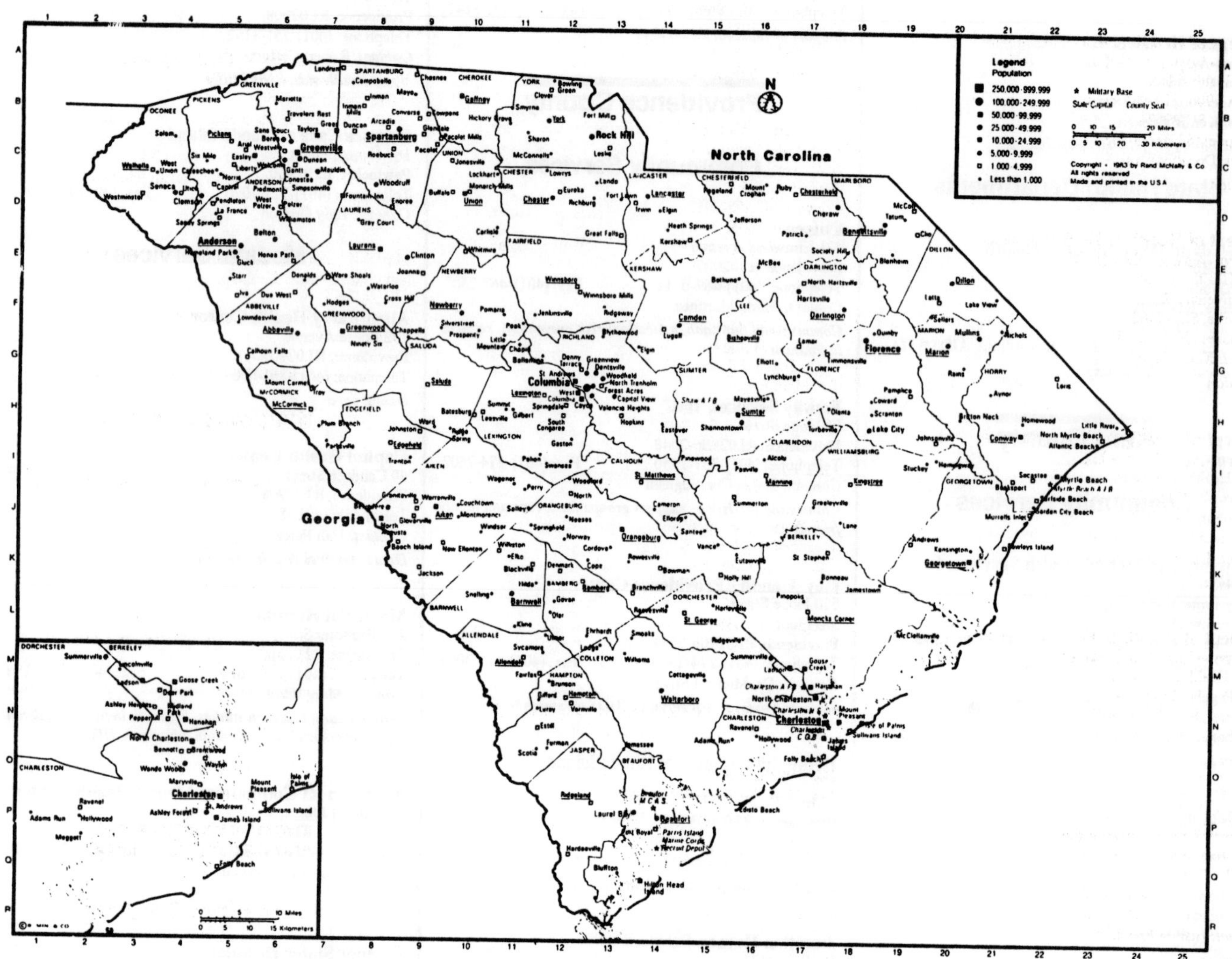

From City/County Planning Atlas Copyright 1989 by Reed McNally & Company, R.L. 90-S-28

South Carolina

General Services

Education

SC Dept of Health & Environmental Control-Appalachia I Dist.
AIDS Health Education
PO Box 1906, 220 McGee Rd
Anderson, SC 29624
Telephone: (803)-225-3731
Contact: Dorothy Willis
Education

SC Dept of Health & Environmental Control-Appalachia II Dist
AIDS Health Education
200 University Ridge
Greenville, SC 29602
Telephone: (803)-467-8991
Contact: Katie Taylor
Education

SC Dept of Health & Environmental Control-Appalachia III
AIDS Health Education
PO Box 4217, 151 E. Wood
Spartanburg, SC 29305
Telephone: (803)-596-3334
Contact: Charlotte Woodall
Education

SC Dept of Health & Environmental Control-Catawba District
AIDS Health Education
1833 Pageland Highway
Lancaster, SC 29720-0817
Telephone: (803)-286-9948
Education

SC Dept of Health & Environmental Control-Low Country Dist.
AIDS Health Education
P.O. Box 229
Walterboro, SC 29488-0229
Telephone: (803)-549-1516
Contact: Juanita Freeman
Education

SC Dept of Health & Environmental Control-Lower Savannah
AIDS Health Education
828 West Richland Avenue
Aiken, SC 29801
Telephone: (803)-642-1603
Contact: Joyce Daniel - AIDS Health Educator
Education

SC Dept of Health & Environmental Control-Trident District
AIDS Health Education
334 Calhoun Street
Charleston, SC 29512
Telephone: (803)-724-5800
Contact: Lori Able
Education

SC Dept of Health & Environmental Control-Trident District
AIDS Health Education
334 Calhoun Street
Charleston, SC 29401
Telephone: (803)-724-5800
Contact: Tony Vaninetti - AIDS Health Educator
Education

SC Dept of Health & Environmental Control-Upper Savannah
AIDS Health Education
1736 S. Main Street
Greenwood, SC 29646
Telephone: (803)-223-8488
Contact: Charles Long
Education, clinic, social work

SC Dept of Health & Environmental Control-Waccamaw District
AIDS Health Education
101 Elm Street
Conway, SC 29526-1206
Telephone: (803)-248-6381
Contact: Cherle Adamson - Dist. Direc. Health Educ.
Education

SC Dept of Health & Environmental Control-Waccamaw District
AIDS Health Education
101 Main Street
Conway, SC 29526-1206
Telephone: (803)-248-6381
Contact: Elaine Russell
Education

SC Dept of Health & Environmental Control-Wateree District
AIDS Health Education
P.O. Box 1628,105 N Magnolia
Sumter, SC 29151
Telephone: (803)-773-5511
Contact: John Canfield
Education

State Health Departments

SC Dept of Health & Environmental Control-Appalachia III Dis
AIDS Health Education
PO Box 4217, 151 E. Wood
Spartanburg, SC 29305-4217
Telephone: (803)-596-3334
Contact: Linda Rogers - AIDS Health Educator
Education - HIV testing

SC Dept of Health & Environmental Control-Catawba District
AIDS Health Education
PO Box 817, Rt 10, Hwy. 9
Lancaster, SC 29721
Telephone: (803)-286-9948
Contact: Susan Collins - AIDS Health Educator
Education

SC Dept of Health & Environmental Control-Edisto District
AIDS Health Education
PO Box 1126,550 Carolina
Orangeburg, SC 29116
Telephone: (803)-536-9060
Contact: John Snell - Health Educator
AIDS Education

SC Dept of Health & Environmental Control-Pee Dee II Dist.
Parsonage Street Extension
Plaza Building
Bennettsville, SC 29512
Telephone: (803)-479-8311
Contact: Dorothy Skitter - RN
HIV testing (confidential), counseling, referals

SC Dept of Health & Environmental Control-Upper Savannah
AIDS Health Education
1736 S. Main Street
Greenwood, SC 29646
Telephone: (803)-942-3646
Contact: Lawri Rhodes - AIDS Health Educator
Education

SC Dept of Health & Environmental Control-Wateree District
AIDS Health Education
PO Bx 1628,105 N Magnolia
Sumter, SC 29151
Telephone: (803)-773-5511
Contact: John Canfield - AIDS Health Educator
Education

South Carolina Department of Health & Environmental Control
HIV/AIDS Division
Robert Mills Bldg., 2600 Bull Street
Columbia, SC 29211
Telephone: (803)-737-4110
Contact: Lynda Kettinger - Director HIV/AIDS

Statewide Services

Palmetto AIDS Life Support Services of S.C., Inc.
P.O. Box 12124
Columbia, SC 29211-2124
Telephone: (800)-723-7257
Practical to Emotional Support

SC Protection and Advocacy System for the Handicapped, Inc.
Region I--Piedmont
1 Chick Springs Rd, #101A
Greenville, SC 29609
Telephone: (803)-235-0273
Protection and Advocacy Services to the Physically Handicapped and MentallyIll

Abbeville County

Community Services

Housing Authority of the City of Abbeville
544 Branch Street
Abbeville, SC 29620-1936
Telephone: (803)-459-4549
Housing Assistance

Testing Sites

Abbeville Health Department, HIV Testing and Counseling
Church and Pinckney
Abbeville, SC 29620
Telephone: (803)-459-2131
HIV Testing, Counseling

Aiken County

Community Services

Housing Authority of the City of Aiken
P.O. Box 889
Aiken, SC 29802-0899
Telephone: (803)-649-6673
Housing Assistance

St. John United Methodist Church
104 Newberry Street, NW
Aiken, SC 29801-3918
Telephone: (803)-648-1595
Contact: Rev. M. Eugene Mullikin
Counseling, Spiritual Support

Home Health Care

SC Dept of Health & Environmental Control-Lower Savannah
Home Health Services
828 W. Richland Avenue
Aiken, SC 29801
Telephone: (803)-642-1603
Home Nursing and Health Aides, Home Therapy, Medical and Social Services

Medical Services

Hartzog Center
SC Dept. of Mental Health
433 Georgia Avenue
N. Augusta, SC 29841
Telephone: (803)-278-0880 Fax: (803)-278-7391
Mental Health Resources

Allendale County

County Health Depts

Allendale Health Department, HIV Testing and Counseling
415 N. Memorial
Allendale, SC 29810-1228
Telephone: (803)-584-3818
HIV Testing, Counseling

Medical Services

Coastal Empire Mental Health Center--Allendale Co. Satellite
SC Dept. of Mental Health
PO Box 514, 213 Water St.
Allendale, SC 29810
Telephone: (803)-584-4636 Fax: (803)-584-5065
Mental Health Services

Low Country Commission on Alcohol and Drug Abuse
Memorial Avenue
Health Department Building
Allendale, SC 29810
Telephone: (803)-584-4238
Substance Abuse Outpatient Services, Referrals, Intervention, Education

Low Country Commission on Alcohol and Drug Abuse
Memorial Avenue
Allendale, SC 29810
Telephone: (803)-584-4238
Contact: Frank Solomon - Prevention Specialist
Substance Abuse Outpatient Services, Referrals, Intervention, Education

Anderson County

Home Health Care

Community Long Term Care, Area 1, Anderson Satellite Office
P.O. Box 5947
Anderson, SC 29623
Telephone: (803)-224-9452 Fax: (803)-225-0871
Contact: Candi Beckley - Social Worker
Nurses, Personal Care Aides, Meals, Counseling; Day, Foster, and Hospice Care

SC Dept of Health & Environmental Control-Appalachia I Dist.
Home Health Services
Anderson, SC 29625
Telephone: (803)-260-5615 Fax: (803)-260-5676
Contact: Barbra Alexander
Home Nursing and Health Aides, Home Therapy, Medical and Social Services

Medical Services

Anderson-Oconee-Pickens Mental Health Center
SC Dept. of Mental Health
200 McGee Road
Anderson, SC 29621
Telephone: (803)-260-2220 Fax: (803)-260-2225
Mental health resources, counseling, support, therapies

Anderson/Oconee Alcohol and Drug Abuse Commission
212 South Main Street
Anderson, SC 29624-1621
Telephone: (803)-260-4168
Contact: Rene Williams
Substance Abuse Outpatient Services, Referrals, Intervention, EducationHIV counseling and seminars.

Bamberg County

County Health Depts

Bamberg Health Department, HIV Testing and Counseling
Log Branch Road
Bamberg, SC 29003
Telephone: (803)-245-5176
Contact: Mary Anne Berry
HIV Testing, Counseling

Medical Services

Tri-County Commission on Alcohol & Drug Abuse (Dawn Center)
Mid Town Office Plaza
608 North Main Street
Bamberg, SC 29003
Telephone: (803)-245-4360
Contact: Perdina Cheeseboro
Outpatient Services, Referrals, Halfway House, Intervention, Education

Barnwell County

County Health Depts

Barnwell Health Department, HIV Testing and Counseling
2100 Calhoun Street
Barnwell, SC 29812-2004
Telephone: (803)-259-3661
Contact: Ann Lancaster
HIV Testing, Counseling

Medical Services

Polly Best Mental Health Center
SC Dept. of Mental Health
2511 Reynolds Road
Barnwell, SC 29812
Telephone: (803)-259-7179
Contact: John Young - Program Director
Mental Health Resources

Beaufort County

Community Services

Department of Social Services, Beaufort County
P.O. Box 1065
Beaufort, SC 29901-1065
Telephone: (803)-525-7361
Social Services

Department of Social Services--Jasper County
P.O. Box 1349
Ridgeland, SC 29936-1349
Telephone: (803)-726-8131
Contact: Lavaughn Nesmith
Social Services

HELP of Beaufort Mobile Meals
H-3 Heritage Woods
Beaufort, SC 29902
Telephone: (803)-524-8681
Contact: Maxine Dunnet - Coordinator
Home Delivered Meals to Disabled People

County Health Depts

Beaufort County Health Department
P.O. Box 235
Bluffton, SC 29910-0235
Telephone: (803)-681-7131
Contact: Vickie Ballard
HIV Testing, Counseling

Beaufort Health Department, HIV Testing and Counseling
600 Wilmington St
Beaufort, SC 29901-4956
Telephone: (803)-525-7615
HIV Testing, Counseling

Jasper County Health Department, HIV Testing and Counseling
113 E. Wilson Street
Ridgeland, SC 29936
Telephone: (803)-726-7788
HIV Testing, Counseling

Home Health Care

Caroline Hospice of Beaufort, Inc.
P.O. Box 1686
Beaufort, SC 29902-1686
Telephone: (803)-525-6257
Contact: Beverly A Porter - RN
Emotional Support, Respite, Home Health Aides, Equipment and Medication Support groups

Medical Services

Coastal Empire Mental Health Center
SC Dept. of Mental Health
P.O. Box 1044
Beaufort, SC 29902
Telephone: (803)-524-3378 Fax: (803)-529-8179
Mental health services, counseling for children and adolescents

Coastal Empire Mental Health Center--Jasper County Satellite
P.O. Box 1216, 113 Wilson
Ridgeland, SC 29936-1216
Telephone: (803)-726-8030 Fax: (803)-726-8207
Contact: Deborah Morris
Mental health services, counseling, referrals

Berkeley County

Community Services

Neighborhood Legal Assistance Program, Moncks Corner
P.O. Box 1418
109 W. Main Street
Moncks Corner, SC 29461-1428
Telephone: (803)-761-8355 Fax: (803)-761-3177
Legal services: domestic matters, Social Security, bankruptcy

County Health Depts

Berkeley County Health Dept., HIV Testing and Counseling
109 West Main Street
Moncks Corner, SC 29461-0566
Telephone: (803)-761-8090
Contact: Lynn Doris
HIV Testing, Counseling

Calhoun County

County Health Depts

Calhoun County Health Department, HIV Testing and Counseling
Lake Inspiration Circle
St. Matthews, SC 29135
Telephone: (803)-874-2037
Contact: Donna Barnes
HIV testing, counseling, home health care

Charleston County

Community Services

Charleston County Housing and Redevelopment Authority
2106 Mt. Pleasant Street
PO Box 6188
Charleston, SC 29405
Telephone: (803)-722-1942
Housing Assistance

County Health Depts

Charleston County Health Department
334 Calhoun Street
Charleston, SC 29401-1188
Telephone: (803)-724-5838
Contact: Pat Stribling
HIV Testing, Counseling

Home Health Care

Caremark Connection Network.
1941 Savage Road
Suite 500AA
Charleston, SC 29407
Telephone: (803)-769-5544 Fax: (803)-769-4300
Toll-Free: (800)-274-4151
Clinical Support and Infusion Therapy: Nutrition, Antimicrobials, Chemo.,Hematopoeti, pain management, antibiotic therapy

Community Long Term Care, Area 10 Charleston
751 A Johnnie Dodds Blvd.
Charleston, SC 29464
Telephone: (803)-887-6600
Contact: Faye Croft
Nurses, Personal Care Aides, Meals, Counseling; Foster, and Hospice Care

Doctors Home Health of Charleston
2440 Mall Drive
Suite #110
Charleston, SC 29405
Telephone: (803)-554-8844
Contact: Sylvia Barnes Green - RN
Nurses and Health Aides; Physical, Speech, Occupational Therapy, Social Workers

Home Health Services, Inc.
P.O. Box 30787
Charleston, SC 29417-0787
Telephone: (803)-763-6767
Contact: Mickey Cook
Intermittent Skilled Nursing, Physical and Speech Therapy, Personal Care Aides

Medical Personnel Pool of Greater Charleston, Inc.
7410 Northside Drive
Suite 101
Charleston, SC 29420-4200
Telephone: (803)-797-2942 Fax: (803)-569-5514
Toll-Free: (800)-951-6877
Contact: Paula Mellichamp
Home Health Care

Saint Francis Home Health Care
1064 Gardner Road, 115
Suite 305
Charleston, SC 29407-5700
Telephone: (803)-556-4044 Fax: (803)-556-5079
Toll-Free: (800)-456-5079
Contact: Cathy Therrell, R.N.
Skilled Nursing, Physical Therapy, Speech Therapy, Home Health Aides

SC Dept of Health & Environmental Control-Trident District
1914 Savage Road
Suite 300 East
Charleston, SC 29407
Telephone: (803)-724-5850 Fax: (803)-724-5858
Home Nursing and Health Aides, Home Therapy, Medical and Social Services

SC Dept of Health & Environmental Control-Trident District
1941 Savage Road
Suite 300E
Charleston, SC 29407-2590
Telephone: (803)-724-5850 Fax: (803)-724-5858
Contact: Cansas Moore
Home Nursing and Health Aides, Home Therapy, Medical and Social Services

Medical Services

Chaps Baker Treatment Center
2741 Speissegger Drive
Suite 201
N. Charleston, SC 29405-8290
Telephone: (803)-745-4268
Contact: Dr. Lamkin - Medical Director, Terry Jorgensen - Program Director
Recovery Program for Substance Dependent Persons and Families in & outpatient

Franklin C. Fetter Center
51 Nassau Street
Charleston, SC 29403-5500
Telephone: (803)-722-4112 Fax: (803)-722-4802
Contact: Dr. Lenes
Medical Services

Cherokee County

County Health Depts

DEHEC Cherokee County Health Department, HIV Testing & Counseling
400 S. Logan St
Gaffney, SC 29342-1609
Telephone: (803)-487-2705
HIV Testing, Counseling

Chester County

County Health Depts

DEHEC Chester County Health Department, HIV Testing and Counseling
129 Wylie
Chester, SC 29706-1786
Telephone: (803)-385-6152
Contact: Nancy Van Dyke
HIV testing, counseling, home health care

Medical Services

Hazel Pittman Center
P.O. Box 636
130 Hudson Street

Chester, SC 29706
Telephone: (803)-377-8111
Contact: Vivan Y. Wiley
Outpatient services, referrals, intervention, prevention, education,counseling

Chesterfield County

Community Services

Legal Services of the Fourth Judicial Circuit, Chesterfield
114 South Page Street
PO Box 87
Chesterfield, SC 29709-1522
Telephone: (803)-623-6077
For low income

County Health Depts

Chesterfield County Health Dept., HIV Testing and Counseling
Scotch Road
Chesterfield, SC 29709
Telephone: (803)-623-2117
Contact: Judy Oliver
HIV Testing, Counseling

Clarendon County

Community Services

Department of Social Services, Clarendon County
South Church Street
Manning, SC 29102
Telephone: (803)-435-4303
Contact: Anderson B. Thomas - Director
Social Services

County Health Depts

Clarendon County Health Department, HIV Testing & Counseling
21 E. Hospital Street
Manning, SC 29102-3152
Telephone: (803)-435-8168
Contact: Anna Morris
HIV Testing, Counseling

Medical Services

Clarendon County Commission on Alcohol and Drug Abuse
14 North Church Street
Manning, SC 29102-3502
Telephone: (803)-435-2121
Contact: Ann Kirven - Director
Outpatient services, referrals, intervention, prevention, education& counseling

Colleton County

Community Services

Neighborhood Legal Assistance Program--Low Country
22 Wichman Street
Walterboro, SC 29488
Telephone: (803)-549-9581 Fax: (803)-549-6931
Legal services, civil cases

County Health Depts

Colleton County Health Department, HIV Testing & Counseling
P.O. Box 229
Walterboro, SC 29488-0229
Telephone: (803)-549-1516
HIV Testing, Counseling

Darlington County

County Health Depts

Darlington County Health Dept., HIV Testing and Counseling
305 Russell Street
Darlington, SC 29532-3323
Telephone: (803)-393-4511 Fax: (803)-398-4400
HIV Testing, Counseling

Darlington County Health Dept., HIV Testing and Counseling
402 S. 4th Street
Hartsville, SC 29550-5718
Telephone: (803)-332-7303
HIV Testing, Counseling

Dillon County

Community Services

Department of Social Services, Dillon County
P.O. Box 1307
Dillon, SC 29536-1307
Telephone: (803)-774-8284 Fax: (803)-814-0253
Social services, aid to family with dependant children, food stamps, adultchild protection services

Legal Services of the Fourth Judicial Circuit Inc.
P.O. Box 1489
Dillon, SC 29536-1489
Telephone: (803)-774-6917
Legal Services

County Health Depts

Dillon County Health Department, HIV Testing and Counseling
1st Avenue and Hampton
Dillon, SC 29536
Telephone: (803)-774-5611
HIV Testing, Counseling

Dorchester County

County Health Depts

Dorchester County Health Dept., HIV Testing and Counseling
201 Gavin Street
St. George, SC 29477-2404
Telephone: (803)-821-1624
HIV Testing, Counseling

Dorchester County Health Dept., HIV Testing and Counseling
505 N. Cedar
Summerville, SC 29483-6409
Telephone: (803)-873-1241
HIV Testing, Counseling

Medical Services

Department of Social Services, Dorchester County
P.O. Box 906
St. George, SC 29477-0906
Telephone: (803)-563-9524 Fax: (803)-563-5587
Social Services

Dorchester County Commission on Alcohol and Drug Abuse
1450 Boone Hill Road
Suite B
Summerville, SC 29483-6409
Telephone: (803)-871-4790 Fax: (803)-871-8579
Contact: Richards Lawson
Outpatient services, referrals, intervention, prevention, education, AIDSeducation (both staff & client)

Edgefield County

County Health Depts

Edgefield County Health Department, HIV Testing & Counseling
300 Gray Street
Edgefield, SC 29824-1128
Telephone: (803)-637-3159
HIV Testing, Counseling

Fairfield County Health Dept., HIV Testing and Counseling
321 By-Pass
Edgefield, SC 29824
Telephone: (803)-635-6481
HIV Testing, Counseling

Fairfield County

Community Services

Department of Social Services, Fairfield County
P.O. Box 210
Winnsboro, SC 29180
Telephone: (803)-635-5502 Fax: (803)-635-2322
Adult services, child protection, food stamps, Medicaid

Florence County

Community Services

Department of Social Services--Florence County
2685 S. Irby St., Box A
Florence, SC 29505
Telephone: (803)-669-3354
Food stamps, human services, aid to families with dependent children

SC Protection and Advocacy System for the Handicapped, Inc.
Region III--Pee Dee
520 West Palmetto Street
Florence, SC 29501-4428
Telephone: (803)-662-0752 Fax: (803)-662-0786
Protection and Advocacy Services to the Handicapped and Mentally Ill

County Health Depts

Florence County Health Department, HIV Testing & Counseling
145 East Cheves Street
Florence, SC 29506-2526
Telephone: (803)-661-4835
HIV Testing, Counseling

Home Health Care

Community Long Term Care-Area 8-Florence
1831 West Evans Street
Suite 201
Florence, SC 29502-5302
Telephone: (803)-667-8718 Fax: (803)-667-9354
Contact: Mona Sechrest - Director
Personal Care Aides, Meals, Counseling, Nursing; Day, Foster and Hospice Care, Case management

McLeod Hospice of the Pee Dee
555 E. Cheves Street
Florence, SC 29506
Telephone: (803)-667-2564 Fax: (803)-678-5135
Contact: Joan Harrison-Pavy - Director
Hospice Care

Visiting Nurses Association of Florence, Inc.
P.O. Box 4598
Florence, SC 29502-4598
Telephone: (803)-667-1515 Fax: (803)-667-0076
Contact: Ellen Williams
Home Health Services

Medical Services

Florence County Commission on Alcohol and Drug Abuse
604 Gregg Avenue
Florence, SC 29502-4317
Telephone: (803)-664-0808 Fax: (803)-667-1615
Contact: Jim Canup
Outpatient Services, Referrals, Halfway House, Intervention, Education

Pee Dee Mental Health Center
SC Dept. of Mental Health
2100 West Lucas Street
Florence, SC 29501
Telephone: (803)-661-4874
Contact: Olin Cross
Mental Health Services

Georgetown County

Community Services

Department of Social Services, Georgetown County
330 Dozier Street
Georgetown, SC 29440-0445
Telephone: (803)-546-5134 Fax: (803)-546-0617
Social services, food stamps, Medicaid, adult & child protection service,AIDS waiver

Neighborhood Legal Assistance Program, Georgetown
201 King Street
Georgetown, SC 29440-3535
Telephone: (803)-546-2491
Legal services, civil cases

County Health Depts

Georgetown County Health Dept., HIV Testing and Counseling
303 Hazard Street
Georgetown, SC 29440-3292
Telephone: (803)-546-5593
HIV Testing, Counseling

Home Health Care

Hospice of Georgetown County, Inc.
P.O. Box 1436
Georgetown, SC 29442-1436
Telephone: (803)-546-3410 Fax: (803)-527-6964
Contact: Marsha Bachtel - R.N.
Skilled Nursing, Social Work, Bereavement Care, Pastoral Counseling

Greenville County

Community Services

Department of Social Services, Greenville County
P.O. Box 10887
Greenville, SC 29603-0887
Telephone: (803)-232-8703
Social Services

Legal Services Agency of Western Carolina--Greenville
P.O. Box 10706, Fed. Sta.
1 Pendleton Street
Greenville, SC 29603-0706
Telephone: (803)-467-3232 Fax: (803)-467-3260
Legal services, civil cases

County Health Depts

Greenville County Health Dept., HIV Testing and Counseling
200 University Ridge
Greenville, SC 29602-3635
Telephone: (803)-240-8800
HIV Testing, Counseling

Home Health Care

Professional Home Nursing
1021 Grove Road
Suite C
Greenville, SC 29605
Telephone: (803)-235-0608 Fax: (803)-370-5472
Contact: Cindy Hoxie - Administrative Assistant
Skilled Nursing, Home Health Aides for AIDS patients referred by doctor.

SC Dept of Health & Environmental Control-Appalachia II
PO Bx 2507, 200 Univ. Rd
Greenville, SC 29601
Telephone: (803)-240-8800
Contact: Dr. Ronald Rolett
Home Nursing and Health Aides, Home Therapy, Medical and Social Services

Medical Services

Family Counseling Service
301 Univ. Ridge
Suite 5500
Greenville, SC 29601-3674
Telephone: (803)-467-3266 Fax: (803)-467-3571
Toll-Free: (803)-467-3636
Contact: Kathleen Howard - Director

Piedmont Center for Mental Health Services
Sc Dept. of Mental Health
207 North Maple Street #12
Simpsonville, SC 29681
Telephone: (803)-963-3421 Fax: (803)-967-8617
Contact: Joe James
Mental Health Services

Piedmont Mental Health Center, S.C. Dept. of Mental Health
64 Main Street
Piedmont, SC 29673
Telephone: (803)-845-7597
Mental Health Services

Psychotherapy Services of Greenville
3575 Rutherford Road Ext
Suite A
Taylors, SC 29687-4153
Telephone: (803)-268-1050
Contact: Francis V. Pate - MSW, ACSW
Individual and Family Counseling; Specializes in People with Long-Term Illness

Resource One, Inc.
Seven Pointe Circle
Greenville, SC 29615-3555
Telephone: (803)-233-5639 Fax: (803)-370-3966
Toll-Free: (800)-327-5509
Contact: Tammy Keelnney; Nuala Browne -
Drug Testing, Employee Assistance Programs, Outpatient Treatment Programs

Greenwood County

Community Services

Department of Social Services--Greenwood County
P.O. Box 1096
Greenwood, SC 29648-1096
Telephone: (803)-229-5258 Fax: (803)-229-4613
Social Services, child protection services, Medicaid, Medicare, adultprotective services

Legal Services Agency of Western Carolina, Greenwood
803 Grier Building
Greenwood, SC 29646
Telephone: (803)-223-4879
Toll-Free: (800)-922-3114
Legal services, civil cases

County Health Depts

Greenwood County Health Dept., HIV Testing and Counseling
1736 S. Main Street
Greenwood, SC 29646-4124
Telephone: (803)-223-8488
HIV Testing, Counseling

Home Health Care

Community Long Term Care, Area 3-Greenwood
State Health & Human Services
PO Box 3088
Greenwood, SC 29648
Telephone: (803)-223-8622
Contact: Richard Copeland - Area Administrator

SC Dept of Health & Environmental Control-Upper Savannah Health Dis.
Home Health Services
P.O. Box 3227
Greenwood, SC 29648
Telephone: (803)-223-8488 Fax: (803)-942-3690
Contact: Shirley Hollis - District Director
Home Nursing and Health Aides, Home Therapy, Medical and Social Services,Family Planning

Medical Services

Piedmont Internal Medicine
104 Liner Drive
Greenwood, SC 29646-2401
Telephone: (803)-227-1115 Fax: (803)-227-4026
Contact: John W. Holman, MD - Infectious Disease
Medical Services

Hampton County

County Health Depts

Department of Social Services, Hampton County
201 Jackson Street, West
Hampton, SC 29924-2567
Telephone: (803)-943-3641
Social Services; food stamps, Medicaid

Hampton County Health Department, HIV Testing and Counseling
Highway 278
Varnville, SC 29924
Telephone: (803)-943-3878
HIV Testing, Counseling

Home Health Care

Community Long Term Care, Area 10-Yemassee Satellite Office
State Health and Human Svcs
P.O. Box 596
Yemassee, SC 29945
Telephone: (803)-726-4149 Fax: (803)-521-9193
Contact: Janet McCray - Office Supervisor
Personal Care Aides, Meals, Counseling, Nursing; Day, Foster, and Hospice Care

Medical Services

New Life Center
Courthouse Annex
Hampton, SC 29924
Telephone: (803)-943-2800 Fax: (803)-943-7538
Contact: Frank Soloman
Outpatient Services, Referrals, Intervention, Education, Prevention

Horry County

Community Services

Department of Social Services, Horry County
P.O. Drawer 1465
Conway, SC 29526-1465
Telephone: (803)-365-5565 Fax: (803)-365-9512
Social Services, adult protective services, child protective services,Medicaid, food stamps

HOPE Support Groups
P.O. Box 8364
Myrtle Beach, SC 29578-8364
Telephone: (803)-448-4881
Contact: Les Williamson
Support Groups for HIV+ Persons

Horry County Task Force on AIDS
800 21st Avenue North
Myrtle Beach,, SC 29577
Telephone: (803)-448-8407 Fax: (803)-448-7499
Contact: Sandra Carmichael
Task force, referrals

Housing Authority of Atlantic Beach
P.O. Box 1721
N. Myrtle Beach, SC 29598-1721
Telephone: (803)-272-4189
Housing Assistance

Housing Authority of the City of Myrtle Beach
P.O. Box 2468
Myrtle Beach, SC 29578-2468
Telephone: (803)-448-3262 Fax: (803)-626-9083
Contact: Jane Hilburn
Housing Assistance

Neighborhood Legal Assistance Program, Conway
P.O. Box 1819
607 Main Street
Conway, SC 29526-1819
Telephone: (803)-248-6376 Fax: (803)-248-6378
Legal Services, civil cases

County Health Depts

Horry County Health Department, HIV Testing and Counseling
101 Elm Street
Conway, SC 29526
Telephone: (803)-248-6381
HIV Testing, Counseling

Horry County Health Department, HIV Testing and Counseling
3811 Walnut Street
Loris, SC 29569
Telephone: (803)-756-4027
HIV Testing, Counseling

Home Health Care

Community Long Term Care, Area 9-Conway
State Health and Human Services
P.O. Box 2150 C
Conway, SC 29526
Telephone: (803)-248-7249 Fax: (803)-248-3809
Contact: Worth Dudley - Area Administrator
AIDS waiver, personal care aides, meals, counseling, nursing; day, foster,and hospice care

SC Dept of Health & Environmental Control-Waccamaw District
Home Health Services
800 21st Avenue North
Myrtle Beach, SC 29577
Telephone: (803)-448-8407 Fax: (803)-448-7499
Contact: David Lowe - Team Leader HIV
Home Nursing and Health Aides, Home Therapy, Medical and Social Services, AIDS intervention & counseling

Kershaw County

Community Services

Department of Social Services--Kershaw County
816 DeKalb Street
Camden, SC 29020-4225
Telephone: (803)-432-7676 Fax: (803)-425-7195
Contact: Bill Bradshaw
Social Services

Legal Services of the Fourth Judicial Circuit, Camden
2 Lafayette Court
Camden, SC 29020-3500
Telephone: (803)-425-1195
Contact: Eileen Marquis
Legal Services

County Health Depts

Kershaw County Health Department, HIV Testing and Counseling
1116 Church Street
Camden, SC 29020-3502
Telephone: (803)-432-1426
HIV Testing, Counseling

Lancaster County

Community Services

Department of Social Services, Lancaster County
P.O. Box 1719
Lancaster, SC 29721
Telephone: (803)-286-6914
Social services, food stamps

County Health Depts

Lancaster County Health Dept., HIV Testing and Counseling
P.O. Box 817
Lancaster, SC 29720-0817
Telephone: (803)-286-9948
HIV Testing, Counseling

Home Health Care

SC Dept of Health & Environmental Control-Catawba District
Home Health Services
Bx 817, Rt 10 Pageland Hwy
Lancaster, SC 29720
Telephone: (803)-286-9948 Fax: (803)-286-1258
Contact: Richard Thunderburk
Home Nursing and Health Aides, Home Therapy, Medical and Social Services

Medical Services

Catawba Mental Health Center--Lancaster Satellite
SC Dept. of Mental Health
210 North Pine Street
Lancaster, SC 29720
Telephone: (803)-285-7456 Fax: (803)-285-5514
Contact: Kathy Wilds
Mental health services, counseling

Laurens County

Community Services

Department of Social Services, Laurens County
P.O. Box 986
Laurens, SC 29360-0986
Telephone: (803)-984-0551
Social Services

Housing Authority of the City of Laurens
P.O. Box 749
Laurens, SC 29360-0749
Telephone: (803)-984-6568
Housing Assistance

County Health Depts

Laurens County Health Department, HIV Testing and Counseling
Route 3 Box 789
Laurens, SC 29325
Telephone: (803)-833-0000
HIV Testing, Counseling

Medical Services

Laurens County Commission on Alcohol and Drug Abuse
Industrial Park
Clinton, SC 29325
Telephone: (803)-833-6500
Contact: Luvenia Johnson
Outpatient Services, Referrals, Halfway House, Intervention, Education

Laurens Mental Health Center
SC Dept. of Mental Health
314 Owings Street
Laurens, SC 29360
Telephone: (803)-984-2568
Contact: Ken Madewell
Mental health referral & counseling

Lee County

Community Services

Department of Social Services, Lee County
P.O. Box 389
Bishopville, SC 29010-0389
Telephone: (803)-484-5376 Fax: (803)-484-6435
Contact: Fanny Watson - Director
Social Services

Legal Services of the Fourth Judicial Circuit, Bishopville
119 South Nettles
Bishopville, SC 29010
Telephone: (803)-484-5341
Contact: Ilene Marquis - Intake Specialist
Legal Services

County Health Depts

Lee County Health Department, HIV Testing and Counseling
810 Brown Street
PO Box 307
Bishopville, SC 29010-1726
Telephone: (803)-484-6612
Contact: Judy Laney
HIV Testing, Counseling

Medical Services

Lee County Commission on Alcohol and Drug Abuse
108 East Church Street
Bishopville, SC 29010
Telephone: (803)-484-5341 Fax: (803)-484-5043
Contact: Christie Huggins
Outpatient Services, Referrals, Halfway House, Education; Phone Extension 51

Lexington County

Community Services

Department of Social Services, Lexington County
P.O. Drawer 430
Lexington, SC 29071-0430
Telephone: (803)-957-7333 Fax: (803)-359-2278
Social Services

County Health Depts

Lexington County Health Dept., HIV Testing and Counseling
112 West Hospital Drive
West Columbia, SC 29169-3406
Telephone: (803)-791-3580
HIV Testing, Counseling

Lexington County Health Dept., HIV Testing and Counseling
P.O. Box 27
Batesburg, SC 29006-0027
Telephone: (803)-532-6326
HIV Testing, Counseling

Medical Services

Charter Rivers Hospital
2900 Sunset Blvd.
West Columbia, SC 29169
Telephone: (803)-796-9911 Fax: (803)-791-7622
Contact: Regina B. King - Patient Care Svcs. Coord.
Comprehensive treatment for drug and alcohol rehabilitation, inpatient andoutpatient level

Testing Sites

SC Dept of Health & Environmental Control-West Midlands
AIDS Health Education
112 West Hospital Drive
West Columbia, SC 29169
Telephone: (803)-791-3580
Contact: Patsy Jacobs - RN
HIV Testing (confidential), counseling, referrals

Marion County

Community Services

Department of Social Services, Marion County
180 Airport Road
Suite A
Mullins, SC 29574-9566
Telephone: (803)-423-4623 Fax: (803)-423-2419
Contact: Joe Baldwin
Social Services

County Health Depts

Marion County Health Department, HIV Testing and Counseling
180 Airport Rd.
Suite H
Marion, SC 29574
Telephone: (803)-423-8295
HIV Testing, Counseling

Marlboro County

Community Services

Department of Social Services, Marlboro County
P.O. Drawer 120
Bennettsville, SC 29512-0120
Telephone: (803)-479-7181 Fax: (803)-479-6254
Social services, child protection services, referrals, Medicaid, AFDC

Legal Services of the Fourth Judicial Circuit, Marlboro
115 Market Street
Bennettsville, SC 29512-0266
Telephone: (803)-479-6014

County Health Depts

Marlboro County Health Dept., HIV Testing and Counseling
Parsonage St. Extension
Bennettsville, SC 29512
Telephone: (803)-479-6801
Contact: Carolyn Millsaps
HIV Testing, Counseling

Home Health Care

Community Long Term Care, Area 8 Bennettsville Satellite
P.O. Box 372
Bennettsville, SC 29512-0372
Telephone: (803)-479-9075
Personal care, meals, counseling, nursing; day, foster, and hospice care, AIDS waiver

Pee Dee Public Health District-Bennettsville Anex
Home Health Services
Plaza Bldg., Market St.
Bennettsville, SC 29512
Telephone: (803)-479-8311 Fax: (803)-479-6781
Home Nursing and Health Aides, Home Therapy, Medical and Social Services

SC Dept of Health & Environmental Control-Pee Dee II Dist.
Home Health Services
Plaza Bldg., Market St.
Bennettsville, SC 29512
Telephone: (803)-479-8311 Fax: (803)-479-6781
Contact: Harold Gowdy,M.D.
Home Nursing and Health Aides, Home Therapy, Medical and Social Services

SC Dept of Health & Environmental Control-Pee Dee II Dist.
Home Health Services
Plaza Bldg., Market St.
Bennettsville, SC 29512
Telephone: (803)-479-8311
Home Nursing and Health Aides, Home Therapy, Medical and Social Services

Mc Cormick County

County Health Depts

McCormick County Health Dept., HIV Testing and Counseling
Main at Highway 28
McCormick, SC 29835
Telephone: (803)-465-2511
HIV Testing, Counseling

Newberry County

County Health Depts

Newberry County Health Dept.
1308 Hunt Street
Newberry, SC 29108-3036
Telephone: (803)-276-4155 Fax: (803)-321-2170
HIV Testing, Counseling

Medical Services

Newberry County Commission on Alcohol and Drug Abuse
P.O. Box 738
Newberry, SC 29108
Telephone: (803)-276-5690 Fax: (803)-321-2234
Outpatient Svcs., Detox., Halfway House, Residential Family Care, Education

Newberry Mental Health Center
P.O. Box 464
Newberry, SC 29108-0464
Telephone: (803)-276-8000 Fax: (803)-276-6669
Mental Health Services

Oconee County

Community Services

Department of Social Services--Oconee County
PO Box 739
Walhalla, SC 29691-0458
Telephone: (803)-638-5882
Social Services

County Health Depts

Oconee County Health Department, HIV Testing and Counseling
200 South Broad
Walhalla, SC 29691
Telephone: (803)-638-3639
HIV Testing, Counseling

Oconee County Health Department, HIV Testing and Counseling
107 East North Second St.
Seneca, SC 29678-3201
Telephone: (803)-882-2245
HIV Testing, Counseling

Medical Services

Anderson/Oconee Alcohol and Drug Abuse Commission
302 North Pine Street
Seneca, SC 29678-3108
Telephone: (803)-882-7563 Fax: (803)-882-7388
Contact: David Winn
Substance Abuse Outpatient Services, Referrals, Intervention, Education

Orangeburg County

County Health Depts

Orangeburg County Health Dept., HIV Testing and Counseling
550 Carolina, NE
Orangeburg, SC 29115-4926
Telephone: (803)-536-9060
Contact: Kathy Johnson
HIV Testing, Counseling

Home Health Care

Community Long Term Care, Area 6-Orangeburg
State Health and Human Services
564 Joe Jefferts Highway
Orangeburg, SC 29115
Telephone: (803)-536-0122
Personal Care Aides, Meals, Counseling, Nursing; Day, Foster, and Hospice Care

SC Dept of Health & Environmental Control-Edisto District
Home Health Services
550 Carolina Avenue
Orangeburg, SC 29116
Telephone: (803)-536-9117 Fax: (803)-536-9118
Home Nursing and Health Aides, Home Therapy, Medical and Social Services

Medical Services

Orangeburg Area Mental Health Center
SC Dept. of Mental Health
Drawer 1929, 550 Carolina
Orangeburg, SC 29115
Telephone: (803)-536-1571 Fax: (803)-534-1463
Mental Health Services

Orangeburg Area Mental Health Center
SC Dept. of Mental Health
Drawer 1929, 550 Carolina
Orangeburg, SC 29115
Telephone: (803)-536-1571 Fax: (803)-536-1463
Mental Health Services

Orangeburg Area Mental Health Center, Holly Hill Satellite
SC Dept. of Mental Health
PO Box 505, 700 Gilway Avenue
Holly Hill, SC 29059
Telephone: (803)-496-3410 Fax: (803)-496-3234
Mental Health Services

Pickens County

Community Services

Department of Social Services, Pickens County
P.O. Box 158
Pickens, SC 29671-0158
Telephone: (803)-878-2451
Contact: John M. Bond - Director
Social Services

S.H.A.R.E. (Sunbelt Human Advancement Resources, Inc.)
121 East First Street
P.O. Box 1628
Easley, SC 29641-1628
Telephone: (803)-859-2989
Contact: Anne C. Holliday - Projects Coordinator
Relief Assistance: Housing, Medical, Food, Fuel, Jobs, Counseling, Education

County Health Depts

Pickens County Health Department, HIV Testing and Counseling
McDaniel Avenue
Pickens, SC 29671
Telephone: (803)-898-5965 Fax: (803)-898-5568
HIV Testing, Counseling

Medical Services

Pickens County Mental Health Center
SC Dept. of Mental Health
314 W. Main Street
Pickens, SC 29671
Telephone: (803)-878-6830 Fax: (803)-878-5396
Mental Health Services

Richland County

Community Services

Family Services Center
1800 Main Street
Columbia, SC 29201
Telephone: (803)-733-5450
Contact: Russell Rawls
Supportive services/counseling

Housing Authority of the City of Cayce
1917 Harden Street
Columbia, SC 29240
Telephone: (803)-254-3886 Fax: (803)-376-6114
Contact: Nancy Stoydenmire - Director of Personnel
Housing Assistance

Palmetto Legal Services, Columbia
P.O. Box 2267
2109 Bull Street
Columbia, SC 29202
Telephone: (803)-799-9668
Toll-Free: (800)-273-1200
Legal services, civil cases, Social Security, domestic cases

PFLAG, Parents and Friends of Lesbians and Gays
493 Hickory Hill Drive
Columbia, SC 29210
Telephone: (803)-772-7396
Contact: Harriet Hancock
Lesbian and Gay Support Organization

South Carolina Legal Services Association
P.O. Box 7187
2109 Bull Street
Columbia, SC 29202-7187
Telephone: (803)-252-0034 Fax: (803)-252-0034
Contact: Mary Williams
Legal Services

South Carolina State Housing Authority
1710 Gervais Street
Suite 300
Columbia, SC 29201-3416
Telephone: (803)-734-8831 Fax: (803)-734-8758
Contact: Dave Leopard
Housing Assistance

University of South Carolina Counseling Center
Close Business Admin. Bldg.
Second Floor
Columbia, SC 29208
Telephone: (803)-777-5223 Fax: (803)-777-9076
Contact: Roger Dowersock
Counseling to Students, Staff, and Faculty Only

County Health Depts

Richland County Health Dept., HIV Testing and Counseling
2000 Hampton Street
Columbia, SC 29204-1059
Telephone: (803)-748-4621
HIV Testing, Counseling

Home Health Care

Caremark Connection Network.
720 Gracem Road
Suite 123
Columbia, SC 29210
Telephone: (803)-731-5076 Fax: (803)-731-4979
Contact: Harriet Fetner - Branch Manager; Alvin Martin - Operations Manager
Clinical Support and Infusion Therapy: Nutrition, Antimicrobials, Chemo.,Hematopoeti

Medical Services

CHAPS Recovery Program
7020 Two Notch Road
Columbia, SC 29223-7523
Telephone: (803)-738-1500 Fax: (803)-738-8111
Contact: Carolyn Rickenbaker - Director
Substance Abuse Services: Inpatient and Outpatient Treatment, Detoxification

Columbia Area Mental Health Ctr-Northeast Richland Satellite
SC Dept. of Mental Health
1801 Sunset Drive
Columbia, SC 29203
Telephone: (803)-737-5500
Mental Health Services

Columbia Oncology Associates
Taylor at Marian Street
Suite 410
Columbia, SC 29220
Telephone: (803)-771-5721 Fax: (803)-771-5741
Contact: William M. Butler, MD - Hematology/Oncology
Medical Services

Community Health Nursing, Preventive Medicine Service
Moncrief Army Comm. Hospital
Box 201
Fort Jackson, SC 29207-5720
Telephone: (803)-751-5251

Lexington/Richland Alcohol and Drug Abuse Council
1325 Harden Street
Columbia, SC 29204-1850
Telephone: (803)-256-3100 Fax: (803)-733-1395
Contact: David Jameson
Outpatient Services, Referrals, Intervention, Education, Halfway House, Detox, AIDS Intervention

Providence Family Practice, Columbia
2750 Laurel Street
Columbia, SC 29204-2038
Telephone: (803)-254-5171 Fax: (803)-254-7411
Contact: Frampton Henderson, MD - Family Practice
Medical Services: Will Accept Referrals of PWAs at Early Stages of Disease

Univ of SC School of Medicine, Children's Immunology Clinic
5 Richland Medical Park
Columbia, SC 29203-6805
Telephone: (803)-765-7020
Contact: Dr. Tanya Reid - Pediatrics
Pediatric AIDS clinic

Saluda County

Community Services

Department of Social Services, Saluda County
P.O. Box 276
Saluda, SC 29138-0276
Telephone: (803)-445-8151 Fax: (803)-445-7088
Contact: Darrow Wilson
Social services, referrals

County Health Depts

Saluda County Health Department, HIV Testing and Counseling
405 West Butler Ave
Saluda, SC 29138-1311
Telephone: (803)-445-2141
HIV Testing, Counseling

Spartanburg County

Community Services

Department of Social Services, Spartanburg County
P.O. Drawer 3548
Spartanburg, SC 29304-3548
Telephone: (803)-596-3001 Fax: (803)-596-3141
Contact: Gaynell West
Social Services

Greater Spartanburg Ministries
680 Asheville Highway
Spartanburg, SC 29303-2946
Telephone: (803)-585-9371
Contact: Rev. W.R. Yown
Relief Assistance: Food, Clothing, Fuel; Spiritual and Emotional Support

Housing Authority of the City of Spartanburg
P.O. Box 4534, Station B
Spartanburg, SC 29305-4534
Telephone: (803)-585-8252 Fax: (803)-585-8040
Contact: Mary Louise Battisti
Housing rental assiatance

Mental Health Association of Piedmont
4 Catawba Street Suite 205
Spartanburg, SC 29303-3036
Telephone: (803)-582-3104
Contact: Sharon Field McCormick - Executive Diretor
Mental Health Services

Mobile Meal Service of Spartanburg County
P.O. Box 461
Spartanburg, SC 29304-0461
Telephone: (803)-573-7684
Contact: Jayne C. McQueen
Home Delivered Meals

Piedmont Community Actions, Inc.
P.O. Box 5374
Spartanburg, SC 29304-5374
Telephone: (803)-585-8133 Fax: (803)-585-8183
Contact: Nancy Knuckles
Emergency food, fuel, medicial, child care, head start

Piedmont Legal Services--Spartanburg
Main Street Mall
148 E. Main Street
Spartanburg, SC 29301
Telephone: (803)-582-0369
Contact: Grant Lanford
Legal Services; Toll-Free Number: 800-922-8176

County Health Depts

Spartanburg County Health Dept., HIV Testing and Counseling
151 East Wood Street
Spartanburg, SC 29305-3016
Telephone: (803)-596-3337
HIV Testing, Counseling

Home Health Care

SC Dept of Health & Environmental Control-Appalachia III
Home Health Services
PO Box 4217, 151 E. Wood
Spartanburg, SC 29305
Telephone: (803)-596-3334
Home Nursing and Health Aides, Home Therapy, Medical and Social Services

Spartanburg Regional Home Health and Hospice Services
101 East Wood Street
Spartanburg, SC 29303-3072
Telephone: (803)-591-6380Fax: (803)-560-6338
Nurses; Occupational, Speech, Physical Therapy; Health Aides; Social Services

Sumter County

Community Services

Department of Social Services--Sumter County
P.O. Box 68
Sumter, SC 29151-0068
Telephone: (803)-778-2778
Contact: Ronald H. Smith
Social Services

County Health Depts

Sumter County Health Department, HIV Testing and Counseling
P.O. Box 1628
Sumter, SC 29151-1628
Telephone: (803)-773-5511
HIV testing, counseling, partner notification

Home Health Care

Community Long Term Care-Area 7-Sumter
St. Health and Human Svcs
213 West Hampton
Sumter, SC 29150
Telephone: (803)-778-5413
Personal Care Aides, Meals, Counseling, Nurses; Day, Foster, and Hospice Care

SC Dept of Health & Environmental Control-Wateree District
STD/HIV Program
P.O. Box 1628
Sumter, SC 29151-1628
Telephone: (803)-773-5511 Fax: (803)-773-6366
Contact: Helen Walters
HIV testing & counseling; partner notification

SC Dept of Health & Environmental Control-Wateree District
Home Health Services
105 N. Magnolia P.O. 1628
Sumter, SC 29151-1628
Telephone: (803)-773-5511
Contact: Helen Walters
Home Nursing and Health Aides, Home Therapy, Medical, Social Services,Testing, Counseling, Referrals

Medical Services

Santee-Wateree Mental Health Center
215 North Magnolia
P.O. Box 1946
Sumter, SC 29151-1946
Telephone: (803)-775-9364 Fax: (803)-773-6615
Contact: Dr. Jacqueline Francis
Mental Health Services HIV and AIDS Support Group for Patients Family, andFriends

Union County

Community Services

Housing Authority of the City of Union
201 Porter Street
Union, SC 29379-2854
Telephone: (803)-427-9679 Fax: (803)-427-9679
Contact: Randy Penland
Housing Assistance

County Health Depts

Union County Health Department, HIV Testing and Counseling
PO Box 500
Thompson Boulevard
Union, SC 29379-0500
Telephone: (803)-429-1690 Fax: (803)-429-1697
Contact: Jane Hammet - Supervisor
HIV Testing, Counseling

Williamsburg County

Community Services

Department of Social Services, Williamsburg County
PO Box 389
Kingstree, SC 29556-2519
Telephone: (803)-354-5411 Fax: (803)-354-3021
Contact: Viloa M. Frazier
Social services: medication, counseling, transportation

County Health Depts

Williamsburg County Health Dept., HIV Testing and Counseling
203 East Brook Street
Kingstree, SC 29556-3411
Telephone: (803)-354-9927
HIV Testing, Counseling

York County

Community Services

Department of Social Services, York County
P.O. Box 261
York, SC 29745
Telephone: (803)-684-2315 Fax: (803)-684-8103
Contact: Art Stephenson
Social services, counseling

Department of Social Services, York County
18 West Liberty Street
York, SC 29745-1454
Telephone: (803)-684-2315
Social Services, food stamps, AFDC, AIDS assistance program

Housing Authority of Fort Mill
105 Bozeman Drive
Fort Mill, SC 29715-2503
Telephone: (803)-547-6787 Fax: (803)-548-2125
Contact: Louise Stams
Housing Assistance

Housing Authority of the City of Rock Hill
P.O. Box 11579
Rock Hill, SC 29730-1579
Telephone: (803)-324-3060 Fax: (803)-324-5857
Housing Assistance

Housing Authority of the City of York
P.O. Box 687
York, SC 29745-0687
Telephone: (803)-684-7359 Fax: (803)-684-0895
Contact: Edwina Barnett
Housing Assistance

Piedmont Legal Services, Rock Hill
P.O. Box 10591
214 Johnson Street
Rock Hill, SC 29731-0591
Telephone: (803)-327-9001
Toll-Free: (800)-922-3853
Legal Services; Toll-Free Number: 800-922-3853

Piedmont Legal Services--Rock Hill
P.O. Box 10591
214 Johnson Street
Rock Hill, SC 29731-0591
Telephone: (803)-327-9001 Fax: (803)-327-7105
Toll-Free: (800)-922-3853
Contact: Lynne Wagner
Legal services

County Health Depts

York County Health Department, HIV Testing and Counseling
P.O. Box 3057
Rock Hill, SC 29731
Telephone: (803)-324-7521
HIV Testing, Counseling

York County Health Department, HIV Testing and Counseling
North Congress Street
PO Box 149
York, SC 29745
Telephone: (803)-684-7004
HIV Testing, Counseling

Home Health Care

Community Long Term Care, Area 4-Rock Hill
State Health and Human Services
219 Hampton Street, Box 109
Rock Hill, SC 29731
Telephone: (803)-327-9061
Personal Care Aides, Meals, Counseling, Nurses; Day, Foster, and Hospice Care

Medical Personnel Pool of Metrolina
1365 Ebenezer Road
Rock Hill, SC 29732-2336
Telephone: (803)-324-4166

Private Duty Nursing, Intermittent Home Health Services

York County Hospice - Home Health Care
P.O. Box 2472
Rock Hill, SC 29731-6068
Telephone: (803)-329-4663 Fax: (803)-329-5935
Toll-Free: (800)-895-2273
Contact: Tamra N. West
Home health care, counseling

Medical Services

Keystone, York County
P.O. Box 4437
Rock Hill, SC 29732
Telephone: (803)-324-1800 Fax: (803)-328-3831
Contact: John Hart
Outpatient Services, Referrals, Intervention, Prevention, Education

SOUTH DAKOTA

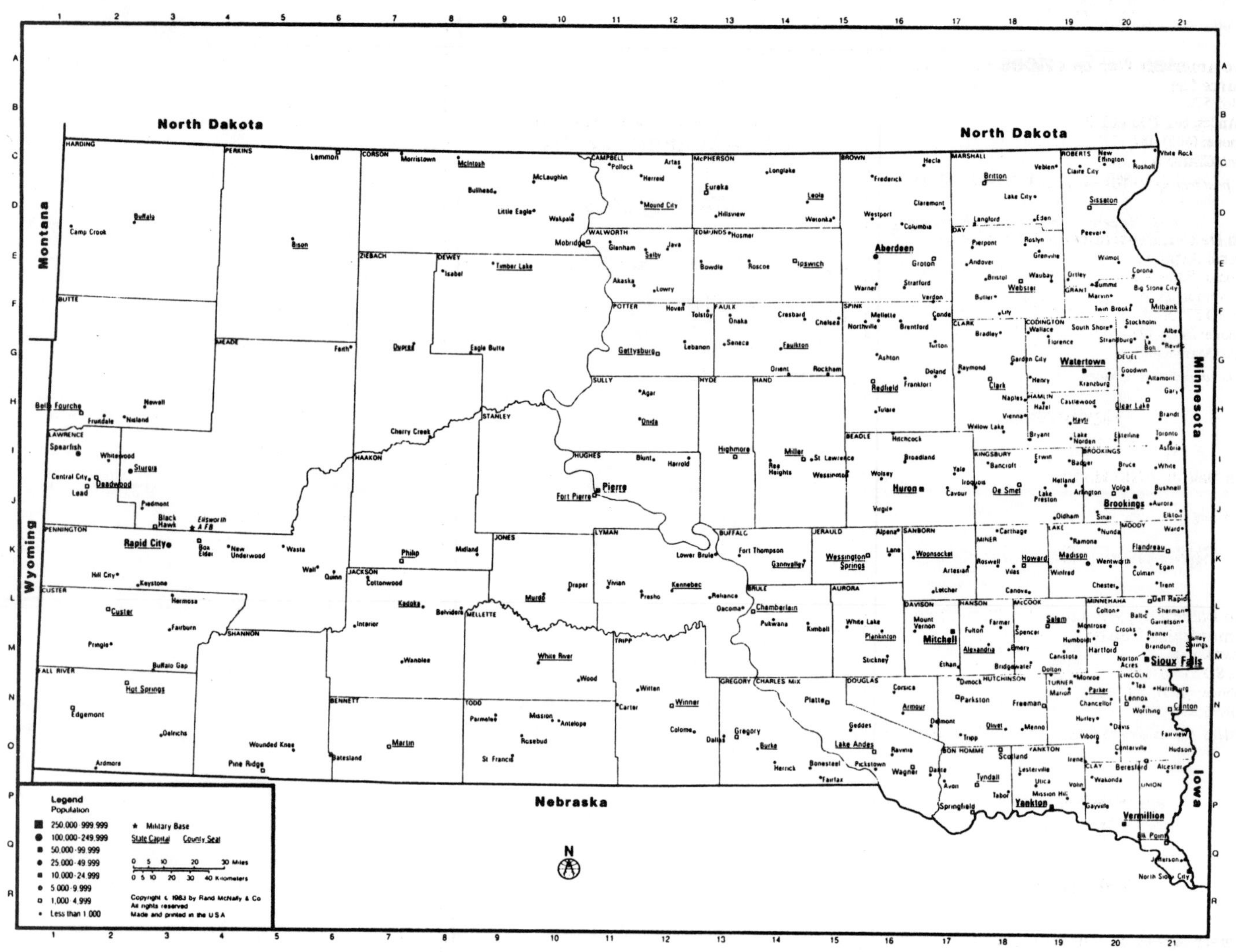

From City/County Planning Atlas Copyright 1989 by Reed McNally & Company, R.L. 90-S-28

South Dakota

General Services

Education

Native American Women's Health Education Resource Center
P.O. Box 572
Lake Andes, SD 57356-0572
Telephone: (605)-487-7072
Contact: Charon Asetoyer
Pre & post testing for HIV workshop, education material

South Dakota Department of Education and Cultural Affairs
Division of Education
700 Governors Drive
Pierre, SD 57501
Telephone: (605)-773-4681
Contact: Marianne Carr
Various educational services

Hotlines

South Dakota AIDS Hotline

In state only (800)-592-1861

State Health Departments

South Dakota Department of Health, Office of Communicable Disease
523 East Capitol
Pierre, SD 57501-3182
Telephone: (605)-773-3364
Contact: Steve Volk
HIV/AIDS Counseling, Testing, Referrals/Free & Anonymous

Brown County

Testing Sites

Aberdeen Area Communicable Disease Control
402 South Main Street
Aberdeen, SD 57401
Telephone: (605)-622-2373
Free counseling & testing

Hughes County

Testing Sites

Pierre Area Communicable Disease Control
412 W Missouri
Pierre, SD 57501-4549
Telephone: (605)-773-5348
Free counseling & testing

Minnehaha County

Testing Sites

Sioux Falls Area Communicable Disease Control
817 West Russell
Room 202
Sioux Falls, SD 57104-1372
Telephone: (605)-335-5020
Free counseling & testing

Pennington County

Testing Sites

Rapid City Area Communicable Disease Control
725 LaCrosse
Rapid City, SD 57701-3007
Telephone: (605)-394-2289
Free counseling & testing

TENNESSEE

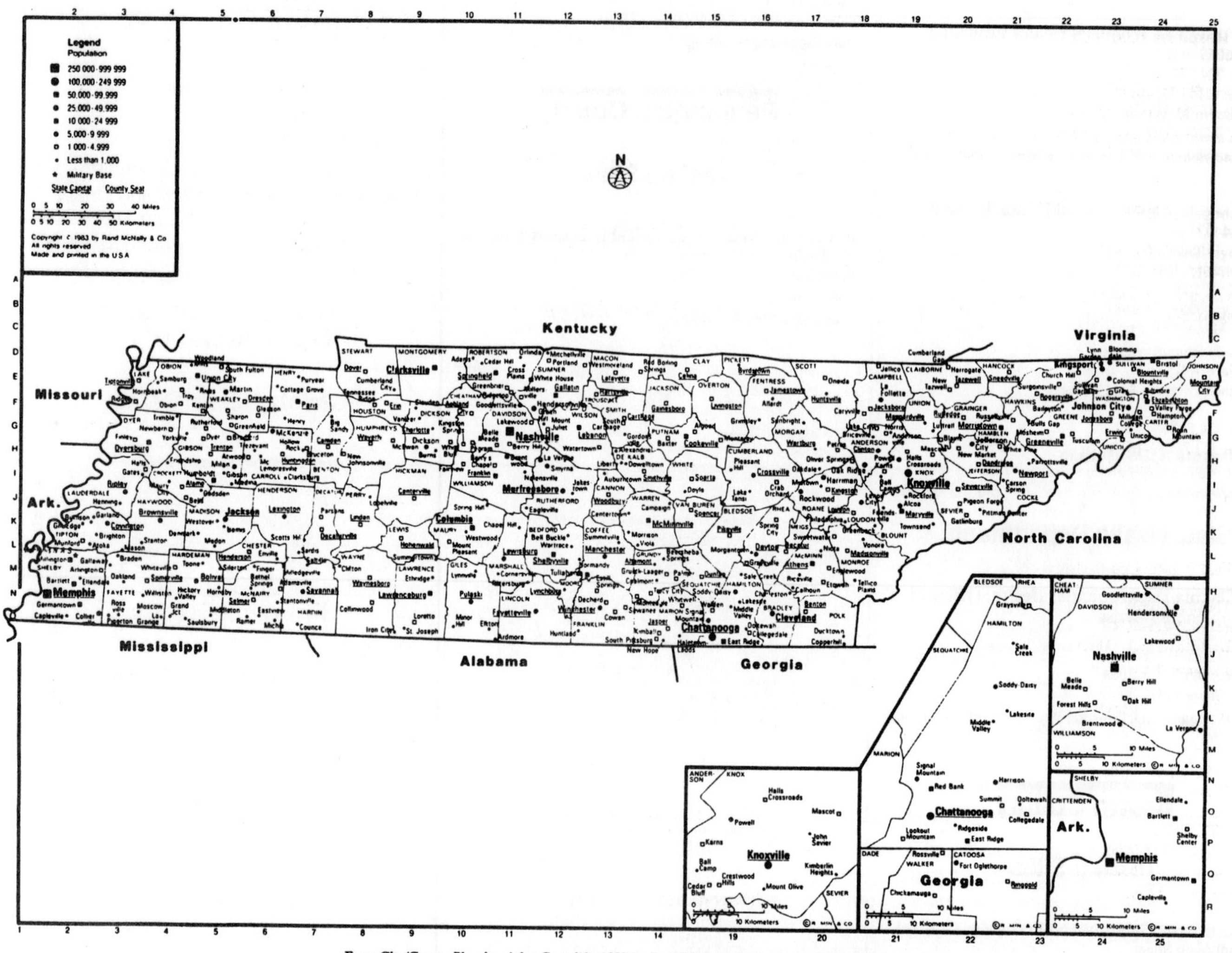

From City/County Planning Atlas Copyright 1989 by Reed McNally & Company, R.L. 90-S-28

Tennessee

General Services

Education

A.I.D.S. Response Knoxville
P.O. Box 6069
Knoxville, TN 37914-6069
Telephone: (615)-523-2437
Contact: Dawn Mickoloff - Director
Education about AIDS and HIV infection; Direct Service to families and victims

Chattanooga CARES
P.O. Box 4497
Chattanooga, TN 37405-0497
Telephone: (615)-265-2273
Education about AIDS and HIV infection; Direct Service to families and victims

Nashville CARES
700 Craighead Street
Suite 200
Nashville, TN 37204-2254
Telephone: (615)-385-1510
Contact: Joseph Bodenmiller
Printed Information, Direct Services to PWA's and familes, Education

South West Tennessee Regional Health Office
295 Summar
Jackson, TN 38301-3905
Telephone: (901)-423-6600
Contact: Barbara Callery - Director
AIDS Information & Services

Hotlines

Meharry Medical College
1005 DB Todd Blvd
PO Box 74-A
Nashville, TN 37208
Telephone: (615)-327-6000
Contact: Maryann Southiams - MADS Educator, ext 6238
HIV hotline, testing clinic

In state only (800)-525-2437

State Health Departments

Central Tennessee Regional Health Office
140 University Drive
Cookeville, TN 38501-6076
Telephone: (615)-528-7531
Contact: Barbara Burchett
Counseling & Testing

First Tennessee Regional Health Office East
1233 Southwest Avenue
Johnson City, TN 37604-6519
Telephone: (615)-929-5928
Contact: Carolyn Sliger - HIVS Director
Counseling & Testing: Monday-Friday, by appointment. 5 counties.

Northwest Tennessee Regional Health Office
1010 Mt. Zion Road
Union City, TN 38261
Telephone: (901)-885-7700
Contact: Debbie White - AIDS Project Director
Counseling & Testing

Southeast Tennessee Regional Health Office
540 McCallie Avenue
Suite 450
Chattanooga, TN 37402
Telephone: (615)-624-9921
Contact: Don Taylor - Regional AIDS Prog Dir
AIDS Information & Services

Tennessee Department of Health, STD/HIV Division
Tennessee Tower, 13th Floor
312 8th Avenue North
Nashville, TN 37247
Telephone: (615)-741-7500
Contact: Dan Burke - Program Director; Laurel Wood - Comm. Disease Program Dir.

Bradley County

County Health Depts

Bradley County Health Department
201 Dooley Street, S.E.
P.O. Box 1398
Cleveland, TN 37364
Telephone: (615)-476-0568
Counseling & Testing: Wed, 9:00 A.M. to 3:00 P.M.

Cheatham County

County Health Depts

Cheatham County Health Department
199 Court Street
Ashland City, TN 37015
Telephone: (615)-792-4318
Contact: Linda Carney
Counseling and Testing: M - F, 8:30 A.M. to 4:00 P.M.

Cumberland County

County Health Depts

Cumberland County Health Department
P.O. Box 1010
Crossville, TN 38557
Telephone: (615)-484-6196
Contact: Barbara Burchett
Counseling & Testing: Fridays only

Davidson County

County Health Depts

HIV Plus Program, Davidson County Health Department
311 23rd. Avenue, North
Metro-Nashville, Rm.116
Nashville, TN 37203-1503
Telephone: (615)-340-5676
Post test care, appointment requested

Nashville/Davidson County Health Department
311 23rd Avenue, North
Nashville, TN 37203-1503
Telephone: (615)-327-9313
Contact: Dan McEachem - Director
Counseling & testing

Home Health Care

Dickson County

County Health Depts

Dickson County Health Department
117 Academy Street
Dickson, TN 37055-2013
Telephone: (615)-446-2839
Counseling & Testing: M-F 8:30 A.M. to 4:00 P.M.

Franklin County

County Health Depts

Franklin County Health Department
1025 Dinah Shore Blvd.
Winchester, TN 37398-1103
Telephone: (615)-967-3826
Contact: Don Taylor
Counseling & Testing: Second and Fourth Tues., 8:30 A.M. to 2:00 P.M.

Hamilton County

County Health Depts

Chattanooga/Hamilton County Health Department
921 East Third Street
Chattanooga, TN 37403-2146
Telephone: (615)-757-2078
Contact: Irby Rowland
HIV testing

Medical Services

Homeless Health Care Center
717 East 11th Street
Chattanooga, TN 37403
Telephone: (615)-265-5708
Contact: Marty Smith
Medical services, mental & substance abuse counseling, HIV testing &counseling

Haywood County

County Health Depts

Haywood County Health Department
950 East Main Street
Bronsville, TN 38012-2628
Telephone: (901)-772-0463 Fax: (901)-772-3377
Contact: Janice Brown
Counseling & Testing

Houston County

County Health Depts

Houston County Health Department
PO Box 370
Erin, TN 37061
Telephone: (615)-289-3463
Contact: Bill Leech
Counseling & Testing: Mon-Fri, 8:30 A.M. to 4:00 P.M.

Humphreys County

County Health Depts

Humphreys County Health Department
208 Wyly
Waverly, TN 37185
Telephone: (615)-296-2231
Contact: Bill Sugg
Counseling & testing

Knox County

County Health Depts

Knoxville/Knox County Health Department
Cleveland Place, N.W.
Knoxville, TN 37917
Telephone: (615)-544-4100 Fax: (615)-544-4295
Contact: Mark Miller
Counseling & Testing: Monday through Friday, 8:00 A.M. to 3:00 P.M.

Home Health Care

Testing Sites

East Tennessee Regional Health Office
PO Box 59019
Knoxville, TN 37950-9019
Telephone: (615)-546-9221
Contact: Frank R. Bristow
Counseling & Testing: Thurs., 9:00 A.M. to 3:30 P.M.

Madison County

County Health Depts

Jackson/Madison County Health Department
745 West Forrest
Jackson, TN 38301-3901
Telephone: (901)-423-3020
Contact: David Argo
Counseling & Testing: Monday through Friday, 8:30 A.M. to 3:30 P.M.

Mc Minn County

County Health Depts

McMinn County Health Department
P.O. Box 665 Showbarn Rd
Athens, TN 37303-0665
Telephone: (615)-745-7431
Contact: Gale Smithers
Counseling & Testing: Thurs. 9:00 A.M. to 3:00 P.M.

Montgomery County

Community Services

Montgomery County Health Department
1606 Haynes
Clarksville, TN 37043-4544
Telephone: (615)-648-5758
Contact: Leslie Dupliessis
Counseling & Testing: M-W-T-F, 8:00 A.M. to 3:30 P.M.

Robertson County

County Health Depts

Robertson County Health Department
800 Brown Street
Springfield, TN 37172
Telephone: (615)-384-4504
Contact: Susan Orman
Counseling & Testing: Mon-Fri 8:30am-4pm

Rutherford County

County Health Depts

Rutherford County Health Department
303 North Church
PO Box 576
Murfreesboro, TN 37133-0573
Telephone: (615)-898-7880
Contact: Bob Moore
Counseling & Testing: Monday through Friday, 8:00 A.M. to 3:00 P.M.

Shelby County

County Health Depts

Memphis/Shelby County Health Department
814 Jefferson
Memphis, TN 38105-5099
Telephone: (901)-576-7600 Fax: (904)-576-7832
Contact: Delois Bolden - Regional AIDS Program Dir
AIDS Testing, Counseling & Services

Home Health Care

Caremark Connection Network
1680 Century Center Pky
Suite #12
Memphis, TN 38134-8849
Telephone: (901)-386-3738 Fax: (901)-388-3992
Contact: Robin Ward - Branch Manager
Clinical Support and Infusion Therapies: Nutrition, Antimicrobials, Chemo.,Hematopoe

Medical Services

Adult Speciality Care Clinic
Regional Med. Cntr. Rm408
42 North Dunlap
Memphis, TN 38103
Telephone: (901)-575-7446 Fax: (901)-575-7446
HIV counseling & treatment

Stewart County

County Health Depts

Stewart County Health Department
1021 Spring Street
PO Box 497
Dover, TN 37058
Telephone: (615)-232-5329
Contact: Donna Parchman - RN
Counseling & Testing: Mon-Fri 8:30am-4pm

Sullivan County

County Health Depts

Sullivan County Health Department
1324 Midland Drive
Kingsport, TN 37664-3099
Telephone: (615)-245-5165
Contact: Bill Devault - Director
Counseling & Testing

Sullivan County Health Department
29 Midway Street
Bristol, TN 37620-1705
Telephone: (615)-968-2511
Contact: Bill Devault - Director
Counseling & Testing: Tues & Fri 9-11:30am

Testing Sites

Sullivan County Regional Health Office
3193 Highway 126
Blountville, TN 37617-0630
Telephone: (615)-323-7131
Contact: Gloria Lewis - AIDS Region Program Dir
HIV testing & counseling

Sumner County

County Health Depts

Sumner County Health Department
411 South Water Street
Gallatin, TN 37066-3310
Telephone: (615)-452-4811
Contact: Jerry Kopce
Counseling & Testing: Mon, Tues, & Thurs 9am-5pm, referrals

Trousdale County

County Health Depts

Trousdale County Health Department
Damascus Avenue
Hartsville, TN 37074-1499
Telephone: (615)-374-2112
Contact: Velma Cathcart
Counseling & Testing: Mon-Fri 8:30am-4pm

Washington County

Home Health Care

Caremark Connection Network
1904 Lark Street
Suite 2
Johnson City, TN 37604-1724
Telephone: (615)-282-1406
Contact: Terry Billingsby - Branch Manager
Clinical Support and Infusion Therapies: Nutrition, Antimicrobials, Chemo.,Hematopoeti

Williamson County

County Health Depts

Williamson County Health Department
1324 West Main
Franklin, TN 37064-3789
Telephone: (615)-794-1542
Contact: Jerry Lewis
Counseling & Testing: Mon-Fri, 8:00 A.M. to 3:30 P.M.

Wilson County

County Health Depts

Wilson County Health Department
400 East Spring Street
Lebanon, TN 37087-3637
Telephone: (615)-444-5325
Contact: Carol Hall
Counseling & Testing: Mon & Fri 8am-Noon

TEXAS

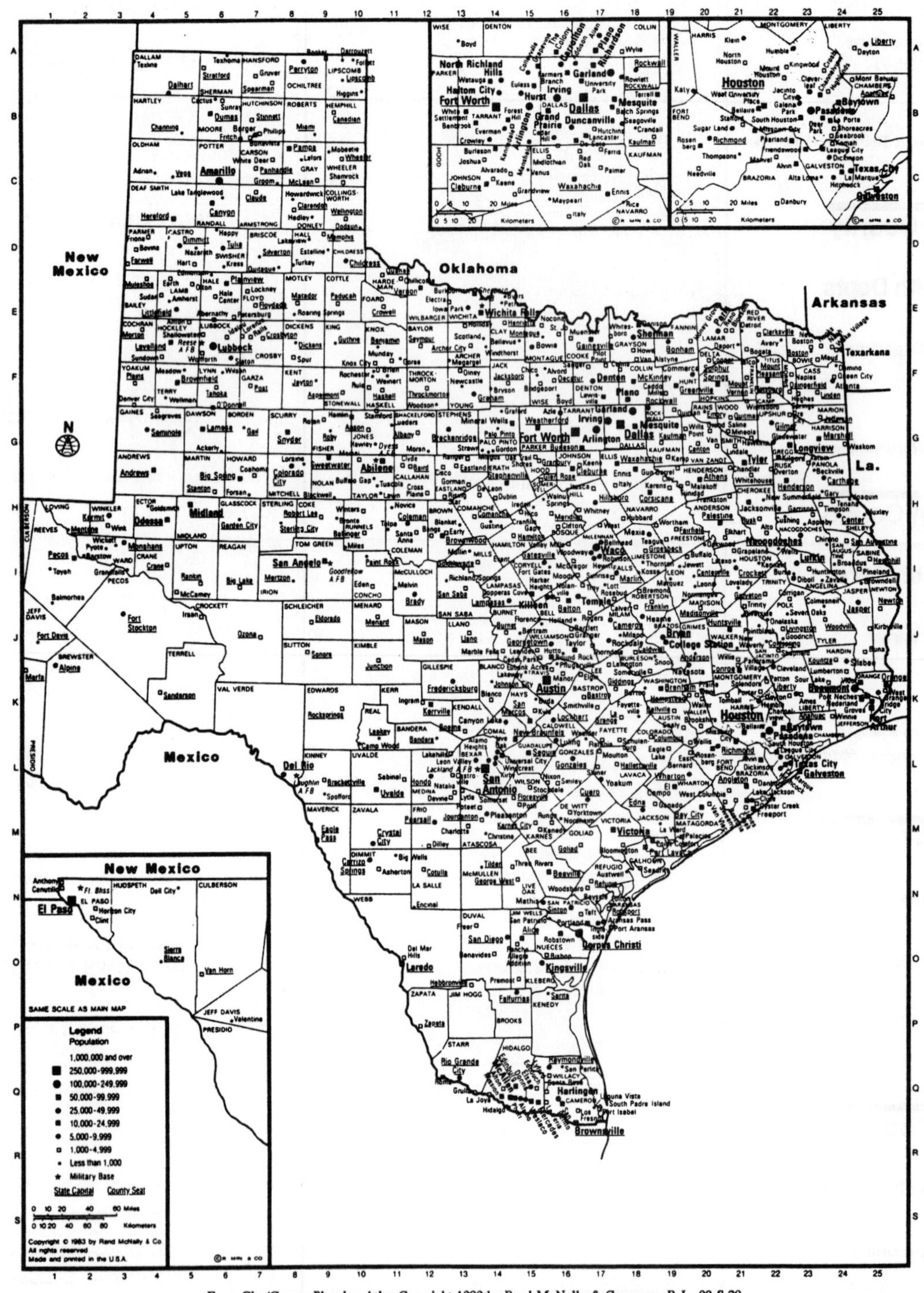

From City/County Planning Atlas Copyright 1989 by Reed McNally & Company, R.L. 90-S-28

Texas

General Services

Education

American Red Cross
2511 North Laurent Street
Victoria, TX 77901
Telephone: (512)-573-2671
Contact: Beverly Hall
AIDS information, education, referral, instruction

American Red Cross
136 Grand Avenue
P.O. Box 593
Paris, TX 75460-5817
Telephone: (214)-784-4690
Contact: Donna Rounsaville
AIDS education.

American Red Cross - Collin County Chapter
1450 Redbud Blvd.
McKinney, TX 75069
Telephone: (214)-422-4282
Contact: Cynthia Walters - Executive Director
In-school education programs, workplace programs, lectures, information.

American Red Cross - Concho Valley Chapter
P.S.C Box 7379
Goodfellow AFB
San Angelo, TX 76908
Telephone: (915)-653-5907
Contact: Roland A. Born
AIDS Education

American Red Cross - Smith County Chapter
P.O. Box 8588
Tyler, TX 75711-8588
Telephone: (214)-581-7981
AIDS educational materials.

American Red Cross - Tarrant County Chapter
1515 S. Sylvania Avenue
Fort Worth, TX 76111-1057
Telephone: (817)-335-9137
Contact: Barbara Paul
Information, referral, programs for general public, workplace andadolescents

American Red Cross, Centex Chapter
2218 Pershing Drive
Austin, TX 78723-5849
Telephone: (512)-928-4271
Contact: Lauri Montgomery
Public and community education programs

American Red Cross-Brazoria County Chapter
135 Hospital Drive
Angleton, TX 77515-4449
Telephone: (409)-869-6439
Contact: Toni Hodges - Director
AIDS education

Baylor Teen Clinic
5656 Kelley Parkway
Houston, TX 77026
Telephone: (713)-636-5612
Contact: Teresa Johnson
AIDS education andfamily planning services

Family Planning
306 East Wallace Street
P.O. Box 846
San Saba, TX 76877-4623
Telephone: (915)-372-5781
Contact: Tama Shaw
AIDS education and risk assessment, Texas Dept. of Health pamphlets andvideos

Hill Country Community Action Association, Inc.
133 North Main Street
P.O. Box 735
Rockdale, TX 76567-0735
Telephone: (512)-446-6112
Contact: Wilmer Green
AIDS education and risk assessment.

Hill Country Community Action Association, Inc.
411 East 1st Street
P.O. Box 603
Cameron, TX 76520-0603
Telephone: (817)-697-3101
Contact: Shirley Young
AIDS education and risk assessment

Hill Country Community Action Association, Inc.
122 Rose Street
P.O. Box 45
Marlin, TX 76661-3053
Telephone: (817)-883-6601
Contact: Louise Welch
AIDS education and risk assessment.

Hill Country Community Action Association, Inc.
409 S. Hill
P.O. Box 867
Meridian, TX 76665-0867
Telephone: (817)-435-2911
Contact: Jan James
AIDS education and risk assessment.

Pan American University
1201 West University Dr.
Edinburg, TX 78539-2999
Telephone: (512)-381-2511
Contact: Erik Svenkervd
Education for individuals and groups, counseling, public speaking

Planned Parenthood Association of Cameron/Willacy Counties
370 Old Port Isabel Road
Brownsville, TX 78521-3547
Telephone: (210)-546-4574 Fax: (210)-544-1292
Contact: Terry Oliver
HIV education, referrals

Planned Parenthood of Austin
1209 Rosewood
Austin, TX 78702
Telephone: (512)-472-0868 Fax: (512)-472-8824
Contact: Fiona Rose
AIDS education and community speaking

Project Reach - Houston Tillotson College
900 Chion
Austin, TX 78702-2762
Telephone: (512)-474-5219
Contact: Gloria Black; Roselee Windgate -
Education and training, speaker's bureau, assistance with school curriculum

Paul Quinn College
3837 Simpson Stuart Road
Dallas, TX 75241
Telephone: (817)-753-6415
Contact: Van S. Allen
AIDS information and education.

Rural Area Eight County Family
P.O. Box 748
415 South Mitchell
San Marcos, TX 78666
Telephone: (512)-392-1161
Contact: Adell Hurst
Community and school education; public speaking.

State Health Departments

Texas Department of Health, HIV Prevention Section
1100 West 49th Street
Austin, TX 78756-3199
Telephone: (512)-458-7400
Contact: Sylvia Watson - Director

Statewide Services

Lynn King - Social Security Region VI
1200 Main Tower
Room 1540
Dallas, TX 75202
Telephone: (214)-767-1348 Fax: (800)-772-1213
Contact: Lynn King - Coordinator

Texas Education Agency
1701 North Congress
Austin, TX 78701-1494
Telephone: (512)-463-9501
Contact: Maryann Ricketson
AIDS education to school district

Texas Rehabilitation Commission
Disability Determination
P.O. Box 2913
Austin, TX 78769
Telephone: (512)-445-8681
Contact: Dennis Neitsch
Medical determinations on Social Security disability claims

Andrews County

County Health Depts

Andrews City County Health Department
County Courthouse #117
2111 Northwest 1st Street
Andrews, TX 79714
Telephone: (915)-524-1434
Contact: Deb McCullough - B.S.N., F.N.P., M.Ed.
HIV testing site& and counseling

Angelina County

County Health Depts

Angelina County and City Health District
202 South Bynum
Lufkin, TX 75901-3750
Telephone: (409)-632-1139
Contact: Michael Lockhart
HIV testing and counseling; AIDS education, primary care

Austin County

Testing Sites

Texas Department of Health - PHR 6 - Field Office
P.O. Box 309
Bellville, TX 77418
Telephone: (409)-865-5211
Contact: Holly Wise - R.N.
HIV testing site

Bailey County

Testing Sites

Texas Department of Health, PHR 1 - Field Office
118 West Ave C
Muleshoe, TX 79347
Telephone: (806)-272-5561
Contact: Judy Jacobs
HIV testing and counseling

Bastrop County

County Health Depts

Bastrop Family Planning
1002 Chesnut Street
P.O. Box 718
Bastrop, TX 78602
Telephone: (512)-321-5539
Contact: Peggy Morales
HIV counseling and testing site.

Testing Sites

Texas Department of Health - Field Office Region 7
104 Loop 150 West
Suite 102
Bastrop, TX 78602
Telephone: (512)-321-3982
Contact: Mary Ryan
HIV testing site, TB testing

Bell County

County Health Depts

Bell County Health Department
509 South 9th Street
Temple, TX 76504
Telephone: (817)-778-4766
Contact: Linda Boggs
Testing, counseling.

Bell County health Department
119 West Avenue D
P.O. Box 306
Killeen, TX 76540
Telephone: (817)-526-8371
Contact: B. Mark
HIV counseling and testing site.

Testing Sites

Texas Department of Health, PHR 7 - Field Office
2408 S. 37th Street
Temple, TX 76504-7168
Telephone: (817)-778-6744
AIDS education, information, consultation, HIV testing, referral services

Bexar County

Home Health Care

Caremark Connection Network
12000 Network Blvd.
Suite 200
San Antonio, TX 78249
Telephone: (210)-618-5550 Fax: (210)-690-8036
Contact: Cathy Jurzek - Pharmacy Manager
Clinical Support and Infusion Therapies: Nutrition, Antimicrobials, Chemo.,Hematopoe

nmc HOMECARE
12500 Network, Suite 307
San Antonio, TX 78249
Telephone: (210)-561-8800
Fax: (210)-561-8817
Contact: Bret Barnett
National JCAHO-Accredited company providing a full range of Infusion and Respiratory therapies and specializing in the care of HIV/AIDS patients. National Case Manager is also available at 800-445-1188

Medical Services

South Texas Children's AIDS Center-UTHSCSA
Department of Pediatrics
7703 Floyd Curl
San Antonio, TX 78284-7818
Telephone: (210)-692-3641 Fax: (210)-615-0658
Contact: James A. Moa - Executive Director, John Mangos, MD -
Diagnostic, treatment, medical, social, dental, psychological, and nutrition.

University of Texas Health Science Center at San Antonio
7703 Floyd Curl Drive
San Antonio, TX 78284-0001
Telephone: (210)-567-7000
Contact: P. Kay Sharky - Director HIV clinic; John Graybill - Cheif of Staff
Medical care to AIDS patients with a malignant disease such as cancer. HIVinpatient & outpatient clinic.

Testing Sites

South Texas Comprehensive Hemophilia Center
Santa Rosa Medical Ctr.
519 W. Houston
San Antonio, TX 78207
Telephone: (512)-228-2191
Testing, counseling and medical services

Texas Department of Health - PHR 6
San Antonio Chest Hosp.
PO Box 23340
San Antonio, TX 78223
Telephone: (210)-534-8857
Contact: Mary M. Martinez
Coordinates activities between Texas Department of Health and local agencies.

Bosque County

Testing Sites

Texas Department of Health, PHR 7 - Field Office
409 South Hill Street
Meridian, TX 76665
Telephone: (817)-675-6122
HIV testing site

Texas Department of Health, Region- Field Office
409 South Hill
Meridian, TX 76665
Telephone: (817)-435-6331
Contact: Martha Payne - R.N.
HIV testing site

Bowie County

Home Health Care

Hospice of Texarkana
803 Spruce Street
Texarkana, TX 75501
Telephone: (903)-794-4263 Fax: (501)-774-1108
Skilled nursing, home health aide, volunteers, social worker.

Brazoria County

County Health Depts

Brazoria County Health Department
432 East Mulberry
Angelton, TX 77515
Telephone: (409)-849-5711
Contact: Gertrude Wright
HIV counseling and testing site.

Home Health Care

Visiting Nurses Association of Brazoria County
201 East Mulberry St
Angleton, TX 77515-4700
Telephone: (409)-849-6476
Skilled nurse; physical, occupational, speech therapy; home health aide

Testing Sites

University of Texas Medical Branch Family Planning
ACHE Clinic
1111 West Adove
Alvin, TX 77511
Telephone: (713)-331-6101
HIV counseling and testing site.

Brazos County

Community Services

Brazos Valley Community Action
111 Main Street
Bryan, TX 77802
Telephone: (409)-260-1386
Contact: Tonya Canattella
AIDS counseling and education

Brazos Valley Community Action Agency
P.O. Box 2730
Bryan, TX 77805
Telephone: (409)-690-2437
Educational services, case management, psychological, Counseling

County Health Depts

Brazos County Health Department
201 North Texas Avenue
First Floor
Bryan, TX 77803-5317
Telephone: (409)-361-4440
Contact: Ursula Idlebird
HIV testing and counseling, education, information

Brewster County

Testing Sites

Texas Department of Health, PHR 9-10 Field Office
205 N. Cockrell St
Alpine, TX 79830-5003
Telephone: (915)-837-3877
Contact: Drunne Mills
HIV testing

Brown County

County Health Depts

Brownwood County Health Department
510 East Leaf
Brownwood, TX 76801
Telephone: (915)-646-1514
Contact: Tanya Boyd
HIV counseling and testing site.

Burleson County

Testing Sites

Texas Department of Health, PHR 1 - Field Office
365 W. Buck Street
Caldwell, TX 77836-0969
Telephone: (409)-567-4539
Contact: Margaret Turnn
HIV testing

Caldwell County

Testing Sites

Texas Department of Health - PHR 1 - Field Office
505 East Fannin St
Luling, TX 78648-2325
Telephone: (210)-875-2609
Contact: Monte Frederick, RN
HIV testing

Cameron County

County Health Depts

Cameron County Health Department
1150 East Madison St
Brownsville, TX 78520-5854
Telephone: (210)-548-9550
Contact: Elma Abrego; Maria Santos San Pedro -
HIV testing and counseling

Cameron County Health Department
100 Hockaday Drive
Port Isabel, TX 78578-2409
Telephone: (210)-943-1300
Contact: Irma Hockaday
HIV testing site

Chambers County

County Health Depts

Chambers County Health Department
P.O. Box 670
Anahuac, TX 77514-0670
Telephone: (409)-267-6679
Contact: Glenda Pearce - R.N., B.S.
HIV testing site

Childress County

Testing Sites

Texas Department of Health - PHR 2 - Field Office
801 Commerce
Childress, TX 79201
Telephone: (817)-937-8225
HIV counseling/testing

Cochran County

Testing Sites

Texas Department of Health, PHR 2 - Field Office
220 West Washington
Morton, TX 79346
Telephone: (806)-266-8813
HIV testing

Collingsworth County

Testing Sites

Texas Department of Health - PHR 2 - Field Office
Collingsworth Courthouse
Wellington, TX 79095
Telephone: (806)-447-2358
Contact: Fraya Hammons
HIV testing, counseling

Colorado County

Testing Sites

Texas Department of Health, PHR 4 - Field Office
514 Washington St.
Columbus, TX 78934
Telephone: (409)-732-3662
Contact: Bernice Richter
HIV testing site

Comal County

Home Health Care

Hospice New Braunfels
613 North Walnut
New Braunfels, TX 78130-5050
Telephone: (512)-625-7500
Contact: Katie Gordon
Support group for HIV +

Coryell County

Testing Sites

Texas Department of Health, PHR 1 - Field Office
1216 Phil Street
Copperas Cove, TX 76522-2330
Telephone: (817)-547-8383
Contact: Connie Patterson
HIV testing

Crockett County

Testing Sites

Texas Department of Health - PHR 3 - Field Office
701 Nineth Street
Ozona, TX 76943
Telephone: (915)-392-2996
Contact: Karen K. Huffman
HIV testing site

Crosby County

Testing Sites

Texas Department of Health - PHR 2 - Field Office
711 Main Street
Ralls, TX 79357
Telephone: (806)-253-2502
Contact: Bettye King
HIV testing site

Culberson County

Testing Sites

Texas Department of Health - PHR 3 - Field Office
704 W. Broadway Ave.
Van Horn, TX 79855-9999
Telephone: (915)-283-2948
Contact: Rose Guevara
HIV testing site

Dallam County

Testing Sites

Texas Department of Health - PHR 2 - Field Office
407 Denver
Dalhart, TX 79022
Telephone: (806)-249-6090
HIV counseling/testing

Dallas County

Community Services

AIDS Interfaith Network
1005 West Jefferson
Suite 30
Dallas, TX 75208
Telephone: (214)-941-7697 Fax: (214)-941-7739
Contact: Michael Konow
Counseling, respite care, and spiritual support services, education,referrals

Dallas Urban League, Inc.
3625 North Hall Street
Suite # 700
Dallas, TX 75219-5118
Telephone: (214)-528-8038 Fax: (214)-443-7663
Contact: Shirley Walker
AIDS education and outreach; presentations, seminars, and workshops

Home Health Care

Caremark, Inc.
7805 Mesquite Bend Blvd.
Irvington, TX 75063
Telephone: (817)-924-1177
Contact: Zee Robb - Director
Clinical Support and Infusion Therapies: Nutrition, Antibiotics, Chemo.,Hematopoe

Curaflex Infusion Services
701 East Plano Parkway
Suite 305
Dallas, TX 75247-4548
Telephone: (214)-424-7060 Fax: (214)-424-8329
Contact: John Harkins - General Manager
Home IV therapy: TPN, Enteral, IV Antibiotics, Aerosolized/IV Pentamidine

Hospice Care Incorporation of Dallas
5001 L.B.J. Parkway
Suite #1050
Dallas, TX 75244
Telephone: (214)-661-2004 Fax: (214)-661-3474
Patient with prognosis of 6 months or less to live

Medical Services

ARMS Clinic
1935 Motor Street
Childrens Medical Center
Dallas, TX 75235
Telephone: (214)-640-2776
Contact: Mary Mallory
Children at risk and babies born to HIV infected mothers.

Greater Dallas Maternal Health and Family Planning Program
UT/SW Medical Center
2330 Butler #103
Dallas, TX 75235
Telephone: (214)-905-2100 Fax: (214)-688-5217
Contact: Emily West
HIV risk assessment for family planning client

Nexus
8733 La Prada Drive
Dallas, TX 75228-5097
Telephone: (214)-321-0156
Contact: Beca Crowell
Residential treatment for chemically dependent women. Counseling, education

Testing Sites

DARCO Drug Services, Inc.
2608 Inwood Road
Dallas, TX 75235
Telephone: (214)-956-7181 Fax: (214)-956-9257
Contact: Joyce Walters
Outpatient drug maintenance; counseling, HIV testing & counseling

Planned Parenthood of Dallas
Red Bird Clinic
4343 W.Camp Wisdom Rd 213
Dallas, TX 75237
Telephone: (214)-709-0081
Contact: Mary Ann Turmer
HIV counseling and testing site.

De Witt County

Community Services

Cuero-DeWitt County Health Department
106 North Gonzales Street
Cuero, TX 77954
Telephone: (512)-275-3461
Contact: Carol Badee
Counseling & testing

Deaf Smith County

Testing Sites

Texas Department of Health - PHR 2 - Field Office
206 West 4th
Suite B
Hereford, TX 79045
Telephone: (806)-364-2401
HIV counseling/testing

Dickens County

Testing Sites

Texas Department of Health - PHR 2 - Field Office
224-B West Harris
Spur, TX 79370-2328
Telephone: (806)-271-3450
HIV testing site

Ector County

Medical Services

Planned Parenthood of West Texas, Inc.
910-B South Grant
Odessa, TX 79762
Telephone: (915)-332-8258
Contact: Carla Holeva
Counseling on all methods of birth control, safer sex practices, HIV testing.

El Paso County

Community Services

Texas Rehabilitation Commission
6585 Montana, Bldg. R
Suite 600
El Paso, TX 79925
Telephone: (915)-778-7714 Fax: (915)-778-2758
Counseling and guidance, job placement, training

County Health Depts

Centro de Salud Familiar La Fe, Inc.
700 South Ochoa Street
P.O. Box 10640
El Passo, TX 79901
Telephone: (915)-545-4550

HIV counseling, testing & case management for residents of El Paso county

Falls County

Testing Sites

Texas Department of Health - PHR 1 - Field Office
2408 South 37th Street
Marlin, TX 76661
Telephone: (817)-883-9206
Contact: Melanie Lockwood
HIV testing site

Fort Bend County

County Health Depts

Fort Bend County Health Department
P.O. Box 668
Rosenberg, TX 77471
Telephone: (713)-342-6414
HIV testing site

Frio County

Testing Sites

Texas Department of Health - PHR 6 - Field Office
402 South Pecan St
Pearsall, TX 78061-3136
Telephone: (210)-334-4104
Contact: Lucresia Vinton, RN - HIV Counselor
HIV testing site, counseling & referrals

Galveston County

Testing Sites

Planned Parenthood of Houston & Southeast Texas
Galveston County Clinic
3315 Gulf Freeway
Dickinson, TX 77539
Telephone: (713)-337-4618
Contact: Denny Selby
HIV counseling and testing site.

Garza County

Testing Sites

Texas Department of Health - PHR 2 - Field Office
Dept. of Human Res. Bldg.
Snyder Highway
Post, TX 79356
Telephone: (806)-495-3996
Contact: Shirley LeBlanc - Advanced Nurse Pratictioner
HIV testing site; counseling & referrals

Gray County

Testing Sites

Texas Department of Health - PHR 2 - Field Office
400 W. Kings Mill
Suite 100, Hughes Bldg
Pampa, TX 79065
Telephone: (806)-665-0746
Contact: Carol Hall RN - HIV Coordinator
HIV counseling and testing; referrals

Gregg County

Home Health Care

Hospice Longview, Inc.
802 Medical Circle
Longview, TX 75601
Telephone: (214)-753-7870
Contact: Mildred Brown - Director
Medical services, nursing care, social services, home health aide services.

Grimes County

Testing Sites

Texas Department of Health - PHR 1 - Field Office
202 South Judson
Navasota, TX 77868
Telephone: (409)-825-7476
Contact: Susan Wright - R.N.
HIV testing site

Hale County

County Health Depts

Plainview-Hale County Health District
1001 Ash Street
Plainview, TX 79072-7331
Telephone: (806)-293-1359
Contact: Esther Banks - RN
HIV testing site, pre and post counseling

Hall County

Testing Sites

Texas Department of Health - PHR 2 - Field Office
Hall County Hospital
1800 N. Boykin
Memphis, TX 79245
Telephone: (806)-259-3747
Contact: Rita Anderson
HIV testing site

Hansford County

Testing Sites

Texas Department of Health, PHR 2 - Field Office
720 S Archer
Spearman, TX 79081
Telephone: (806)-659-3996
Contact: Joan McClellan - RN
HIV testing, counseling, follow-up for HIV positive patients; referrals

Harris County

Community Services

AIDS Foundation Houston
3202 Weslayan Annex
Houston, TX 77027
Telephone: (713)-623-6796 Fax: (713)-623-4029
Social services and education

Casa de Esperanza
P.O. Box 66581
Houston, TX 77006-6581
Telephone: (713)-529-0639 Fax: (713)-529-9079
Contact: Sister Kathy
Parent and family services for families with HIV, counseling for parentswith children in their care

United Way of the Texas Gulf Coast
2200 North Loop West
Houston, TX 77018
Telephone: (713)-685-2300 Fax: (713)-956-2868
Contact: Judith Craven - Director
Non-profit organization

County Health Depts

Harris County Health Department
2501 Dunstan Street
Houston, TX 77005
Telephone: (713)-526-1841
Contact: Neoma Harris
Information and referrals, disease reporting, HIV testing, and educationalprograms

Harris County Health Department
Humble Health Center
1730 Humble Place Drive
Humble, TX 77396
Telephone: (713)-441-4664
Contact: Letcia Vallejo - HIV Counselor
HIV counseling and testing site.

Harris County Health Department
1000 Lee Drive
Baytown, TX 77520
Telephone: (713)-427-5195
Contact: Sally Statler
HIV counseling and testing site.

Home Health Care

HealthCare Planners, Inc.
P.O. Box 300247
Houston, TX 77230-0247
Telephone: (713)-741-0355 Fax: (713)-741-0357
Contact: Paul Pendleton; Mary Arnold -

Skilled nursing, PT, OT, ST, MSW, RT, private duty, home health aides

New Age Hospice
1905 Holcomb Blvd.
Houston, TX 77030-4123
Telephone: (713)-467-7423 Fax: (713)-799-9227
Contact: Lars Egede Nissen - Executive Director
Hospice home care, inpatient unit, and bereavement services

nmc HOMECARE
9315 Kirby Drive
Houston, TX 77054
Telephone: (713)-795-4343
Fax: (713)-795-0711
Contact: Dorothy Christman
National JCAHO-Accredited company providing a full range of Infusion and Respiratory therapies and specializing in the care of HIV/AIDS patients. National Case Manager is also available at 800-445-1188

Nursefinders of Houston I
41001 Westheimer Road
Suite 113
Houston, TX 77027
Telephone: (713)-961-1001 Fax: (713)-961-7736
Contact: Cheryl Duke
Licensed home health agency

Omega House, Inc.
602 Branard Raod
Houston, TX 77006-2714
Telephone: (713)-523-1139 Fax: (713)-526-8144
Contact: Margot Morris - Director
AIDS hospice for terminally ill patients

Visiting Nurse Association of Houston
2905 Sackett Street
Houston, TX 77098
Telephone: (713)-520-8115
Toll-Free: (800)-375-6877
Home hospice, home health care, and medical equipment

Medical Services

Bering Dental Clinic
1440 Harold St
Houston, TX 77006-3798
Telephone: (713)-524-7933 Fax: (713)-524-7995
Contact: Dr. Mark Nichol
Dental clinic for HIV/AIDS persons, by emergency or appoin

Bering Dental Clinic
1440 Harold Street
Houston, TX 77006-3798
Telephone: (713)-524-7933 Fax: (713)-524-7995
Contact: Michael Collins
Dental clinic for HIV/AIDS persons, by emergency or appointment

Casa, A Special Hospital
1803 Old Spanish Trail
Houston, TX 77054-2001
Telephone: (713)-796-2272 Fax: (713)-790-1865
Contact: Gretchen Thorp
In-patient facility, home health, outpatient treatment

Neighborhood Centers Inc.
720 Fairmont Parkway
Pasadena, TX 77504
Telephone: (713)-944-9186 Fax: (713)-944-6128
Contact: Lee Medina
AIDS education primarily in the minority community. Individual or group.

Park Plaza Hospital - AMI
1313 Hermann Drive
Houston, TX 77004-7092
Telephone: (713)-527-5000
Contact: Bobby King
Counseling, psychosocial support groups, referrals for home care, physicianreferrals

Texas Childrens Hospital Project Share
Baylor College of Medicine, Department of Pediatrics
One Baylor Plaza
Houston, TX 77030
Telephone: (713)-770-3440 Fax: (713)-770-2045
Contact: Susan Hirtzhacko - Coordinator
Region VI

Thomas Street Clinic
2015 Thomas Street
Houston, TX 77009
Telephone: (713)-546-5733
Contact: Marlene Jones - Manager
Full service clinic, social service, physical therapy

University of Houston College of Optometry
4901 Calhoun Road
Houston, TX 77204
Telephone: (713)-743-1917 Fax: (713)-743-2053
Contact: Ralph Herring - O.D.
Vision and eye care for persons with AIDS and ARC

Testing Sites

ACT Health Services
Fannin Medical Plaza
7505 Fannin, Suite 212
Houston, TX 77054
Telephone: (713)-795-4590
HIV testing, counseling

Texas Department of Health - PHR 6
10500 Forum Place Drive
Suite 123
Houston, TX 77036-8599
Telephone: (713)-995-1112
Contact: Judy Spong
Public information, teacher inservices, testing, counseling

Veteran's Administration Medical Center
2002 Holcombe
Houston, TX 77030
Telephone: (713)-791-1414 Fax: (713)-794-7806
HIV testing, medications and treatment for ARC, AIDS; AZT program

Hidalgo County

County Health Depts

Hidalgo County Health Department
1304 South 25th
Edinburg, TX 78539-7205
Telephone: (210)-383-6221
Contact: Lyva Sema - RN
HIV testing, pre/post counseling, and public speaking

Hidalgo County Health Department Field Office
300 East Hackberry
McAllen, TX 78501-9220
Telephone: (210)-682-6155
Contact: Helen Schmidt - RN
HIV testing, counseling, medical services

Medical Services

Tropical Texas MHMR
1409 South 9th Street
P.O. Box 1108
Edinburg, TX 78540
Telephone: (210)-383-0121
Contact: Olga LePere
Substance abuse HIV postive

Howard County

Testing Sites

Texas Department of Health
201 Lancaster
Big Spring, TX 79720
Telephone: (915)-263-7261
Contact: Linda Norman - RNC
Medical services, HIV testing and counseling

Hutchinson County

Testing Sites

Texas Department of Health - PHR 2 - Field Office
600 South Cedar
Borger, TX 79007-4656
Telephone: (806)-274-5213
HIV testing and counseling

Jackson County

County Health Depts

Jackson County Health Department
411 N. Wells
Edna, TX 77957-2734
Telephone: (512)-782-5221
Contact: Lisa Larkin - RNC
Health care, HIV testing and counseling

Jasper County

Medical Services

Deep East Texas Regional Health Center
Rt. 2 Box 317
Jasper, TX 75951
Telephone: (409)-384-6839
Contact: Suzanne Woods - Director

Jeff Davis County

Testing Sites

Texas Department of Health - PHR 3 - Field Office
101 Court Street
P.O. Box 824
Fort Davis, TX 79734
Telephone: (915)-426-3551
Health services, HIV testing and counseling, womens infant and childrenprogram

Jefferson County

Community Services

Triangle AIDS Network
P.O. Box 12279
Beaumont, TX 77726
Telephone: (409)-832-8338
Contact: Sheridan Tutl - Director
Support groups, respite care, education, speakers bureau, case management,legal, rent & utility assistance transportation for AIDSpatients, foodpantry, nutritional & dental care, home health care

Kerr County

Home Health Care

Heart of the Hills Hospice
P.O. Box 950
Kerrville, TX 78029-0950
Telephone: (512)-896-7770
Home nursing services, counseling, equipment, medication, personal care

Lubbock County

Community Services

South Plains AIDS Resource Center (SPARC)
4204 B 50th Street
Hotline: 806-792-7783
Lubbock, TX 79413
Telephone: (800)-288-9058
Contact: David Crader
HIV testing (confidential), food & financial support, shelter

Home Health Care

Hospice of Lubbock, Inc.
P.O. Box 53276
Lubbock, TX 79453-3276
Telephone: (806)-795-2751 Fax: (806)-795-8468
Toll-Free: (800)-658-2648
Contact: Lee Battey
Hospice care to the terminally ill, PWA's/families, bereavement support

Matagorda County

Medical Services

Matagorda County General Hospital District
1115 Avenue G
Bay City, TX 77414-3544
Telephone: (409)-245-6383
Contact: Nancy Godsui
Primary care, HIV testing, referrals, home care

Mc Lennan County

Community Services

Planned Parenthood of Central Texas
1121 Ross
P.O. Box 1518
Waco, TX 76703-1755
Telephone: (817)-752-8301 Fax: (817)-752-4707
Contact: Sue Havens Drake
HIV/STD testing

Home Health Care

Community Hospice of Waco - HBMC
P.O. Box 5100
Waco, TX 76708-0100
Telephone: (817)-756-8649
Nursing, personal care, social work, chaplain, therapy, terminal care.

Testing Sites

Waco-McLennan County Public Health District
225 West Waco Drive
Waco, TX 76707
Telephone: (817)-750-5450 Fax: (817)-750-5663
Toll-Free: (800)-756-2437
Contact: Joyce Nelson - AIDS Director
AIDS testing anonymous, case management, disease intervention, Ryan Whitefund, educational services, coordination with school nursing, volunteers,support groups

Milam County

County Health Depts

Milam County Health Department
209 South Houston Street
P.O. Box 469
Cameron, TX 76520
Telephone: (817)-697-3411
HIV testing, well child clinic

Nueces County

Home Health Care

nmc HOMECARE
4639 Corona Dr. #55
Corpus Christi, TX 78411
Telephone: (512)-854-1414
Fax: (512)-854-0907
Contact: Robert Humphrey

National JCAHO-Accredited company providing a full range of Infusion and Respiratory therapies and specializing in the care of HIV/AIDS patients. National Case Manager is also available at 800-445-1188

Spohn Home and Health Hospice
1300 3rd Street
Corpus Christi, TX 78404
Telephone: (512)-881-3159 Fax: (512)-888-7405
Hospice and in-home services

Orange County

Home Health Care

Southeast Texas Hospice
912 West Cherry
P.O. Box 2385
Orange, TX 77630-5017
Telephone: (409)-886-0622 Fax: (409)-886-0623
Home health with volunteers, clergy, and physician.

Randall County

Community Services

Metropolitan Community Church
2123 S. Polk Street
Amarillo, TX 79109-2651
Telephone: (806)-372-4557
Contact: Reverend Bob Finch
Spiritual counseling, informational services, referrals

San Patricio County

Community Services

San Patricio County Health Department
401 San Angelo
Ingleside, TX 78362
Telephone: (512)-776-3591 Fax: (512)-364-4518
Contact: Edith Rollinson
HIV testing, counseling

San Saba County

Community Services

Hill Country Community Action Association, Inc./ Family Planning
2005 W. Wallace
P.O. Box 846
San Saba, TX 76877
Telephone: (915)-372-5781 Fax: (915)-372-3526
Contact: Frances Gamboa
AIDS education and risk assessment.

Smith County

Community Services

Community Assistance foir AIDS Relief (C.A.R.E.)
3006 Tower Drive
Tyler, TX 75701
Telephone: (903)-566-3539
Contact: Louise Caraway
Educational

East Texas Crisis Center, Inc.
3027 S. South Loop
Suite 23
Tyler, TX 75701
Telephone: (903)-595-3199 Fax: (903)-535-9117
Contact: Don Franks
HIV crisis referrals

Tarrant County

Community Services

Agape Metropolitan Community Church
4615 California Parkway
Fort Worth, TX 76119
Telephone: (817)-535-5002
Contact: Reverend Brenda Hunt
Pastoral counseling, some daily assistance, support groups

AIDS Outreach Center
1125 West Petersmith
Fort Worth, TX 76104-2183
Telephone: (817)-335-1994 Fax: (817)-335-3617
Toll-Free: (800)-836-0066
Contact: Thomas Bruner
Advocacy, financial assistance, nutrition center, counseling, legalservices; info-line, education

Home Health Care

Family Service Hospice
1424 Hemphill
Fort Worth, TX 76104-4790
Telephone: (817)-927-8884
Contact: Nancy Thurman
HIV nursing care, IV therapy, injections

HNS, Inc.
4108 Amon Carter Blvd
Suite #204
Ft. Worth, TX 76155
Telephone: (817)-267-1696 Fax: (817)-685-6063
Toll-Free: (800)-872-4467
Contact: Susan Radolf
Home Infusion Therapy, in-home nursing and attendant care, social workers, dietitians

Naurse House Calls
1200 Summit Avenue
Suite 620
Fort Worth, TX 76102-4462
Telephone: (817)-877-1777
Contact: Dixie Launius; Shirley Garrett -
Home health; private duty, RN's, LVN's and CHHA's

Nursefinders of Arlington
944 N. Cooper Street
Arlington, TX 76011-5778
Telephone: (817)-469-1058
Licensed home health agency

Nursefinders of Fort Worth
909 West Magnolia Avenue
Suite #6
Fort Worth, TX 76104-4594
Telephone: (817)-924-8331
Contact: Gay Kelly
Licensed home health agency and supplemental facility staffing service;in-services for HIV patients

Taylor County

County Health Depts

Abilene-Taylor County Health Department
P.O. Box 6489
2241 South 19th Street
Abilene, TX 79605-6489
Telephone: (915)-692-5600
Contact: Maria David, RN - HIV Coordinator
Health services, HIV testing and counseling

Testing Sites

Big Country AIDS Support Group
317 B Pecan
P.O. Box 6489
Abilene, TX 79608-6489
Telephone: (915)-676-7825
Contact: Maria David
HIV testing, pre and post test counseling, AIDS education

Terry County

Testing Sites

South Plains Public Health District
919 East Main Street
P.O. Box 112
Brownfield, TX 79316
Telephone: (806)-637-2164
Contact: Gloria McNabb
HIV counseling and testing site.

Tom Green County

County Health Depts

San Angelo-Tom Green County Health Department
P.O. Box 1751
2 City Hall Plaza
San Angelo, TX 76903
Telephone: (915)-657-4214
Contact: Jean Richey - R.N.
HIV testing site

Travis County

Community Services

AIDS Services of Austin, Inc. (ASA)
P.O. Box 4874
Austin, TX 78765-4874
Telephone: (512)-451-2273 Fax: (512)-452-3299
Contact: Janna Zumbrun - 512-459-DEAF (TDD)
Direct services, case management, pentamidine clinic

Allgo, Inc./Infornesida
P.O. Box 13501
Austin, TX 78711-3501
Telephone: (512)-472-2001 Fax: (512)-472-6301
Contact: Jose Orta
Bilingual information and referral, emergency medical fund for people ofcolor PWA'S

Social Security Administration
611 East 6th Street
Austin, TX 78701-3788
Telephone: (800)-234-5772
Contact: Josie Palacios
Assistance in applying for retirement/disability/survivor benefits

Waterloo Counseling Center
2525 Wallingwood Street
Suite 1500
Austin, TX 78746
Telephone: (051)-232-2963
Contact: Kieth Arrington - Director
Free individual, couple, and group counseling for AIDS, ARC, or HIV

County Health Depts

Austin-Travis County Health Department
15 Waller Street
Austin, TX 78702-5240
Telephone: (512)-469-2132
HIV testing, AIDS education, information, out-patient care, case management

Home Health Care

Caremark Connection Network
4200 Marathon
Ste. 200
Austin, TX 78756
Telephone: (512)-451-0877
Contact: Judi McNeel - General Manager; Mark Loescher - Director
Clinical Support and Infusion Therapies: nutrition, antimicrobials, chemo.,Hematopoti

Caremark Connection Network
4030 W Braker Lane
Suite 500
Austin, TX 78759-5329
Telephone: (512)-338-9600 Fax: (512)-338-0713
Contact: Judy McNeel - Sales Director, Kim Stelly - Pharmacy/Ops Manager
Clinical Support and Infusion Therapies: Nutrition, Antimicrobials, Chemo.,Hematopoeti

Curaflex Infusion Services
2201 Denton
Suite 100
Austin, TX 78758-1240
Telephone: (512)-250-3924
Contact: Sarah Harrington - Director
Home IV therapy: TPN, Enteral, IV Antibiotics, Aerosolized/IV Pentamidine,pain management, chemotherapy, antiviral/antinfectines

Hospice Austin
3710 Cedar Street
Suite 300
Austin, TX 78705
Telephone: (512)-458-3261
Contact: Peg O. McCuistion
Nursing, social service, spiritual care, therapy, volunteer support

Nursefinders of Austin
1500 West 38th, Suite 28
Austin, TX 78731-6395
Telephone: (512)-454-6777
Licensed home health care

Project Transitions
PO Box 4826
Suite 501
Austin, TX 78765-6926
Telephone: (512)-443-2555
Contact: Charlotte Hale - Director
Hospice services

Testing Sites

ALLGO/Informe SIDA
1715 East 6th Street
Austin, TX 78702
Telephone: (512)-472-2001
HIV counseling and testing site for the Hispanic population.

Peoples Community Clinic
2909 North IH 35
Austin, TX 78722
Telephone: (512)-478-8924
Contact: Sandy Welles
HIV counseling and testing site.

The C.A.R.E. Program
1631-B East 2nd Street
Austin, TX 78702
Telephone: (512)-473-2273 Fax: (512)-476-0217
Contact: Patricia Garrett - Unit Manager
HIV counseling and testing site for general public and IVDU's.

The University of Texas Student Health Center
105 West 26th Street
P.O. Box 7339
Austin, TX 78713
Telephone: (512)-471-4955 Fax: (512)-471-0898
Contact: Scott Spear
HIV counseling and testing site for University of Texas students.

Uvalde County

Medical Services

Uvalde County Clinic, Inc.
1009 Garnerfield Road
Uvalde, TX 78801
Telephone: (210)-278-7173 Fax: (210)-278-1836
Contact: Rachel A. Gonzales
HIV testing and counseling, primary health care.

Val Verde County

Testing Sites

Texas Department of Health - Region #8 Office
Del Rio-Val Verde Dept.
1401 Las Vegas Avenue
Del Rio, TX 78840-6112
Telephone: (210)-774-8673 Fax: (210)-774-8683
Contact: Judy Phinesmith - R.N.
Health services, HIV testing and counseling, referrals, education

Waller County

Testing Sites

Texas Department of Health - PHR 6 - Field Office
911 Otto Street
Brookshire, TX 77423
Telephone: (713)-934-8112
Contact: Dorothy Towns - R.N.
Health services, HIV testing and counseling

Texas Department of Health - PHR 6 - Field Office
911 Atto Street
Brookshire, TX 77423
Telephone: (713)-934-8112
Contact: Dorothy Towns - R.N.
Health services, HIV testing and counseling

Washington County

Testing Sites

Texas Department of Health - PHR 1 - Field Office
P.O. Box 2329
Brenham, TX 77834-7329
Telephone: (409)-836-1740
Contact: Bonnie Lokey
Health services, HIV testing and counseling

Texas Department of Health, Field Office - PHR 7
P.O. Box 2329
Brenham, TX 77834-7329
Telephone: (409)-836-1740
Contact: Bonnie Lokey
Health services, HIV testing and counseling

Webb County

County Health Depts

City of Laredo Health Department
2600 Cedar Street
P.O. Box 2337
Laredo, TX 78044-2337
Telephone: (210)-722-2437
Contact: Arturo Diaz
HIV testing, AIDS Hotline Information, AIDS Education/Awareness presentations

Wharton County

Testing Sites

Texas Department of Health - PHR 4 - Field Office - PHR 6
2407 North Richmond
Suite 1
Wharton, TX 77488-2403
Telephone: (409)-532-5336
Contact: Tamora Morris, RNC - Nurse Practitioner
Health services, HIV testing and counseling

Texas Department of Health, PHR 4 - Field Office - PHR 6
601 E. Calhoun St
El Campo, TX 77437-4613
Telephone: (409)-543-7414
Contact: Pat Korenek
Health services, HIV testing and counseling

Wheeler County

Testing Sites

Texas Department of Health - PHR 2 - Field Office
118 West 2nd Street
Shamrock, TX 79079
Telephone: (806)-256-2147
HIV counseling/testing

Wichita County

County Health Depts

Wichita Falls-Wichita County Health Department
1700 Third Street
Wichita Falls, TX 76301-2113
Telephone: (817)-761-7800
Contact: Edward Matelski
Health services, HIV testing and counseling

Home Health Care

Hospice of Wichita Falls, Inc.
4909 Johnson Road
P.O. Box 4804
Wichita Falls, TX 76310
Telephone: (817)-322-8268
Contact: Jan Banta
Hospice care.

Williamson County

Medical Services

Family Planning
109 West 3rd Street
Taylor, TX 76574-3516
Telephone: (512)-352-7697
Women's health services

Wilson County

County Health Depts

Wilson County Health Department
P.O. Box 276
Floresville, TX 78114-0276
Telephone: (210)-393-7350
Contact: Georgie A. Thies - R.N.
Health services, HIV testing and counseling

Wood County

County Health Depts

Wood County Health Department
P.O. Box 596
Quitman, TX 75783-0596
Telephone: (903)-763-5406
Contact: David Murley, M.D.
Information and referral.

UTAH

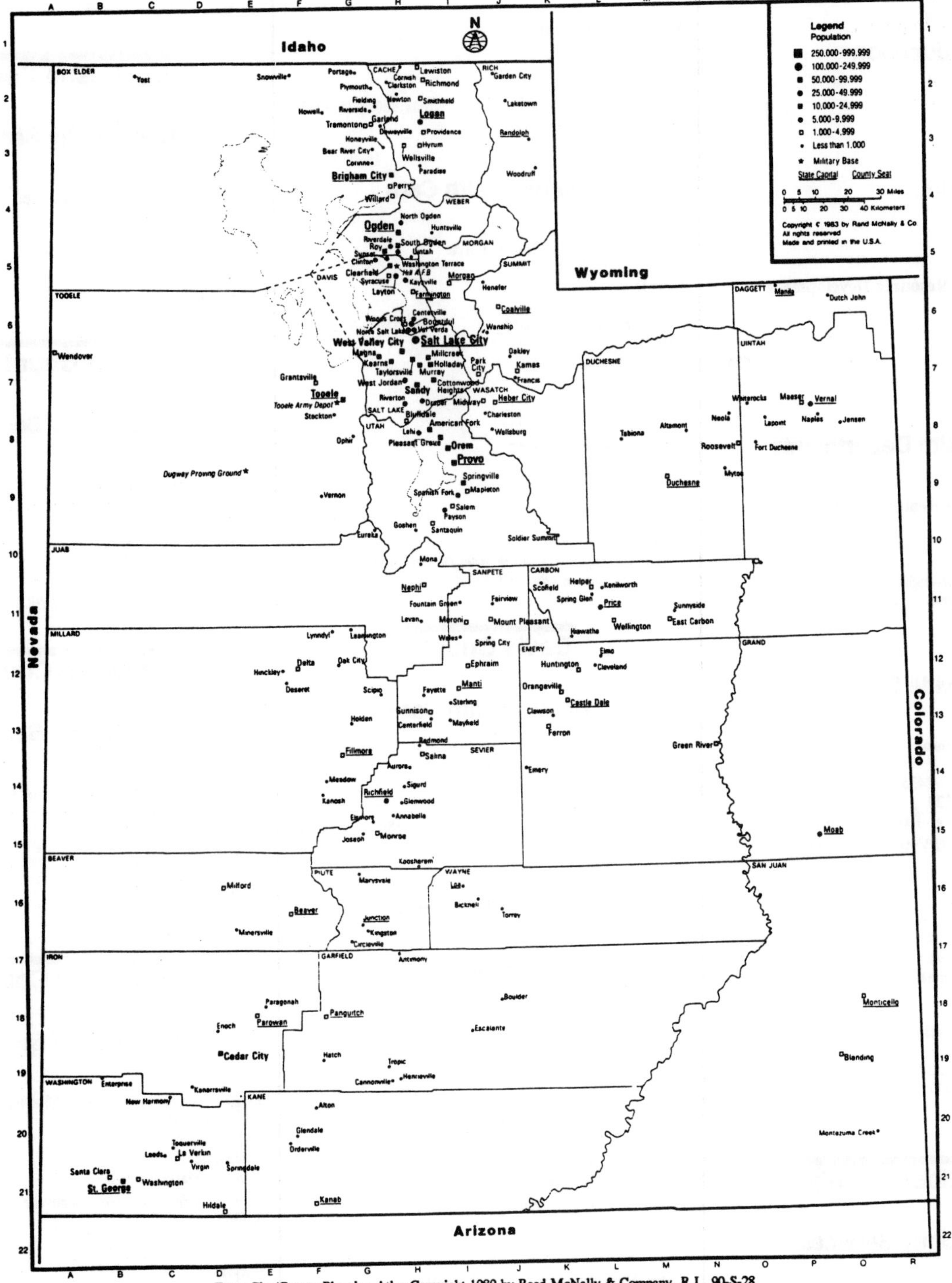

From City/County Planning Atlas Copyright 1989 by Reed McNally & Company, R.L. 90-S-28

Utah

General Services

Education

American Red Cross
Salt Lake Chapter
1391 Park Street
Salt Lake City, UT 84105
Telephone: (801)-467-7339
Contact: Lois Barker
HIV education

Institute of Human Resource Development
205 West 7005
Suite 301
Salt Lake City, UT 84101
Telephone: (801)-521-4473 Fax: (801)-521-6242
Contact: Marc Hoenig
Prevention education

State Health Departments

Utah Department of Health, Bureau of HIV/AIDS
P.O. Box 16660
288 North 1460 West
Salt Lake City, UT 84116-0660
Telephone: (801)-538-6096
Contact: Shari Shubert
Counseling & testing

Statewide Services

Utah AIDS Foundation
1408 South 1100 East
Salt Lake City, UT 84105-2435
Telephone: (801)-487-2323
Contact: La Donna Moore - Executive Director
Statewide services to all HIV/AIDS, education, outreach

Utah Legal Services
124 South 400 East
Salt Lake City, UT 84111-2135
Telephone: (801)-328-8891
Contact: Anne Milne - Director

Utah Medical Association
540 East 500 South
Salt Lake City, UT 84102-2775
Telephone: (801)-355-7477
Physician referral

Box Elder County

Community Services

Department of Human Services office of Family Support
1050 South 500 West
Brigham City, UT 84302-3020
Telephone: (801)-723-8591 Fax: (801)-723-7829
Contact: Jill Bingham
Welfare, child protective services, alcohol, drug treatment prevention

Cache County

Community Services

Planned Parenthood
550 North Main Street
Suite #117
Logan, UT 84321-3957
Telephone: (801)-753-0724 Fax: (801)-753-0724
Contact: Debbie Moosman
Referrals

Home Health Care

Creekside Home Health Care
395 East 1400 North
Suite D
Logan, UT 84321-6533
Telephone: (801)-753-8833 Fax: (801)-753-6058
Toll-Free: (800)-789-4000
Contact: Bonnie James
In home health care

Home Health Services
1400 North 550 East
Suite G
Logan, UT 84321
Telephone: (801)-752-2050 Fax: (801)-750-5361
Contact: Neil Perkes
Skilled nursing; home health aides for personal care; social services;physical medicine & rehab

Davis County

Home Health Care

Community Nursing Services
1190 East 1450 South
Clearfield, UT 84015-1630
Telephone: (801)-776-4445 Fax: (801)-776-4450
Contact: Kathie Korth
Home health care

Medical Services

Benchmark Regional Hospital
592 West 1350 South
Woods Cross, UT 84087-2240
Telephone: (801)-298-2844 Fax: (801)-299-5309
Contact: George Mitchell
Counseling, support for families

Davis County Mental Health
470 East Medical Drive
Bountiful, UT 84010-4928
Telephone: (801)-298-3446
Contact: Dr. Harold Ogihuie
Counseling

Davis Hospital and Medical Center
1600 West Antelope Drive
Layton, UT 84041-1182
Telephone: (801)-825-9561 Fax: (801)-774-7045
Contact: Karla Johnson - Educational Director
HIV education, referral, medical service

Davis Mental Health
Addictions Recovery Ctr
860 South State Street
Clearfield, UT 84015
Telephone: (801)-776-4188
Referral

Lakeview Hospital
630 East Medical Drive
Bountiful, UT 84010-4996
Telephone: (801)-292-6231

Duchesne County

Community Services

Uintah Basin Counseling, Inc.
510 West 200 North
P.O. Box 1524
Roosevelt, UT 84066-2652
Telephone: (801)-722-4625
Counseling

Iron County

Community Services

Legal Center for People with Disability
216 South 200 West
Cedar City, UT 84720-3207
Telephone: (801)-586-2773 Fax: (801)-586-0844
Toll-Free: (800)-824-9311
Contact: Ann Bames
Advocates for people with disabilities

Madison County

Community Services

Charter Counseling Center of Ogden
4155 Harrison Blvd.
Suite 105
Ogden, UT 40403
Telephone: (801)-392-0915
Contact: Darlene Kirson
Counseling

Salt Lake County

Community Services

Dept of Veterans Affairs Medical Center
500 Foothill Blvd
Salt Lake City, UT 84148
Telephone: (801)-363-6101 Fax: (801)-582-1565
Contact: Marlene Finch
Primary care, dental care, home care, nutrition, counseling & HIV testing

Northwest Passage
432 North 300 West
Salt Lake City, UT 84103-1219
Telephone: (801)-364-3138 Fax: (801)-364-3151
Contact: Craig L. Hansen
Drug & alcohol treatment program

Planned Parenthood Association of Utah
654 South 900 East
Salt Lake City, UT 84102-3430
Telephone: (801)-532-1586 Fax: (801)-322-0065
Contact: Karrie Galloway
Education services HIV testing (Park City)

Volunteers of America
252 West Brooklyn Avenue
Salt Lake City, UT 84101-3024
Telephone: (801)-363-9400
Contact: Karen Dodd
Counseling, referrals, AIDS education

Wasatch Youth Support System
3540 South 4000 West
Suite 550
W. Valley City, UT 84120
Telephone: (801)-969-8841 Fax: (801)-969-8898
Contact: Michelle Wilcox
Teens educational AIDS/HIV program

County Health Depts

Southwest Utah District Health Department
288 North 1460 West
Salt Lake City, UT 84116
Telephone: (801)-538-6101 Fax: (801)-538-6036
Contact: 801-673-4180
HIV referrals/counseling

Home Health Care

Caremark
1149 West - 2240 South
Suite A
West Valley, UT 84119
Telephone: (801)-972-6512 Fax: (801)-973-7533
Toll-Free: (800)-245-2463
Contact: Kirby Ryan
Clinical Support and Infusion Therapy: Nutrition, Antimicrobials, Chemo.,Hemat

CNS Home Health Plus
1370 South West Temple
Salt Lake City, UT 84115-3552
Telephone: (801)-486-5588 Fax: (801)-485-3428
Contact: Carol Robey
Home health care

Community Nursing Service Hospice
2970 South Main
Salt Lake City, UT 84115-3553
Telephone: (801)-486-5131 Fax: (801)-486-2193
Contact: Grant Howarth
Home health care

Critical Care America
150 Wright Brothers Dr
Suite 540
Salt Lake City, UT 84116
Telephone: (801)-575-6787 Fax: (801)-575-6795
Toll-Free: (800)-888-2055
Contact: Liz Tucker
Coordinate & integrate all clinical & psychosocial services for HIV+, homeIV therapy

Intermountain Home Health Hospice
1245 East Brickyard Road
Salt Lake City, UT 84106-2559
Telephone: (801)-484-8700 Fax: (801)-466-1135
Home health care

Odyssey Adolescent Facility
623 South 200 East
Salt Lake City, UT 84111-3801
Telephone: (801)-363-0203 Fax: (801)-359-3864
Contact: Steve Sawyer
Residential treatment for adolescents & adults

Odyssey House of Utah
68 South 600 East
Salt Lake City, UT 84102-1007
Telephone: (801)-322-1001 Fax: (801)-359-3864
Contact: Val Fritz
Drug & alcohol treatment program

VA Hospital Based Home Care Program
500 Foothill Boulevard
Salt Lake City, UT 84148-0001
Telephone: (801)-582-1565 Fax: (801)-539-1251
Contact: Rebecca Burrage
In home nursing; social services, dietitian

Medical Services

Central City Community Health Center
461 South 400 East
Salt Lake City, UT 84102
Telephone: (801)-539-8617 Fax: (801)-537-7238
Contact: Sherry Padderson
Early prevention, HIV testing, pre-post counseling, Ryan White fund foreligible recipients

Charter Counseling Center of Midvale
195 West 7200 South
Midvale, UT 84047-3722
Telephone: (801)-562-9440
Contact: Susanne Wheaton - Director
Theraputic support: group, individual, HIV/AIDS

Department of Veterans Affairs
Medical Center
500 Foothill Boulevard
Salt Lake City, UT 84148-3003
Telephone: (801)-582-1565 Fax: (801)-584-1251
AIDS clinic, education, inpatient and outpatient services

Highland Ridge Hospital
4578 South Highland Drive
Salt Lake City, UT 84117-4200
Telephone: (801)-272-9851
Testing & education

Mountain States Hemophilia Center
50 North Medical Drive
IC26
Salt Lake City, UT 84132-0001
Telephone: (801)-581-7914 Fax: (801)-581-2759
Testing, counseling (pre-post testing and bereavement for hemophiliacs &t heir families)

Primary Children's Outpatient Clinic
100 N Medical Drive
Salt Lake City, UT 84113-1100
Telephone: (801)-588-2700
Testing

Redwood Community Health Center
3060 Lester Street
W. Valley City, UT 84119-3026
Telephone: (801)-972-8638
HIV testing & counseling

San Juan County

Community Services

San Juan Community Social Services
117 South Main, Crthouse
P.O. Box 127
Monticello, UT 84535-0127
Telephone: (801)-587-2015 Fax: (801)-587-3451
Contact: Gerry Eberhart
Medicaid, food stamps, financial aid, counseling

Summit County

Community Services

Summit County Valley Mental Health
1753 Sidewinder Drive
P.O. Box 680308
Park City, UT 84068
Telephone: (801)-649-8347 Fax: (801)-649-2157
Contact: Robert Gorelik - Unit Manager
Out patient individual therapy

County Health Depts

Summit City/County Health Department
1753 Sidewinder Drive
P.O. Box 680166
Park City, UT 84060-7322
Telephone: (801)-649-9072
Contact: Diane Maxwell
Testing, counseling; referrals, group education

Tooele County

County Health Depts

Tooele County Health Department
47 South Main, Room 220
Tooele, UT 84074-2194
Telephone: (801)-882-9240 Fax: (801)-882-8138
STD testing, family planning

Uintah County

Community Services

Unitah Basin Counseling, Inc.
559 North 1700 West
Vernal, UT 84078-8200
Telephone: (801)-781-0743
Contact: Russ Stevenson - Doctor
Counseling, referrals

County Health Depts

Uintah Basin District Health Department
147 East Main
Vernal, UT 84078
Telephone: (801)-781-0770
HIV testing, counseling

Medical Services

Ute Tribe - Alcohol and Drug Program
3-A Main Street
Fort Duchesne, UT 84026
Telephone: (801)-722-5141 Fax: (801)-722-2374
Contact: Mary Lee Longhair
Counseling, alcohol and drug abuse, educational program for high risk

Utah County

Community Services

Planned Parenthood
1840 Columbia Lane
Orem, UT 84057
Telephone: (801)-226-5246 Fax: (801)-226-5246
Contact: Cindy Greenland - Manager
Literature & education

Utah County Council on Drug Abuse Rehabilitation
555 South State
Suite 203
Orem, UT 84058-6398
Telephone: (801)-226-2255
Contact: Dennis Hansen
Counseling & referrals

County Health Depts

City/County Health Department of Utah County
589 South State Street
Provo, UT 84606-2430
Telephone: (801)-370-8715
Testing/Counseling site.

Home Health Care

Community Nursing Services - Hospice of Utah County
893 South Arn Blvd.
Orem, UT 84058
Telephone: (801)-224-8138
Contact: Cathy Gillmore
In home nursing

Medical Services

Utah Valley Regional Medical Center
1034 North 500 West
Provo, UT 84604-3377
Telephone: (801)-373-7850 Fax: (801)-371-7186
HIV testing & education

Wasatch County

Community Services

Wasatch County Prevention Services
805 West 100 South
P.O. Box 126
Heber City, UT 84032-2442
Telephone: (801)-654-3003 Fax: (801)-654-2705
Contact: Rod Hopkins - Program Director
Counseling for HIV risk drug users & support for family members

County Health Depts

Wasatch City/County Health Department
805 West 100 South
P.O. Box 246
Heber City, UT 84032-2442
Telephone: (801)-654-2700
Referral, testing, counseling

Washington County

Community Services

Brightway At St. George
115 West 1470 South
St. George, UT 84770-6799
Telephone: (801)-673-0303 Fax: (801)-673-8420
Contact: Pauls Bell - Director
Alcohol & substance abuse counseling

Home Health Care

Nurses House Call
676 South Bluff
Suite 207
St. George, UT 84770-3568
Telephone: (801)-628-5277 Fax: (801)-673-0432
Toll-Free: (800)-660-0337
Contact: Carrie Morrell
In home nursing; companion, respite

Weber County

Community Services

Odgen Rescue Mission
2781 Wall Avenue
Ogden, UT 84401-3539
Telephone: (801)-621-4360 Fax: (801)-621-4361
Contact: Howard Langston - Executive Director
Shelter, food boxes, medical clinic, substance abuse, rehabilitation

Ogden Rescue Mission
2781 Wall Avenue
Ogden, UT 84401
Telephone: (801)-621-4360
Contact: Howard Landston
Shelter; meals, food pantry

Home Health Care

Continuing Care Home Health Agency
St. Benedict's Hospital
5475 South 500 East
Ogden, UT 84405
Telephone: (801)-479-2111
Contact: Danielle Warburton
In home nursing

Medical Services

McKay-Dee Hospital
3939 Harrison Boulevard
Ogden, UT 84409
Telephone: (801)-625-2040 Fax: (801)-629-5434
Contact: Roberta Dixon

Utah Alcoholism Foundation - Northern Division
529 25th Street
Ogden, UT 84401-2406
Telephone: (801)-392-5971
Contact: Mike Sutton
Alcohol & drug treatment center

VERMONT

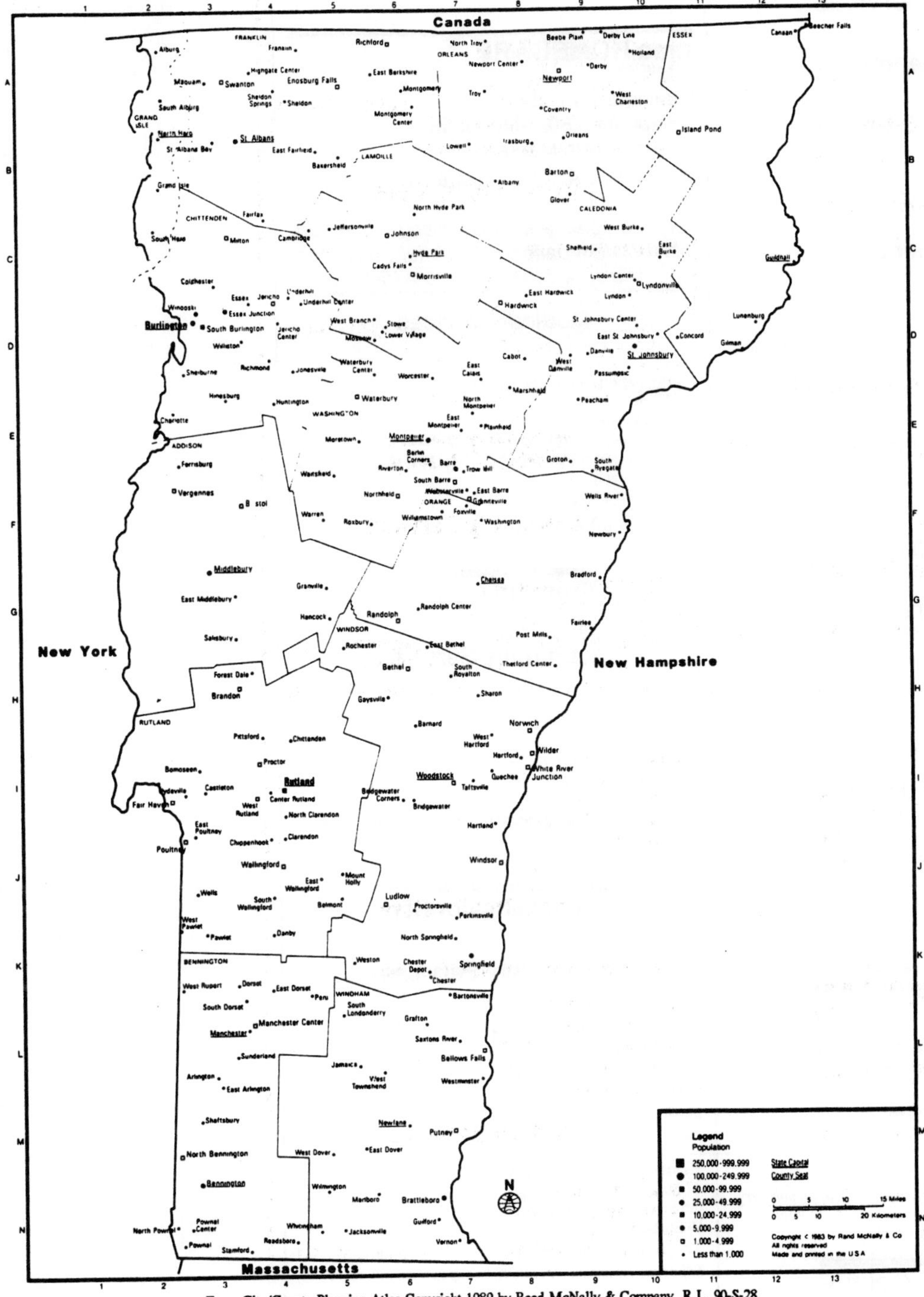

From City/County Planning Atlas Copyright 1989 by Reed McNally & Company, R.L. 90-S-28

Vermont

General Services

Education

AIDS Community Awareness Project (ACAP)
PO Box 608
St Johnsbury, VT 05819
Telephone: (802)-748-1149
Education, speakers, support, info

Hotlines

Vermont AIDS Hotline

In state only (800)-882-2437

Vermont CARES
PO Box 5248
Burlington, VT 05402
Telephone: (802)-863-2437
Contact: Kate Hill
AIDS/HIV education, direct services

State Health Departments

Vermont Department of Health
PO Box 70
Burlington, VT 05402
Telephone: (802)-863-7280
Contact: Shari Brenner - HIV/AIDS Education Coord.
Education, testing, counseling, referrals

Statewide Services

Vermont AIDS Council
PO Box 275
Montpelier, VT 05601
Telephone: (802)-229-2557
Contact: Erica Garfin
AIDS service network

Bennington County

Community Services

Bennington Area AIDS Project
PO Box 1066
Bennington, VT 05201
Telephone: (802)-442-4481
Emergency financial assistance, service coord, support services, advocacy

Caledonia County

Community Services

AIDS Community Awareness Project (ACAP)
PO Box 608
St Johnsbury, VT 05819
Telephone: (802)-748-1149
Emergency financial assistance, support groups, buddies, advocacy & phoneline

Chittenden County

Home Health Care

nmc HOMECARE
1 Mill St.
Burlington, VT 05401
Telephone: (802)-865-9563
Contact: Tom Markert
National JCAHO-Accredited company providing a full range of Infusion and Respiratory therapies and specializing in the care of HIV/AIDS patients. National Case Manager is also available at 800-445-1188

Medical Services

Comprehensive Care Clinic
5th Floor
1 South Prospect
Burlington, VT 05401
Telephone: (802)-656-4594 Fax: (802)-656-1982
Toll-Free: (800)-358-1144
Contact: Dr. Christopher Grace
Services for HIV+ persons

Franklin County

Community Services

Franklin/Grand Isle AIDS Task Force
PO Box 241
St Albans, VT 05478
Telephone: (802)-524-7742
Contact: John Smiley
Emergency financial assistance, service coord, support services, advocacy

Windham County

Community Services

Brattleboro AIDS Project
P.O. Box 1486
Brattleboro, VT 05302-1486
Telephone: (802)-254-8263
Services for HIV+ persons only

Brattleboro AIDS Project
67 Main Street
4th Floor
Brattleboro, VT 05302
Telephone: (802)-254-4444
Support, counseling education, buddy system, outreach

VIRGINIA

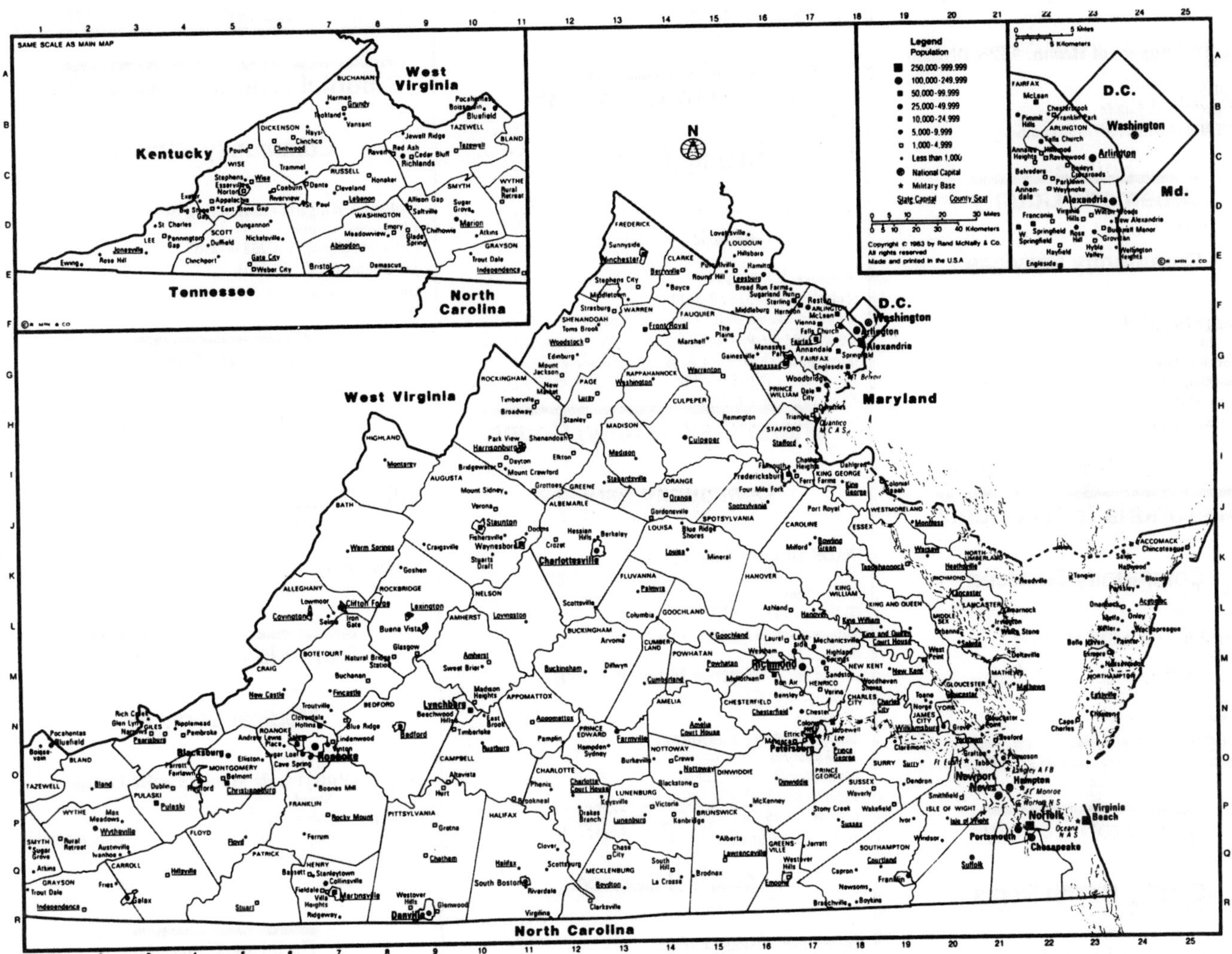

From City/County Planning Atlas Copyright 1989 by Reed McNally & Company, R.L. 90-S-28

Virginia

General Services

State Health Departments

Virginia Department of Health, AIDS Division

Richmond, VA 23219
Telephone: (804)-225-4844
Contact: Elaine Martin - AIDS Coordinator

Albemarle County

Community Services

Blue Ridge Hospital
Univ of Virginia
Mental Health Dept.
Charlottesville, VA 22901
Telephone: (804)-924-2251
Contact: Penny Drumheller, R.N.
Out patient psychiatary, AIDS support group

Alexandria (city) County

Community Services

Northern Virginia AIDS Ministry
413 Duke Streetoad
Alexandria, VA 22314
Telephone: (703)-751-5520
Contact: Barry Goodinson
Transportation, emergency financial assistance, children's services,pastoral counseling, support groups, education

Arlington County

County Health Depts

Arlington County Division of Human Services
Division of Social Srvcs
800 South Walter Reed Dr.
Arlington, VA 22204
Telephone: (703)-358-5590
Emergency partial financial assistance. Prescription Medication Program.

Home Health Care

Arlington Department of Human Services AIDS Bureau
Home Health Nursing
1810 North Edison Street
Arlington, VA 22207
Telephone: (703)-358-4940 Fax: (703)-358-5233
Contact: Bonnie Kiessling - Nursing Supervisor
Nurses provide assessment, teaching and consultation. Limited home services.

Hospice of Northern Virginia
4715 North 15th Street
Arlington, VA 22205-2699
Telephone: (703)-525-7070 Fax: (703)-538-2162
Contact: Jo Turner - Director of Marketing & Public; - Relation
Servicing Northern Virginia. Home/inpatient care

Visiting Nurse Association of Northern Virginia
2775 South Quincy Street
Suite # 200
Arlington, VA 22206
Telephone: (703)-379-6800 Fax: (703)-379-5496
Contact: Emily Deaby - President
Servicing Northern Virginia, home care, medical and social services

Botetourt County

Home Health Care

Caremark
6711 Peters Creek Road
Suite 206
Roanoke, VA 24019
Telephone: (703)-362-5411
Contact: Steven Holt - General Manager
CLINICAL SUPPORT AND INFUSION THERAPY: Nutrition, Antimicrovirals, Chemo.,Hematopoeti

Charlottesville (city) County

Community Services

AIDS Support Group, Inc.
P.O. Box 2322
Charlottesville, VA 22902-2322
Telephone: (804)-979-7714
Contact: Emily Dreyfus

Home Health Care

Hospice of the Piedmont
1002 East Jefferson St.
Charlottesville, VA 22902
Telephone: (804)-971-3995
Contact: Victoria Todd - Executive Director
Home and inpatient services.

Medical Services

Infectious Disease Clinic
Univ of Virginia Hospital
Charlottesville, VA 22908-0001
Telephone: (804)-924-0257
Contact: Dr. Brian Wistelwey
Medical care for PWAs and HIV infected.

Chesterfield County

County Health Depts

Chesterfield County Health Department
P.O. Box 100
Chesterfield, VA 23832-0100
Telephone: (804)-751-4359
Screening & counseling, intermittent care

Home Health Care

nmc HOMECARE
1800 Coyote Drive
Chester, VA 23831
Telephone: (804)-768-1200
Fax: (804)-748-3551
Contact: Peggy Trible
National JCAHO-Accredited company providing a full range of Infusion and Respiratory therapies and specializing in the care of HIV/AIDS patients. National Case Manager is also available at 800-445-1188

Colonial Heights (city) County

Community Services

Colonial Heights Counseling Services
130 James Avenue
Colonial Heights, VA 23834-2802
Telephone: (804)-520-7210
Ouypatient counseling

Culpeper County

Community Services

Rappahannock-Rapidan Community Services
401 South Main Street
Culpeper, VA 22701-3117
Telephone: (703)-825-3100
Servicing Fauquier, Madison, Rappahannock and Orange; substance abuse,mental health services

Danville (city) County

Medical Services

Danville-Pittsylvania Mental Health Center
245 Hairston Street
Danville, VA 24540-4137
Telephone: (804)-793-4922 Fax: (804)-793-4201
Contact: Cheryl Chittum
Crisis counseling, case management, referrals

Fairfax County

Community Services

Haven of Northern Virginia
4606 Ravensworth Road
Annandale, VA 22003-5641
Telephone: (703)-941-7000
Support groups for the terminally ill & bereaved

County Health Depts

Fairfax County Health Department
Falls Church District
7115 Leesburg Pike
Falls Church, VA 22043
Telephone: (703)-246-7100
Case management, clinic, HIV/STD testing & counseling

Fairfax County Health Department
Mt Vernon District
6301 Richmond Highway
Alexandria, VA 22306
Telephone: (703)-660-7100

Family services & HIV,STD testing.

Fairfax County Health Department
Springfield District
5700 Hanover Avenue
Springfield, VA 22150
Telephone: (703)-569-1031
HIV testing & counseling, case management

Fairfax County Health Department Alexandria District
6301 Richmond Highway
Alexandria, VA 22306
Telephone: (703)-660-7100
STD & AIDS testing

Home Health Care

Caremark Connection Network
3701 Concorde Parkway
Suite 800
Chantilly, VA 22021
Telephone: (703)-631-4790
Contact: Jonathon Cooper - Branch Manager
Clinical Support and Infusion Therapy: Nutrition, Antimicrobials, Chemo.,Hematopoeti

Hispanic Resource Center
8027 Leesburg Pike
Suite 702
Vienna, VA 22182
Telephone: (703)-827-8666
Contact: Adolfo Arsuaga - District Manager
Medical Case Management, Vocational Rehab., Life Care Plans, Expert Testimony

Inova Home Care
8003 Forbes Place
Springfield, VA 22151
Telephone: (703)-321-7979
Contact: Linda Scott
Home care, private duty, therapy and home health aides

Resource Opportunities, Inc.
8027 Leesburg Pike
Suite 604
Vienna, VA 22182
Telephone: (703)-893-4600
Contact: Linda Szalay - District Manager
Medical Case Management, Vocational Rehab., Life Care Plans, Expert Testimony

Medical Services

Northwest Center for Community Mental Health
1850 Cameron Glen Drive
Reston, VA 22091-3310
Telephone: (703)-481-4100
Contact: Betty Giller - Emergency Srvcs; Libby Jenkins -
Crisis counseling, Case management, Support Group.

Hanover County

Medical Services

Hanover Mental Health/Substance Abuse Center
P.O. Box 2182
Ashland, VA 23005-5182
Telephone: (804)-798-3279 Fax: (804)-798-0658
Crisis counseling, Case management. Mental Health and Substance Abusecounseling

Henrico County

Community Services

Department of Social Services
1604 Santa Rosa Road
Suite 103, Wythe Bldg.
Richmond, VA 23229-5008
Telephone: (804)-662-9743 Fax: (804)-662-7023
Contact: Jack Richardson - Regional AIDS Coordinator

Home Health Care

HNS, Inc.
1632 East Parham Road
Richmond, VA 23228
Telephone: (804)-266-0677
Toll-Free: (800)-659-0672
Contact: Bob Corvin
Home Infusion Therapy, In-home Nursing and Attendant Care, P.T. Services, Pentamidine

Resource Opportunities, Inc.
4124 Inns Lake Drive
Glenn Allen, VA 23060
Telephone: (804)-527-0100
Contact: Linda McIinley - District Manager
Medical Case Management, Vocational Rehab., Life Care Plans, Expert Testimony

Resource Opportunities, Inc.
4122 Inns Lake Drive
Glenn Allen, VA 23060
Telephone: (804)-527-1100
Toll-Free: (800)-438-4764
Contact: Alice T. Hall,RN, MS, CRC - Executive Vice President
Medical Case Management, Vocational Rehab., Life Care Plans, Expert Testimony

Medical Services

Richmond Memorial Hospital
1300 Westwood Avenue
Richmond, VA 23227-4699
Telephone: (804)-254-6000 Fax: (804)-355-3952
Contact: Ronald Artz, MD
Internal Medicine.

Lynchburg (city) County

Medical Services

Lynchburg Mental Health Center
2235 Landover Place
Lynchburg, VA 24501-0497
Telephone: (804)-847-8000 Fax: (804)-847-6099
Contact: David Baer
Crisis counseling, Case management.

Mecklenburg County

Medical Services

Chase City Mental Health
22 North Main Street
Chase City, VA 23924
Telephone: (804)-372-2168 Fax: (804)-372-2170
Counseling, referrals

Montgomery County

Home Health Care

Home Health Plus of the New River Valley
203 Roanoke Street
Christiansburg, VA 24073
Telephone: (703)-382-5484
Contact: Nancy R. Root
Home health, physical/speech therapy; also servicing Floyd, Pulaski, andGiles; general services includes AIDS

Norfolk (city) County

Community Services

AIDS Network
3309 Gramby Street
Norfolk, VA 23517-1807
Telephone: (804)-622-0837
Supply day care for children with AIDS & support groups

Tidewater AIDS Crisis Taskforce (TACT)
740 Duke Street
Suite #520
Norfolk, VA 23510-1515
Telephone: (804)-626-0127 Fax: (804)-627-4641
Contact: Pat Barner
Task force, counseling, education

Home Health Care

Caremark Connection Network
2550 Ellsmere Ave
Suite C
Norfolk, VA 23513
Telephone: (804)-853-7212
Clinical Support and Infusion Therapy: general Nutrition, Antimicrobials,Chemo., Hematopoeti

Norfolk Department of Public Health/Home Health
401 Colley Avenue
Norfolk, VA 23507
Telephone: (804)-683-2783 Fax: (804)-683-8878
Contact: Louellen C. Rowe
STD, clinic

Petersburg (city) County

Community Services

Crater Family Counseling Services
24 South Adams Street
Petersburg, VA 23803-4525
Telephone: (804)-733-1030 Fax: (804)-861-8123
Children & family counseling

District 19 Alcohol and Drug Services
116 S. Adams Street
Petersburg, VA 23803-4511
Telephone: (804)-861-0242 Fax: (804)-861-3122
Counseling services; case management.

District 19 Community Services Board
24 South Adams Street
Petersburg, VA 23803-4511
Telephone: (804)-861-6606 Fax: (804)-861-3122
Crisis counseling, Case management.

Sycamore Center
314 S. Sycamore Street
Petersburg, VA 23803-5401
Telephone: (804)-861-5856
Rehabilitation center

Richmond (city) County

Community Services

Commonwealth Professional Services
12 S. Auburn Street
Richmond, VA 23221-2910
Telephone: (804)-353-1169
Contact: Stephen Lenton, Ph.D; Frances Stewart, Ph.D; Donnie Connor, Ed.D
HIV/AIDS for gay & bisexual men, individual counseling

Richmond AIDS Information Network (RAIN)
Fan Free Clinic, Inc.
1721 Hanover Avenue
Richmond, VA 23220
Telephone: (804)-358-6343
Contact: Jim Beckner - Executive Director
Support Groups and Advocacy, Case Mgt, educ, referral, testing

Medical Services

Medical College of Virginia Infectious Disease Clinic
P.O. Box 445
MCV Station
Richmond, VA 23298
Telephone: (804)-371-6163 Fax: (804)-371-0816
Contact: Vicky Watson
Clinical evaluation and care of persons with HIV.

Roanoke County

Testing Sites

Parkway Physicians
204 Maple Street
Vinton, VA 24179
Telephone: (703)-982-6886 Fax: (703)-982-6928
Contact: Dr. Henry R. Ivey
Testing

Roanoke (city) County

Community Services

Council of Community Services
AIDS Council of West VA
502 Campbell Avenue Southwest
Roanoke, VA 24016
Telephone: (703)-696-4653
Contact: Fraser Nelson
Support services for PWAs, PWARCs, HIV positive; education services, case management

Department of Social Services
Roanoke Regional Office
210 Church Avenue SW, 100
Roanoke, VA 24011-1779
Telephone: (703)-857-7972 Fax: (703)-857-7363
Contact: Page McAllister - Regional AIDS Coordinator
Social services

County Health Depts

Roanoke City Health Department
515 8th Street SW
Roanoke, VA 24016-3529
Telephone: (703)-857-7600 Fax: (703)-857-7987
Contact: Lee Radecke
Examination and follow-up of HIV Positive persons.

Home Health Care

Abbey Foster Medical Corporation
5151 B Starkey Road
Roanoke, VA 24014
Telephone: (703)-772-0725
Contact: Sylvia Broukhiyan
Servicing 45 mile radius of Roanoke. Medical equip, & oxygen.

Medical Services

Community Hospital of Roanoke Valley
101 Elm Avenue SE
Roanoke, VA 24014-2230
Telephone: (703)-985-8200 Fax: (703)-224-4405
Contact: Donna McMillen - Director
Education and Information for Professional who work with HIV Patients.

Internal Medicine Association of Roanoke, Inc.
1310 Third Street SW
Roanoke, VA 24016-5299
Telephone: (703)-345-4946 Fax: (703)-343-7693
Contact: Gerald Roller, MD
Internal Medicine.

Salem (city) County

Testing Sites

Veteran's Administration Medical Center
1970 Roanoke Blvd.
Salem, VA 24153-6483
Telephone: (703)-982-2463 Fax: (703)-983-1028
Contact: Charles Schleupner, MD
VA eligible patients only; HIV testing, counseling

Virginia Beach (city) County

Home Health Care

Medical Care Plus
5760 North Hampton Blvd.
Suite 100
Virginia Beach, VA 23455
Telephone: (804)-468-0557
Contact: Narlie Amarasinghe
Servicing Peninsula, Richmond. Home care. IV services.

Resource Opportunities, Inc.
5041 Corporate Woods Dr.
Suite 185
Virginia Beach, VA 23462
Telephone: (804)-671-8400
Contact: Mark G. Willis - District Manager
Medical Case Management, general vocational Rehab., Life Care Plans, Expert Testimony

York County

Community Services

Family Resources, Inc.
7142 Duffie Drive
Williamsburg, VA 23185-5301
Telephone: (804)-253-1459
Contact: James W. Reilly, Psy.D.
Individual, family and couple therapy.

WASHINGTON

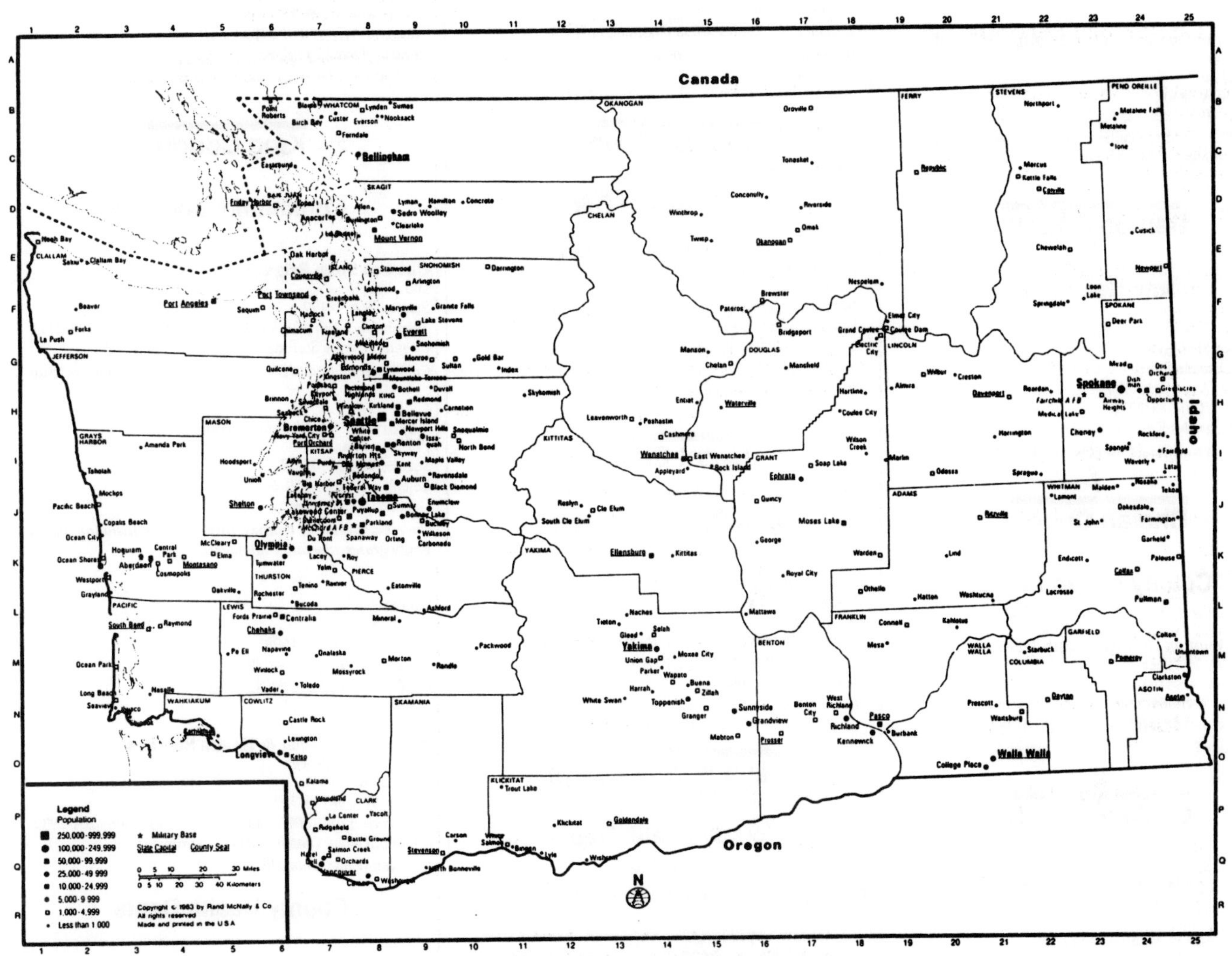

From City/County Planning Atlas Copyright 1989 by Reed McNally & Company, R.L. 90-S-28

Washington

General Services

State Health Departments

Washington Department of Health, Office of AIDS/STD
PO Box 47840
Olympia, WA 98504
Telephone: (206)-464-5457
Contact: Deenie M.T. Dudley - Clearinghouse Manager; Mary Cummings - Office Director

Benton County

Home Health Care

O.P.T.I.O.N. Care
21 South Cascade Street
Kennewick, WA 99336-3849
Telephone: (509)-783-2273 Fax: (509)-586-0327
Contact: Roger McKinnon
Home IV and Nutritional Services

Chelan County

County Health Depts

Chelan-Douglas County Health District
316 Washington Street
Wenatchee, WA 98801
Telephone: (509)-664-5306
Contact: Terri Steckmest
HIV Antibody Testing, Counseling Services

Clallam County

County Health Depts

Clallam County Health Department
223 East Fourth Street
Port Angeles, WA 98362-3098
Telephone: (206)-417-2431 Fax: (206)-452-0470
Contact: Chris Borchers - Program Coordinator
HIV antibody testing, counseling services

Clark County

Testing Sites

Southwest Washington Health District, Vancouver-Clark County
2000 Fort Vancouver Way
P.O. Box 1870
Vancouver, WA 98663-3503
Telephone: (206)-695-9215
HIV Antibody Testing, Counseling Services

Cowlitz County

County Health Depts

Cowlitz-Wahkiakum Health District
1516 Hudson Street
Longview, WA 98632-3006
Telephone: (206)-425-7400
Contact: Clark Geer - AIDS Coordinator
HIV antibody testing, counseling, support groups, outreach, education

Garfield County

County Health Depts

Garfield County Health District
P.O. Box 130
(10th and Columbia)
Pomeroy, WA 99347-0130
Telephone: (509)-843-3412
Contact: Patty Appel
HIV Antibody Testing, Counseling Services

Grant County

County Health Depts

Grant County Health District
County Courthouse
P.O. Box 37
Ephrata, WA 98823
Telephone: (509)-754-2011
Contact: Kirsten Sweet
HIV Antibody Testing, Counseling Services

Grays Harbor County

County Health Depts

Grays Harbor County Health Department
2109 Sumner Avenue
Aberdeen, WA 98520-3600
Telephone: (206)-532-8631
Contact: Pat Meldrich
HIV Antibody Testing, Counseling Services

Island County

County Health Depts

Island County Health Department
HIV/AIDS Project
P.O. Box 5000
Coupeville, WA 98239-5000
Telephone: (206)-679-7351
Contact: Gary Childers
HIV counseling/testing, education, Case Management

Jefferson County

County Health Depts

Jefferson County Health Department
Castle Hill Mall
615 Sheridan
Port Townsend, WA 98368
Telephone: (206)-385-0722
Contact: Denis Langlois
HIV antibody testing, counseling, case management

King County

Community Services

Chicken Soup Brigade
1002 East Seneca
Seattle, WA 98122
Telephone: (206)-328-8979 Fax: (206)-328-0171
Contact: Carole Sterling
Community-based AIDS services, prepares & delivers foods

Northwest AIDS Foundation
127 Broadway E
Seattle, WA 98102-5711
Telephone: (206)-329-6923
Contact: Lilliam Rea
Case management, housing insurance continuation, emergency grants,education volunteers

Shanti
P.O. Box 20698
Seattle, WA 98102-1698
Telephone: (206)-322-0279
Community-Based AIDS Services

WA Dept of Social & Health Services
1610 NE 150th Street
Mailstop K-17-9
Seattle, WA 98155-7224
Telephone: (206)-361-2888 Fax: (206)-261-2932
Contact: Danny Daniel - AIDS Coordinator
HIV testing and counseling

County Health Depts

Seattle King County Department of Health
400 Yesler Building
3rd Floor
Seattle, WA 98104-2614
Telephone: (206)-296-4568 Fax: (206)-296-4803
Contact: Kurt Wuellner - Program Coordinator; Pamela J. Ryan - Program Supervisor
HIV testing and counseling

Seattle-King Cty. Dept. of Pub Health, AIDS Prevention Proj.
2124 4th Avenue
4th Floor
Seattle, WA 98121
Telephone: (206)-296-4649 Fax: (206)-296-4895
Contact: Tim Burak - AIDS Project Manager
Publisher of: Advice About AIDS for Pub. Safety, Health and Emergency Personnel

Seattle-King Cty. Dept. of Pub. Health, AIDS Prevention Proj.
1116 Summitt Ave.
Ste. 200
Seattle, WA 98101-2831
Telephone: (206)-296-4755

Contact: Patricia McInturff
Publisher of: Advice about AIDS for pub. safety, health and emergencypersonnel

Home Health Care

Caremark
6645 185th Ave. NE
Suite 151
Redmond, WA 98052
Telephone: (206)-885-5938
Toll-Free: (800)-727-1415
Contact: Joe Fazio
Clinical Support and Infusion Therapy: nutrition, antimicrobiels,chemotherapy, hematopoeti

Critical Care America
11711 N Creek Pkwy So
Suite 112
Bothell, WA 98011
Telephone: (206)-485-4112 Fax: (206)-487-0353
Toll-Free: (800)-288-7177
Coordinate & integrate all clinical & psychosocial services for HIV& AIDS patients.

HNS, Inc.
1331 118th Ave SE
Suite 100
Bellevue, WA 98004
Telephone: (206)-453-1988 Fax: (206)-453-1887
Contact: Todd Feider
Home Infusion Therapy, In-home Nursing and Attendant Care

Homedco Infusion Inc.
14935 North East 87th Street
Redmond, WA 98052-3863
Telephone: (206)-881-8500 Fax: (206)-881-8779
Toll-Free: (800)-452-8137
Nationwide experience inproviding home infusion therapy to AIDS patients,respiratory services, home medical equipment services.

Kitsap County

County Health Depts

Bremerton-Kitsap County Health District
109 Austin Drive
Bremerton, WA 98312-1805
Telephone: (206)-478-5235
Contact: Paul Chen
HIV testing, counseling, TB & STD clinic, family services

Kittitas County

County Health Depts

Kittitas County Health Department
507 Nanum Street
Ellensburg, WA 98926-2898
Telephone: (509)-962-6811
HIV Antibody Testing, Counseling Services

Lewis County

County Health Depts

Lewis County Health District
360 N.W. North Street
P.O. Box 706
Chehalis, WA 98532-0706
Telephone: (206)-748-9121 Fax: (206)-740-1472
Contact: Ext. 368
HIV Antibody Testing, Education & Counseling, Case Management

Lincoln County

County Health Depts

Lincoln County Health Department, Nursing Office
507 7th Street
P.O. Box 215
Davenport, WA 99122-0215
Telephone: (509)-725-1001
Contact: Diane A. Martin - Director
HIV Antibody Testing, Counseling Services

Mason County

County Health Depts

Mason County Health Department, Nursing Division
303 North 4th Street
Shelton, WA 98584-3417
Telephone: (206)-427-9670
Contact: Carol Oliver
HIV Antibody Testing, Counseling Services

Okanogan County

County Health Depts

Okanogan County Health District
Administration Building
P.O. Box 231
Okanogan, WA 98840-0231
Telephone: (509)-422-3867
Contact: Ken Brown
HIV Antibody Testing, Counseling Services, outreach case management

Pacific County

County Health Depts

Pacific County Health Department
P.O. Box 26
South Bend, WA 98586-0026
Telephone: (206)-875-9343
Contact: Lorrie Ashley
HIV Antibody Testing, Counseling Services

Pierce County

Home Health Care

Homedco Infusion Inc.
2008 48th Avenue Court E
Tacoma, WA 98424-2653
Telephone: (206)-922-3200 Fax: (206)-922-3481
Toll-Free: (800)-638-0140
Nationwide experience inproviding home infusion therapy to AIDS patients,respiratory services, home medical equipment services.

San Juan County

County Health Depts

San Juan County Health Department
145 Rhone
P.O. Box 607
Friday Harbor, WA 98250-0607
Telephone: (206)-378-4474
Contact: Joan Campbell
HIV Antibody Testing, Counseling Services, Education, Case Management

Skagit County

County Health Depts

Skagit County Health Department
Admin. Bldg., Room 301
700 South 2nd Street
Mount Vernon, WA 98273
Telephone: (206)-336-9380
Contact: Kay Van Stralen
HIV Antibody Testing, Counseling Services, Case Mgt, support group

Snohomish County

Community Services

Helpers of Persons with AIDS
1918 Everett Avenue
Everett, WA 98201-3607
Telephone: (206)-259-9188
Community-Based AIDS Services

Spokane County

Community Services

Spokane AIDS Network
1613 West Gardner
Spokane, WA 99201
Telephone: (509)-326-2467
Community-Based AIDS Services

County Health Depts

Spokane County Health District
West 1101 College Avenue
Spokane, WA 99204
Telephone: (509)-456-3640

HIV Antibody Testing, Counseling Services

Home Health Care

HNS, Inc.
329 East Sprague
Spokane, WA 99202
Telephone: (509)-838-0140 Fax: (509)-838-1079
Toll-Free: (800)-872-4467
Contact: Todd Feider - General Manager
Home Infusion Therapy

Stevens County

County Health Depts

Northeast Tri-County Health District
240 E. Dominion
P.O. Box 270
Colville, WA 99114
Telephone: (509)-684-5048
Contact: Maureen Considine
HIV antibody testing, counseling services, & case management

Thurston County

County Health Depts

Thurston County Health Department
529 4th Avenue West
Olympia, WA 98501-8200
Telephone: (206)-786-5581
Contact: Diana Johnson
Anonymous HIV antibody testing, counseling services, & outreach.

Walla Walla County

County Health Depts

Walla Walla County-City Health Department
310 West Poplar
P.O. Box 1753
Walla Walla, WA 99362-2857
Telephone: (509)-527-3290
Contact: Joan Perry
HIV Antibody Testing, Counseling Services

Whitman County

County Health Depts

Whitman County Health Department
NE 235 Olsen
Pullman, WA 99163
Telephone: (509)-332-6752
Contact: Fran Martin
Case Management, Education

Whitman County Health Department
Public Service Building
North 310 Main Street
Colfax, WA 99111
Telephone: (509)-397-3471
HIV Antibody Testing, Counseling Services, Case Management

Yakima County

Home Health Care

O.P.T.I.O.N. Care
103 N 7th Avenue
Yakima, WA 98902
Telephone: (509)-575-0867 Fax: (509)-452-3710
Contact: Judy Beck - Branch Manager
Home IV and Nutritional Services

WEST VIRGINIA

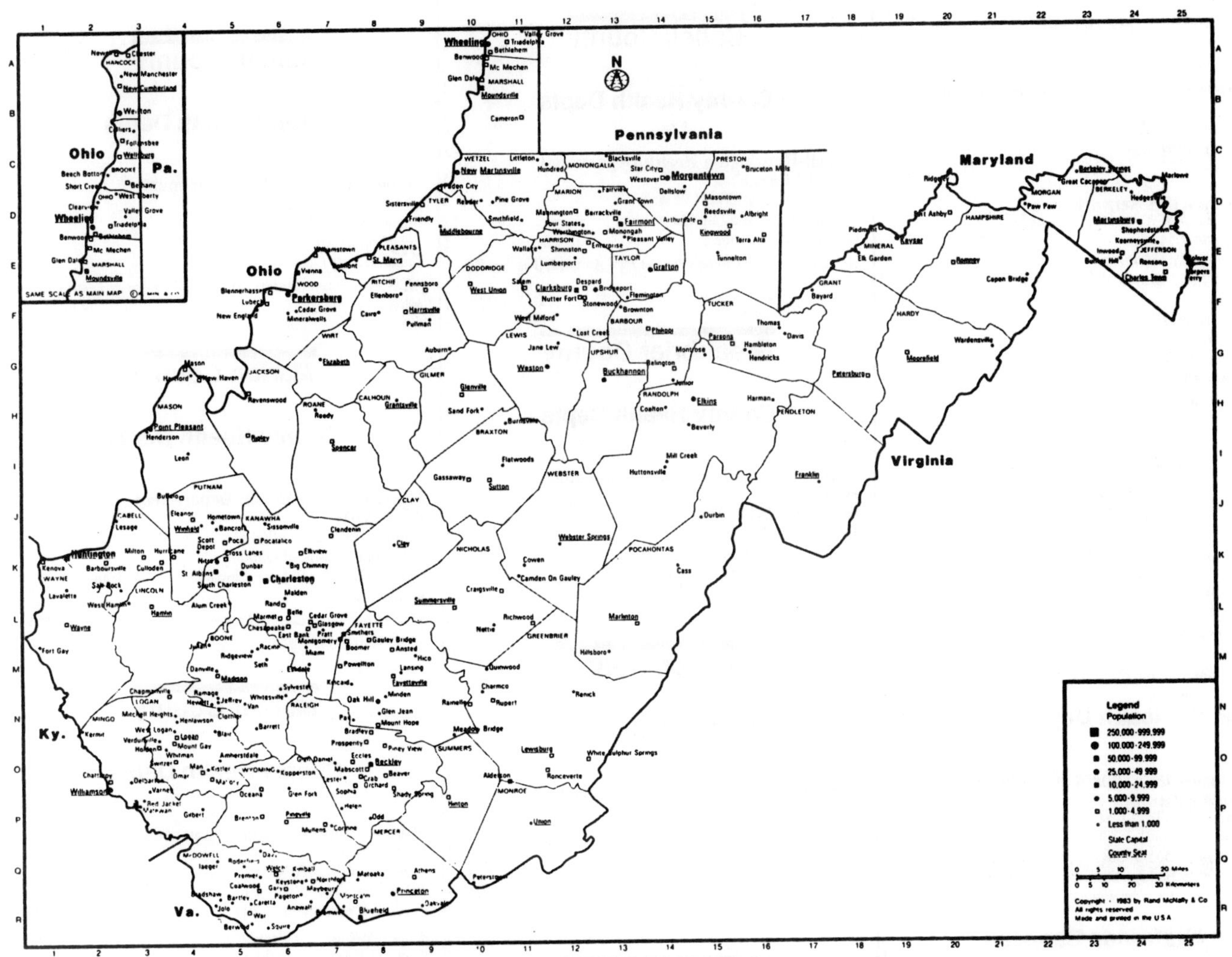

From City/County Planning Atlas Copyright 1989 by Reed McNally & Company, R.L. 90-S-28

West Virginia

General Services

Hotlines

AIDS Task Force of the Upper Ohio Valley

Wheeling, WV 26003
Telephone: (304)-232-6822

Charleston AIDS Network

Charleston, WV 25324
Telephone: (304)-345-4673

Huntington AIDS Task Force
P.O. Box 2981
Huntington, WV 25728-2981
Telephone: (304)-696-7132
Referrals-counseling-buddy support

Mid-Ohio Valley AIDS Task Force

Parkersburg, WV 26102
Telephone: (304)-428-4488

Mountain State AIDS Network
235 High Street
Suite 306
Morgantown, WV 26505
Telephone: (304)-599-9726
Support-buddy system-education-speakers

State Health Departments

West Virginia Department of Health, AIDS Prevention Program
1422 Washington Street East
Charleston, WV 25301
Telephone: (304)-558-5358 Fax: (304)-558-6335
Contact: Loretta Haddy - Director, AIDS Prevention; Robert Johnson - Coordinator HIV

Statewide Services

Mountain State AIDS Network
PO Box 576
Morgantown, WV 26505-0576
Telephone: (304)-292-5789
AIDS Information & Services

Berkeley County

County Health Depts

Berkeley County Health Department
800 S. Queen Street
Martinsburg, WV 25401
Telephone: (304)-263-5131
Contact: Elaine Renner; Kimberly Cleaver -
AIDS Prevention Centers for the HIV Antibody Testing Program

Medical Services

Shenandoah Community Health Center
East Moler Ave.
P.O. Box 3236
Martinsburg, WV 25401
Telephone: (304)-263-4956 Fax: (304)-263-0984
Contact: Tina Burns - Migrant Director; Carolyn Clarke, PAC -
Servicing Winchester, Frederick, Shenandoah. Care service to migrant workers

Cabell County

County Health Depts

Cabell-Huntington Health Department
1336 Hal-Greer Blvd
Huntington, WV 25701-3804
Telephone: (304)-523-6483
Contact: Martha Pierce
AIDS Prevention Centers for the HIV Antibody Testing Program

Greenbrier County

County Health Depts

Greenbrier County Health Department
PO Box 890
Fairlea, WV 24902-0890
Telephone: (304)-645-1787
Contact: Gay Sebert
AIDS Prevention Centers for the HIV Antibody Testing Program

Harrison County

County Health Depts

Harrison-Clarksburg Health Department
Courthouse
Clarksburg, WV 26301
Telephone: (304)-624-8570
Contact: Margaret Howe; Agtha Sigley, R.N. -
STD clinic referrals, AIDS prevention center for the HIV Antibody Testing Program.

Kanawha County

Community Services

Charleston AIDS Network
PO Box 1024
Charleston, WV 25324-1024
Telephone: (304)-345-4673
Contact: Brian Henry
AIDS Task Force (Hotline 6-8pm), buddy program, referrals for financial and medical assistance

County Health Depts

Kanawha-Charleston Health Department
108 Lee Street East
Charleston, WV 25323-1506
Telephone: (304)-348-8069 Fax: (304)-348-6821
Contact: Donald Rosenberg - Medical Director
AIDS Prevention Centers for the HIV Antibody Testing Program

Public Health Unit, CAMC (Mem. Div.)
3101 MacCorkle Avenue SE
Charleston, WV 25304-1200
Telephone: (304)-348-8160
Contact: Libby Boggess
AIDS Prevention Centers for the HIV Antibody Testing Program

Logan County

County Health Depts

Logan County Health Department
Courthouse, Room 203
Logan, WV 25601
Telephone: (304)-752-2000
Contact: Judy Cope
AIDS Prevention Centers for the HIV Antibody Testing Program

Marion County

County Health Depts

Marion County Health Department
P.O. Box 649
Fairmont, WV 26555-0649
Telephone: (304)-366-3360
Contact: Barbara Balmer; Linda Rutherford; Jean Wadsworth
STD clinic referrals, AIDS prevention center for the HIV antibody testingprogram.

Mercer County

County Health Depts

Mercer County Health Department
Route 2, Box 382
Bluefield, WV 24701-0382
Telephone: (304)-325-3621
Contact: Cheryl Gaither, RN
AIDS Prevention Centers for the HIV Antibody Testing Program, HIV testing(confidential & anonymous), pre & post counseling, referrals

Monongalia County

Community Services

Mountain State AIDS Network
235 High Street
Suite 306
Morgantown, WV 26505
Telephone: (304)-292-9000
Contact: Christopher Morrison - Executive Director
AIDS Task Force (Hotline 304-599-9726, 7-11pm), counseling, education,speakers bureau

County Health Depts

Monongalia County Health Department
453 VanVoorhis Road
Morgantown, WV 26505-3408
Telephone: (304)-598-5100
Contact: Linda Bennett
AIDS Prevention Centers for the HIV Antibody Testing Program

Ohio County

County Health Depts

Wheeling-Ohio Health Department
1500 Chapline Street
City-County Building
Wheeling, WV 26003
Telephone: (304)-234-3682 Fax: (304)-234-3889
Contact: Patty Owens
AIDS Prevention Centers for the HIV Antibody Testing Program

Home Health Care

Homedco Infusion
22 National Road
Triadelphia, WV 26059
Telephone: (304)-242-1938
Contact: Steve Fortunato
Nationwide experience in providing home infusion therapy to AIDS patients

Raleigh County

County Health Depts

Raleigh County Health Department
1602 Harper Road
Beckley, WV 25801
Telephone: (304)-252-8531
Contact: Yvonne Boumer
AIDS Prevention Centers for the HIV Antibody Testing Program, TB skintesting & Hepatitis screening

Randolph County

County Health Depts

Randolph County Health Department
201 Henry Avenue
Elkins, WV 26241-3892
Telephone: (304)-636-0396
Contact: Jill Dailer
AIDS Prevention Centers for the HIV Antibody Testing Program

Wood County

County Health Depts

Mid-Ohio Valley Health Department
211 Sixth Street
Parkersburg, WV 26101
Telephone: (304)-485-7374
Contact: Dixie Showalter; Bernie Kessel -
AIDS Prevention Centers for the HIV Antibody Testing Program

WISCONSIN

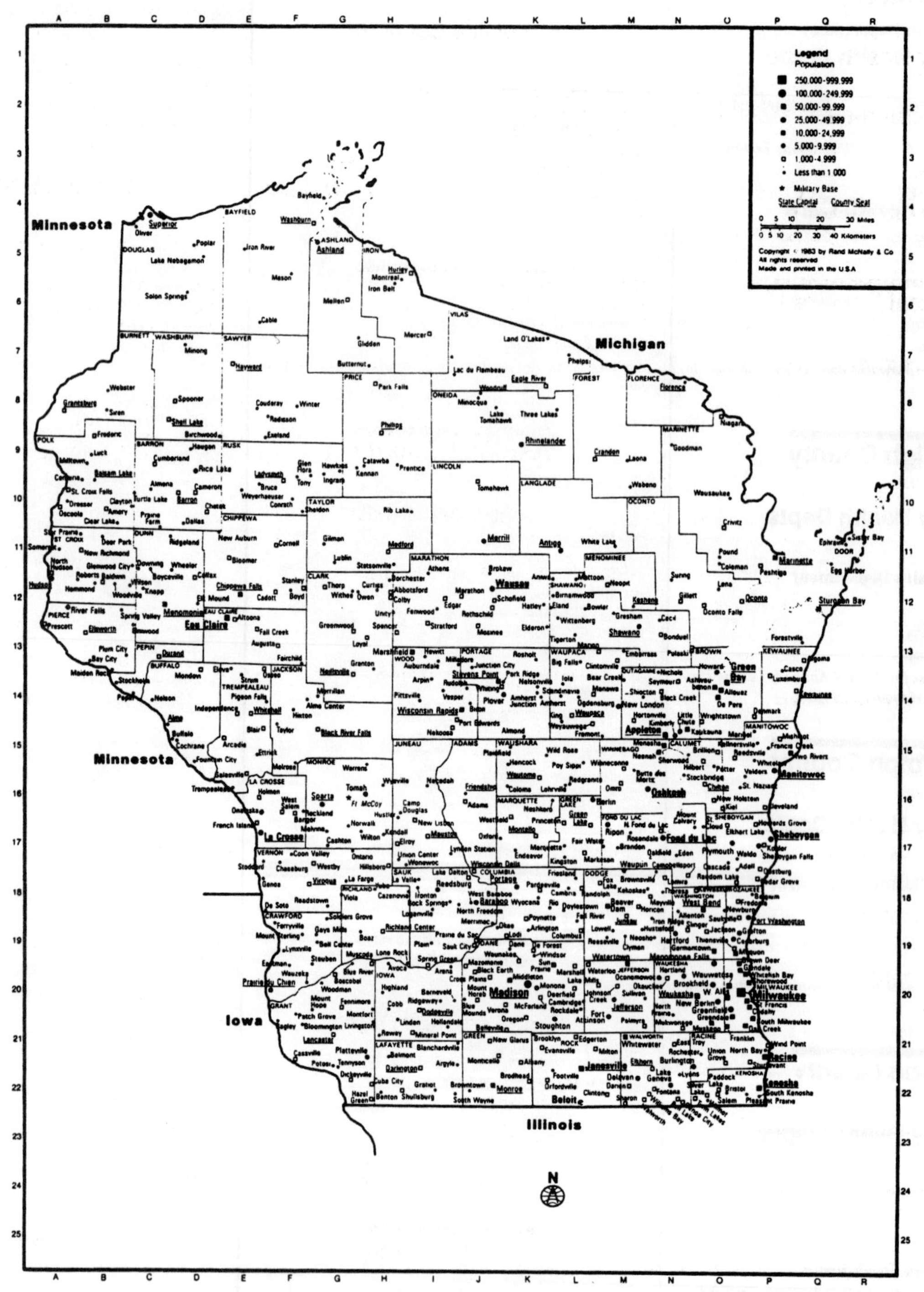

From City/County Planning Atlas Copyright 1989 by Reed McNally & Company, R.L. 90-S-28

Wisconsin

County

County Health Depts

Central Wisconsin AIDS Network - Marathon C.H.D.
1200 Lake View Drive
Wausau, WI 54403-6797
Telephone: (715)-848-9060 Fax: (715)-848-9060
Contact: Peggy Kurtzes - HIV Coordinator
Case Mgt, support group, education, free loan library

General Services

Education

Blue Bus Clinic
1552 University Avenue
Madison, WI 53705-4084
Telephone: (608)-262-7330
Contact: Tim Tillotson
Peer Educators

North Central Health Care
Out Patient Department
1100 Lakeview Drive
Wausau, WI 54401
Telephone: (715)-848-4455
Contact: Peter DeSantis
AIDS education and family planning services

Red Cross - Madison
4860 Sheboygan Avenue
Madison, WI 53705-2906
Telephone: (608)-263-9300
Contact: Margaret A. Sutinen - Program Manager
Community & industrial education, literature for hemophilia population with/without HIV

Hotlines

Milwaukee AIDS Project
P.O. Box 92505
Milwaukee, WI 53202
Telephone: (414)-273-1991
Contact: Douglas Nelson
HIV testing, counseling, legal, financial & case management

The Underground Helpline Switchboard
P.O. Box 92455
Milwaukee, WI 53202
Telephone: (414)-271-3123
A Program of Milwaukee Council on Drug Abuse. Hotline. TDD# 414-271-6039

State Health Departments

Wisconsin Department of Health & Social Services, AIDS Program
1414 East Washington Avenue
Madison, WI 53703-3041
Telephone: (608)-267-5287
Contact: James Vergeront - M.D.

Wyoming Department of Health, AIDS Education & Prevention Program
Hathaway Bldg., 4th Floor
Cheyenne, WI 82002
Telephone: (307)-777-5800
Contact: Terry Foley - Program Mgr.

Statewide Services

Great Lakes Hemophilia Foundation
8739 Watertown Plank Road
Milwaukee, WI 53226
Telephone: (414)-344-0772
Contact: Janis Hand
Information, testing and support for persons with hemophilia only.

Great Lakes Hemophilia Foundation
8739 Water Town Road
Wanwatosa, WI 53213-0217
Telephone: (414)-344-0772
Contact: Janice Hand
Provides supportive services for a variety of different audiences

Ashland County

Home Health Care

Ashland Co. Public Health Nursing
301 Ellis Avenue
Ashland, WI 54806-1629
Telephone: (715)-682-7028
Contact: Ruth Johnson - Administrator
Home health care, counseling; education, referrals

Testing Sites

Health Care Clinic
522 Chapple Avenue
Ashland, WI 54806-1417
Telephone: (715)-682-9596
Contact: Joann Zlfko
Family Planning Providers. Confidential HIV Antibody Test Site

Barron County

County Health Depts

Barron Co. Public Health Agency
1443 E. Division Ave.
Barron, WI 54812-1230
Telephone: (715)-537-6230
Contact: Kathleen Newman, R.N. - Director
HIV testing & counseling, education (confidential)

Brown County

Community Services

Alpha Home Health Agency
1600 Shawano Avenue
Green Bay, WI 54303-3246
Telephone: (414)-497-2111
Contact: Jimmy Alewine
Social services

Catholic Social Services of the Green Bay Diocese
1825 Riverside Drive
Green Bay, WI 54305-3825
Telephone: (414)-437-7531 Fax: (414)-437-0694
Contact: Paul Grimm
Support, counseling, AIDS, information, referrals

Lutheran Social Services - Green Bay
424 South Monroe Street
Green Bay, WI 54301-4401
Telephone: (414)-437-8914 Fax: (414)-437-3750
Counseling, education

Home Health Care

Caregivers Home Health Care
2626 S. Oneida Street
Green Bay, WI 54304-5302
Telephone: (414)-498-0606 Fax: (414)-498-9421
Contact: Lynn Koivisto, R.N.
Home health care

Unity Hospice
801 East Walnut Street
P.O. Box 22395
Green Bay, WI 54305-1700
Telephone: (414)-433-7470 Fax: (414)-437-1934
Contact: Donald Seibel; Sue Koller
Hospice

Medical Services

N.E.W. Community Clinic
622 Bodart Way
Green Bay, WI 54301
Telephone: (414)-437-9773
Care for uninsured

Webster Clinic SC
900 South Webster Street
Green Bay, WI 54301
Telephone: (414)-437-0431
Referrals

Testing Sites

De Pere Health Department
335 S. Broadway
De Pere, WI 54115-2526
Telephone: (414)-336-8868
Contact: Shirley Rok, R.N.
Mobile testing site, anonymous

Deckner Medical Center
1751 Deckner Avenue
Green Bay, WI 54302-2690
Telephone: (414)-468-5621
Contact: Raymond Bachhuber, M.D.
HIV testing

Buffalo County

Community Services

Buffalo Co. Dept of Human Services
Health Unit-Courthouse
407 S. 2nd Street
Alma, WI 54610
Telephone: (608)-685-4412
Nursing services, social workers, home care, medical & financial assistance

Burnett County

County Health Depts

Burnett Co. Health Services
7410 County Road K.
#114
Siren, WI 54872-9786
Telephone: (715)-349-2141
Referrals

Clark County

County Health Depts

Clark County Health Deptartment
Clark Co. Courthouse
517 Court Street
Neillsville, WI 54456
Telephone: (715)-743-3241
Contact: Allan Berrett - Director

Dane County

Community Services

Counseling/Consultation Services
905 University Avenue
Room 401
Madison, WI 53715-1005
Telephone: (608)-262-1744 Fax: (608)-265-4572
UW - Madison Students Only

Family Service
128 E Olin Ave, #100
Madison, WI 53713
Telephone: (608)-251-7611 Fax: (608)-251-4665
Individual & family counseling

Family Therapy Center of Madison
700 Rayovac Drive
Suite 220
Madison, WI 53711-2476
Telephone: (608)-276-9191
Contact: Vincent Fish, M.S.S.W.
Mental health services

Wisconsin Institute
1906 Monroe Street
Madison, WI 53711-2027
Telephone: (608)-256-6205 Fax: (608)-256-0973
Contact: Dorothy Helman, M.S.S.W.
Mental Health, psychotherapy, counseling, therapy

County Health Depts

Dane Co. Public Health Department
1206 Northport Dr.
Room 211
Madison, WI 53704-2047
Telephone: (608)-242-6520
Counseling & referrals to AIDS clinics

Madison Department of Public Health
City-County Bldg, Rm 507
210 Martin Luther King Jr
Madison, WI 53710-0001
Telephone: (608)-266-4821
HIV testing & counseling, nursing services

Home Health Care

Hospicecare Inc.
2802 Coho Street
Suite 100
Madison, WI 53713-4235
Telephone: (608)-271-5222 Fax: (608)-276-4672
Home health care and hospice

Visiting Nurse Service
128 Olin Avenue
Suite 200
Madison, WI 53713-1466
Telephone: (608)-257-6710 Fax: (608)-257-8706
Contact: Colleen Pyle
Home health care

Medical Services

Associated Physicians
4410 Regent Street
Madison, WI 53705-4994
Telephone: (608)-233-9746

Jackson Clinic
345 W. Washington Ave.
Madison, WI 53703-2720
Telephone: (608)-252-8510
Contact: Richard M. Reich, M.D.; Carl Silverman, M.D. -

Meadowood Family Physicians
5722 Raymond Road
Madison, WI 53711-4298
Telephone: (608)-271-2333
Contact: Victoria Vullrath. M.D.
General family practice

Odana Medical Center-Physicians Plus
5714 Odana Road
Madison, WI 53719-1278
Telephone: (608)-274-1100 Fax: (608)-274-1101
Contact: Richard Schmelzer, M.D.
General family practice

University Hospital & Clinics
600 Highland Avenue
Madison, WI 53792-0001
Telephone: (608)-263-7022 Fax: (608)-263-0946
Contact: Bradford S. Schwartz, M.D.
HIV/AIDS pre post testing counseling, education, prevention care

Veterans Administration
Wm. S. Middleton Hospital
2500 Overlook Terrace
Madison, WI 53705
Telephone: (608)-262-7055 Fax: (608)-262-7047
Contact: Rose Birkholz

Testing Sites

Madison Department of Public Health
2713 East Washington Ave.
Madison, WI 53704-5002
Telephone: (608)-246-4516
Contact: Mary Jo Hussey
HIV testing & counseling

Door County

Home Health Care

Door Co. Public Health Nurs Serv
421 Nebraska Street
Sturgeon Bay, WI 54235-1499
Telephone: (414)-743-5511 Fax: (414)-746-2330
Contact: Mary Lindhorst
Hospice, home care

Douglas County

Community Services

Human Resource Center
39 North 25th Street E
Superior, WI 54880-5269
Telephone: (715)-392-8216 Fax: (715)-392-6055
Contact: Shirley 'Hara M.D.; Gene Johnson, R.N. -
Mental health agency, counseling, testing

Lutheran Social Service
2231 Catlin
Superior, WI 54880-5137
Telephone: (715)-394-4173 Fax: (715)-394-9182
Contact: John Ball, M.S.W.
Counseling, referrals

County Health Depts

Douglas County Health Department
1409 Hammond Avenue
Superior, WI 54880-1674
Telephone: (715)-394-0404
Contact: Judith Walker - HHC Coordinator
HIV testing & counseling

Medical Services

Douglas County Community Health Care Clinic, Inc.
2231 Catlin Avenue
Superior, WI 54880-5137
Telephone: (715)-394-4117 Fax: (715)-394-5711
Contact: Lynda Wilsoxin - Director
Family Planning Providers. Confidential HIV Antibody Test Site

Dunn County

County Health Depts

Dunn Co. Public Health Nurs Serv
800 Wilson Ave.
Menomonie, WI 54751-2734
Telephone: (715)-232-2388
Contact: Karen Levandoski, P.H.N. - Director

Eau Claire County

Community Services

Eau Claire Department of Human Services & Social Workers
202 Eau Claire Street
Eau Claire, WI 54702-3620
Telephone: (715)-833-1977
Contact: Mike Campbell - Adult Disabilities; Neil Hovind - Income Maintenance
Social services

County Health Depts

Eau Claire City-County Health Department
720 Second Ave.
Eau Claire, WI 54703-5413
Telephone: (715)-839-4718
Contact: Jim Ryder - Director
HIV testing

Home Health Care

Combined Nursing Service
720 Second Avenue
Eau Claire, WI 54703
Telephone: (715)-839-4995 Fax: (715)-839-1674
Contact: Mary Ann Murphy, R.N.
Home nursing care

Medical Services

Family Medicine GHC
Highland Clinic
2119 Heights Drive
Eau Claire, WI 54701-3879
Telephone: (715)-836-8540
Contact: James Volk, MD
Acute care clinic

Midelfort Clinics, Ltd.
733 West Clairemont Ave
Eau Claire, WI 54701-6101
Telephone: (715)-839-5238
Contact: Phillip J. Happe, M.D. - Internist; William C. Rupp, M.D. - Oncologist-Hematologist
Treatment of infectious diseases

Florence County

Home Health Care

Florence County Nurses Office
433 Florence Ave
P.O. Box 17
Florence, WI 54121-0017
Telephone: (715)-528-4837
Contact: Karen Wertanen
Home visits, home health care

Fond Du Lac County

County Health Depts

Fond du Lac County Public Health Nursing Service
160 South Macy Street
Fond Du Lac, WI 54935-4241
Telephone: (414)-929-3085
Contact: Diane Cappozzo - R.N.
HIV Positive Support Group

Testing Sites

St. Agnes Hospital
430 East Division Street
Fond Du Lac, WI 54935-4597
Telephone: (414)-922-6531
Contact: Gayle Rosenberg, R.N.
General health-HIV testing

Forest County

Home Health Care

Forest Co. Nursing Service
Forest Co. Courthouse
Crandon, WI 54520
Telephone: (715)-478-3371
Contact: Judy Hitcock - Administrator
Home health care, education

Grant County

County Health Depts

Grant County Department of Health
Courthouse Annex
111 S. Jefferson St.
Lancaster, WI 53813
Telephone: (608)-723-6416
Contact: Linda Adrian
Hospice home nursing, personal care

Medical Services

Grant Community Clinic
235 North Madison
Lancaster, WI 53813-1349
Telephone: (608)-723-2131 Fax: (608)-723-2707
Contact: Robert M. Railey, M.D.
Family Practice

Southwest Family Planning
165 West Pine Street
Platteville, WI 53818-3145
Telephone: (608)-348-9766
Contact: Billee Bayou - Director
Family Planning Providers. Confidential HIV Antibody Test Site

Green County

County Health Depts

Green Co. Health Department
3150 Higway 81
Monroe, WI 53566
Telephone: (608)-328-9390

Iron County

County Health Depts

Iron Co. Public Health Nurs Serv
Courthouse
300 Taconite Street
Hurley, WI 54534
Telephone: (715)-561-2191
Anonymous HIV testing, counseling, referrals

Jackson County

Medical Services

Jackson Co. Public Health Nursing
227 S. 11th Street
P.O. Box 310
Black River Fls, WI 54615-0310
Telephone: (715)-284-9622
Contact: Karen Bums - Director
Personal & home care

Jefferson County

Home Health Care

Jefferson Co. Health Agency
Courthouse Rm 111
320 S. Main Street
Jefferson, WI 53549-1799
Telephone: (414)-674-7275 Fax: (414)-674-7368
Home health care

Juneau County

Medical Services

Juneau Co. Public Health Nurse
Courthouse Annex
220 Lacrosse Street
Mauston, WI 53948-9744
Telephone: (608)-847-9373
Contact: Barb Theis - Coordinator
Educational information, contact follow-up; resource center

Kenosha County

County Health Depts

County Health Department
714 52nd Street
Kenosha, WI 53140-3480
Telephone: (414)-656-8170

Contact: Esther Alexanian

Home Health Care

Olsten Kimberly Quality Care
625 57th Street
Suite 418
Kenosha, WI 53140
Telephone: (414)-886-4714
Contact: Joan Anderson
RN, LPN, home health aide, speech therapy, physical therapy, home IV,pediatric program

Medical Services

Kenosha Counseling and Psychiatric Clinic
7505 Sheridan Road
Kenosha, WI 53143-1517
Telephone: (414)-652-5555
Contact: Steve Goldberg, MSW ASCW
Counseling

Testing Sites

Planned Parenthood
618 - 55th St., Ste 1
Kenosha, WI 53140-3753
Telephone: (414)-654-0491
Contact: Mary Collins, R.N. - CA
Family Planning Providers. Confidential HIV Antibody Test Site

Kewaunee County

Medical Services

Kewaunee Co. Public Health Department
510 Kilbourn Street
Kewaunee, WI 54216-1344
Telephone: (414)-388-4410
Contact: Kaye Shillin - Administrative Assistant
Communicable disease follow-up

La Crosse County

Community Services

Family and Childrens Center
1707 Main Street
La Crosse, WI 54601-6897
Telephone: (608)-785-0001
Mental health, counseling, education

Human Development Association
110 North 17th Street
3rd floor
La Crosse, WI 54601
Telephone: (608)-784-8688
Contact: Pat B. Richgels, M.S.S.W
Outpatient counseling

Lutheran Social Services
2350 South Avenue
La Crosse, WI 54601-6292
Telephone: (608)-788-5090 Fax: (608)-788-6623
Contact: Paul Ranum, M.S.W.
Counseling

Riverdale Clinic
128 South 6th Street
La Crosse, WI 54601-4104
Telephone: (608)-782-0704 Fax: (608)-782-0702
Financial counseling, therapy

County Health Depts

La Crosse Co. Health Department
County Office Building
300 North 4th Street
La Crosse, WI 54601
Telephone: (608)-785-9723
Contact: Al Graewin
Case management, educational services, counseling & testing, Ryan White Fund

Medical Services

Coulee Region Family Planning Center
312 State Street
La Crosse, WI 54601-3222
Telephone: (608)-784-5730
AIDS testing & counseling

Gunderson Clinic
1836 South Avenue
Guderson
La Crosse, WI 54601-5429
Telephone: (608)-782-7300 Fax: (608)-782-7343
Contact: William Agger, M.D.; James Glasser, M.D.; William Morgan, M.D.
General family practice; testing

Skemp Clinic
800 West Avenue South
La Crosse, WI 54601-8806
Telephone: (608)-782-9760 Fax: (608)-782-9898
Contact: Dr. Micheal O'Brien
Urgent care clinic: supportive care, pre-post HIV, education, medical care.

St. Francis Medical Center
700 West Avenue South
La Crosse, WI 54601-4783
Telephone: (608)-785-0940 Fax: (608)-791-9548
Counseling, outpatient, HIV testing

University of Wisconsin - La Crosse
Student Health Services
1725 State Street
La Crosse, WI 54601
Telephone: (608)-785-8559
Contact: Peggy Agger
Education, testing (pre & post), referral, medical clinic, outpatient(University students only)

Lafayette County

Home Health Care

Lafayette Co. Community Health Nursing Agency
740 East Street
P.O. Box 118
Darlington, WI 53530-0118
Telephone: (608)-776-4895
Contact: Mary Oechslin
Home health care

Langlade County

Home Health Care

Langlade County Public Health Nursing Service
1225 Langlade Road
Antigo, WI 54409-2762
Telephone: (715)-627-6250 Fax: (715)-627-6295
Contact: Pat Galarowicz
Home health care

Lincoln County

Home Health Care

Lincoln Co. Nursing Service
1106 E. 8th Street
Merrill, WI 54452-1199
Telephone: (715)-536-0307
Contact: Greta Rusch
Home health care, public health

Manitowoc County

Community Services

Family Service Association of Manitowoc County
1228 South ninth Street
Manitowoc, WI 54220-5047
Telephone: (414)-682-8869
Contact: Tom Aronson
Home Health Counseling

Lutheran Social Services-Manitowoc
721 Park Street
Manitowoc, WI 54220-3947
Telephone: (414)-682-3332
Contact: Rev. James McClurg
Counseling

Medical Services

Two Rivers Clinic, Ltd.
2219 Garfield Street
Two Rivers, WI 54241-2498
Telephone: (414)-793-2281 Fax: (414)-793-3669
Referral, medical services for HIV+

Testing Sites

Manitowoc Co. Public Health Nursing
823 Washington Street
Manitowoc, WI 54220-4528
Telephone: (414)-683-4155
Contact: Kerri Arrievedo
Anonymous testing, case management, referrals, education

Marathon County

Medical Services

Family Planning Health Services, Inc.
908 Grand Avenue
Schofield, WI 54476-1120
Telephone: (715)-359-8300 Fax: (715)-359-8301
Contact: Lon Newman - Director

Family Planning Providers. Confidential HIV Antibody Test Site

Marinette County

Medical Services

Marinette-Menominee Clinic
1510 Main Street
Marinette, WI 54143-1397
Telephone: (715)-735-7421
Contact: Willi Martens, M.D.
Referrals, counseling, HIV testing, confidential pre/post counseling

Milwaukee County

Community Services

Family Service America
11700 West Lake Park Drive
Milwaulkee, WI 53224
Telephone: (414)-359-1040 Fax: (414)-359-1074
Toll-Free: (800)-221-2681
HIV referrals

Milwaukee AIDS Project (MAP)
315 W. Court Street
PO Box 92505
Milwaukee, WI 53202
Telephone: (414)-273-1991 Fax: (414)-273-2357
Contact: Douglas Nelson - Executive Director
Provides supportive services for AIDS patients

United Migrant Opportunity Services, Inc.
929 West Mitchell Street
PO Box 04129
Milwaukee, WI 53204-4129
Telephone: (414)-671-5700 Fax: (414)-671-4833
Contact: Mary Ann Borman
Minority services under grant AIDS education and counseling

County Health Depts

Brown Deer Health Department
4800 W. Green Brook Dr.
Brown Deer, WI 53223-2406
Telephone: (414)-357-0138

Cudahy Health Department
5050 S. Lake Dr.
Cudahy, WI 53110-1744
Telephone: (414)-769-2239
Home visits

South Milwaukee Health Department
2424 Fifteenth Ave
South Milwaukee, WI 53172-2499
Telephone: (414)-764-5060 Fax: (414)-762-3272
Contact: Marcia Meilicke - Administrator
Home visits, education

Wauwatosa Health Department
7725 W. North Ave.
P.O. Box 13068
Wauwatosa, WI 53213-0068
Telephone: (414)-471-8400 Fax: (414)-471-8414
Contact: Kathy Scott - Administrator
Home visits, education services

West Alice Health Department
7120 West National Avenue
West Alice, WI 53214-3517
Telephone: (414)-645-1822
Contact: Rita Lichterman - Administrator
STD anonymous testing (HIV)

Home Health Care

Visiting Nurse Association of Milwaukee
11333 West National Ave
Milwaukee, WI 53227
Telephone: (414)-327-2295
Home health care

Medical Services

Brady East STD Clinic
1240 East Brady Street
Milwaukee, WI 53202-1603
Telephone: (414)-272-2144
Contact: Robert Ambelang
HIV Positive Support Group

East Side Community Clinic
Suite 608
2266 North Prospect
Milwaukee, WI 53202
Telephone: (414)-278-0955
Contact: Randy Ness
Group counseling, referrals, research

Glendale Health Department
5909 N. Milwaukee Rv Pkwy
Glendale, WI 53209
Telephone: (414)-228-1704
Contact: Jane Lyne
Referrals, counseling

Greendale Health Department
6500 Northway
P.O. Box 257
Greendale, WI 53129-1815
Telephone: (414)-423-2100
Contact: Joan Lietz
Referrals

Harwood Medical Associates
7400 Harwood Avenue
Milwaukee, WI 53213-2655
Telephone: (414)-771-8228 Fax: (414)-771-1095

Issac Coggs Clinic
2779 North 5th Street
Milwaukee, WI 53212-2325
Telephone: (414)-226-8880 Fax: (414)-278-3887
Contact: Roy Troutman, M.D.
Mental health, phsychiatrist

Marquette University
Student Health Services
Schroeder Complex
Milwaukee, WI 53233
Telephone: (414)-288-7184 Fax: (414)-288-5681
Contact: Julie Jagemann, M.D.
General health for Marquette University students only.

Marquette University Dental School
604 North 16th Street
Milwaukee, WI 53233-2188
Telephone: (414)-288-6790
Contact: Kenneth Zakariasen, DDS
Dental service including AIDS

Medical Complex
P.O. Box 117
Milwaukee, WI 53226-0117
Telephone: (414)-257-6151 Fax: (414)-257-7801
Toll-Free: (800)-472-3660
Contact: Dr. Peter Sohnle

Residential Treatment Center
2105 North Booth Street
Milwaukee, WI 53212-3400
Telephone: (414)-264-4481 Fax: (414)-263-4188
Contact: Kathy Bryant
HIV Testing

Sixteenth Street Community Clinic
1036 South 16th Street
Milwaukee, WI 53204-2203
Telephone: (414)-672-1353
Contact: Isle Soriano

STD Specialties Clinic, Inc.
3251 N. Holton Street
Milwaukee, WI 53212-2126
Telephone: (414)-264-8800
Contact: Douglas Johnson
Anonymous HIV Counseling and Testing Site

Testing Sites

John L. Doyne Hospital
P.O. Box 117
8700 W. Wisconsin Ave.
Milwaukee, WI 53226-0117
Telephone: (414)-257-5684
Contact: Dr. Barry Biernstein
HIV testing, treatment center

Milwaukee Medical Clinic
3003 West Good Hope Road
Milwaukee, WI 53217
Telephone: (414)-352-3100
Contact: Karen Maclay
HIV testing, therapy

South Side Health Center
1640 South 24th Street
Milwaukee, WI 53204-2507
Telephone: (414)-286-8620 Fax: (414)-286-5480
Anonymous HIV Counseling and Testing Site

West Allis Health Department
7120 W. National Ave.
West Allis, WI 53214-4774
Telephone: (414)-256-8400
Contact: Terry Brandenburg
HIV anonymous testing, home visits for high risk mothers

Oconto County

Testing Sites

NEWCAP, Inc.
Family Planning Program
1201 Main Street
Oconto, WI 54153
Telephone: (414)-834-4621 Fax: (414)-834-4887
Contact: Sharon Fellion
Family Planning Providers. Confidential HIV Antibody Test Site

Oneida County

County Health Depts

Oneida County Health Department
Courthouse
P.O. Box 400
Rhinelander, WI 54501-0400
Telephone: (715)-369-6111
Contact: Kathryn Sutliff, R.N.

Medical Services

Psychological Associates
203 Schiek Plaza
Rhinelander, WI 54501-3450
Telephone: (715)-362-5150 Fax: (715)-362-1254
Contact: Mike Galli, Ph.D.; Gina Koeppl, Ph.D.; Robert Spensberg, A.C.S.W.
Mental health

Outagamie County

Community Services

Outagamie Co. Dept of Human Service
Courthouse
410 S. Walnut Street
Appleton, WI 54911-5936
Telephone: (414)-832-5100
Contact: Virginia Betley
Referrals to hotline, home care

St. Elizabeth Hospital
1506 South Oneida
Appleton, WI 54915
Telephone: (800)-223-7332
Contact: Sue Fritz; Jackie Kobierecki
Fox Valley AIDS Project, staff education, referrals

Home Health Care

Outagamie County Public Health Services
410 South Walnut
Appleton, WI 54911
Telephone: (414)-735-5100
Contact: Virginia Betley, R.N.
Counseling, home health care visits

Visiting Nurses Association of Appleton
2003 N Meade Street
Appleton, WI 54911-3110
Telephone: (414)-733-8562
Contact: Sue Kostka, R.N.
Home health care & hospice

Testing Sites

Appleton Family Health Center
229 S. Morrison
Appleton, WI 54911
Telephone: (414)-832-2783
Contact: Robert Garrett, M.D.
HIV testing

Fox Valley AIDS Project
120 N. Morrison Street
#201
Appleton, WI 54911-5472
Telephone: (414)-733-7950
HIV testing, education, case management

Planned Parenthood - Appleton
508 West Wisconsin Ave
Appleton, WI 54911-4358
Telephone: (414)-731-6304
Contact: Jean Nolan
HIV testing

Ozaukee County

County Health Depts

Ozaukee Co. Public Health Department
Administration Building Room 246
121 W. Main St, P.O. Box 994
Port Washington, WI 53074-0994
Telephone: (414)-284-9411
Contact: Caroline Voss - Director
Home care, physical therapy

Pepin County

County Health Depts

Pepin Co. Nursing Service
740 Seventh Avenue West
P.O. Box 39
Durand, WI 54736-0039
Telephone: (715)-672-5961
Contact: Sharon Prissel
Home care, referrals

Pierce County

Home Health Care

Pierce Co. Community Health Services
412 West Kinne
P.O. Box 238
Ellsworth, WI 54011-0238
Telephone: (715)-273-3531
Contact: Raymond Cink - Director
Skilled nursing, home health aide

Polk County

County Health Depts

Polk Co. Public Health Nurs Serv
300 Polk County Plaza
P.O. Box 545
Balsam Lake, WI 54810
Telephone: (715)-485-3938
Contact: Beverly Larson, R.N., M.P.H. - Director
Home care, HIV testing

Portage County

Medical Services

Plover Family Practice
2831 Post Road
Plover, WI 54467
Telephone: (715)-345-0990 Fax: (715)-345-2099
Contact: Steven Bahrke, M.D.; Peter Sanderson, M.D.

Rice Clinic
2501 Main
Stevens Point, WI 54481-4098
Telephone: (715)-344-4120
Contact: Steve Bergin, M.D. - Ob-Gyn; William Jean, M.D. - Internal Medicine; Egbert Kamstra, M.D. - Psychiatrist
Obstetrics & gynecology

University of Wisconsin-Stevens Point
Student Health Service
Delzell Hall
Stevens Point, WI 54481
Telephone: (715)-346-4646
Contact: John Betinis, M.D.; Jim Zach, M.D.
Medical care available to UWSP students only

Racine County

Community Services

Crossroads Consultants
3308 Washington Avenue
Racine, WI 53405-3039
Telephone: (414)-632-2420
Contact: Mary Tampsett
Outpatient clinic, support, counseling, groups

Lutheran Social Services
2711 - 19th Street
Racine, WI 53403-2330
Telephone: (414)-637-3886 Fax: (414)-637-9080
Contact: Dr. Virginia Thome
Counseling

County Health Depts

Racine Health Department
730 Washington Avenue
Racine, WI 53403-1184
Telephone: (414)-636-9498
Contact: Michele Breheim
Testing, counseling & referrals

Town of Norway Health Care Provider
156 East State Road
Burlington, WI 53105
Telephone: (414)-895-6335
Contact: Sheryl Mazmanin

Village of Waterford Health Officer
228-C N. Milwaukee Ave.
Waterford, WI 53185-4312
Telephone: (414)-534-4100

Home Health Care

Daily Nursing Service, Inc.
4000 Spring Street
Racine, WI 53405-1691
Telephone: (414)-633-9444
Contact: Debra Lass, R.N.
Home health care & hospice

Olsten Kimberly Quality Care
1300 South Green Bay Road
Suite 205
Racine, WI 53406
Telephone: (414)-886-0606
Contact: Laura Mesenbrink
Skilled nursing, homemaker assistance

Visiting Nurses Association & Hospice of Racine
4000 Spring St.
P.O. Box 4045
Racine, WI 53404
Telephone: (414)-633-9444 Fax: (414)-635-7598
Contact: Vicki Taylor - Director of Clinical Services
Skilled nursing care, therapy, social & chaplain services

Medical Services

Southeastern Wisconsin Medical & Social Services, Inc.
1055 Prairie Drive
Racine, WI 53406-3971
Telephone: (414)-886-6575 Fax: (414)-886-6875
Toll-Free: (800)-832-2286
Contact: Joyce S. Degenhart, PhD
Mental health

Westwind Treatment Center
P.O. Box 081098
Racine, WI 53408-1098
Telephone: (414)-886-9020 Fax: (414)-886-7567
Toll-Free: (800)-252-8973
Contact: Dan Wrensch, PA-C - Intake Dept.
Inpatient/residential & outpatient drug & alcohol abuse program

Testing Sites

City of Racine Health Department
City Hall
730 Washington Ave.
Racine, WI 53403
Telephone: (414)-636-9498
Contact: Michele Breheim - Epidemiologist
HIV testing & counseling; partner, referrals to other providers

Richland County

County Health Depts

Richland Co. Health Center
Courthouse
P.O. Box 404
Richland Center, WI 53581
Telephone: (608)-647-2166
Contact: Maryanne Stanek

Rock County

Community Services

Janesville Counseling Center
3506 Hwy 51 North
Janesville, WI 53545-0351
Telephone: (608)-757-5215 Fax: (608)-757-5010
Contact: George M. Kerbs, PhD

Home Health Care

Credible Care, Inc.
2004 West Court Street
Janesville, WI 53545-3470
Telephone: (608)-755-0592
Home health care

Janesville Visiting Nurses Association
20 East Court Street
Janesville, WI 53545-3919
Telephone: (608)-754-2201 Fax: (608)-754-1147
Contact: Bonnie Brikowski; Jessica Cooper -
Therapy-counseling-education

Testing Sites

Beloit Stateline Clinic
1430 4th Street
Beloit, WI 53511-4442
Telephone: (608)-364-6630
Contact: Maureen Churchill, PHN
Anonymous HIV counseling and testing site, educational programs

Saint Croix County

County Health Depts

St. Croix Co. Human Serv-Public Health
1445 North 4th Street
New Richmond, WI 54017-6004
Telephone: (715)-243-8181
Contact: Kris Ylikopsa, R.N.
HIV testing, counseling, education

Sauk County

County Health Depts

Sauk Co. Public Health Nurs Service Commission
515 Oak Street
Baraboo, WI 53913
Telephone: (608)-356-5581
Contact: Carol Jeffers

Sawyer County

Home Health Care

Sawyer Co. Public Health Agency
109 E. Fifth St.
P.O. Box 528
Hayward, WI 54843-0528
Telephone: (715)-634-4874 Fax: (715)-634-3580
Contact: Della Schuck, R.N., B.S.N. - Director
Public & home health care

Taylor County

Home Health Care

Taylor Co. Nursing Service
Courthouse G50
224 S. Second St.
Medford, WI 54451-1899
Telephone: (715)-748-1410 Fax: (715)-748-1415
Contact: Patricia Krut RN
Homecare, infusion therapy, chemotherapy

Trempealeau County

Home Health Care

Trempealeau Co. Public Health Nurs Serv
Courthouse
PO Box 67
Whitehall, WI 54773-0067
Telephone: (715)-538-2311
Home care, public health, HIV testing

Vernon County

County Health Depts

Vernon Co. Health Services
R. 3, Co. BB
P.O. Box 209
Viroqua, WI 54665-0209
Telephone: (608)-637-2233
Contact: Elizabeth Johnson
AIDS referrals, education

Vilas County

County Health Depts

Vilas County Public Health
Courthouse
P.O. Box 369
Eagle River, WI 54521
Telephone: (715)-479-3656
AIDS education-referrals

Walworth County

Medical Services

Walworth Co. Public Health Nurse
W3929 County Road NN
P.O. Box 1002
Elkhorn, WI 53121
Telephone: (414)-741-3140

Washburn County

Home Health Care

Washburn Co. Nursing Agency
222 Oak Street
Spooner, WI 54801-1493
Telephone: (715)-635-7616
Contact: Billie LaBumbard - Director
HIV testing & counseling, home care

Washington County

Home Health Care

Washington Co. Community Health Nursing
333 East Washingotn Street
Suite 1100

West Bend, WI 53095-7986
Telephone: (414)-338-4462
Home care, nursing

Testing Sites

Planned Parenthood
2361 West Washington
West Bend, WI 53095-2144
Telephone: (414)-338-1303
Contact: Wendie Winkler
Family Planning Providers. Confidential HIV Antibody Test Site

Waukesha County

County Health Depts

Waukesha Co. Department of Health
325 E. Broadway
Waukesha, WI 53186-5079
Telephone: (414)-549-3012
HIV testing & counseling, infectious disease clinic

Home Health Care

Caremark Connection Network
17012 West Victor Road
New Berlin, WI 53151-4137
Telephone: (414)-785-9318 Fax: (414)-785-0484
Contact: Michael Taylor - Branch Manager
Clinical Support and Infusion Therapies: Nutrition, Antimicrobials, Chemo.,Hematopoe

Visiting Nurse Assoc. of the Greater Waukesha Area
419 Fredrick Street
Waukesha, WI 53186-5605
Telephone: (414)-542-0724
Home care & hospice

Medical Services

Medical Associates
W 180 N 7950 Town Hall Rd
Menomonee Falls, WI 53051
Telephone: (414)-255-2500 Fax: (414)-255-2434
Contact: Michael P. Dailey, M.D.
General clinic

Women and Family Psychotherapy Resources
707 West Moreland Blvd
Suite 7
Waukesha, WI 53188-2400
Telephone: (414)-542-0123 Fax: (414)-542-1199
Contact: Ramona Powers
Out-patient

Waupaca County

County Health Depts

Waupaca Co. Department of Human Serv/Health Serv Division
811 Harding St. #Bldg
Waupaca, WI 54981-2087
Telephone: (715)-258-6300
Home care

Home Health Care

Alpha Home Care Agency
112 South Main Street
Suite 2
Waupaca, WI 54981
Telephone: (715)-258-2130
Contact: Marlys Meier
Home helath care & hospice

Waushara County

County Health Depts

Waushara Co. Health Service
230 West Park Street
P.O. Box 837
Wautoma, WI 54982
Telephone: (414)-787-4661

Winnebago County

Community Services

Lutheran Social Services
420 South Koeller
Suite 208
OshKosh, WI 54901-4958
Telephone: (414)-235-4307 Fax: (414)-235-7853
Contact: Audrey Aardappel
Counseling

Neenah-Catholic Social Services
201 Ceape Avenue
Oshkosh, WI 54901-5066
Telephone: (414)-235-6002
Contact: Daniel Lange
Counseling

County Health Depts

Neenah Department of Public Health
211 Walnut Street
P.O. Box 426
Neenah, WI 54957-0426
Telephone: (414)-751-4650 Fax: (414)-751-4640

Oshkosh Health Department
215 Church Ave.
P.O. Box 1130
Oshkosh, WI 54902-4747
Telephone: (414)-236-5030
Communicable disease follow ups

Preferred Home Health Care
36 Jewelers Park Drive
Suite 120
Neenah, WI 54956-3000
Telephone: (414)-325-4326 Fax: (414)-725-1146
Contact: Wendy Marquardt; Olivia Desmond
Home care services

Winnebago County Public Health Dept.
725 Butler Avenue
Winnebago, WI 54985-9999
Telephone: (414)-235-5100
Contact: Kathy Lloyd
HIV Positive Parent Support Groups

Home Health Care

Neenah-Menasha Visiting Nurses Association
406 E. Wisconsin Avenue
Neenah, WI 54956-2965
Telephone: (414)-727-5555
Contact: Judy Eberhardy
Home health care & hospice

Supportive Home Care
704 North Main
Oshkosh, WI 54901-4445
Telephone: (414)-426-1931
Contact: Diane Schmude
Home health service

Winnebago County Public Health Nurses
725 Butler Avenue
Winnebago, WI 54985
Telephone: (414)-235-5100

Medical Services

University of Wisconsin-Oshkosh
Student Health Services
777 Algoma Boulevard
Oshkosh, WI 54901
Telephone: (414)-424-2424 Fax: (414)-424-7317
Contact: Penny McElroy
Student health care

Testing Sites

Nicolet Clinic
411 Lincoln Street
Neenah, WI 54956
Telephone: (414)-727-4425 Fax: (414)-727-2743
Contact: F.L. Hildebrand, M.D.
Counseling, HIV testing

Wood County

County Health Depts

Wood County Health Department Annex
604 East Fourth Street
Marshfield, WI 54449-4868
Telephone: (715)-387-8646
Contact: Ann Reusch, R.N., B.S.N.

Home Health Care

Caremark Connection Network
611 St Joseph Avenue
South Wing
Marshfield, WI 54449-1832
Telephone: (715)-387-0755 Fax: (715)-387-0345
Contact: Judy Geil - General Manager
Clinical Support and Infusion Therapies: Nutrition, Antimicrobials, Chemo.,Hematopoe

Health Care at Home
4011 8th St South
Wisconsin Rapids, WI 54494-7827
Telephone: (715)-421-2323
Contact: Darcy Stephens, RN
Home care, speakers

Medical Services

Marshfield Clinic
1000 North Oak
Marshfield, WI 54449-5772
Telephone: (715)-387-5511
Contact: Bruce M. Hathaway, M.D.
Referrals, staff education

WYOMING

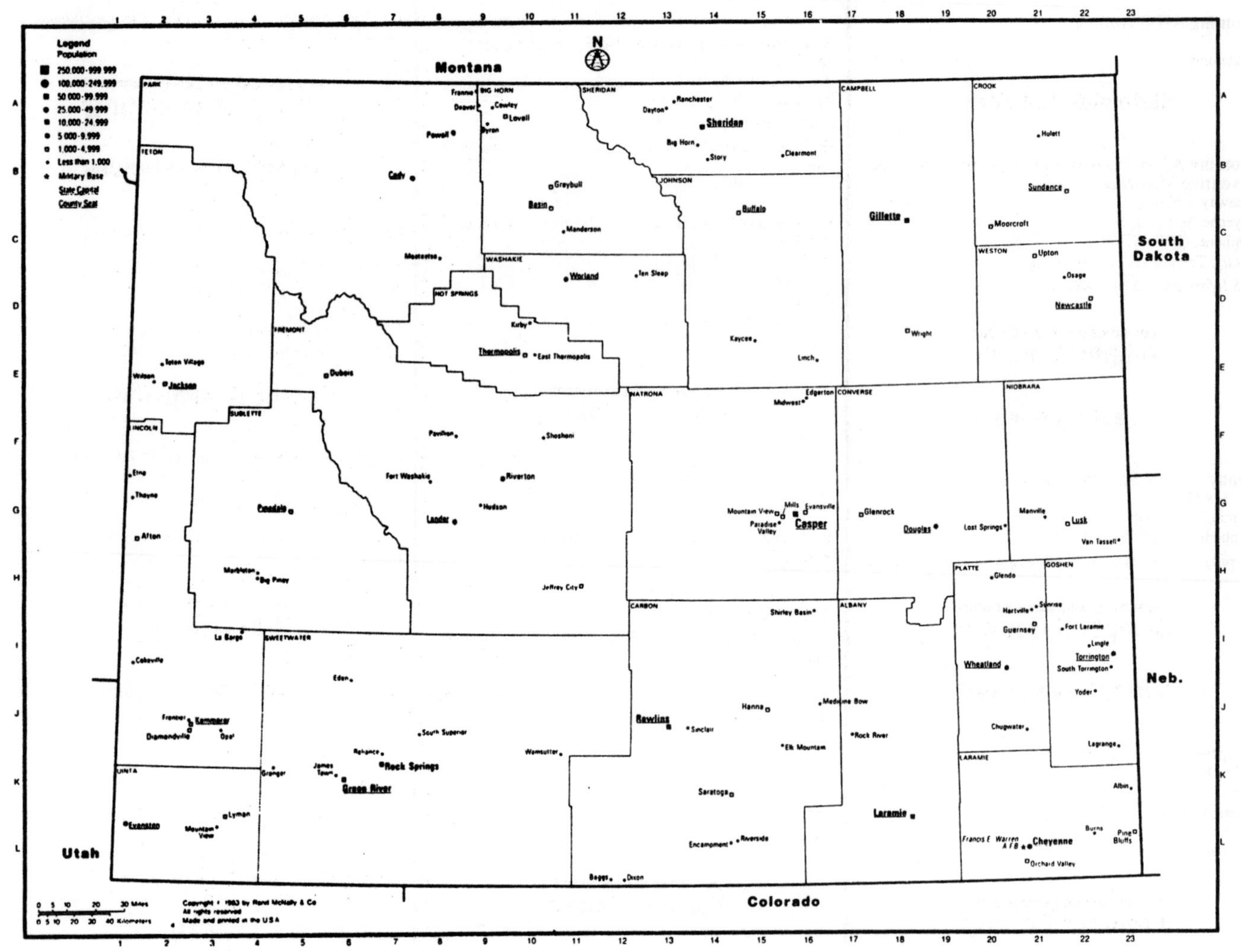

From City/County Planning Atlas Copyright 1989 by Reed McNally & Company, R.L. 90-S-28

Wyoming

General Services

Hotlines

Wyoming AIDS Hotline

In state only (800)-327-3577

Statewide Services

Wyoming AIDS Prevention Program/Division of Preventive Medicine
Hathaway Building
Cheyenne, WY 82002
Telephone: (307)-777-5800
Contact: Terry Foley - Program Mgr.
AIDS Information & Resource Referrals

Albany County

Testing Sites

Albany County Family Planning
P.O. Box 1145
Laramie, WY 82070
Telephone: (307)-745-5364
Wyoming Counseling & Testing Site/Appointment Requested

Campbell County

County Health Depts

Campbell County Public Health
416 W. Juniper Lane
PO Box 3420
Gillette, WY 82716-5341
Telephone: (307)-682-7275
Counseling & Testing Site Information/Appointment Only

Fremont County

County Health Depts

Fremont County Public Health
County Courthouse, #203
450 N 2nd Street
Lander, WY 82520
Telephone: (307)-332-2573
Wyoming Counseling and Testing Site/Appointment Required

Fremont County Public Health
County Office Center
818 South Federal
Riverton, WY 82501
Telephone: (307)-857-3620
Wyoming Counseling and Testing Site/Appointment Required

Medical Services

PHS Indian Health Center
Bldg 29, Washakie Street
Ft Washakie, WY 82514
Telephone: (307)-332-9416
Contact: Bob Sivert - AIDS Coordinator

Testing Sites

Arapahoe Health Facility/Native Americans
14 Great Plains Road
Arapahoe, WY 82510
Telephone: (307)-856-9281
Contact: Robert Sivret, RN
Wyoming Counseling and Testing Site/Appointment Required

Ft. Washakie Health Facility/Native Americans
Box 128
Ft. Washakie, WY 82514-0128
Telephone: (307)-332-7300
Contact: Robert Sivert, RN
Wyoming Counseling and Testing Site/Appointment Required

Laramie County

Testing Sites

Pathfinder, Inc./Cheyenne Community Drug Abuse Treatment
803 W. 21st Street
Cheyenne, WY 82001-3413
Telephone: (307)-635-0256
Wyoming Counseling and Testing Site/Appointment Required

Veterans Administration/Cheyenne/AIDS Prevention Program
V.A. Medical Center
2360 E Pershing
Cheyenne, WY 82001-0001
Telephone: (307)-778-7550
Medical, counseling, and testing services

Natrona County

County Health Depts

Natrona County Health Department
1200 E. 3rd Street
Casper, WY 82601-2990
Telephone: (307)-235-9280
Wyoming Counseling and Testing Site/Appointment Required

Home Health Care

Continue Care of Wyoming
111 S. Jefferson
Suite 120
Casper, WY 82601
Telephone: (307)-577-7112
Contact: Chris Tice
Home Infusion Therapy, In-home Nursing and Attendant Care, PhysicalTherapy, Pentamidine, Pharmacy

Sheridan County

County Health Depts

Sheridan County Community Health Service
41 W. Whitney
Sheridan, WY 82801-4742
Telephone: (307)-672-9791
Wyoming Counseling and Testing Site/Appointment Required

Sweetwater County

Community Services

Sweetwater County AIDS Corps Groups
PO Box 956
Memorial Hospital
Rock Springs, WY 82902-0956
Telephone: (307)-362-3711
Contact: Nancy Hickerson
AIDS Information & Resource Referrals

County Health Depts

Sweetwater County Community Nursing Service
731 C Street
Rock Springs, WY 82901-6202
Telephone: (307)-362-7423
Wyoming Counseling and Testing Site/Appointment Required

Uinta County

Home Health Care

Uinta County Rehabilitation Center
350 City View Drive
Suite 303
Evanston, WY 82930-5327
Telephone: (307)-789-3710

Human Resources & Training Administration-Education-Training

AIDS Education and Training Center for Southern CA
University of Southern CA
1975 Zonal Avenue KAM200
Los Angeles, CA 90033
Telephone: (213)-342-1846 Fax: (213)-342-2051
Contact: Dr. Jerry Gates

AIDS Education and Training Center for Texas and Oklahoma
University of Texas
P.O. Box 20186
Houston, TX 77225
Telephone: (713)-794-4705
Contact: Dr. Richard M. Grimes, PhD
Oklahoma, Texas

AIDS ETC Program
Bureau of Health Prof.
Fishers Lane,Rm 4C-03
Rockville, MD 20857
Telephone: (301)-443-6364 Fax:301-443-8890
Primary care provider throughout U.S.

AIDS Program
Boston Public Health Department
1010 Massachusetts Avenue
Boston, MA 02118
Telephone: (617)-534-4559 Fax: (617)-534-5358
Contact: Jack Vondras - Director

AIDS Program Office
600 S. Commonwealth
6th Floor
Los Angeles, CA 90005
Telephone: (213)-351-8000 Fax: (213)-738-0825
Contact: John Schunoff
Referrals, counseling, training, education

Board of Commissioners of Fulton County
County Government Center
141 Pryor Street, 10th Floor
Atlanta, GA 30303
Telephone: (404)-730-8239
Contact: Michael Lomax - Chairman
Atlanta/Fulton County

Chicago Department of Health
333 South State Street
Room 200
Chicago, IL 60604
Telephone: (312)-747-9430 Fax: (312)-747-9694
Contact: Erica Salem - Assistant Director for Program; - Development
HIV primary care, mental health services, case management

Contra Costa County AIDS Program
Suite 200
597 Center Avenue
Martinez, CA 94553
Telephone: (510)-313-6770
Oakland/Alameda County

Dallas County Department of Human Services, STD Clinic
4917 Harry Hines Boulevard
Dallas, TX 75235
Telephone: (214)-920-7845
Contact: Jon R. Cameron

Delta Region AIDS Education and Training Center
Louisiana State Univ.
1542 Tulane Avenue
New Orleans, LA 70112
Telephone: (504)-568-3855 Fax: (504)-568-7893
Toll-Free: (800)-548-4659
Contact: Dr. William R. Brandon, MD - Project Director
HIV/AIDS training for health care providers

District of Columbia AIDS ETC
Howard Univ Hosp, Med Dept.
2112 Georgia Ave. NW
Washington, DC 20060
Telephone: (202)-865-6249
Contact: Margaret Kadree, MD Fax:202-865-1983
Training, for home care professionals in care of AIDS/HIV patients;research materials

East Central AIDS Education & Training Center
Area 300 Research Center
1314 Kinnear Rd
Columbus, OH 43212
Telephone: (614)-292-1400
Contact: James A. Pearsol
AIDS education and training

Emory AIDS Training Network
Emory University
735 Gatewood Road NE
Atlanta, GA 30322
Telephone: (404)-727-2929 Fax: (404)-727-4562
Contact: Ira Schwartz, MD
Alabama, Georgia, North Carolina, South Carolina: AIDS/HIV trainingfor health providers

HIV Planning & Management Organization
150 West Flagler Street
Suite 2650
Miami, FL 33130
Telephone: (305)-374-8422
Contact: Juan Kourt - Executive Director
Technical assistance for providers, funded by Ryan White Title I

Mid-Atlantic AIDS Education and Training Center
Med College of Virginia
PO Box 49, MCV Station
Richmond, VA 23298-0049
Telephone: (804)-786-2210 Fax: (804)-371-0495
Contact: Lisa Kaplowitz, MD
Training for health care providers

Medicaid AIDS Coordinator

Casey Jones
75 Hawthorne Street
5th Floor
San Francisco, CA 94105
Telephone: (415)-744-3600 Fax: (415)-744-3761

Dept. of Health & Human Services, Health Care Financing Administration
101 Marietta Street
Suite 602
Atlanta, GA 30323
Telephone: (404)-331-0070
Contact: Michael McDaniel
Administers Medicaid program

Health Care Financing Administration, Region VII
601 East 12th Street
Room 227
Kansas City, MO 64106
Telephone: (816)-426-6477
Contact: Toni Cordry
Identify state needs for technical assistance, encourage state outreachactivities, protect Medicaid rights of HIV+ persons

Health Financing Administration
1200 Main Tower
Room 2000
Dallas, TX 75202
Telephone: (214)-767-3693
Contact: Jack Ashcraft - HIV Coord.
Administers Medicaid program for Arkansas, Texas, Oklahoma, Louisiana andNew Mexico

Jack Ashcraft
1200 Main Tower
Dallas, TX 75202
Telephone: (816)-426-6477

Janice Cekan
105 W. Adams Street
Chicago, IL 60603
Telephone: (312)-353-1670

Liz Trias
2201 6th Avenue
Mailstop RX-43
Seattle, WA 98121
Telephone: (206)-615-2340

Michael McDaniel
101 Marietta Street
Atlanta, GA 30323
Telephone: (404)-730-2733

Sarah Taylor-Charvis
JFK Federal Bldg.
Room 2375
Boston, MA 02203
Telephone: (617)-565-1198

Stephen Blake
1961 Stout Street
Room 1185
Denver, CO 80294-3538
Telephone: (303)-844-6216 Fax: (303)-844-3753

Steve Shaw
26 Federal Plaza
Room 38-130
New York, NY 10278
Telephone: (212)-264-2775

Theresa Rubin
PO Box 7760
Philadelphia, PA 19101
Telephone: (215)-596-1300

Toni Coudry
601 East 12th Street
Room 227
Kansas City, MO 64106
Telephone: (816)-426-6477 Fax: (816)-426-3851

Pediatric/Family Projects

AIDS Institute, Pediatric HIV/AIDS Comprehensive Center
Empire State Plaza, Tower Bldg.
Room 321
Albany, NY 12237
Telephone: (518)-473-8427
Contact: Gloria C. Maki - Ph.D.
Primary care, AIDS drug assistance program

Albert Einstein College of Medicine, Bronx Pediatric AIDS Consortium
B-PAC
1300 Morris Park Avenue
Bronx, NY 10461
Telephone: (718)-430-2940
Contact: William Caspe, M.D.

Association for the Care of Children's Health
7910 Woodmont Avenue
Room 300
Bethesda, MD 20814
Telephone: (301)-654-6549
Contact: Linda Crites
Region III; education and advocacy related to children with special healthcare needs

Brooklyn Pediatric AIDS Demonstration Project
SUNY Health Science Center, Box 48
450 Clarkson Avenue, Box 49
Brooklyn, NY 11203
Telephone: (718)-270-3825
Contact: Herman Mendez - M.D.
Pediatric care, maternal care, adolescent program

Catholic Charities, Diocese of Ft. Worth
1300 South Lake Drive
Ft. Worth, TX 76104
Telephone: (817)-534-0814
Contact: Dolores Barkovsky - Director
Region VI residential treatment center for children

Chicago Pediatric HIV Care Project
Hektoan Institute for Medical Research
627 South Wood Street
Chicago, IL 60612
Telephone: (312)-633-5080
Contact: Mardge Cohen - Director
Inpatient care, support groups, classes, nutrition

Children's Hospital - New Orleans
200 Henry Clay Avenue
New Orleans, LA 70117
Telephone: (504)-524-4611 Fax: (504)-523-2084
Contact: Michael Kaiser - Director
Case management

Comprehensive Pediatric AIDS Project (CPAP)
North Broward Hospital Dist., Children's Diagnostic & Treatment Center, 417 South Andrews Avenue
Ft. Lauderdale, FL 33301
Telephone: (305)-779-1400
Contact: Susan M. Widmayer - Ph.D.

Connecticut Primary Care Association, Inc.
30 Arbor Street North
Hartford, CT 06106
Telephone: (203)-232-3319
Contact: Richard Jacobsen - Ph.D.
Region I; recipient of pediatric AIDS grant, statewide association ofcommunity health centers

D.C. Pediatric AIDS Health Care Demonstration Project
Dept. of Human Services, Comm. of Public Health
Office of Maternal & Child Health, 1660 L Street, N.W.
Washington, DC 20036
Telephone: (202)-673-4551
Contact: Linda Jenstrom Fax: 202-727-9021
Family centered case management, education and training for health careprofessionals, program developmentfor at risk adolescents

Dimock Community Health Center
Pediatric AIDS Project
55 Dimock Street
Roxbury, MA 02119
Telephone: (617)-442-8802 Fax: (617)-445-0091
Contact: Ruthie Leberman
Respite care, workshops

Dom. Sisters Family Health Service, Inc.
278 Alexander Avenue
Bronx, NY 10454
Telephone: (718)-665-6557
Contact: Margaret J. Sweeney

Expanding LAPAN: Providing Comprehensive Care to HIV
Children's Hospital of Los Angeles
4650 Sunset Blvd., Box 30
Los Angeles, CA 90027
Telephone: (213)-669-5616
Contact: Marcy Kaplan
Case management

Family AIDS Center for Treatment & Support
18 Parkis Avenue
Providence, RI 02907
Telephone: (401)-461-6330
Contact: Paul Fitzgerald
Cae management, care for HIV+ children and families, education, servicesfor substance abuse

Family Planning Council of Southeastern PA
Suite 1900
210 South Broad Street
Philadelphia, PA 19102
Telephone: (215)-985-2600
Contact: Alioia Beatty-Tee

Family-Centered, Community-Based, Coordinated HIV Care Progam
Children's Hospital Research Foundation
Children's Hospital, 700 Children's Drive
Columbus, OH 43205
Telephone: (614)-722-4451
Contact: Michael Brady - M.D.

Foundation for Children with AIDS
1800 Columbus Avenue
Roxbury, MA 02119
Telephone: (617)-442-7442 Fax: (617)-442-1705
Group meetings, counseling, day care & early intervention

Georgia Department of Human Resources, Division of Public Health
2 Peachtree Street, NE
Atlanta, GA 30303
Telephone: (404)-679-4771
Contact: Wyndelyn Bell - M.D.
Administrative office for Georgia pediatric AIDS demonstration project

Georgia Division of Public Health, Maternal Child Health Branch
2 Peachtree Street N.W.
Suite 8-113
Atlanta, GA 30303
Telephone: (404)-657-2850 Fax: (404)-657-7307
Contact: Virginia D. Floyd, M.D.
Pediatric AIDS demonstration project.

Maryland Dept. of Health, Pediatric AIDS Health Care Project
201 West Preston Street
Baltimore, MD 21201
Telephone: (410)-225-6804
Contact: Julie Hidalgo - Sc.D.
Primary care, case management

Model Comprehensive Health Care Program for HIV Adolescents
Montefiore Medical Center
111 E. 210th Street
Bronx, NY 10426
Telephone: (718)-920-6612
Contact: Karen Hein - M.D.

Multicity Training of Outpatient Caregivers of HIV Children
Children's Hospital National Medical Center
111 Michigan Avenue, N.W.
Washington, DC 20010
Telephone: (202)-884-5000
Contact: Dr. Robert Parrott

National Center for Youth Law
114 Sansome Street
Suite 900
San Francisco, CA 94104
Telephone: (415)-543-3307

Northern Manhattan Women & Children HIV Demo. Project
Columbia Univ. School of Public Health
600 West 168th Street, 7th Floor
New York, NY 10032
Telephone: (212)-305-3971
Contact: Debra Bartelli Fax: 212-305-6832

Pediatric AIDS Demo: Collaborative Model Project
University of Texas, SW Medical Center
5323 Harry Hines Blvd.
Dallas, TX 75235
Telephone: (214)-640-2329
Contact: Janet Squires - Director

Pediatric AIDS Health Care Demo. Project for the State of AL
University of Alabama at Birmingham
Department of Pediatrics
Birmingham, AL 35294
Telephone: (205)-934-7883 Fax: (205)-934-8658
Contact: Marilyn Crain - Principle Investigator

Pediatric AIDS Health Care Demonstration Project
PO Box 016960
Mailstop D53
Miami, FL 33101
Telephone: (305)-547-5658
Contact: Jo Nell Efantis-Potter
Care and treatment, case management for HIV+ pregnant women

Pediatric AIDS Health Care Financing Study
NY State Dept. of Health and Health Research, Inc.
Empire State Plaza
Albany, NY 10032
Telephone: (518)-474-6034
Contact: Herbert Fillmore

Pediatric AIDS Program (PAP)
Children's Hospital - New Orleans
200 Henry Clay Avenue
New Orleans, LA 70118
Telephone: (504)-524-4611 Fax: (504)-523-2084
Contact: Michael Kaiser - Director
Case management

Project AHEAD
Larkin Street Youth Center
1044 Larkin Street
San Francisco, CA 94109
Telephone: (415)-673-0911

Statewide Family Srvc. Ntwk. for Children & Families w/HIV
New Jersey Dept. of Health
Special Child Health Services, CN 364
Trenton, NJ 08625
Telephone: (609)-984-0755 Fax: (609)-292-3580
Contact: Diane DiDonato
Pediatric HIV/AIDS treatment center network provides arranges for care ofHIV children

Tampa Bay Pediatric AIDS Project
University of So. Florida Hospital
4202 Fowler Avenue
Tampa, FL 33620
Telephone: (813)-972-7210
Contact: Jay Wolfson - Dr. P.H.

United Hospital Medical Center, Children's Hospital AIDS Program
15 South 9th Street
Newark, NJ 07107
Telephone: (201)-268-8273
Contact: Mary Boland
Region II; social services for HIV+ women, national pediatric HIV resourcecenter

University of Texas Health Science Center
7703 Floyd Curl Drive
San Antonio, TX 78284-7818
Telephone: (512)-567-5202
Contact: John Moa - Admin. Director
Primary medical care for children and adults; social service advocacy

Yale University School of Medicine Child Study Center
333 Cedar Street
New Haven, CT 06520-7900
Telephone: (203)-785-2546
Contact: Melvin Lewis - M.D.
Programs for infected and uninfected children of HIV infected families

Youth and AIDS Prevention Program
University of Minnesota
Box 721 - UMHC Harvard Street
nneapolis, MN 55455
Telephone: (612)-627-6824
Contact: Gary Remafedi - M.D., M.P.H.; Judith Kahn - Coord.

Ryan White-Title I

AIDS Program
Boston Public Health Department
1010 Massachusetts Avenue
Boston, MA 02118
Telephone: (617)-534-4559 Fax: (617)-534-5358
Contact: Jack Vondras - Director

AIDS Program Office
600 S. Commonwealth
6th Floor
Los Angeles, CA 90005
Telephone: (213)-351-8000 Fax: (213)-738-0825
Contact: John Schunoff
Referrals, counseling, training, education

Baltimore City Helath Dept., Preventive Medicine and Epidemiology
Baltimore City Health Department
303 East Fayette Street, 5th Floor
Baltimore, MD 21202
Telephone: (410)-396-4438 Fax: 410-625-0688
Contact: John N. Lewis - MD,MPH, Asst.Commissioner
Baltimore

Board of Commissioners of Fulton County
County Government Center
141 Pryor Street, 10th Floor
Atlanta, GA 30303
Telephone: (404)-730-8239
Contact: Michael Lomax - Chairman
Atlanta/Fulton County

Broward County HIV/AIDS Support Services
1323 Southeast 4th Ave.
Ft. Lauderdale, FL 33316
Telephone: (305)-357-6385
Contact: Wayne Sheppard - Assistant to the Director
Housing and medical treatment

Chicago Department of Health
333 South State Street
Room 200
Chicago, IL 60604
Telephone: (312)-747-9430 Fax: (312)-747-9694
Contact: Erica Salem - Assistant Director for Program; - Development
HIV primary care, mental health services, case management

Contra Costa County AIDS Program
Suite 200
597 Center Avenue
Martinez, CA 94553
Telephone: (510)-313-6770
Oakland/Alameda County

Dallas County Department of Human Services, STD Clinic
4917 Harry Hines Boulevard
Dallas, TX 75235
Telephone: (214)-920-7845
Contact: Jon R. Cameron

Hudson County Department of Human Services
114 Clifton Place
Murdock Hall
Jersey City, NJ 07304
Telephone: (201)-309-1524 Fax: 201-432-1188
Contact: Cindy Vitone - AIDS Coordinator
Ryan White funding

Management Services Division
140 W. Flagler Street
Suite 1107
Miami, FL 33130
Telephone: (305)-375-5494
Contact: Dan Wall - Project Director
Miami/Dade county; administrative agent for Ryan White Title I funding

New York City Department of Health
125 Worth Street
Room 331
New York, NY 10013
Telephone: (212)-788-5250 Fax: 212-788-4734
Contact: Margaret Hamburg - M.D., Commissioner
AIDS contract programs, AIDS program service administration

Newark Department of Health and Human Services
110 William Street
Newark, NJ 07102
Telephone: (201)-733-5310
Contact: Bobi Ruffin - Acting Director
Medical services for STDs, dental clinic, free testing, shelter, foodpickup

Patient Svcs. Div., Office of AIDS Activities, Comm. of Public Health
1660 L Street, N.W.
Suite 700
Washington, DC 20036
Telephone: (202)-673-6888
Contact: Steve Havenner
Washington, D.C.

San Diego Dept. of Health Services, Office of AIDS Coordination
1700 Pacific Hwy.
San Diego, CA 92186-5524
Telephone: (619)-236-2254 Fax: (619)-236-2660
Contact: Bonnie Callendar
HIV testing & counseling

San Francisco Dept. of Public Health, Health Svcs. Branch AIDS Office
25 Van Ness
Suite 500
San Francisco, CA 94102
Telephone: (415)-554-9017
Contact: M.D., Chief
San Francisco

Ryan White-Title II

Arizona Department of Health Services
Division of Disease Prevention
3008 North 3rd Street
Phoenix, AZ 85012
Telephone: (602)-230-5808

Arkansas Department of Health
4815 West Markham Street
Little Rock, AR 72205-3867
Telephone: (501)-661-2408 Fax: (501)-661-2082
Contact: AIDS Prevention Program
Three day HIV counselor training course. Hotline 1-800-445-7720

California Dept. of Health Services, Office of AIDS
830 S Street
Sacramento, CA 95814
Telephone: (916)-323-7415
Contact: Wayne Sauseda
HIV testing and counseling

Connecticut Department of Health Services AIDS Section
Bureau of Health Promotion
150 Washington Street
Hartford, CT 06106
Telephone: (203)-566-1157
Contact: Beth Wienstein - Chief of AIDS Section

District of Columbia Commission of Public Health
Office of AIDS Activities
1660 L Street, N.W., Suite 700
Washington, DC 20036
Telephone: (202)-673-6888 Fax: (202)-727-2386
Long term care, preventive health services, agency for HIV/AIDS referralsto services in DC

Division of Public Health
Federal and Water Streets
Dover, DE 19903
Telephone: (302)-739-4724
Contact: Paul Silverman - Ph.D.
Delaware

Florida Department of Health and Rehabilitative Services
Office - HRSA AIDS Program
1317 Winewood Blvd., Building E, Room 117
Tallahassee, FL 32399-0700
Telephone: (904)-487-2478 Fax: (904)-488-1899
Contact: James Jackson

Georgia Dept of Human Resources, Epidemiology & Prevention Branch
2 Peach Tree Street NW
Atlanta, GA 30303
Telephone: (404)-894-5304
Contact: Dr. Katheen Tooney
AIDS education for community worksites, schools and professional groups

Hawaii State Dept. of Health, AIDS Research & Seroprevalence
Leahi Hospital
3675 Kilauea Avenue
Honolulu, HI 96816
Telephone: (808)-735-0440
Contact: Lanette Shizuru - PhD
Coordinates CDC & State prevalence and incidence for State planningcoordination

HIV/AIDS Treatment and Care Program Coordination
Bureau of Chronic Disease Control
P.O. Box 16660
Salt Lake City, UT 84116-0660
Telephone: (801)-538-6225
Contact: Edie Sidle
AIDS information & referral line

Idaho Department of Health and Welfare
Bureau of Communicable Disease Prevention
STD/AIDS Program, 450 West State Street
Boise, ID 83720
Telephone: (208)-334-5932 Fax: (208)-334-6581
Contact: John Glaza - Supervisor

Indiana State Board of Health
Division of HIV/AIDS
1330 West Michigan Street
Indianapolis, IN 46202
Telephone: (317)-633-0893
Contact: Dennis Stover - Director

Iowa Department of Public Health
AIDS Prevention Program
Lucas State Office Building, 321 East 12th Street
Des Moines, IA 50319-0075
Telephone: (515)-281-4938
Contact: Carolyn Jacobson - Program Manager

Kansas Department of Health & Environment
Bureau of Disease Control, Suite 605
Mills Building, 109 S.W. 9th
Topeka, KS 66612-1271
Telephone: (913)-296-6036
Contact: Sally Finney-Brazier - Director, AIDS Section

Kentucky Cabinet for Human Resources
Department of Health Services
275 East Main Street
Frankfort, KY 40621
Telephone: (502)-564-7647
Contact: Reginald Finger, M.D., M.P.H. - Dir.,Div. of Epidemiology

Louisiana Department of Health & Hospitals
HIV Program Office
1542 Tulane Avenue
New Orleans, LA 70112
Telephone: (504)-568-7041
Contact: Ted Wisniewski - M.D.

Maine Department of Human Services
State House Station 11
Augusta, ME 04333
Telephone: (207)-287-5060
Contact: Tom Bancroft - AIDS Coordinator
Advocacy, acute care, home health, income assistance, mental health, other

Maryland Dept. of Health and Mental Hygiene, STD Section
201 West Preston Street
Baltimore, MD 20201
Telephone: (410)-225-6688
Contact: Eric Fine, M.D., M.P.H.

Massachusetts Department of Public Health
150 Tremont Street
Boston, MA 02111-1126
Telephone: (617)-727-0368
Contact: John Auerbach - AIDS Program Director
Alternative Testing and Seropositive support

Michigan Department of Public Health, Div. of Disease Control
3500 N. Logan, Martin Luther King Blvd.
P.O. Box 30035
Lansing, MI 48909
Telephone: (517)-335-8063
Contact: David Johnson - M.D., Chief

Minnesota Department of Health, AIDS/STD Prevention Services
717 SE Delaware Street
P.O. Box 9441
Minneapolis, MN 55440-9441
Telephone: (612)-623-5698 Fax: (612)-623-5743
Contact: Jill DeBoer
Information & disease prevention services for HIV/STD infected and relatedpersons

Mississippi State Department of Health
HIV/AIDS Prevention Program
P.O. Box 1700
Jackson, MS 39215-1700
Telephone: (601)-960-7723
Contact: Mary Jane Coleman - R.N., Director

Montana Department of Health and Environmental Services
AIDS Program
1400 Broadway
Helena, MT 59620
Telephone: (406)-444-2454 Fax: (406)-444-2606
Contact: Bruce Desonia - AIDS/STD Program Mgr.

Nebraska Department of Health, AIDS Prevention Program
Craft State Office Bldg.
200 South Silber Street
North Platte, NE 69101
Telephone: (308)-535-8134
Contact: Virginia Wilkinson - AIDS Program Director
Confidential AIDS testing site, counseling.

Nevada State Health Department
Division of STD/AIDS
505 East King Street
Carson City, NV 89710
Telephone: (702)-687-4804
Contact: Dr. John Yacenda - Program Manager, HIV/AIDS; Bill Hill - Surveillance Coord.; Pam Walton - Ryan White Care Coord.
Drug assistance, home health care

New Hampshire Division of Public Health
HIV/AIDS Program
6 Hazen Drive
Concord, NH 03301
Telephone: (603)-271-4576

New Jersey State Department of Health
Division of AIDS Prevention and Control
363 West State Street, CN 363
Trenton, NJ 08625
Telephone: (609)-984-5888
Contact: Carmine Grasso - Active Service Director

New Mexico Department of Health HIV/AIDS Prev. & Services Bureau
1190 St. Francis Drive
P.O. Box 26110
Santa Fe, NM 87502
Telephone: (505)-827-0086
Contact: Francesca Estrada - Administrator for Bur. Chief

New York State Department of Health
AIDS Institute
Corning Tower, Room 342, Empire State Plaza
Albany, NY 12237
Telephone: (518)-473-7542
Contact: Dennis Whelan - Acting Director

North Carolina Dept. of Environment, Health & Natural Resources
Division of Adult Health, HIV Service Unit
P.O. Box 27687
Raleigh, NC 27611-7687
Telephone: (919)-733-7081
Contact: Hope K. Lucas - Program Manager
Ryan White Program & Housing Program.

North Dakota State Dept. of Health and Consolidated Labs
Division of Disease Control
600 East Boulevard
Bismarck, ND 58505-0200
Telephone: (701)-224-2370
Contact: Susan Pederson - HIV/AIDS Project Director

Ohio Department of Health, AIDS Unit
Bureau of Preventive Medicine
246 North High Street, PO Box 118
Columbus, OH 43266-0118
Telephone: (614)-466-5480

Oklahoma Department of Health, AIDS Division
1000 NE 10th Street, Mail Drop 0308
Oklahoma City, OK 73152
Telephone: (405)-271-4636
Contact: Janet Richey - Administrative Dir. AIDS/HIV

Rhode Island Department of Health
3 Capitol Hill
Cannon Building
Providence, RI 02908
Telephone: (401)-277-2320
Contact: MaryLou DeCiantis - Chief Admin. AIDS/STD
AIDS educators, HIV testing

South Carolina Department of Health & Environmental Control
HIV/AIDS Division
Robert Mills Bldg., 2600 Bull Street
Columbia, SC 29211
Telephone: (803)-737-4110
Contact: Lynda Kettinger - Director HIV/AIDS

South Dakota Department of Health, Office of Communicable Disease
523 East Capitol
Pierre, SD 57501-3182
Telephone: (605)-773-3364
Contact: Steve Volk
HIV/AIDS Counseling, Testing, Referrals/Free & Anonymous

State of Alaska, AIDS/STD Program
PO Box 240249
3601 C Street, Suite 576
Anchorage, AK 99524-0249
Telephone: (907)-561-4406 Fax: (907)-562-7802
Training for counselors, technical assistance to various agencies

Tennessee Department of Health, STD/HIV Division
Tennessee Tower, 13th Floor
312 8th Avenue North
Nashville, TN 37247
Telephone: (615)-741-7500
Contact: Dan Burke - Program Director; Laurel Wood - Comm. Disease Program Dir.

Texas Department of Health, HIV Prevention Section
1100 West 49th Street
Austin, TX 78756-3199
Telephone: (512)-458-7400
Contact: Sylvia Watson - Director

Vermont Department of Health
PO Box 70
Burlington, VT 05402
Telephone: (802)-863-7280
Contact: Shari Brenner - HIV/AIDS Education Coord.
Education, testing, counseling, referrals

Virginia Department of Health, AIDS Division

Richmond, VA 23219
Telephone: (804)-225-4844
Contact: Elaine Martin - AIDS Coordinator

Washington Department of Health, Office of AIDS/STD
PO Box 47840
Olympia, WA 98504
Telephone: (206)-464-5457
Contact: Deenie M.T. Dudley - Clearinghouse Manager; Mary Cummings - Office Director

West Virginia Department of Health, AIDS Prevention Program
1422 Washington Street East
Charleston, WV 25301
Telephone: (304)-558-5358 Fax: (304)-558-6335
Contact: Loretta Haddy - Director, AIDS Prevention; Robert Johnson - Coordinator HIV

Wisconsin Department of Health & Social Services, AIDS Program
1414 East Washington Avenue
Madison, WI 53703-3041
Telephone: (608)-267-5287
Contact: James Vergeront - M.D.

Wyoming Department of Health, AIDS Education & Prevention Program
Hathaway Bldg., 4th Floor
Cheyenne, WI 82002
Telephone: (307)-777-5800
Contact: Terry Foley - Program Mgr.

SS AIDS Coord

Coy Short - Region IV
101 Marietta Tower, Suite 1902
Atlanta, GA 30323
Telephone: (404)-331-2475

Dan Farrow - Region X
2901 Third Avenue
Mail Stop 301
Seattle, WA 98121
Telephone: (206)-615-2105

Fran Scott - Region VIII
1961 Stout Street, Room 834
Denver, CO 80294
Telephone: (303)-844-3346

Frank Horn - Region IX
DBP, 3rd Floor
75 Hawthorne Street
San Francisco, CA 94105
Telephone: (415)-744-4511

Karen Brach - Social Security Region V
600 West Madison
Chicago, IL 60680
Telephone: (312)-353-1733 Fax: (312)-353-0781
Contact: Richard Rouse - Deputy Regional Public Affairs

Kate Thornton - Region III

Philadelphia, PA 19191
Telephone: (215)-597-2818

Kurt Czarnowski - Region I
Room 1100 JFK Bldg., Government Center
Boston, MA 02203
Telephone: (617)-565-2881

Linda Griffin - Region V
PO Box 8280
Chicago, IL 60880-8280
Telephone: (312)-886-3419

Lynn King - Region VI
1200 Main Tower, Room 1500
Dallas, TX 75202
Telephone: (214)-767-4468

Maureen O'Connor - Region II
26 Federal Plaza, Room 40-112
New York, NY 10278
Telephone: (212)-264-7317

Social Security Region I
JFK Federal Bldg.
Room 1900
Boston, MA 02203
Telephone: (617)-565-2881
Contact: Kurt Czarnowski
(CT, ME, MA, NH, RI, VT)

Social Security Region IV
101 Marietta Tower
Suite 1904
Atlanta, GA 30323
Telephone: (404)-331-2475
Contact: Coy A. Short
Regional Social Security office

Social Security Region VIII - Fran Scott
1961 Stout Street
Room 834
Denver, CO 80294
Telephone: (303)-844-3346
Contact: Fran Scott; Jim Dittmann
Answers SS policy questions in CO, MT, ND, SD, UT and WY

Social Security/Disability Program
26 Federal Plaza
Room 40-112
New York, NY 10278
Telephone: (212)-264-7299
Contact: Maureen O'Conner
Regional office overseeing disability programs in NY, NJ, PR and VI

Thomas Swain - Region VII
601 East 12th Street
Room 436
Kansas City, MO 64106
Telephone: (816)-374-7257

Addiction Research and Treatment Corporation
22 Chapel Street
Brooklyn, NY 11201
Telephone: (718)-260-2917 Fax: (718)-522-3186
Contact: Stanley John, MD
Community Program for Clinical Research on AIDS

AIDS Clincal Trials
PO Box 6421
Rockville, MD 20849
Telephone: (301)-217-0023 Fax: (301)-738-6616
Toll-Free: (800)-874-2572
Research projects; information on AIDS clincal studies

AIDS Community Research Consortium
1048 El Camino Real
Suite A3
Redwood City, CA 94063
Telephone: (415)-364-6563 Fax: (415)-364-9001
Contact: Susan Burton
Community based AIDS research

AIDS Research Consortium of Atlanta, Inc.
131 Ponce de Leon
Suite 130
Atlanta, GA 30308
Telephone: (404)-876-2317 Fax: (404)-872-1701
Contact: Amy Morris - Administrative Director
Community Program for Clinical Research on AIDS

AIDS Resource Center/Nelson-Tebedo Community Clinic
P.O. Box 190712
Dallas, TX 75219
Telephone: (214)-521-5124 Fax: (214)-522-4604
Contact: Gil Flores - Office Adminstration
American Foundation for AIDS Research

Albert Einstein College of Medicine
Adult AIDS Clinical Trial Unit
Forchheimer 418, 1300 Morris Park Avenue
Bronx, NY 10461
Telephone: (718)-430-3099 Fax: (718)-597-5814
Contact: Gayle Keinak
Adult AIDS Clinical Trial Unit

Baltimore Community Research Initiative
22 South Green Street
Box 202
Baltimore, MD 21201
Telephone: (410)-328-3588 Fax: (410)-328-4430
American Foundation for AIDS Research

Bay Area AIDS Consortium
2655 Swann Avenue
Suite 107
Tampa, FL 33609
Telephone: (813)-877-5696 Fax: (813)-877-6593
American Foundation for AIDS Research

Boston City Hospital, Boston University School of Medicine
Department of Pediatrics
818 Harrison Avenue
Boston, MA 02118
Telephone: (617)-534-5000 Fax: (617)-534-7475
Contact: Stephen Ira Pelton, M.D. - Principal Investigator
AIDS Pediatric Clinical Trials Unit

Case Western Reserve University
School of Medicine, #W-106
2061 Cornell Road
Cleveland, OH 44106
Telephone: (216)-844-8175 Fax: (216)-844-5356
Contact: ; Michael M. Lederman, M.D. - Principal Investigator
Adult AIDS Clinical Trial Unit

Chicago Community Program for Clinical Research on AIDS
711 W North Avenue
Chicago, IL 60610-1042
Telephone: (312)-266-0227 Fax: (312)-266-0306
Contact: Jeff Zuklinden
Coordinates clinical trials

Chicago Community Program for Clinical Research on AIDS
711 West North Avenue
Suite 201
Chicago, IL 60610
Telephone: (312)-266-0227 Fax: (312)-266-0306
Contact: Jeff Zurlinden
AIDS research

Chicago Community Program for Clinical Research on AIDS
711 West North Avenue
Suite 201
Chicago, IL 60610
Telephone: (312)-266-0227 Fax: (312)-266-0306
Contact: Jeffrey Zurlinden, MS, RN - Director; Roberta Luskin, M.D. - Principal Investigator
Community Program for Clinical Research on AIDS

Children's Hospital
Division of Infectious Disease
300 Longwood Avenue
Boston, MA 02115
Telephone: (617)-735-6832 Fax: (617)-730-0660
Contact: Kenneth McIntosh, M.D. - Principal Investigator
AIDS Pediatric Clinical Trials Unit

Children's Hospital and Medical Center
AIDS Pediatric Clinical Trials Unit
4800 Sand Point Way N.E.
Seattle, WA 98105
Telephone: (206)-526-2073 Fax: (206)-527-3780
Contact: Ann Melvin
AIDS Pediatric Clinical Trials Unit

Children's Hospital of New Jersey
United Hospitals Med. Ctr
15 South 9th Street
Newark, NJ 07107-2147
Telephone: (201)-268-8009
Contact: Mary Boland - RN
Experimental Drug Treatment

Children's Hospital of New Jersey
AIDS Program
15 South Ninth Street
Newark, NJ 07107
Telephone: (201)-268-8298 Fax: (201)-268-7769
Contact: Joseph Picordi - RN; Edward M. Connor, M.D. - Principal Investigator
AIDS Pediatric Clinical Trials Unit

Children's Memorial Hospital
Northwestern University Medical School
Div. Infectious Disease 2300 Children's Pl.
Chicago, IL 60614
Telephone: (312)-880-4757 Fax: (312)-880-3208
Contact: Dr Ram Yogeu - Directorr
AIDS Pediatric Clinical Trials Unit

Children's Memorial Medical Center
2300 Children's Plaza
Box 20
Chicago, IL 60614
Telephone: (312)-880-4757 Fax: (312)-880-3208
Contact: Dr. Ram Yogen
HIV testing, family counseling, AIDS clinical trials group, social workers & psychologists

Colorado AIDS Clinical Trials Group
4200 East Ninth Avenue
Box B-163
Denver, CO 80262
Telephone: (303)-270-8551
Contact: Graham Ray, R.N.
Research program

Columbia University College of Physicians and Surgeons
Dept. of Pediatrics, Black Bldg., Rm.427
650 West 168th Street
New York, NY 10032
Telephone: (212)-305-7222 Fax: (212)-305-2284
Contact: Mercy Lipton; Anne A. Gershon, M.D. - Principal Investigator
AIDS Pediatric Clinical Trials Unit

Community Consortium
San Francisco General Hospital
3180 18th Street, Suite 201
San Francisco, CA 94110
Telephone: (415)-476-9554 Fax: (415)-476-4734
Contact: Program Director - Donald I. Abrams, M.D.; Principal Investigator
Community Program for Clinical Research on AIDS

Community Research Initiative of New England
320 Washington Avenue
3rd Floor
Boston, MA 02115
Telephone: (617)-566-4004 Fax: (617)-566-8226
Independent AIDS Research

Community Research Initiative of South Florida
1508 San Franscico Ignacio Avenue
Suite 200
Corah Gables, FL 33146
Telephone: (305)-576-1081 Fax: (305)-667-9296
AIDS research

Community Research Initiative/New England
320 Washington Street
Third Floor
Brookline, MA 02146
Telephone: (617)-566-4004 Fax: (617)-566-8226
Contact: Mary Dugan - Clinical Nurse
Community based clinical trials

Comprehensive AIDS Alliance of Detroit
Wayne State University
Harper-Grace Hospital
Detroit, MI 48201
Telephone: (313)-745-9131 Fax: (313)-745-9173
Community based clinical trials center

Comprehensive AIDS Alliance of Detroit/Wayne State Univ.
Detroit Medical Center/ID Dept.
4201 St. Antoine
Detroit, MI 48201
Telephone: (313)-993-0934 Fax: (313)-745-9173
Contact: Constance Rowley, RN, MSN, MEd - Project Coordinator; Lawrence R. Crane, M.D. - Principal Investigator
Community based clinical research on AIDS

Cornell University Medical Center
1300 York Avenue
24th Floor
New York, NY 10021
Telephone: (212)-746-4177

Contact: Michael Giordano; Henry W. Murray, M.D. - Principal Investigator
Adult AIDS Clinical Trials Unit

Delaware Community Program for Clinical Research on AIDS
Medical Center of Delaware
501 West 14th Street
Wilmington, DE 19801
Telephone: (302)-428-4281 Fax: (302)-428-4548
Contact: Arlene Bincsik, RN, MS - AIDS Research Pgm. Dir.; William J. Holloway, M.D. - Principal Investigator
Community Program for Clinical Research on AIDS

Department of Medical Microbiology/Creighton University
School of Medicine
California & 24th Street
Omaha, NE 68178-0001
Telephone: (402)-280-2921
Contact: Dr. Marvin Bittner
AIDS Medical Referral & Research Center

Duke University Medical Center
428 Jones Building, Research Drive
Box 3499
Durham, NC 27710
Telephone: (919)-684-6335 Fax: (919)-684-8514
Contact: Catherine Wilfert, M.D. - Principal Investigator
AIDS Pediatric Clinical Trials Unit

Georgetown University Department of Medicine, ID
Kober-Cogan, Room 210
3750 Reservior Road, N.W.
Washington, DC 20007
Telephone: (202)-687-1079 Fax: (202)-687-6476
Adult AIDS Clinical Trials Unit

HEMACARE
4954 Van Nuys Boulevard
Sherman Oaks, CA 91403-1719
Telephone: (818)-986-3883 Fax: (818)-986-1417
Contact: Joann Stover
HIV testing, clinical trials

Henry Ford Hospital
2799 West Grand Boulevard
Detroit, MI 48202
Telephone: (313)-876-2573 Fax: (313)-876-2993
Contact: Diann Mastropolak
Community based clinical trials center

Henry Ford Hospital, Infectious Diseases Division
Hospital Epidemiology
2799 West Grand Boulevard
Detroit, MI 48202
Telephone: (313)-876-7664 Fax: (313)-876-2993
Contact: Dr. Louis Saravolatz - Project Coordinator
Community Program for Clinical Research on AIDS

Milton M. Hershey Medical Center
Dept. of Medicine/Division of Hematology
500 University Drive, P.O. Box 850
Hershey, PA 17033
Telephone: (717)-531-7488 Fax: (717)-531-5461
Contact: Fran Damianos
Adult AIDS Clinical Trials Unit

Hill Health Center
428 Columbus Avenue
New Haven, CT 06519-1233
Telephone: (203)-776-9594 Fax: (203)-787-4912
Contact: Marian Holmes - Director of Nursing
Community based clinical trials

Hill Health Corporation
428 Columbus Avenue
New Haven, CT 06519
Telephone: (203)-776-9594 Fax: (203)-787-5510
Community program for clinical research on AIDS

HIV Care - Saint Francis Memorial Hospital
900 Hyde Street
San Francisco, CA 94109-4806
Telephone: (415)-775-4321 Fax: (415)-353-6594
Toll-Free: (415)-807-5774
Contact: Mark Bouer
Clinical research

HIV Study Group/Central Texas Medical Foundation
4614 North IH-35
Austin, TX 78751
Telephone: (512)-450-1866 Fax: (512)-459-0838
Community-based AIDS research

Indiana University School of Medicine
Adult AIDS Clinical Trial Unit
Emerson Hall 435, 545 Barnhill Drive
Indianapolis, IN 46202
Telephone: (317)-274-8456 Fax: (317)-274-1876
Contact: Beth Zwickl; Robert B. Jones, M.D., Ph.D. - Principal Investigator
Adult AIDS Clinical Trial Unit

Johns Hopkins Center for Immunological Research
624 North Broadway St
Room 114
Baltimore, MD 21205
Telephone: (410)-955-7283 Fax: (410)-955-1622
AIDS research

Johns Hopkins Hospital
Johns Hopkins Univ. School of Medicine
Ross Bldg., Room 1159, 600 North Rutland
Baltimore, MD 21205
Telephone: (410)-955-4370 Fax: (410)-614-0691
Contact: : John G. Bartlett, M.D. - Principal Investigator
Adult AIDS Clinical Trials Unit

Johns Hopkins University (Pediatrics)
600 North Wolfe Street
Baltimore, MD 21287-4933
Telephone: (410)-955-3271 Fax: (410)-614-1491
Contact: Robert Livingston
Clinical trials

Johns Hopkins University, School of Medicine
1830 East Monument
Room 8071
Baltimore, MD 21205
Telephone: (410)-955-2898 Fax: (410)-614-0691
Contact: John G. Bartlett, MD
AIDS clinical trials unit, education, referrals

The Joseph Stokes Jr. Research Institute
Children's Hospital of Philadelphia
34th Street & Civic Center Blvd.
Philadelphia, PA 19104
Telephone: (215)-590-3800
Contact: Stuart Starr, M.D. - Principal Investigator
AIDS Pediatric Clinical Trials Unit

Kaiser Permanente
HIV Research Unit
2590 Geary Blvd
San Francisco, CA 94115
Telephone: (415)-202-3480 Fax: (415)-202-3483
Contact: W. Jennifer Sessel
AIDS Clinical trials, funded by NIAID

Lakeshore Infectious Disease Assoc. Ltd., St. Joseph Hospital
St. Joseph Hospital
2900 N. Lake Shore Drive
Chicago, IL 60657
Telephone: (312)-665-3261 Fax: (312)-665-3384
Contact: Dr. Roberta Luskin-Hawk
Community based clinical trials site

Los Angeles County - University of Southern California
1175 N. Cummings
Bldg. 5P21
Los Angeles, CA 90033
Telephone: (213)-343-8288 Fax: (213)-226-2083
Contact: John Leedom, MD - Principal Investigator
Adult AIDS Clinical Trial Unit

Los Angeles Pediatric AIDS Network, Children's Hospital
4650 Sunset Boulevard
Los Angeles, CA 90027-6016
Telephone: (213)-660-2450 Fax: (213)-663-6896
Experimental medication to children with HIV

Louisiana Community AIDS Research Program
Tulane Univ. Medical Ctr.
1430 Tulane Avenue
New Orleans, LA 70112
Telephone: (504)-584-1976 Fax: (504)-584-1972
Toll-Free: (800)-233-8967
Contact: Janice Walker
AIDS clinical trials & research

Louisiana Community AIDS Research Program
Tulane University Medical Center
1430 Tulane Avenue
New Orleans, LA 70112
Telephone: (504)-584-1971 Fax: (504)-584-1972
Contact: Janice Walker, M.S. - Project Coordinator; C. Lynn Besch, M.D. - Principal Investigator
Community Program for Clinical Research on AIDS

Massachusetts General Hospital
Infectious Disease Unit
55 Fruit Street
Boston, MA 02114
Telephone: (617)-726-5596 Fax: (617)-726-7653
Contact: Martin S. Hirsch, M.D. - Principal Investigator
Adult AIDS Clinical Trial Unit

Minnesota AIDS Clinical Trials Unit
Box 437
Mayo Building
Minneapolis, MN 55455
Telephone: (612)-625-1462 Fax: (612)-626-2337
NIH/AIDS clinical trials group

Minority Outreach Project
2121 West Taylor
Room 553
Chicago, IL 60612
Telephone: (312)-996-5523 Fax: (312)-996-0064
Contact: Dr. Wayne Wieble
AIDS research for experimental cures, case management, AIDS education/outreach

Mount Sinai Medical Center
One Gustave, Levy Place
New York, NY 10029
Telephone: (212)-241-0433 Fax: (212)-860-4607
Contact: Eileen Chusid; Henry S. Sacks, M.D., Ph.D. - Principal Investigator
Adult AIDS Clinical Trials Unit

Mount Sinai School of Medicine
19 East 98th Street
New York, NY 10029
Telephone: (212)-241-8902 Fax: (212)-860-4607
Contact: Eileen Chusid, PhD - Contact person
AIDS clinical trials unit, research

Mt. Sinai Medical Center, Clinical Trials Unit
1 Gustave Levy Place
New York, NY 10029
Telephone: (212)-241-8254
Contact: Dr. Gustave Levy
Medical services, clinical trials research

National Institute of Health NCI Pediatric Branch
Building 10-13N 240
Clinical Center
Bethesda, MD 20892
Telephone: (301)-496-4256 Fax: (301)-402-3327
Contact: Susan Sandelli - HIV Clinical Trials Coordinato
AIDS clinical trials program

National Institutes of Health, Clinical Center
Patient Referral Service
Building 10, Room 1C-255
Bethesda, MD 20892
Telephone: (301)-496-4891 Fax: (301)-402-2984
Research, clinical care, and support. AIDS health information protocols.

New York University Medical Center
Dept. of Pediatrics, Div. of Infectious
Diseases & Immunology, 550 First Avenue
New York, NY 10016
Telephone: (212)-263-6426 Fax: (212)-263-7806
Contact: William Borkowsky, M.D. - Principal Investigator
Pediatric AIDS Clinical Trials Unit

New York University Medical Center
Department of Medicine
550 First Avenue
New York, NY 10016
Telephone: (212)-263-6565 Fax: (212)-263-8264
Adult AIDS clinical trials unit

New York University, Medical Center, Bellevue Hospital
5501 1st Avenue
New York, NY 10016
Telephone: (212)-340-6565 Fax: (212)-263-6565
Contact: Fred T. Valentine, MD - Principal Investigator
AIDS clinical trials unit

North Jersey Community Research Initiative
393 Central Avenue
Suite 301
Newark, NJ 07103
Telephone: (201)-483-3444 Fax: (201)-485-7080
Contact: Bill Orr
Experimental drug treatment, clinical trials, social services.

North Jersey Community Research Initiative
393 Central Avenue
Suite 301
Newark, NJ 07103
Telephone: (201)-483-3444 Fax: (201)-485-7080
Contact: Victoria Taylor - Project Coordinator; George Perez, M.D. - Principal Investigator
Community program for clinical research on AIDS, mental health counseling

Northwestern University Medical School
303 E. Superior Street, 8 E. Passavante
Chicago, IL 60611
Telephone: (312)-908-9636 Fax: (312)-908-9630
Contact: John Phair, M.D. - Principal Investigator
Adult AIDS Clinical Trials Unit

Northwestern University, Medical School
AIDS Clinical Trials Unit
303 E. Superior
Chicago, IL 60611-3053
Telephone: (312)-908-9639
Contact: John Phair, M.D.
AIDS Treatment, Evaluation Services; Drug, Pharmaceutical Research

Northwestern University, Medical School
303 East Superior
Chicago, IL 60011
Telephone: (312)-908-8358 Fax: (312)-908-8281
Contact: Lisa Williams - Contact person; John Phair, M.D. - Principal Investigator;
AIDS clinical trials unit

Ohio State Univ., Medical Center
4725 University Hosp. Cln
456 W. 10th Avenue
Columbus, OH 43210
Telephone: (614)-293-8112 Fax: (614)-293-5240
Contact: Judy Neidig - Study Coordinator
AIDS clinical trails unit, evaluation pharmaceutical research

Ohio State University, Medical Center
456 W. 10th Avenue
Columbus, OH 43210
Telephone: (614)-293-8732 Fax: (614)-293-8732
Contact: Judy Neidig - Study Coordinator
AIDS clinical trials unit, treatment, pharmaceutical research

Philadelphia FIGHT
201 N. Broad Street
6th Floor
Philadelphia, PA 19107
Telephone: (215)-557-8265 Fax: (215)-557-8275
Contact: Carol Graeber
American Foundation for AIDS Research

Research Medical Center
2316 E. Meyer Blvd
Kansas City, MO 64132
Telephone: (816)-276-4038 Fax: (816)-276-3763
Contact: David S. McKinsey
Research

Richmond AIDS Consortium
Box 49 MCV Station
Richmond, VA 23298
Telephone: (804)-371-6471 Fax: (804)-371-0570
Contact: Susan DePew - Project Coordinator; Thomas M. Kerkering, M.D. - Principal Investigator
Community Program for Clinical Research on AIDS

San Diego Community Research Group
3800 Ray Street
San Diego, CA 92104
Telephone: (619)-291-2437
Contact: John Connelly
American Foundation for AIDS Research

San Francisco General Hospital
Building 80, Ward 84
995 Potrero Avenue
San Francisco, CA 94110
Telephone: (415)-476-9296
Contact: John Mills, M.D. - Principal Investigator
Adult AIDS Clinical Trial Unit

Search Alliance
7461 Beverly Blvd.
Suite 304
Los Angeles, CA 90036
Telephone: (213)-930-8820 Fax: (213)-934-3919
Non-profit, community-based research

Southwest Community-Based AIDS Treatment Group
1800 North Highland
Suite 610
Los Angeles, CA 90028
Telephone: (213)-469-5888 Fax: (213)-464-4404
Community-based AIDS research

St. Jude Children's Research Hospital
332 North Lauderdale
Memphis, TN 38105
Telephone: (901)-522-0485 Fax: (901)-527-6616
Contact: Walter Hughes, M.D. - Principal Investigator
AIDS Pediatric Clinical Trials Unit

St. Louis University School of Medicine
3635 Vista FDT 8 North
St Louis, MO 63310
Telephone: (314)-577-8649 Fax: (314)-771-3816
Contact: Heide Israel
Vaccine trials (phase I & II): primarily preventive seronegative, alsolimited therapeutic seropositive trials

St. Luke's / Roosevelt Hospital Center
1000 Tenth Avenue
New York, NY 10019
Telephone: (212)-523-6741
Contact: Michael Grieco, M.D. - Principal Investigator
AIDS clinical trials unit, drug reseatch

Stanford University Medical Center
Adult AIDS Clinical Trial
300 Pasteur Drive, S-156
Stanford, CA 94305
Telephone: (415)-723-6231 Fax: (415)-725-2395
Contact: Virginia Talman
Adult AIDS Clinical Trial Unit

Stanford University, School of Medicine
Div of Infectious Disease
Stanford, CA 94305
Telephone: (415)-723-6231 Fax: (415)-725-2395
Contact: Virginia Tallman, RN - Coordinator
AIDS clinical trials unit

State University of New York at Brooklyn
Health Science Center, Box 56
450 Clarkson Avenue
Brooklyn, NY 11203
Telephone: (718)-270-1000 Fax: (718)-270-1628
Adult AIDS Clinical Trials Unit

State University of New York at Stony Brook
Health Sciences Center, T15-080
Division of Infectious Diseases
Stony Brook, NY 11794-8153
Telephone: (516)-444-1658 Fax: (516)-444-7518
Contact: Roy T. Steigbigel, M.D. - Principal Investigator
Adult AIDS clinical trials unit

Texas Children's Hospital
6621 Fannin, A380
Houston, TX 77030
Telephone: (713)-770-1319 Fax: (713)-770-1260
Contact: ; William T. Shearer, M.D. - Principal Investigator
AIDS Pediatric Clinical Trials Unit

The Immune Response Corporation
5935 Darwin Ct.
Carlsbad, CA 92008
Telephone: (619)-431-7080 Fax: (619)-431-8636
Contact: Dr. Dennis Carlo - Senior Research Scientist
Biotech company involved in AIDS research

The Research and Education Group
2701 NW Vaughn Street
Suite 770
Portland, OR 97210
Telephone: (503)-229-8428 Fax: (503)-227-0902
Contact: James Sampson, M.D. - Principal Investigator
Community Program for Clinical Research on AIDS

TREAT (Resources for Experimental AIDS Therapies)
"Bread for the Journey"
1915-A Rosina Street
Santa Fe, NM 87501
Telephone: (505)-983-3633
Access to experimental AIDS therapies, access to drugtrials; research committees.

Tulane University School of Medicine
Pediatric Infectious Diseases
1430 Tulane Avenue
New Orleans, LA 70112
Telephone: (504)-588-5422 Fax: (504)-586-3805
Contact: Jane Price
AIDS Pediatric Clinical Trials Unit

Twin Cities IV Drug/AIDS Research & Demonstration Project
University of Minnesota
1985 Buford Avenue
St. Paul, MN 55108
Telephone: (612)-625-5700
Contact: Tom Flynn
AIDS research

UCLA CARE
10833 Le Conte Drive
BH 412 CHS
Los Angeles, CA 90024
Telephone: (310)-206-3474 Fax: (310)-206-3311
Contact: Dr. W. David Hardy
HIV testing and research

UCLA/Chicano Studies Research Center
405 Hilgard Avenue
Los Angeles, CA 90024-1544
Telephone: (310)-825-2363 Fax: (310)-206-1784
Contact: Executive Director
Clinical studies

University Hospital of Cleveland, Department of Infectious Diseases
2061 Cornell Road
Cleveland, OH 44106
Telephone: (216)-844-8175 Fax: (216)-844-5356
Contact: Michael Chance
AIDS clinical trials unit

University of Alabama at Birmingham
908 South 20th Street
Birmingham, AL 35294
Telephone: (205)-934-3690 Fax: (205)-975-6448
Contact: : Michael Saag, M.D. - Principal Investigator
Adult AIDS Clinical Trial Unit

University of California at Los Angeles
School of Medicine, Dept. of Pediatrics
10833 Le Conte Avenue, 22-442
Los Angeles, CA 90024
Telephone: (310)-206-6369 Fax: (310)-825-9175
Contact: Yvonne J. Bryson, MD
AIDS Pediatric Clinical Trials Unit

University of California at Los Angeles Medical Center
Care Center
10833 Le Conte Avenue, BH 412 CHS
Los Angeles, CA 90024
Telephone: (310)-206-6414 Fax: (310)-206-3311
Contact: Ronald T. Mitsuyasu, MD - Principal Investigator
Adult AIDS Clinical Trial Unit

University of California at San Diego Medical Center
2760 5th Avenue
Suite 300
San Diego, CA 92103
Telephone: (619)-543-8080 Fax: (619)-298-0177
Contact: Stephen A. Spector, MD - Principal Investigator
AIDS Pediatrics Clinical Trials Unit

University of California at San Diego/Pediatrics & Infectious Disease
2760 5th Avenue
Suite 300
San Diego, CA 92103
Telephone: (619)-543-8080 Fax: (619)-298-0177
Contact: Stephen A. Spector, M.D. - Principal Investigator
Adult AIDS Clinical Trials Unit

University of California at San Francisco
Department of Pediatrics, Box 0105
Moffitt Hospital M-601B,
San Francisco, CA 94143
Telephone: (415)-476-1736 Fax: (415)-476-3466
Contact: Diane W. Wara, M.D. - Principal Investigator
AIDS Pediatric Clinical Trials Unit

University of California Los Angeles, School of Medicine
10833 Le Conte Avenue R60-051
Suite BH-412 CHS
Los Angeles, CA 90024
Telephone: (310)-206-6414 Fax: (310)-206-3311
Contact: Ashley Mead
AIDS clinical trials unit, evaluation services; drug, pharmaceuticalresearch

University of Cincinnati, Medical Center
Holmes Hospital Division
Eden and Bethesda Avenues
Cincinnati, OH 45267-0405
Telephone: (513)-558-6977 Fax: (513)-558-6386
Contact: Jill Leonard; Peter T. Frame, M.D. - Principal Investigator
Adult AIDS Clinical Trial Unit

University of Colorado Health Sciences Center
Pediatric Infectious Diseases
4200 E. 9th Avenue, Box C-227
Denver, CO 80262
Telephone: (303)-270-8501 Fax: (303)-270-7909
Contact: Myron Levin, M.D. - Principal Investigator
AIDS Pediatric Clinical Trials Unit

University of Colorado Health Sciences Center
Infectious Disease Division
4200 East 9th Avenue
Denver, CO 80262
Telephone: (303)-270-8551 Fax: (303)-270-6102
Contact: Graham Ray - Head Research Nurse
Adult AIDS clinical trials unit, research

University of Kansas School of Medicine CBCT
1010 North Kansas
Wichita, KS 67214
Telephone: (316)-261-2622 Fax: (316)-261-2672
American Foundation for AIDS Research, phase 3 & 4 drug study

University of Massachusetts Medical Center
Department of Pediatrics
55 Lake Avenue, North
Worchester, MA 01655
Telephone: (508)-856-3947 Fax: (508)-856-5500
Contact: John Sullivan, MD - Principal Investigator
AIDS Pediatric Clinical Trials Unit

University of Massachusetts, Medical School
AIDS Clinical Trials Unit
55 Lake Avenue, N.
Worcester, MA 01655-0001
Telephone: (508)-856-2456 Fax: (508)-856-5981
Contact: Kim Wojnoskski; Neil Blacklow, M.D.
AIDS clinical trials unit, referrals & case management, AIDS treatment,evaluation services, drug and pharmaceutical research

University of Massachusetts, Medical School
55 Lake Avenue, N.
Worcester, MA 01655
Telephone: (508)-856-3158 Fax: (508)-856-5981
Contact: Joan Avato
AIDS clinical trials unit, HIV testing & counseling referrals

University of Miami Medical School-Dept. of Neurology
P.O. Box 016966 (D-9)
Miami, FL 33101
Telephone: (305)-547-5601 Fax: (305)-547-4002
NIH funded Clinical trials, Care and therapy of Neurological Disorders

University of Miami School of Medicine
First Floor Elliott Building
1800 North West 10th Avenue
Miami, FL 33136
Telephone: (305)-547-3838 Fax: (305)-545-6705
Contact: Margaret A. Fischi, M.D. - Principal Investigator
Adult AIDS Clinical Trials Unit

University of Minnesota AIDS Clinical Trial's Unit
Room G 255 Mayo
Box 437
Minneapolis, MN 55455
Telephone: (612)-625-1462 Fax: (612)-626-1923
Contact: Nancy Reed
AIDS clinical trials unit

University of Minnesota Health Sciences Center
Laboratory of Medicine and Pathology
Box 437 UMHC
Minneapolis, MN 55455
Telephone: (612)-625-1462 Fax: (612)-626-1923
Contact: Sue Reaney - Contact Person
Adult AIDS Clinical Trial Unit

University of Pennsylvania
Infectious Disease Section
536 Johnson Pavilion
Philadelphia, PA 19104-6073
Telephone: (215)-349-8091 Fax: (215)-349-8011
Contact: ; Harvey Friedman, M.D. - Principal Investigator
Adult AIDS clinical trials unit

University of Puerto Rico, Childrens Hospital
4th Floor, South Wing Gamma Project ACTU
Room 4b-45 Po box 365067

NOTES

NOTES

NOTES

NOTES

Advertisers Index

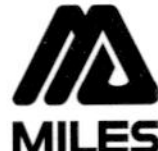

MYCELEX®

(clotrimazole) TROCHE

FOR TOPICAL ORAL ADMINISTRATION

PZ100717 2147

DESCRIPTION Each Mycelex® Troche contains 10mg clotrimazole [1-(o-chloro-α,α-diphenylbenzyl) imidazole], a synthetic antifungal agent, for topical use in the mouth.

Structural Formula:

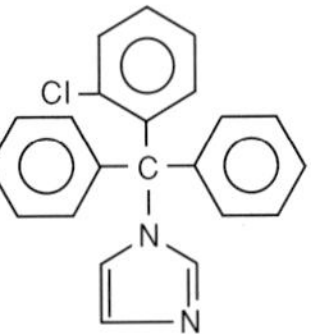

Chemical Formula:

$C_{22}H_{17}ClN_2$

The troche dosage form is a large, slowly dissolving tablet (lozenge) containing 10 mg of clotrimazole dispersed in dextrose, microcrystalline cellulose, povidone, and magnesium stearate.

CLINICAL PHARMACOLOGY Clotrimazole is a broad-spectrum antifungal agent that inhibits the growth of pathogenic yeasts by altering the permeability of cell membranes. The action of clotrimazole is fungistatic at concentrations of drug up to 20 mcg/mL and may be fungicidal *in vitro* against *Candida albicans* and other species of the genus *Candida* at higher concentrations. No single-step or multiple-step resistance to clotrimazole has developed during successive passages of *Candida albicans* in the laboratory; however, individual organism tolerance has been observed during successive passages in the laboratory. Such *in vitro* tolerance has resolved once the organism has been removed from the antifungal environment.

After oral administration of a 10 mg clotrimazole troche to healthy volunteers, concentrations sufficient to inhibit most species of *Candida* persist in saliva for up to three hours following the approximately 30 minutes needed for a troche to dissolve. The long term persistence of drug in saliva appears to be related to the slow release of clotrimazole from the oral mucosa to which the drug is apparently bound. Repetitive dosing at three hour intervals maintains salivary levels above the minimum inhibitory concentrations of most strains of *Candida;* however, the relationship between *in vitro* susceptibility of pathogenic fungi to clotrimazole and prophylaxis or cure of infections in humans has not been established.

In another study, the mean serum concentrations were 4.98 ± 3.7 and 3.23 ± 1.4 nanograms/mL of clotrimazole at 30 and 60 minutes, respectively, after administration as a troche.

INDICATIONS AND USAGE Mycelex® Troches are indicated for the local treatment of oropharyngeal candidiasis.The diagnosis should be confirmed by a KOH smear and/or culture prior to treatment.

Mycelex Troches are also indicated prophylactically to reduce the incidence of oropharyngeal candidiasis in patients immunocompromised by conditions that include chemotherapy, radiotherapy, or steroid therapy utilized in the treatment of leukemia, solid tumors, or renal transplantation. There are no data from adequate and well-controlled trials to establish the safety and efficacy of this product for prophylactic use in patients immunocompromised by etiologies other than those listed in the previous sentence. (See DOSAGE AND ADMINISTRATION.)

CONTRAINDICATIONS Mycelex® Troches are contraindicated in patients who are hypersensitive to any of its components.

WARNING Mycelex® Troches are not indicated for the treatment of systemic mycoses including systemic candidiasis.

PRECAUTIONS Abnormal liver function tests have been reported in patients treated with clotrimazole troches; elevated SGOT levels were reported in about 15% of patients in the clinical trials. In most cases the elevations were minimal and it was often impossible to distinguish effects of clotrimazole from those of other therapy and the underlying disease (malignancy in most cases). Periodic assessment of hepatic function is advisable particularly in patients with pre-existing hepatic impairment.

Since patients must be instructed to allow each troche to dissolve slowly in the mouth in order to achieve maximum effect of the medication, they must be of such an age and physical and/or mental condition to comprehend such instructions.

Carcinogenesis: An 18 month dosing study with clotrimazole in rats has not revealed any carcinogenic effect.

Usage in Pregnancy: Pregnancy Category C: Clotrimazole has been shown to be embryotoxic in rats and mice when given in doses 100 times the adult human dose (in mg/kg), possibly secondary to maternal toxicity. The drug was not teratogenic in mice, rabbits, and rats when given in doses up to 200, 180, and 100 times the human dose.

Clotrimazole given orally to mice from nine weeks before mating through weaning at a dose 120 times the human dose was associated with impairment of mating, decreased number of viable young, and decreased survival to weaning. No effects were observed at 60 times the human dose. When the drug was given to rats during a similar time period at 50 times the human dose, there was a slight decrease in the number of pups per litter and decreased pup viability.

There are no adequate and well-controlled studies in pregnant women. Clotrimazole troches should be used during pregnancy only if the potential benefit justifies the potential risk to the fetus.

PEDIATRIC USE Safety and effectiveness of clotrimazole in children below the age of 3 years have not been established; therefore, its use in such patients is not recommended.

The safety and efficacy of the prophylactic use of clotrimazole troches in children have not been established.

ADVERSE REACTIONS Abnormal liver function tests have been reported in patients treated with clotrimazole troches; elevated SGOT levels were reported in about 15% of patients in the clinical trials (See Precautions section).

Nausea, vomiting, unpleasant mouth sensations and pruritus have also been reported with the use of the troche.

OVERDOSAGE No data available.

DRUG ABUSE AND DEPENDENCE No data available.

DOSAGE AND ADMINISTRATION Mycelex® Troches are administered only as a lozenge that must be slowly dissolved in the mouth. The recommended dose is one troche five times a day for fourteen consecutive days. Only limited data are available on the safety and effectiveness of the clotrimazole troche after prolonged administration; therefore, therapy should be limited to short term use, if possible.

For prophylaxis to reduce the incidence of oropharyngeal candidiasis in patients immunocompromised by conditions that include chemotherapy, radio therapy, or steroid therapy utilized in the treatment of leukemia, solid tumors, or renal transplantation, the recommended dose is one troche three times daily for the duration of chemotherapy or until steroids are reduced to maintenance levels.

HOW SUPPLIED Mycelex® Troches, white discoid, uncoated tablets are supplied in bottles of 70 and 140. Mycelex Troches are also available for institutional use in foil packages of 70 tablets. Each tablet will be identified with the following: Miles 095.

Store below 86°F (30°C).

Avoid freezing.

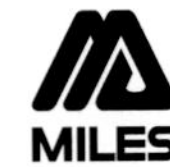

Miles Inc.
Pharmaceutical Division
400 Morgan Lane
West Haven, CT 06516 USA

PZ100717 8/92 BAY 5097 2147
Printed in USA